Transradial Approach for Percutaneous Interventions

Yujie Zhou • Ferdinand Kiemeneij
Shigeru Saito • Wei Liu
Editors

Transradial Approach for Percutaneous Interventions

Springer

Editors
Yujie Zhou
Department of Cardiology
Beijing Anzhen Hospital
Capital Medical University
Beijing
China

Shigeru Saito
Division of Cardiology &
Catheterization Laboratories
Shonan Kamakura General Hospital
Kamakura
Japan

Ferdinand Kiemeneij
Department of Cardiology
Tergooi Hospital
Blaricum
The Netherlands

Wei Liu
Department of Cardiology
Beijing Anzhen Hospital
Capital Medical University
Beijing
China

ISBN 978-94-017-7349-2 ISBN 978-94-017-7350-8 (eBook)
DOI 10.1007/978-94-017-7350-8

Library of Congress Control Number: 2017930223

Printed on acid-free paper

This Springer imprint is published by Springer Nature
The registered company is Springer Science+Business Media B.V.
The registered company address is: Van Godewijckstraat 30, 3311 GX Dordrecht, The Netherlands

Preface

Transradial Approach in China: A Journal for the West

My main goal in cardiovascular diseases intervention is to carry out the most complex procedures through the smallest vessels possible. I have made this goal known to my team and patients. After two decades, my team and I have made great strides in shaping and developing one the best interventional techniques in the world. Above all, I take pride in seeing my patients liberated from the deepest and the darkest abyss of cardiovascular diseases. It is therefore my greatest hope that this book will become the tool for sharing experiences, skills, and techniques of transradial intervention with medical professionals all across the world.

The last decade of the twentieth century records the beginning and the developmental stages of percutaneous coronary intervention in China. Those early years had plenty of unforgettable moments of both joy and pain, as well as sweet and sour moments, and could be simply described as "the best of times and the worst of times." The unforgettable moments were related to the complications resulting from transfemoral access (major hematoma, severe hemorrhage, and retroperitoneal bleeding). I could recall vividly those devastating nights, when I was called by my junior doctors to return to the hospital with urgency for complications of the femoral artery.

The fall of 2002 marks the milestone in our journey. I received a phone call for a patient who had femoral aneurysm after a successful coronary intervention, and then developed femoral venous thrombosis following local compression. A strong feeling of hopelessness descended upon me. On that day, I proposed a new direction for my team: to establish a center for transradial coronary intervention where our hospital (Beijing Anzhen Hospital) would serve as the training center for the whole nation.

Our determination to develop transradial technique was strong; however, devices and equipment presented limitations impeding the pace of our progress. We had to import almost everything and most often we had to wait for days, even months to receive supplies of the required equipment. The only catheters we had were 6F Judkins left and Judkins right. The next hurdle to flip was the puncture technique and the frequency of vasospasm of the radial artery. That was the time when more than half of radial artery spasms in my career were encountered. We continued to explore different ways for increasing the quality and success rate of radial puncture in different kind of patients – (obese, thin, female, atrial fibrillation, etc.). We also made our own "cocktail" (lidocaine, nitroglycerine, and sometimes with verapamil).

Following our initial design, Beijing Anzhen Hospital had become the national and international training center for transradial intervention, and doctors came from across the nation for training. My mobile phone also became a "hotline" for consultation of scenarios such as puncture maneuver, difficulty in catheter withdrawal, and sometimes compartment syndrome.

Moreover, transradial coronary intervention was not widely accepted in China at that time. So it frequently met resistance from experts who were used to traditional transfemoral artery approach. Sometimes we were either greeted with sarcasm or seen by "traditional transfemoral artery operators" as promoting "rectal approach to tonsillectomy." We faced humiliation and withstood mockery but we never gave up, we improved and seized every opportunity to make progress at all cost. I came to know that people are not afraid of change itself but rather are afraid of themselves being changed.

It is said that a friend in need is a friend indeed. I am grateful for friends who stood by me, and fought by my side during the toughest days, such as Prof. Xiang Hua Fu from the Second Hospital of Hebei Medical University, Prof. Guo Sheng Fu from Shao Yi Fu Hospital, and Prof. Ming Yao who is one of the earliest interventionists who had training for the radial intervention from Japan, and many more.

I must admit that the success of transradial coronary intervention in China could not have been achieved without mentioning many international friends. One of them is Prof. Ferdinand Kiemeneij, the first scholar to have successfully performed transradial PCI in the world. I see him as a gift to the world, born for transradial PCI; he told the whole world that the transradial approach is the future of intervention. He also gave me the direction and path in my clinical practice and taught me to be optimistic and confident. Prof. F Kiemeneij supported our transradial conference by driving his old car all the way from the Netherlands to Beijing. As a token to our team, he has given the original poster presentation from 1993, summarizing the results of TRI in the first 100 patients. My interpretation of this token was that he gave us his 100 % trust, approval that encouraged us to do all the best we have in transitioning our goals and dreams into a reality.

The year 2006 marks the golden year when our dream of making transradial technique for coronary intervention became a reality. We finally had transradial dedicated puncture needles, the incidence of radial spasm became dramatically reduced. Apart from the Judkins Guiding catheter, we started to obtain the XB series, then EBU 0.071′ inner diameter catheter. The whole world changed with an increase of 0.001′ inner diameter in that step crush technique, modified T, TAP could be performed with 6 Fr radial approach. More complicated procedures, even left main bifurcations become possible. Our team also developed our own technique for left main bifurcation lesions: ATP (active transfer of plaque). We are looking forward to a good result from the RCT report of the ATP technique. Our dreams become true from femoral to radial artery, from 8 to 5 Fr.

I am happy to see that with all these efforts and heartwarming memories, my team and I have a chance to showcase China to the whole world. Dr. Anthony Demaria the former chief editor of *Journal of the American College of Cardiology* had this written on the editorial page (*JACC* vol. 62, No 21 2013) after paying a historical visit to our hospital, he recognized the work of our team and mentioned that "China has energy and determination to play a leadership role in cardiovascular medicine internationally."

Beijing, China Yujie Zhou

A Memory of Transradial Revolution in China

I still clearly remember the exciting days and my first experiences in China, when I was invited to the first Beijing Medical University, Anzhen Hospital, and Fuwai Hospital to demonstrate balloon coronary angioplasty on mid-December in 1990. It was very cold in Beijing Capital City, where most of the people were walking or riding bicycles while wearing dark green so-called People's Formal Clothes under the temperature of minus 10 Celsius. Next day early morning, I visited the first Hospital of Beijing Medical University, which is now a part of Beijing University. When I reached the catheterization laboratory, Dr. Hu Dayi welcomed me, and several technicians were working hard to restart the cine X-ray machine (French machine, named CGR). We were waiting for the machine to restart for a few hours but failed. We decided to send the patient on the schedule to Anzhen Hospital. While transferring the patient to Anzhen Hospital, I was lucky to have time for my first and short visit at Forbidden City. In the afternoon, I treated several patients by balloon angioplasty in Anzhen Hospital successfully.

Next day, I visited Fuwai Hospital, where Dr. Gao Runlin welcomed me. I treated four patients there. After finishing these cases, I heard that PCI in China was still at the beginning phase, and that the total number of cases all around China ever was less than 500 after the first case of PCI in X'ian in 1983. This visit opened my eyes to China, since then I have decided to devote my life to the development of PCI in China. I have been to so many places all around China to treat many patients and teach PCI. In this long journey, I introduced the first transradial coronary angioplasty case in China. It was in 1998. After this first case, it is amazing to see how quickly TRI and PCI have been growing in China.

This book is a milestone and should be memorized forever in the PCI history in China. With this book in my hands, I will continue to devote myself to further development of PCI in China, and now I will learn much more from China.

Kanagawa, Japan

Shigeru Saito

Acknowledgements

Be grateful to Muzina Akhtar, Madhvi Tandel, Osman Shahid, Arooj Aslam, and Bilal Baran from Capital Medical university Beijing for their contributions in this manuscript.

Contents

Part I

An Introduction to Transradial Intervention

The History and Evolution of Transradial Coronary Interventions

1

Ferdinand Kiemeneij

Abstract

This chapter gives an overview of the development and evolution of transradial coronary access. The history of transradial coronary interventions is a bit artificially divided into the following phases: prehistory, pioneering phase, a phase of international recognition and one of international acceptance.

Transradial coronary interventions (TRI) started as a practical solution to prevent the massive and sometimes fatal groin bleedings in the early years of coronary stenting and will become the global standard of treatment. This evolution from experiment to guideline can be divided into several phases (Table 1.1).

1.1 The Pre-history of TRI

In 1948, Radner [1] was the first to describe transradial catheterization using radial artery cut-down. Probably due to the limitations of this technique and the limited size of the radial artery, use of larger arteries were explored. In 1953 Seldinger reported on non selective coronary angiography by percutaneous femoral approach [2] It was Mason Sones Jr. who introduced selective coronary angiography by cutdown arteriotomy of the brachial artery in the early sixties of the previous century [3]. This technique became the standard approach for decades. The first percutaneous transfemoral selective coronary angiograms were introduced by Ricketts and Abrams in 1961 [4]. By development of a special set of preshaped catheters for percutaneous transfemoral coronary angiography, Melvin Judkins popularized this technique [5].

Lucien Campeau from the Montreal heart Institute reactivated Radner's idea in order to overcome the shortcomings and complications of brachial artery cutdown. In 1964 he reported on radial artery access by arteriotomy of the proximal radial artery [6]. In 1989 Campeau published a paper on percutaneous entry into the distal radial artery for selective coronary angiogiography using a 5 F sheath and pre-shaped catheters in 100 patients [7]. In ten patients radial artery access was impossible and in another two patients the coronary arteries could not be catheterized. This paper was published in those years when the interventional cardiologists worldwide were coping with the serious and frequent bleeding complications associated with transfemoral coronary stenting. Years later, in 1992 another paper on transradial coronary angiography was published by Dr. Otaki, Department of Cardiovascular Surgery, Osaka National Hospital, Japan [8]. Out of 40 patients, 39 patients underwent successful coronary angiography with five Fr catheters.

1.2 1992–1994 Transradial Coronary Interventions: a Pioneering Phase

In the same year of Dr. Campeau's publication, Kiemeneij et al. introduced the coronary use of Palmaz Schatz stents at the Onze Lieve Vrouwe Gasthuis in Amsterdam, which had to be inserted femorally via 8 and 9 F guide catheters. The unacceptable high incidence of severe and sometimes fatal local bleeding complications under aggressive anticoagulation regimens and during and after prolonged bed rest following sheath removal [9] was their major reason to use Dr. Campeau's work as the basis for developing transradial coronary interventions and stent implantation. The superficial course of the radial artery, the ease of compression, the absence of major structures near the radial artery and the double blood supply to the hand, made the radial artery theoretically the most ideal site to introduce

F. Kiemeneij, MD, PhD
Department of Cardiology, Tergooi Hospital, Blaricum, The Netherlands
e-mail: f.kiemeneij@gmail.com

Y. Zhou et al. (eds.), *Transradial Approach for Percutaneous Interventions*, DOI 10.1007/978-94-017-7350-8_1

Table 1.1 The history of transradial coronary interventions

1948–1992 Prehistory	1992–1994 TRI pioneering	1994–2004 Recognition	2004–2014 Acceptation
1948: Radner CAG by radial artery cut down	1992: Kiemeneij First 6 Fr coronary balloon angioplasty by percutaneous transradial approach	1994: Fajadet & Louvard First pioneers to be trained in TRI at OLVG	2004: Agostoni et al.: Meta-analysis TRI CRT shows less bleeding
1953: Seldinger Non-selective CAG by percutaneous femoral approach	1993: Kiemeneij First 6 Fr coronary stent implantation by percutaneous transradial approach	1994: Fajadet performed first TRI live demo from Toulouse to TCT Washington	2008; Chase et al.: MORTAL study shows mortality reduction
1961: Ricketts and Adams Selective CAG by percutaneous femoral approach	1993: Kiemeneij, Laarman, Slagboom and van der Wieken first default radial angioplasters at OLVG	1994: ACCESS study starts as first CRT	2009: Jolly et al. Meta analysis TRI CRT shows less bleeding, better outcome
1962: Sones Selective CAG by brachial cut down	1993: Kiemeneij et al. First TRI poster at ACC followed by international papers	1995: First dedicated TRI course at OLVG	2011: Jolly et al. RIVAL study large CRT shows better outcome and mortality benefit
1964: Campeau CAG by cut down proximal radial artery	1994: Kiemeneij First transradial stent patient on outpatient basis	1995: More international pioneers started to build on the TRI expertise: Saito, Tift Mann, Hilton, Barbeau, Louvard, Fajadet, Spaulding, Hildick Smith, Nolan, Ludwig, Patel, Wang, Zhou, Soon, and many others	2012: Romagnoli et al. RIFLE-STEACS shows mortality benefit in PPCI for STEMI
1989: Campeau Selective CAG by percutaneous transradial approach		2000: After world wide training opportunities a new generation radialists emerged	2013: Hamon et al. Consensus document TRI
1992: Otaki Selective CAG by percutaneous transradial approach			2013: ESC declares TRI Class IIa level B guideline for PPCI 2015: ESC declares TRI Class I, level A guideline for NSTEMI

catheters in patients who required intense postprocedural antiocoagulation strategies. The small size of the artery did not allow use of 8 F guides however. Although at that time it was unthinkable to place stents through 5 F catheters it was just a matter of time before the first 6 F guides became available in the Netherlands in 1992. That year the first patient underwent successful transradial coronary balloon angioplasty for an LAD stenosis. Early 1993 the first (hand crimped) Palmaz Schatz coronary stent was placed successfully via a 6 Fr guide inserted in the radial artery in a patient with an ostial venous bypass graft stenosis. This pioneering phase was characterized as a single operator, and later a single center experiment when Drs Laarman, Slagboom and van der Wieken joined. Much emphasis was placed on training of nursing staff at the catheterization laboratory. There were no dedicated needles, sheaths, catheters and hemostasis devices available and the technique had to be developed from zero. The main goal was to increase safety of coronary stenting. The frontiers and limitations were yet unknown and had to be explored. Radial artery spasm, complex anatomy of the arm vasculature, late radial artery occlusions all had to be overcome. Results however were impressive enough to continue exploration of this technique. A patient could walk immediately after stent placement and nobody needed to worry about access site bleeding complications. These very first results were presented during the 66th scientific sessions of the AHA in 1993 in the form of a poster and early publications [10–12]. Although it drew modest attention, the poster presentation ignited international interest and it was the start of a new "movement" in interventional cardiology. Those who believed the message just started to build up experience, received training at the OLVG or started own training programs.

1.3 1994–2004 International Recognition

The pioneering single center phase now gradually started to internationalize. Dr. Jean Fajadet and Dr. Yves Louvard visited the OLVG early 1994 to see the application of TRI with their own eyes [13]. Only 2 weeks later Dr. Fajadet showed a live demonstration from Toulouse to the TCT Washington. This really ignited the international breakthrough. Thousands of interventional cardiologists witnessed for the first time a transradial coronary stent procedure, followed by immediate mobilization of the patient. The reactions were overwhelming.

Simply based on the attractive applied anatomy of the radial artery, more and more operators started to realize that the great promise of TRI was the reduction of major access site bleeding and thus resulting in less mortality, increased safety and patient comfort and in a reduction of costs. It can be said that in the first 50 papers published from 1992 to 1997, all these promises were demonstrated to hold and initial limitations and barriers were progressively torn down. The ACCESS [14] study was the first randomized study showing equivalence between radial, femoral and brachial access. The technique proved to be applicable for most patient subsets and most forms of coronary pathology. A growing number of radialists started to join, organizing dedicated meetings all over the world, the first one held in Amsterdam in 1995. It resulted in a challenging phase of exploration, education and development of dedicated TRI materials. Opposition, criticism and reluctance to restart a new learning curve by "femoralists" had to be overcome. Radial congresses emerged all over the world and were true reunions, meetings of friends, a perfect mix of exchanging information and experience with celebration of mutual recognition. The "Radial Revolution" became a fact.

There was a huge diversity in acceptance of TRI nationally, internationally and intercontinentally. In Asia, Japan was the front runner, followed by China and later India. Dr. Shigeru Saito, Shonan Kamakura, General Hospital played a pivotal role (and still does) in the spread and acceptance of TRI, not only in Japan, but also far beyond. Many countries developed training programs and research programs initiated by great pioneers like Tift Mann (USA), David Hilton (Canada), Gerald Barbeau (Canada), Yves Louvard, Jean Fajadet, Christian Spaulding (France), David Hildick Smith, Jim Nolan (UK), Josef Ludwig (Germany), Dr. Tejas Patel (India), Dr. Wang (Taiwan), Dr. Yu Jie Zhou (China), and many, many others.

Due to this international cooperation and cooperation with medical device industry, dedicated materials were developed to overcome most of the problems. Availability of radial artery puncture sets, sheaths, dedicated catheters and hemostasis devices did not only result in better outcome but also in lower thresholds to start a radial program.

1.4 2004–2014 International Acceptation

In the last decade evidence started to accumulate that bleeding complications after PCI results in major adverse outcome and mortality [15].

Meta-analysis suggested that TRI, by reducing bleeding complications, is associated with better outcome after PCI [16, 17]. The MORTAL study [18], the RIVAL study [19], the RIFLE STEACS study [20] and MATRIX study [21] demonstrated for the first time that TRI is associated with lower mortality, especially in acute coronary syndromes and primary PCI. It is one of the reasons that today TRI is gaining in popularity, especially in the US where TRI increased from 1.2 % in the first quarter of 2007 to 16.1 % in quarter 3 2012 [22]. A consensus paper of the ESC [23] declared that radial access is the route of choice for coronary interventions. TRI finally received official recognition and matured from experiment to guideline [24]. ESC Guideline 2015 Class I Level B.

1.5 Future Perspectives: A Personal View

Continued validation Much of the promises of transradial access, all related to reduction of bleeding complications are proven to hold. Still we have to demonstrate mortality reduction by TRI in all patient subsets. But the value of TRI is not only determined by major adverse cardiac events. For example, also patient friendliness and cost reduction are issues of great importance. Research should focus on these issues as well. Currently more attention is focused on hand- and arm function after transradial access.

Miniaturization Materials are refined, especially due to all efforts of the Japanese Slender Club, directed by Drs. Fuminobu Yoshimachi and Takashi Matsukage. By making sheaths, catheters and devices smaller and by developing more techniques and manoeuvers, TRI can be offered to all patients, also to patients with very small radial arteries. Miniaturization will make the procedure more comfortable and safe. If all promises of maximal miniaturization come true, patient value will increase because of better outcome at lower cost. But still this trend needs to become validated. In addition, slender TRI does not only require refined materials, it also demand excellent operator skills. Therefore, a lot has to be invested in material development and production and in training. So far the most slender products are exclusively available in Japan. Global availability of the best materials is mandatory. This is only possible by joint efforts and intensive communication between cardiologists and manufactures.

Japanese style Slender Clubs will expand to other countries and continents in order to share knowledge and experience.

Radial artery occlusion We are facing a huge challenge in preservation of radial artery patency for future use. If radial access for coronary angiography and intervention becomes default, more and more patients will suffer from radial artery occlusions. This is a serious complication, despite the benign clinical course. In my perspective, radial artery occlusion is the worst threat for the success of transradial access. Will TRI succumb under its own success? Not if we invest in minimal invasiveness, in proper post-operative care of the radial artery and in proper techniques to prevent and also to treat radial artery occlusions.

Training The transradial catheterization technique certainly is not on easy street. Anatomical variations, spasm, tortuosity, loops, calcifications, all need to be overcome before the guide reaches the coronary ostium. Sometimes this is frustrating, time consuming, painful, especially early in the learning curve. But with proper training, all these difficulties can be overcome, allowing more cardiologists to make this technique their default approach. Until now, training has not been structured nationally and internationally. Transradial access is not a compulsery part of the official training in cardiology. Perhaps an international accreditation program should be established, in order to offer the best, most updated basic and practical training.

An other point of concern is maintenance of proficiency in femoral access. This is mandatory in case of cross-over from radial to femoral and for specific femoral techniques such as insertion of balloon pumps and other left ventricular assist devices and of artificial valves. Thus a proper balance between training in radial and femoral access should be offered to future invasive cardiologists.

Despite these problems and open ends, TRI is here to stay. The technique has matured and has proven itself. Today, a radialist is not someone just being able to reach the heart from the wrist. A radialist is an invasive cardiologist who faces the challenge to reach the coronary arteries via the radial artery in such a way, that it is associated with maximal safety and comfort to the patient and who knows how to preserve the artery for future use. The radial artery belongs to the patient and we should keep it that way.

References

1. Radner S. Thoracal aortography by catheterization from the radial artery; preliminary report of a new technique. Acta Radiol. 1948;29(2):178–80.
2. Seldinger SI. Catheter replacement of the needle in percutaneous arteriography; a new technique. Acta Radiol. 1953;39(5):368–76.
3. Sones Jr FM, Shirey EK. Cine coronary angiography. Mod Concepts Cardiovasc Dis. 1962;31:735–8.
4. Ricketts HJ, Abrams HL. Percutaneous selective coronary cine arteriography. JAMA. 1962;181:620–4.
5. Judkins MP. Selective coronary arteriography.I.A percutaneous transfemoral technique. Radiology. 1967;89:815–24.
6. Campeau L. Entry sites for coronary angiography and therapeutic interventions from the proximal to the distal radial artery. Can J Cardiol. 2001;17:319–25.
7. Campeau L. Percutaneous radial artery approach for coronary angiography. Cathet Cardiovasc Diagn. 1989;16:3–7.
8. Otaki M. Percutaneous transradial approach for coronary angiography. Cardiology. 1992;81:330–3.
9. Serruys PW, de Jaegere P, Kiemeneij F, et al. A cpmparison of balloon expandable stent implantation with balloon angioplasty in patients with coronary artery disease. N Engl J Med. 1994;331:489–95.
10. Kiemeneij F, Laarman GJ, de Melker E. Transradial coronary artery angioplasty. Circulation. 1993;88:I–251. abstract.
11. Kiemeneij F, Laarman GJ, de Melker E. Transradial coronary artery angioplasty. Am Heart J. 1995;129:1–7.
12. Kiemeneij F, Laarman GJ. Percutaneous transradial artery approach for coronary Palmaz-Schatz stent implantation. Am Heart J. 1994;128:167–74.
13. http://www.escardio.org/communities/EAPCI/news/Pages/radial-approach-consensus.aspx
14. Kiemeneij F, Laarman GJ, Odekerken D, Slagboom T, van der Wieken R. A randomized comparison of percutaneous transluminal coronary angioplasty by the radial, brachial and femoral approaches: the ACCESS study. J Am Coll Cardiol. 1997;29:1269–75.
15. Doyle BJ, Rihal CS, Gastineau DA, Holmes Jr DR. Bleeding, bloodtransfusion, and increased mortality after percutaneous coronary intervention: implications for contemporary practice. J Am Coll Cardiol. 2009;53:2019–27.
16. Agostoni P, Biondi-Zoccai GC, de Benedictis ML, et al. Radial versus femoral approach for percutaneous coronary diagnostic procedures; Systematic overview and meta-analysis of randomized trials. J Am Coll Cardiol. 2004;44:349–56.
17. Jolly SS, Amlani S, Hamon M, Yusuf S, Mehta SR. Radial versus femoral access for coronary angiography or intervention and the impact on major bleeding and ischemic events: a systematic review and meta-analysis of randomized trials. Am Heart J. 2009;157(1):132–40.
18. Chase AJ, Fretz EB, Warburton WP, et al. Association of the arterial access site at angioplasty with transfusion and mortality: the M.O.R.T.A.L. Study (mortality benefit of reduced transfusion after percutaneous coronary intervention via the arm or leg). Heart. 2008;94:1019–25.
19. Jolly SS, Yusuf S, Cairns J, Niemelä K, Xavier D, Widimsky P, Budaj A, Niemelä M, Valentin V, Lewis BS, Avezum A, Steg PG, Rao SV, Gao P, Afzal R, Joyner CD, Chrolavicius S, Mehta SR, RIVAL trial group. Radial versus femoral access for coronary angiography and intervention in patients with acute coronary syndromes (RIVAL): a randomised, parallel group, multicentre trial. Lancet. 2011;377(9775):1409–20.
20. Romagnoli E, Biondi-Zoccai G, Sciahbasi A, Politi L, Rigattieri S, Pendenza G, Summaria F, Patrizi R, Borghi A, Di Russo C, Moretti C, Agostoni P, Loschiavo P, Lioy E, Sheiban I, Sangiorgi G. Radial versus femoral randomized investigation in ST-segment elevation acute coronary syndrome: the RIFLE-STEACS (Radial Versus Femoral Randomized Investigation in ST-Elevation Acute Coronary Syndrome) study. J Am Coll Cardiol. 2012;60(24):2481–9.
21. Valgimigli M, et al. Radial versus femoral access in patients with acute coronary syndromes undergoing invasive management: a randomised multicentre trial. Lancet. 2015;385(9986):2465–76.
22. Feldman DN, Swaminathan RV, Kaltenbach LA, Baklanov DV, Kim LK, Wong SC, Minutello RM, Messenger JC, Moussa I,

Garratt KN, Piana RN, Hillegass WB, Cohen MG, Gilchrist IC, Rao SV. Adoption of radial access and comparison of outcomes to femoral access in percutaneous coronary intervention: an updated report from the national cardiovascular data registry (2007-2012). Circulation. 2013;127(23):2295–306.
23. Hamon M, Pristipino C, Di Mario C, et al. Consensus document on the radial approach in percutaneous cardiovascular interventions: position paper by the European Association of Percutaneous Cardiovascular Interventions and Working Groups on Acute Cardiac Care and Thrombosis of the European Society of Cardiology. EuroIntervention. 2013;8:1242–51.
24. The Task Force on the management of ST-segment elevation acute myocardial infarction of the European Society of Cardiology (ESC). ESC Guidelines for the management of acute myocardial infarction in patients presenting with ST-segment elevation. Eur Heart J. 2012;33:2569–619.

Trans-radial and Trans-femoral Intervention

2

Marianna Adamo, Martial Hamon, and Marco Valgimigli

Abstract

The clinical equipoise, or lack thereof, between radial and femoral access site in patients undergoing coronary angiography and/or percutaneous coronary intervention has been extensively debated over the last two decades. Registries, randomized trials and meta-analyses have reported the benefit of the radial use with respect to vascular access site complications and bleeding. As result, expert opinion paper and European and American guidelines have endorsed the preferential use of radial over femoral access, in order to allow minimization of periprocedural bleeding events. Whether trans-radial intervention is also associated to improved patient outcomes beyond vascular and bleeding complications has been a matter of ongoing debate. The RIVAL study failed to provide unquestionable evidence of benefit in favor of radial approach. However, more recently the MATRIX study, which is the largest randomized comparison between radial versus femoral intervention in patients with acute coronary syndromes, provided clear evidence that radial, as compared to femoral intervention, reduces vascular and site-related major bleeding complications, transfusion, need for surgical repair of the arterial access and improves survival at 30 days.

The purpose of this chapter will be to critically revise the existing evidence comparing radial and femoral approaches for percutaneous coronary procedures.

2.1 Earliest Evidence

Campeau introduced the trans-radial approach for the first time in 1989 for diagnostic coronary angiography [1]; few years later Kiemeneij and Laarman reported the radial access use for percutaneous coronary interventions (PCIs) [2]. Since then, overwhelming evidence has been provided regarding its feasibility, safety and efficacy across the literature.

The earliest studies comparing radial and femoral approaches were pooled for the very fist time in 2004 by Agostoni et al. who performed a meta-analysis of 12 studies demonstrating that the radial access for coronary procedures (diagnostic catheterization and PCI) was safe and effective with a similar major adverse cardiovascular events (MACE) rate as compared to femoral access (OR 0.92; 95 % CI 0.57–1.48; $p=0.73$). Moreover, the radial approach drastically reduced the entry site complications (OR 0.20, 95 % CI 0.09–0.42; $p<0.001$), but it was also associated to a higher proportion of procedural failure (7.2 % vs. 2.4 %).

M. Adamo • M. Valgimigli, MD, PhD, FESC (✉)
Erasmus MC, Thoraxcenter Ba 587, Rotterdam, The Netherlands
e-mail: mariannaadamo@hotmail.com; m.valgimigli@erasmus.nl; vlgmrc@unife.it

M. Hamon
University of Caen, Caen, France
e-mail: hamon.martial@wanadoo.fr

Y. Zhou et al. (eds.), *Transradial Approach for Percutaneous Interventions*, DOI 10.1007/978-94-017-7350-8_2

Nevertheless, the observed heterogeneity for procedural failure disappeared when the study population was stratified according to the year of publication, most likely reflecting a possible learning curve effect [3].

2.2 Registries

The Mortality benefit Of Reduced Transfusion after percutaneous coronary intervention via the Arm or Leg (MORTAL) registry, published on 2008 by Chase et al., retrospectively analyzed an unselected PCI population of 38,872 patients underwent procedure either via trans-radial (7,972 patients) or trans-femoral artery (30,900 patients). The results showed that radial approach halved the need for blood transfusion and was associated to 29 % and 17 % reduction of 30-day and 1-year mortality, respectively [4].

A propensity score matched analysis published on 2012 from an observational region-wide registry (REgistro regionale AngiopLastiche dell'Emilia-Romagna - REAL) compared clinical outcome of more than 12,000 patients undergoing trans-radial or trans-femoral primary PCI for ST-elevation myocardial infarction (STEMI). This study reported a lower rate of 2-year mortality (8.8 % vs. 11.4 %; P=0.025) and vascular complication requiring surgery or blood transfusion (1.1 % vs. 2.5 %; P=0.005) in patients treated by radial approach as compared to those treated by femoral access [5].

Recently, Ratib et al. performed a retrospective analysis on a very large mixed PCI population reporting that radial access use was associated, irrespective of the clinical presentation, with a significant reduction of bleeding (stable OR 0.24; non-ST elevation acute coronary syndrome [NSTEACS] OR 0.35; STEMI OR 0.47; all P<0.001) and access site complications (stable OR 0.21; NSTEACS OR 0.19; STEMI OR 0.16; all P<0.001). However, a roughly 30 % risk reduction of MACE (composite of in-hospital mortality, myocardial infarction and repeat revascularization) was observed only in patients with unstable syndrome treated by radial approach. Of note, bleeding events were defined as any gastrointestinal, intra-cerebral or retroperitoneal bleeding, or blood product transfusion [6].

2.3 Randomized Trials

The RadIal Versus femor AL access for coronary intervention (RIVAL) study was the first large-scale randomized trial recruiting 7,021 patients in 32 countries, of which 3,507 patients were randomly assigned to radial access and 3,514 to femoral access. The trial failed to demonstrate the anticipated superiority of the radial approach with respect to the primary endpoint, which was a composite of death, myocardial infarction (MI), stroke and non- coronary artery bypass graft (non-CABG)-related major bleeding at 30 days (3.7 % vs. 4.0 %, HR 0.92, 95 %CI: 0.72–1.17; p=0.50) [7].

However, major vascular access site complications were significantly reduced in the radial arm (1.4 % vs. 3.7 % P<0.0001), whereas non-CABG-related major bleeding (0.5 % vs. 0.5 % P=ns) and access site major bleeding (0.2 % vs. 0.3 % P=ns) were similar in the two groups [7]. Bleeding events were defined according to the Thrombolysis in Myocardial Infarction (TIMI) classification.

This study has suggested a possible gradient in benefit with respect to radial versus femoral access, with STEMI patients deriving benefit for the composite of death, MI and stroke ($P_{int}=0.011$) and for all-cause mortality ($P_{int}=0.001$), whereas no such treatment effect was noted in patients with NSTEACS. A significant interaction for the primary outcome was also noted in the highest tertile volume radial centers (HR 0.49, 95 %CI 0.28–0.87; p=0.015) [7].

When the less stringent Acute Catheterization and Urgent Intervention strategy (ACUITY) bleeding definition was explored, instead of the protocol major bleeding scale, a significant reduction of major bleeding was observed in the radial cohort (1.9 % vs. 4.5 %; p<0.0001) in the RIVAL [7].

The Radial Versus Femoral Randomized Investigation in ST-Segment Elevation Acute Coronary Syndrome (RIFLE-STEACS) trial included 1,001 patients undergoing primary PCI by radial or femoral approach. The primary end-point was a composite of death, MI, target vessel revascularization, stroke or non–CABG-related major bleeding at 30 days. Of note, the trial endorsed the new Bleeding Academic Research Consortium (BARC) definition. A significant reduction of the primary endpoint (13.6 % vs. 21 %; P=0.003), owing to a lower rate of non–CABG-related major bleeding (7.8 % vs. 12.2 %; P=0.026) and death (5.2 % vs. 9.2 % P=0.02) in the radial arm was observed [8].

These apparently striking results need to be interpreted in the context of multiple considerations: (a) The operators in the RIFLE-STEACS performed more than 300 PCI/year; (b) The crossover rate from radial to femoral was almost 10 %, mainly due to shock, peripheral vascular disease and previous thrombolysis [8]; (c) Mortality and bleeding rates of the RIFLE-STEACS population was higher compared with previous STEMI trials, possibly reflecting the high risk profile of the included population allowing for cardiogenic shock and rescue PCIs to be included; (d) The respectively high and low use of glycoprotein IIb/IIIa inhibitors (GPI – 70 %) and bivalirudin in the study has been criticized [8]; (e) Although the access-site bleeding resulted significantly lower in the radial as compared to the femoral group, at a post-hoc analysis performed using the TIMI bleeding definition this benefit was no longer evident [8].

In the ST Elevation Myocardial Infarction treated by RADIAL or femoral approach (STEMI-RADIAL) roughly

700 patients with STEMI were randomly assigned to radial or femoral access before the primary PCI. The primary endpoint was a composite of 30-day major bleeding and vascular access site complications and resulted significantly higher in the femoral as compared to the radial arm (1.4 % vs. 7.2 %; P<0.0001). Trans-radial technique also reduced the rate of net adverse clinical events (NACE) defined as a composite of death, MI, stroke, major bleeding and major vascular complications (4.6 % vs. 11 %; P=0.0028). In contrast with the RIFLE-STEACS, no difference between radial and femoral groups with respect to 30-day mortality was noted in the STEMI-RADIAL (2.3 % vs. 3.1 %; P=0.64) [9].

The recent Minimizing Adverse haemorrhagic events by TRansradial access site and systemic Implementation of AngioX (MATRIX) Access was the largest randomized trial to compare radial and femoral access. 8,404 patients with acute coronary syndrome, with or without ST-segment elevation, were randomly allocatedto radial (4,197) or femoral (4,207) approach for invasive management. The two co-primary 30-day end-points were MACE (all-cause death, myocardial infarction or stroke) and NACE (MACE or BARC type 3 or 5 bleeding). A two-sided alpha was set at 2.5 % in order to reach statistical significance to account for two primary endpoints. A significant reduction of NACE was observed in radial compared with femoral group (9.8 % vs. 11.7 %; RR 0.83; 95 %CI 0.73–0.96; P=0.009), driven by a 28 % and 33 % risk reduction of mortality and bleeding, respectively. On the other hand, MACE rate was tendially lower in the radial arm but it did not reach statistical significance (8.8 % vs. 10.3 %, RR 0.85; 95 % CI 0.74–0.99; P=0.031) [10]. (Fig. 2.1).

No differences were observed with respect to myocardial infarction or stroke between the two groups. Radial approach significantly reduced vascular access complications and red blood cell transfusion compared with femoral access, with similar PCI success rates. Evidence for an interaction between tertiles of the centers' percentage of radial PCI and allocated access site was noted for both two co-primary endpoints (P_{int}=0.0048) with a pronounced benefit of radial access in center that did at least 80 % radial PCI. On the other hand, the anti-thrombin regimen used as per randomization scheme (bivaliridin vs. unfractionated heparin) did

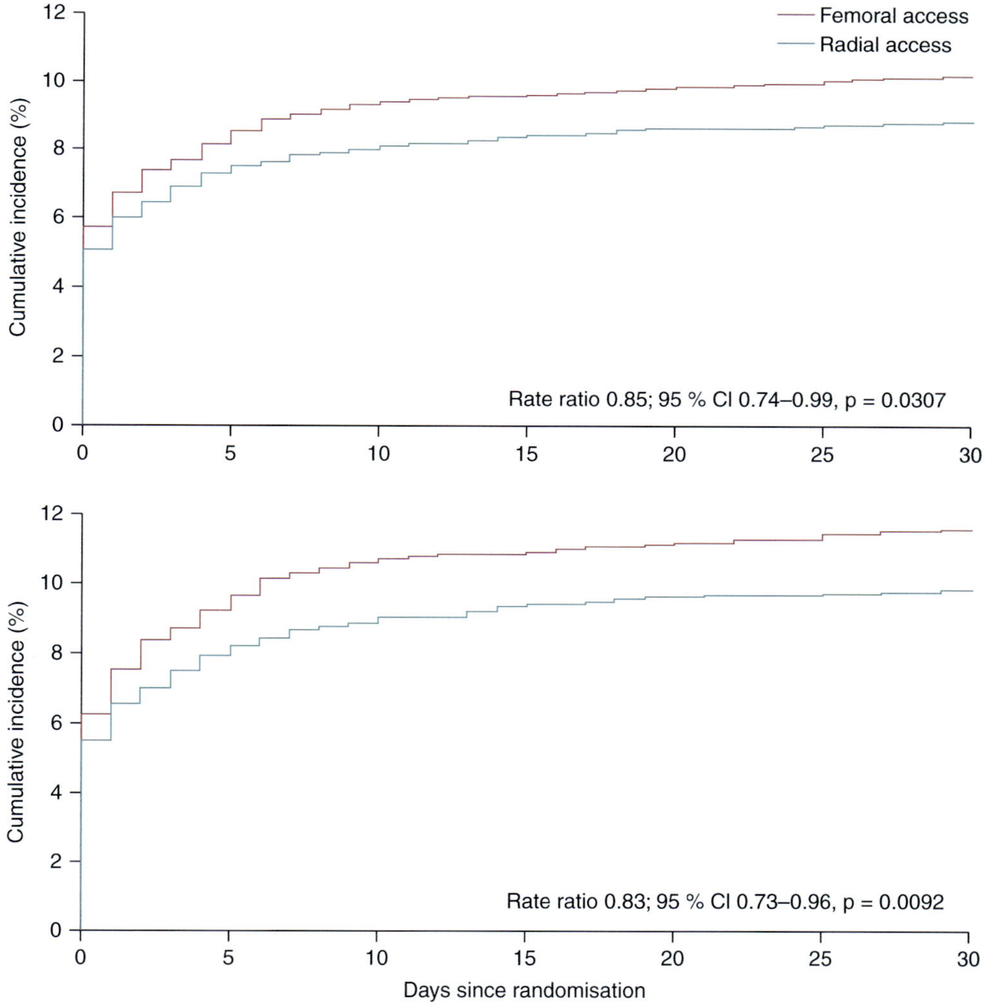

Fig. 2.1 MATRIX Access trial: Kaplan Meier curves for the co-primary end-points (Reprint with permission from Ref. [10])

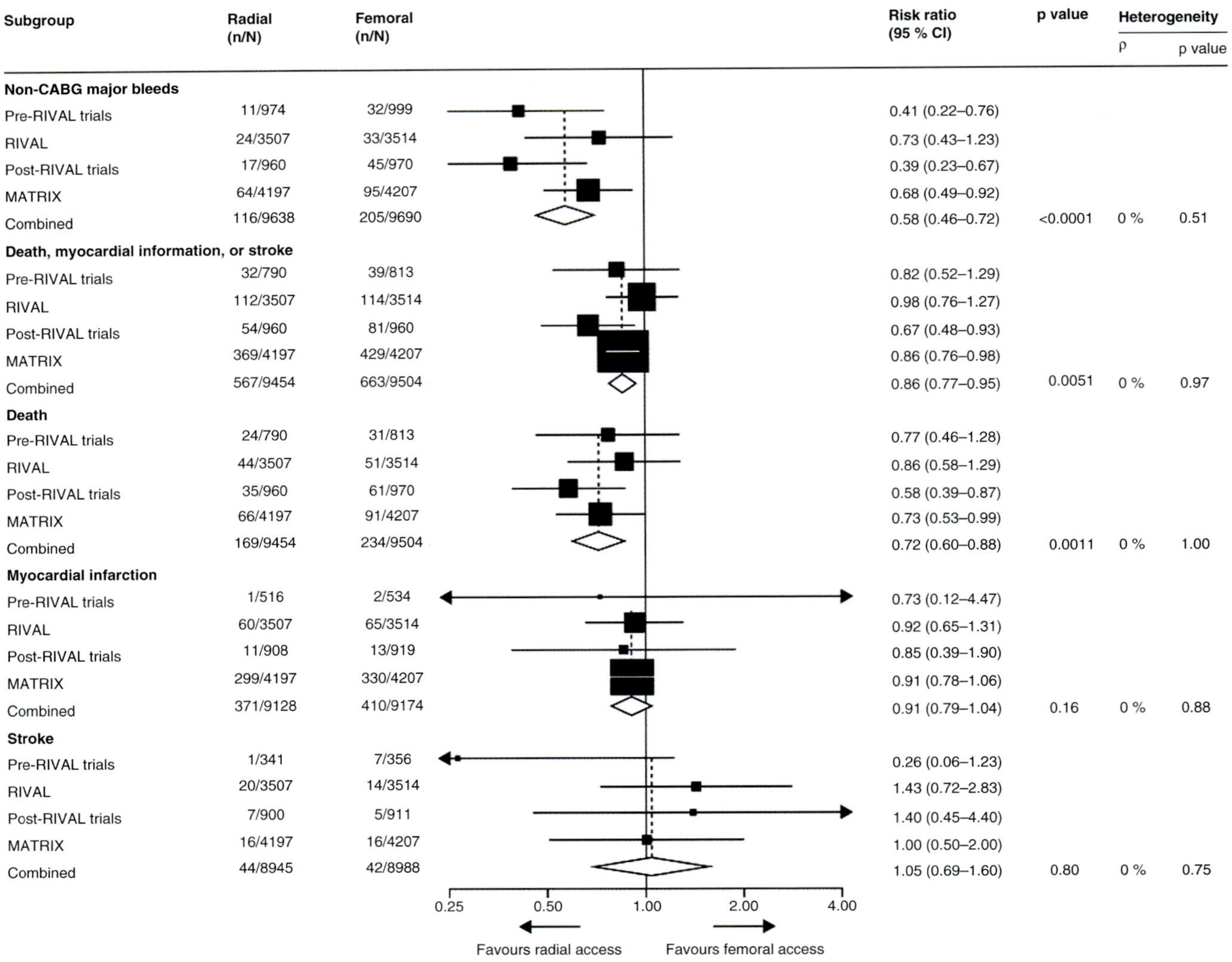

Fig. 2.2 Update meta-analysis from MATRIX Access paper (Reprint with permission from Ref. [10])

not modify the effect of arterial access site. Moreover, in contrast with the RIVAL results, the radial benefit was consistent across ACS patients [10].

In order to put the MATRIX Access results in the context of prior trials, the authors performed a meta-analysis updating those reported by RIVAL investigators, which confirms a significant mortality and MACE reduction in the radial as compared to femoral group [10]. (Fig. 2.2).

Hence, when taken together, the MATRIX Access study and the update meta-analysis suggest that radial access, reducing MACE, major bleeding and mortality, should become the default approach for patients with acute coronary syndrome undergoing invasive management [10].

2.4 Learning Curve and Expertise

Many studies attempted to define the learning curve of the trans-radial approach.

Ball et al. prospectively collected almost 1,700 patients with single vessel disease, undergoing non-urgenttrans-radial PCI by different physicians. The outcomes were stratified according to the time of operators starting trans-radial experience. The control group included only expert radial operators (>300 trans-radial procedures). The study showed that the PCI failure occurrence was inversely associated with the physician experience; about 30 % reduction of PCI failure every additional 50 radial procedures performed was observed [11].

More recently, Hess et al. investigated the learning curve for radial PCI among 54,561 procedures performed at 704 centres. Interestingly, as radial caseload increased, higher-risk patients were chosen (i.e., women, ST-segment elevation myocardial infarction and emergency indications). There was higher use of fluoroscopy time and contrast among newer (<30–50 cases) compared with more experienced (>30–50 cases) operators whereas procedural success rate was linearly associated with greater operator radial

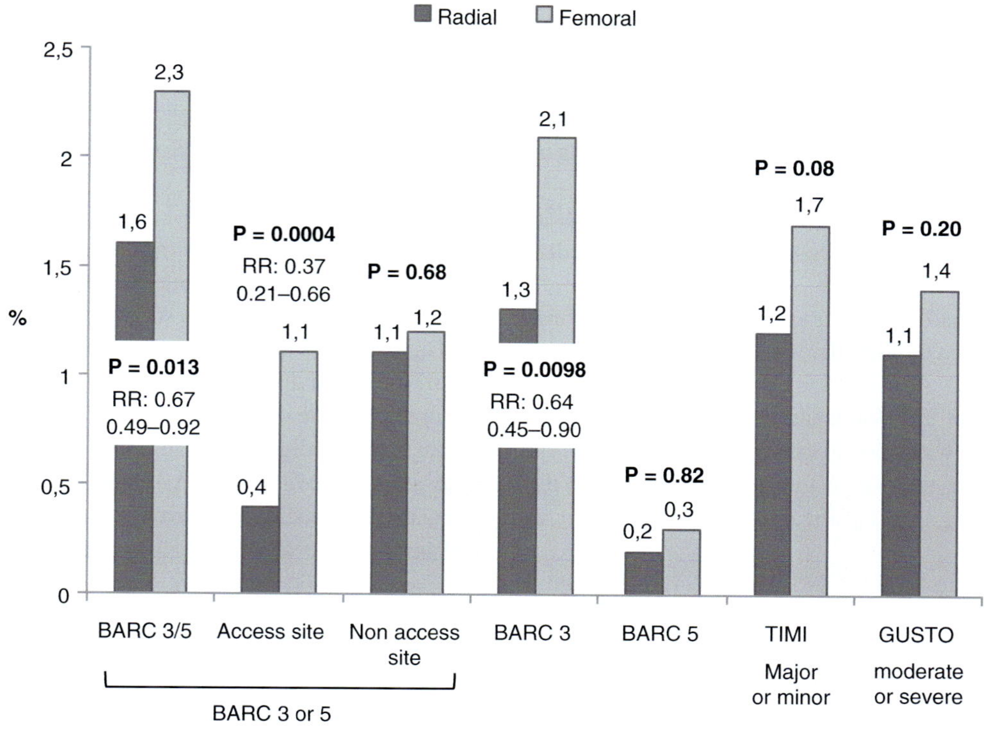

Fig. 2.3 MATRIX Access trial: bleeding events in radial and femoral groups according to BARC, TIMI and GUSTO classifications

experience. The authors concluded that the threshold to overcome the learning curve appears to be approximately 30–50 cases [12].

It has been suggested that left radial approach may have a shorter learning curve compared to the right radial access, owing to a lower impact of subclavian tortuosity in the left radial artery. Moreover, standard diagnostic and procedural catheters have been largely designed for the femoral route and as such may better adapt to left than right radial access site [13].

The radial approach requires expertise of both individual operators and institutional teams. The consensus document performed by the European Association of Percutaneous Cardiovascular Interventions in 2013 reported that, after learning curve, over 50 % radial access in routine practice with a minimum of 80 procedures/year per operator (including diagnostic and interventional procedures) should be a reasonable objective for achieving an average satisfactory proficiency [14].

In the RIVAL study, that included operators who had cumulatively performed at least 50 trans-radial catheterization at the randomization time, a significant interaction between access site and volume radial centers was observed for the primary outcome, with benefit for radial access in highest tertile [7].

Although MATRIX Access trial used a more strict selection of expert radial and femoral operators (at least 75 trans-radial intervention) the center proportion of radial PCI emerged as treatment modifier for both co-primary endpoints and all cause death. When major bleeding was separately appraised, there was no such effect of radial versus femoral access. These observations may suggest that while the bleeding benefit accrues at an earlier stage of the learning curve of trans-radial intervention, high proficiency and superior efficacy as compared to femoral requires high skills which can be met only by high volume radial operators [10].

2.5 Bleeding Issue

Bleeding related to the access site occurred in 30–70 % of PCI [15]. This high variability probably depends on patient's clinical presentation, concomitant medications and employed bleeding definition.

Based on MATRIX results, radial approach is associated to a 63 % reduction of access site related major bleeding, 33 % decrease of non–CABG-related major bleeding (Fig. 2.3) and 38 % reduction of transfusion rates compared with the femoral route [10].

Interestingly, the bleeding benefit of radial approach persisted also when vascular closure devices were employed in the femoral arm [16].

Considering the potential relationship between major bleeding and mortality, the reduction of bleeding events is of paramount importance.

Rao et al. demonstrated, in a large cohort of patients with NSTEACS, that bleeding severity was significantly related to 30-day mortality [17].

A sub-study of the TRITON-TIMI 38 trial that there was a high correlation between serious spontaneous bleeding and mortality within the first month after PCI [18].

Similarly, a sub-analysis of the PLATO trial demonstrated that bleeding related to the procedure strongly affected death at early follow-up [19].

As consequence of these findings, bleeding prevention strategies have been applied demonstrating a better survival in ACS patients.

In the OASIS-5 trial fondaparinux was found to be not inferior compared with enoxaparin in terms of ischemic outcomes and superior with respect to major bleeding at 9 days eventually resulting in a significant decrease of 30-day all-cause death [20].

Moreover, in the HORIZONS AMI the implementation of the bivalirudin compared with unfractionated heparin plus GPI in patients who underwent primary PCI, resulted in a reduction of both major bleeding and mortality at 30 days [21].

Finally, the EUROMAX trial showed that upstream bivalirudin compared with heparin use, in a context of new antiplatelet drugs (i.e., prasugrel and ticagrelor), reduced 30-day mortality or major bleeding [22].

2.6 Does the Radial Approach Reduce the Mortality?

Before the RIVAL study, many registries showed a mortality benefit of trans-radial as compared to the trans-femoral approach [4, 23, 24].

The unexpected results of RIVAL trial tempered the enthusiasm showing a not significant mortality difference between the two access groups. However, in the subgroup of STEMI patients with STEMI a 54 % mortality reduction after the trans-radial treatment was observed. On the other hand, in patients with NSTEACS a trend towards a 66 % higher mortality rate was noted ($P = 0.082$) [7].

In the RIFLE-STEACS trial a significant decrease of 30-day mortality was found in the radial group [8].

In the REAL registry a significant mortality reduction was reported in the radial versus femoral group at both early- and long-term follow-up [5].

Finally, the MATRIX trial showed a 28 % risk reduction of all-cause mortality at 30-day in patients undergoing invasive management through radial approach, irrespective of the clinical presentation. The updated meta-analysis of trials in patients with ACS, reported by MATRIX Investigators (Fig. 2.2), showed a statistically robust and clinically relevant reduction in all-cause death in radial as compared to femoral access, which could not be found in the previous meta-analysis reported in conjunction with the RIVAL paper [10].

When interpreted in the context of available evidence, radial access emerged as the most important single mortality reducer in patients undergoing PCI. Nevertheless, the reason of this impressive impact on survival is not fully explained.

The reduction in access site major bleeding is a clear benefit of the radial approach but it remains to be understood if it can explain the observed mortality benefit. However, non-access site bleeding affects mortality two times more than access site bleeding [15]. As BARC 5 (i.e., fatal haemorrhage event) bleeding were evenly distributed between radial and femoral access in MATRIX, it is tempting to speculate that non-fatal bleeding may trigger a sequence of consequences, ultimately leading to higher mortality risk in the acute setting of ACS. Radial approach allows early mobilization and it has been suggested it can minimize the risk of acute kidney injury as compared to femoral intervention [25]. Yet, the contribution of non-bleeding related benefit in patients undergoing radial intervention remains to be further elucidated.

Anticoagulation strategies with low use of bivalirudin (<10 %) and higher than contemporary use of GPI (30–70 %) might have contributed to the mortality difference in the two groups in STEMI patients included in RIVAL and RIFLEACS studies.

In the MATRIX Access trial bivalirudin was used during PCI in more than 40 % of the patients; less than 14 % of the patients received GPI at the time of intervention and more than 50 % of the patients were treated with ticagrelor or prasugrel, more closely reflecting contemporary clinical practice [10].

Conclusions

The benefit of the radial approach in coronary procedures with respect to vascular access site complications and bleeding has been largely reported. Moreover, strong evidence now supports the use of radial route as factor improving clinical outcome in patients undergoing invasive management for acute coronary syndrome. Given the observed and statistically sound mortality benefit in favor of radial access, a continuous effort should be done to improve the proficiency in this approach and make transradial intervention the default choice across the globe, given its impact on safety, efficacy and costs.

References

1. Campeau L. Percutaneous radial artery approach for coronary angiography. Cathet Cardiovasc Diagn. 1989;16(1):3–7.
2. Kiemeneij F, Laarman GJ. Percutaneous transradial artery approach for coronary stent implantation. Cathet Cardiovasc Diagn. 1993;30(2):173–8.
3. Agostoni P, Biondi-Zoccai GG, de Benedictis ML, Rigattieri S, Turri M, Anselmi M, et al. Radial versus femoral approach for percutaneous coronary diagnostic and interventional procedures; Systematic overview and meta-analysis of randomized trials. J Am Coll Cardiol. 2004;44(2):349–56.
4. Chase AJ, Fretz EB, Warburton WP, Klinke WP, Carere RG, Pi D, Berry B, Hilton JD. Association of the arterial access site at angioplasty with transfusion and mortality: the M.O.R.T.A.L study (mortality benefit of reduced transfusion after percutaneous coronary intervention via the Arm or Leg). Heart. 2008;94(8):1019–25.
5. Valgimigli M, Saia F, Guastaroba P, Menozzi A, Magnavacchi P, Santarelli A, et al.; REAL Registry Investigators. Transradial versus transfemoral intervention for acute myocardial infarction: a propensity score-adjusted and -matched analysis from the REAL (REgistro regionale AngiopLastiche dell'Emilia-Romagna) multicenter registry. JACC Cardiovasc Interv. 2012;5(1):23–35.
6. Ratib K, Mamas MA, Anderson SG, Bhatia G, Routledge H, De Belder M, et al. Access site practice and procedural outcomes in relation to clinical presentation in 439,947 patients undergoing percutaneous coronary intervention in the United kingdom. JACC Cardiovasc Interv. 2015;8(1 Pt A):20–9.
7. Jolly SS, Yusuf S, Cairns J, Niemelä K, Xavier D, Widimsky P, et al. RIVAL trial group. Radial versus femoral access for coronary angiography and intervention in patients with acute coronary syndromes (RIVAL): a randomised, parallel group, multicentre trial. Lancet. 2011;377(9775):1409–20.
8. Romagnoli E, Biondi-Zoccai G, Sciahbasi A, Politi L, Rigattieri S, Pendenza G, et al. Radial versus femoral randomized investigation in ST-segment elevation acute coronary syndrome: the RIFLE-STEACS (Radial Versus Femoral Randomized Investigation in ST-Elevation Acute Coronary Syndrome) study. J Am Coll Cardiol. 2012;60(24):2481–9.
9. Bernat I, Horak D, Stasek J, Mates M, Pesek J, Ostadal P, et al. ST-segment elevation myocardial infarction treated by radial or femoral approach in a multicenter randomized clinical trial: the STEMI-RADIAL trial. J Am Coll Cardiol. 2014;63(10):964–72.
10. Valgimigli M, Gagnor A, Calabró P, Frigoli E, Leonardi S, Zaro T, et al.; MATRIX Investigators. Radial versus femoral access in patients with acute coronary syndromes undergoing invasive management: a randomised multicentre trial. Lancet. 2015; 385(9986):2465–76. pii: S0140-6736(15)60292-6.
11. Ball WT, Sharieff W, Jolly SS, Hong T, Kutryk MJ, Graham JJ, et al. Characterization of operator learning curve for transradial coronary interventions. Circ Cardiovasc Interv. 2011;4(4):336–41.
12. Hess CN, Peterson ED, Neely ML, Dai D, Hillegass WB, Krucoff MW, et al. The learning curve for transradial percutaneous coronary intervention among operators in the United States: a study from the National Cardiovascular Data Registry. Circulation. 2014;129(22):2277–86.
13. Sciahbasi A, Romagnoli E, Trani C, Burzotta F, Pendenza G, Tommasino A, et al. Evaluation of the "learning curve" for left and right radial approach during percutaneous coronary procedures. Am J Cardiol. 2011;108(2):185–8.
14. Hamon M, Pristipino C, Di Mario C, Nolan J, Ludwig J, Tubaro M, European Association of Percutaneous Cardiovascular Interventions; Working Group on Acute Cardiac Care of the European Society of Cardiology; Working Group on Thrombosis on the European Society of Cardiology. Consensus document on the radial approach in percutaneous cardiovascular interventions: position paper by the European Association of Percutaneous Cardiovascular Interventions and Working Groups on Acute Cardiac Care** and Thrombosis of the European Society of Cardiology. EuroIntervention. 2013;8(11):1242–51.
15. Verheugt FW, Steinhubl SR, Hamon M, Darius H, Steg PG, Valgimigli M, et al. Incidence, prognostic impact, and influence of antithrombotic therapy on access and nonaccess site bleeding in percutaneous coronary intervention. JACC Cardiovasc Interv. 2011;4(2):191–7.
16. Mann T, Cowper PA, Peterson ED, Cubeddu G, Bowen J, Giron L, et al. Transradial coronary stenting: comparison with femoral access closed with an arterial suture device. Catheter Cardiovasc Interv. 2000;49(2):150–6.
17. Rao SV, O'Grady K, Pieper KS, Granger CB, Newby LK, Van de Werf F, et al. Impact of bleeding severity on clinical outcomes among patients with acute coronary syndromes. Am J Cardiol. 2005;96(9):1200–6.
18. Hochholzer W, Wiviott SD, Antman EM, Contant CF, Guo J, Giugliano RP, et al. Predictors of bleeding and time dependence of association of bleeding with mortality: insights from the Trial to Assess Improvement in Therapeutic Outcomes by Optimizing Platelet Inhibition With Prasugrel--Thrombolysis in Myocardial Infarction 38 (TRITON-TIMI 38). Circulation. 2011;123(23):2681–9.
19. Ducrocq G, Schulte PJ, Becker RC, Cannon CP, Harrington RA, Held C, et al. Association of spontaneous and procedure-related bleeds with short- and long-term mortality after acute coronary syndromes: an analysis from the PLATO trial. EuroIntervention. 2015;11(7):737–45. pii: 20140908-03.
20. Anderson JA, Hirsh J, Yusuf S, Johnston M, Afzal R, Mehta SR, et al. Comparison of the anticoagulant intensities of fondaparinux and enoxaparin in the Organization to Assess Strategies in Acute Ischemic Syndromes (OASIS)-5 trial. J Thromb Haemost. 2010 Feb;8(2):243–9.
21. Stone GW, Witzenbichler B, Guagliumi G, Peruga JZ, Brodie BR, Dudek D, et al. Bivalirudin during primary PCI in acute myocardial infarction. N Engl J Med. 2008;358(21):2218–30.
22. Steg PG, Van't Hof A, Hamm CW, Clemmensen P, Lapostolle F, Coste P, et al. Bivalirudin started during emergency transport for primary PCI. N Engl J Med. 2013;369(23):2207–17.
23. Pristipino C, Trani C, Nazzaro MS, Berni A, Patti G, Patrizi R, et al. Major improvement of percutaneous cardiovascular procedure outcomes with radial artery catheterisation: results from the PREVAIL study. Heart. 2009;95(6):476–82.
24. Vorobcsuk A, Konyi A, Aradi D, Horvath IG, Ungi I, Louvard Y, et al. Transradial versus transfemoral percutaneous coronary intervention in acute myocardial infarction systematic overview and meta-analysis. Am Heart J. 2009;158(5):814–21.
25. Andò G, Costa F, Boretti I, Trio O, Valgimigli M. Benefit of radial approach in reducing the incidence of acute kidney injury after percutaneous coronary intervention: a meta-analysis of 22,108 patients. Int J Cardiol. 2015;179:309–11.

Part II

Transradial Approach: From Novice to Master

3 Radial Anatomy and Pre-operative Evaluation

Yujie Zhou, Wei Liu, and Zhi Tao Jing

Abstract

Procedures using transradial coronary approach have been challenging technically and include specific characteristics of the route in comparison to the traditional femoral technique, thus carry a prolonged learning curve. However, with the knowledge of route anomalies and the advancement of interventional devices, successful transradial procedures can be performed even with abnormal radial anatomy. The numerous advantages of transradial access have been well discussed in many previous studies for over two decades, justified well enough to be chosen as solid alternative for coronary interventions. However, the disadvantages or difficulties found are restricted to anatomy related challenges, due to the transradial technique having its unique differences in comparison to the transfemoral technique. In this chapter, we start with normal and abnormal radial anatomy then deal with the common problems that hurdle the success in transradial intervention practice.

3.1 The Wrist

The wrist is the joint between the forearm and hand. It consists of 8 bones known as the carpals. The radial, ulnar and interosseous arteries supply the wrist and hand via the deep and superficial palmar arch (Fig. 3.1). At wrist level, the radial artery sits above the scaphoid bone, the trapezium and the external lateral ligament. If the radial artery is cannulised too distal, the retinaculum will be encountered, and it would be found that the artery is diving deep and lateral. It is very important to be precise with the cannulation (approximately 2–3 cm from flexion crease of wrist, 1 cm above radial styloid process) due to the minor superficial branches of the radial artery exiting in the same area.

Y. Zhou (✉) • W. Liu
Department of Cardiology, Beijing Anzhen Hospital, Capital Medical University, Beijing, China
e-mail: Azzyj12@163.com; Liuwei525@hotmail.com

Z.T. Jing
PLA Rocket General Hospital, Chaoyang Qu, Beijing, China

3.2 Deep and Superficial Palmar Arch

Moving closer towards the hand, the radial artery makes its way into the palm by going through the gap between the metacarpal bones of the thumb and index finger, which then passes the little finger metacarpal bone, where the terminal parts of the radial artery meet with the ulnar artery's deep palmar branch to form the deep palmar arch (Deep vola arch). The deep palmer arch is formed mainly by terminal parts of radial artery and gives branch of the palmar metacarpal arteries which serve the fingers but not the thumb,latter is supplied by princeps pollicis artery (Fig. 3.1). The palmar metacarpal arteries terminate at finger clefts by joining the common digital branches of the superficial palmer arch. Dorsally, the deep palmer arch also gives off three perforating arteries (proximally) in connecting the digital branches of the superficial palmar arch with dorsal metacarpal arteries.

In completion of the superficial palmer arch (superficial vola arch), the superficial palmer branch of the radial artery links with the terminal branch of ulnar artery at the palmar region. The superficial palmer arch gives branch to 4

Y. Zhou et al. (eds.), *Transradial Approach for Percutaneous Interventions*, DOI 10.1007/978-94-017-7350-8_3

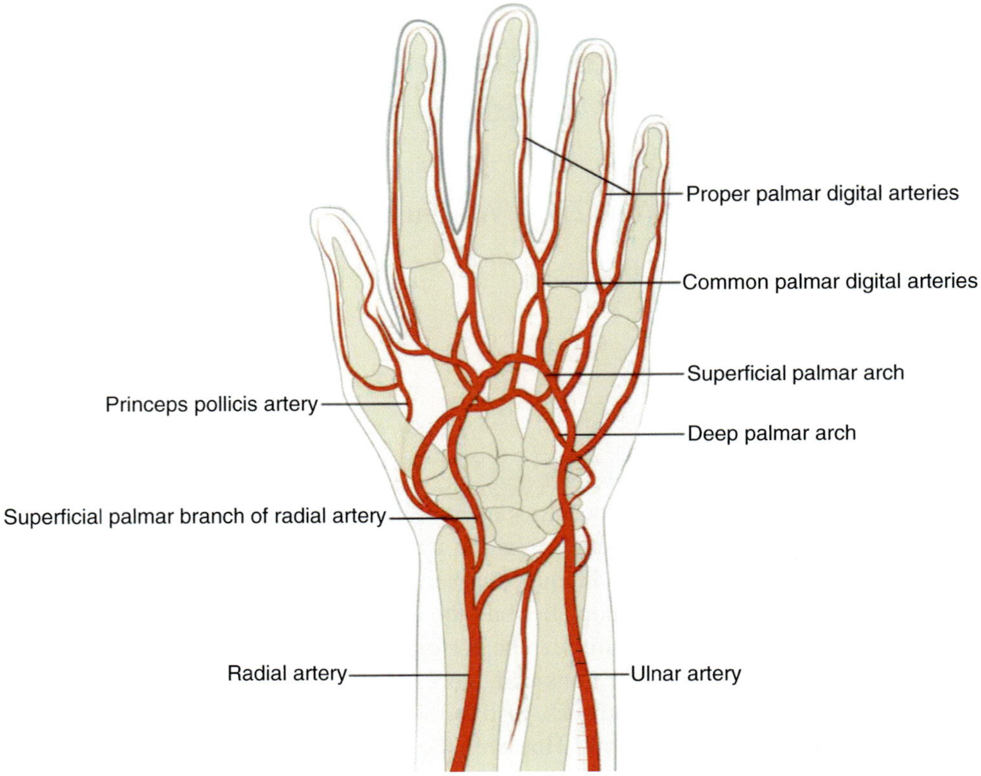

Fig. 3.1 Deep and superficial palmar arches formed by radial and ulnar artery

common palmer digital arteries supplying the medial 3 1/2 fingers. The superficial palmar arch is formed predominantly by the ulnar artery, with a contribution from the superficial palmar branch of the radial artery. However in some individuals the contribution from the radial artery might be absent, and instead anastomoses with either the princeps pollicis artery, the radialis indicis artery, or the median artery, the former two of which are branches from the radial artery.

The presence of variations in the superficial palmer arch is of great surgical importance. The anatomic variation of palmer arch has been described by many previous papers with different results and percentages. However, most paper suggest that majority hand showed complete superficial palmer arch which implies that collateral circulation is present in majority of cases [1]. In addition, studies also showed that there were no cases of an incomplete superficial and deep palmar arch being present in the same hand. Such as in the case of the incomplete deep palmar arch, all these hands had complete superficial palmar arches [2]. This would result in least number of complications considering radial artery harvesting for coronary bypass or transradial cannulation, thus provides a rational for performing these procedures. However, since all specimen in these studies were free of atherosclerosis disease, the authors from those studies still recommend testing the hand (by using the modified Allen test, Doppler ultrasonography, photoplethysmography, or oximetric techniques) before performing an arterial intervention to identify the occasional case in which collateral circulation is compromised by the presence of arterial disease [2].

In conclusion : Both the radial and ulnar arteries sub branch in such a manner that blood is sufficiently provided to the entire hand, allowing dual blood supply which also gives a critical advantage to transradial intervention in rivalry to transfemoral intervention.

3.3 Allen's Test

The aim of the Allen's test is to inspect the superficial and deep palmar arches. Acute vascular disease is indicated by presence of abnormal arches. The superficial and deep palmar arches provide the blood supply to the fingers. The radial artery and the ulnar artery supplies the deep palmar arch and superficial palmar arch, respectively. Allen's test had been performed prior to radial puncture interventions.

The examiner performs the test by initially palpating and applying pressure on the radial and ulnar arteries by using three fingers on each artery. This act occludes the blood supply to the entire hand. The patient is then asked to clinch then open his/her hand tightly 10 times, ending with an open hand position. The patient should not over extend the fingers and wrist as this could cause the soft tissues to appear white due to tension, leading to a false positive result. The palmar region of the hand should then appear white or pale. Then the examiner releases the pressure applied from one of the arteries. A positive result is noted when it takes >5 s for palmar blood supply to return (note colour). Repeat these same tests to assess the unexamined artery (Fig. 3.2).

Because Allen's test is more subjective, in some labs, patients who are considered for transradial catheterization should be tested by the modified Allen's test by means of a pulse oximeter, also known as the Barbeau test. The modified Allen's test involves a few alterations. After the patient is asked to close the fist, the examiner massages blood out of the hand. The pressure to both arteries will then be given by using the thumb rather than three fingers. After the patient opens his/her hand paleness should be noted around the thenar. The examiner will then release the thumb off the ulnar artery and observe the thenar eminence. If the normal colour returns within 15 s, it indicates intact blood flow. The same steps should be repeated for the radial artery however, the pressure applied by the thumb should first be released off the radial artery [4] (Fig. 3.3).

This is a great method to test adequate blood flow, because with the pressure applied occlusion is formed within the arteries limiting the blood to enter the hand. Clinching the hand repetitively pushes the blood out of the hand which justifies the white/pale colour. At the time when the examiner releases the pressure from one of the arteries and normal colour is visible self-explains adequate blood circulation from that particular artery.

The sensor clamp is preferably applied to the thumb. The presence of a pulse tracing during radial artery compression, as in types A and B, represents uninterrupted pulsatile arterial blood filling. Because the radial artery pulse could be present with a patent palmar arch in several cases of radial artery occlusion (RAO), that is occasionally seen in the type A pattern; in which, pulsatile blood flow to the thumb is not reduced. RAO can then be suspected when ulnar artery compression produces a type D reading, enabling pre- and post-procedural evaluation of radial artery patency.

In type C, pulsatile blood flow, and pulse oximetry, is abolished temporarily by radial artery compression, but it reappears within a pre-specified amount of time, arbitrarily chosen to be 2 min. When radial artery compression is repeated within approximately 1 min, a type C pattern is often changed into a type B pattern, suggesting collaterals recruitment induced by relative hand ischemia. In type D, pulsatile blood flow, and pulse oximetry, is abolished by radial artery compression and does not reappear within 2 min. The type D pattern was considered to be a contra-indication for the transradial approach.

Whether the Allens test is still a valid method to examine both the radial and ulnar blood flow for transradial interventions?

According to studies till date, it has been a rather controversial topic predicting whether the Allens test is sufficient to certify that ischemic complications post transradial access will not occur. According to readings from earlier studies, after 30 min of radial artery occlusion patients with a negative Allens test result proved to have an inadequate amount of blood circulation to the thumb, and an increased thumb capillary lactate, which is suggestive of ischemia. This suggested that patients with an abnormal Allens test should not undergo procedure via the transradial route. On the contrary, a more recent RADAR study suggests that the Allens test and oximetry-plethysmography are not scientifically reliable and predictive for noting rises in lactate levels, weakness in the hand, or persistent discomfort for transradial interventions. Thus, the study concluded that completely denying radial access due to a negative Allens test result is not a solid enough justification. Currently, many transradial centres have come very close to completely nullifying the Allens test for pre-procedure tests for TRA. However, emphasis on techniques such as oximetry-plethsmography for patent hemostasis along with other techniques should be strengthened to minimise potential RAO complication [5, 6].

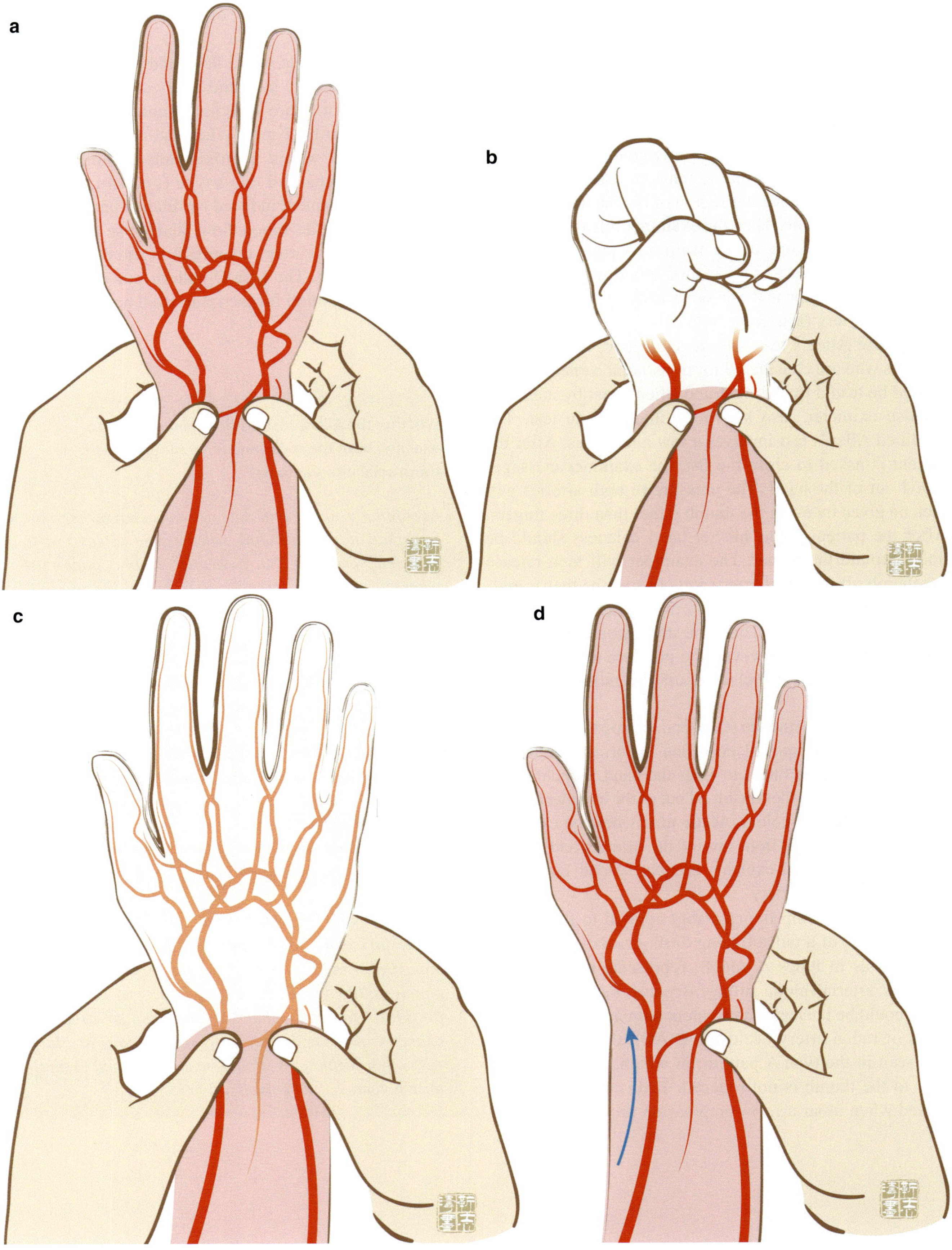

Fig. 3.2 (**a**) Palpation of the radial and ulnar arteries. (**b**) Manual compression of the radial and ulnar artery upon clenching the fist (**c**) Palmar blanching upon opening the fist. (**d**) The ulnar artery pressure is released; if the colour returns to *pink*, it is indication of positive test; if the colour does not return to *pink*, it indicates a negative test [3]

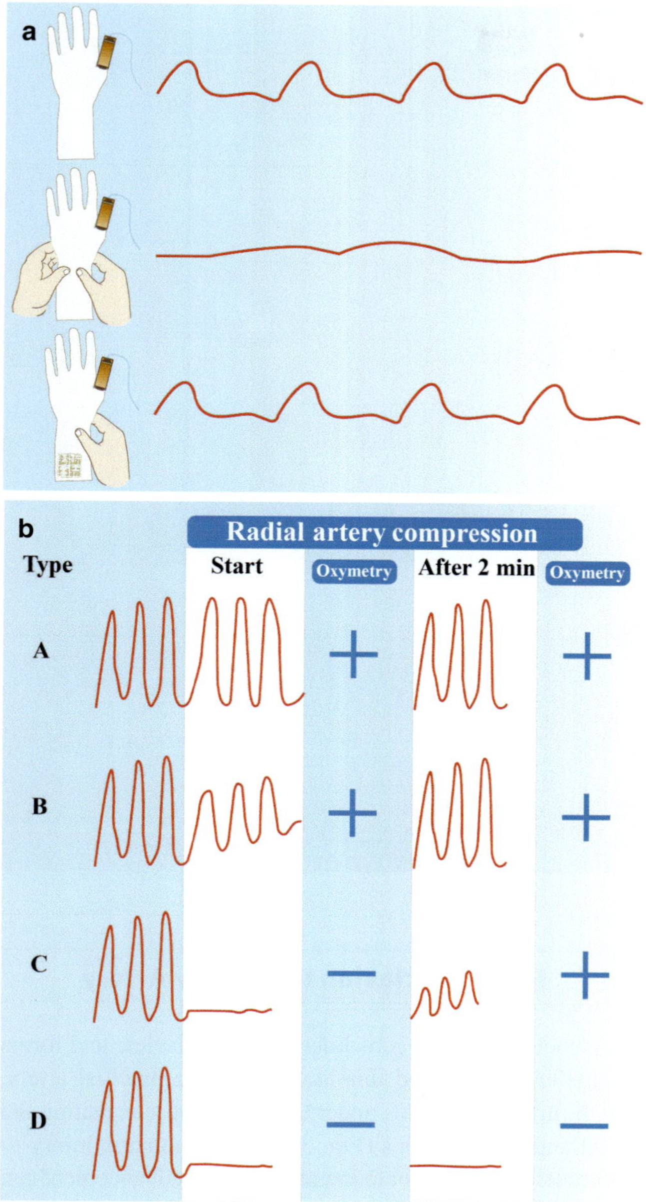

Fig. 3.3 (**a**) Modified Allen's test by means of a pulse oximeter, also known as the Barbeau test; (**b**) Type A: No damping of pulse tracing immediately after radial artery compression, Type B: Damping of pulse tracing, Type C: Loss of pulse tracing followed by recovery of pulse tracing within 2 min Type D: Loss of pulse tracing without recovery within 2 min

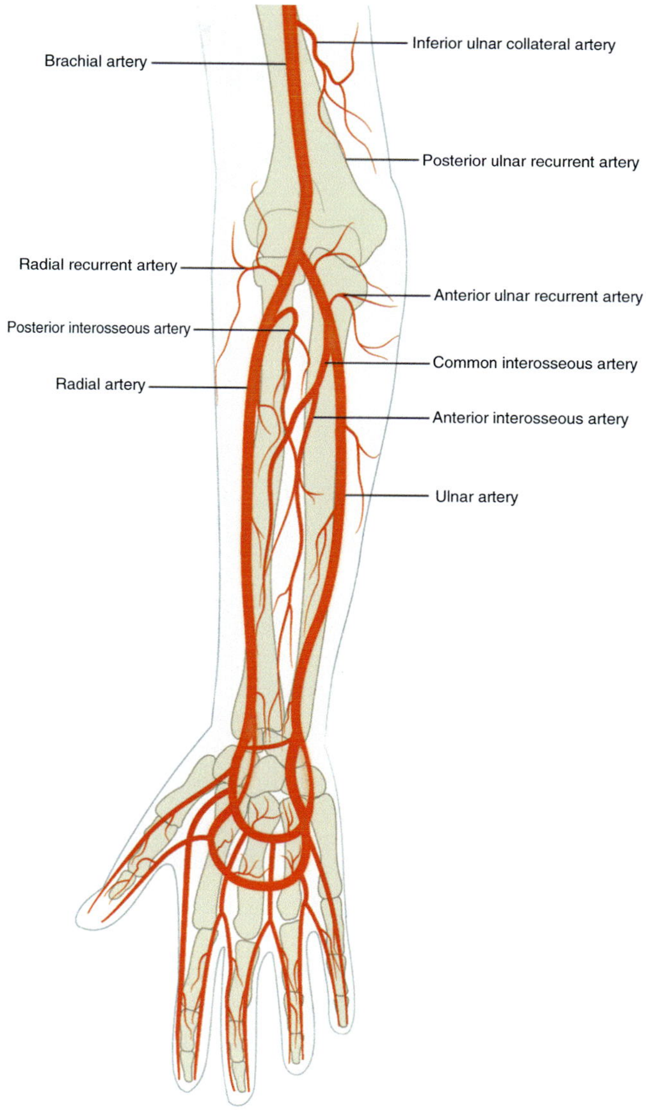

Fig. 3.4 An artwork illustrates anatomic course of the right radial/ulnar artery from elbow (brachial bifurcation) to wrist (palm arch)

3.4 Anatomic Anomalies at Brachial Bifurcation

The radial and ulnar arteries both run through either side of the forearm to the wrist. Proximally, they both form recurrent arteries that complete the arterial anastomosis at the elbow. In addition, the ulnar artery gives off an intraosseous branch that bifurcates to form anterior, posterior and recurrent branches. Anatomic anomalies are frequently encountered at brachial bifurcation which impede the successful cannulation (Fig. 3.4).

Radial recurrent artery The radial current or pseudo radial artery is a small artery that branches of the radial artery just below the elbow. Its incidence rate is 8.3 % [1]. It runs next to the brachial artery then joins the brachial artery close to the axillary artery. During catheterization in TRI, the wire could possibly travel up the radial recurrent artery instead of the brachial artery (Fig. 3.5a). This could be problematic as the lumen of the radial recurrent artery is small, leading to wiring challenges and possible perforation (Fig. 3.5b).

Radial loop The radial loop is a tight bend forming a 360° loop which occurs in the radial artery, distal to the bifurcation of the brachial artery. Occurring in approximately 2 % [2] of patients, the radial loop poses a higher chance of technical failure. The radial loop has a tendency to avert the straight tipped wire up the side to the recurrent radial artery,

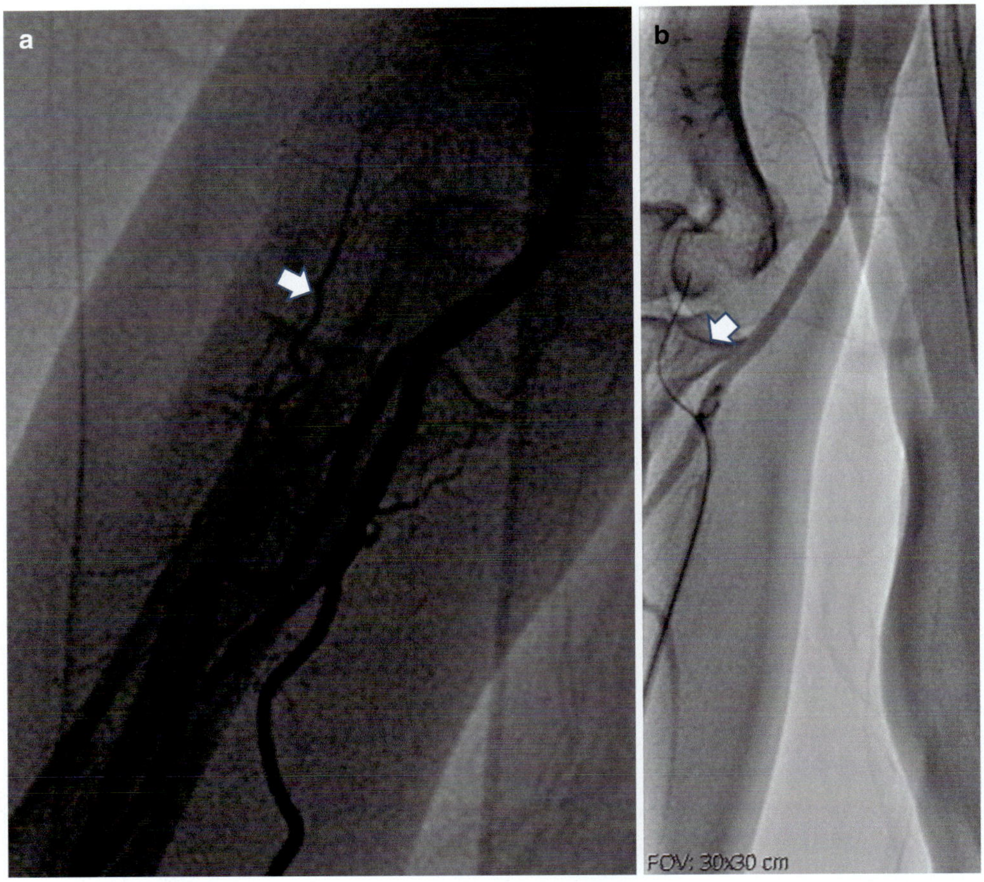

Fig. 3.5 (**a**) Radial recurrent artery (*white arrow*) (**b**) Hydrophilic wire entering into the radial recurrent branch

which runs parallel to the brachial artery. Patients with a radial loop have a high tendency of having a recurrent radial artery branch or pseudo radial artery. This puts the patient at risk of avulsion and wire perforation as well as causing wiring challenges (Fig. 3.6).

High bifurcation Around 7 % of patients have their radial arteries bifurcating off the brachial artery above the antecubital fossa. This is an abnormally high bifurcation point of the brachial artery as most bifurcate below the elbow joint. Although this phenomenon does not lead to a high incidence of TRI failure, it can lead to a radial artery that is tortuous and has a small lumen, making it difficult for the catheter wire to pass through smoothly (Fig. 3.7).

Tortuous artery Tortuous arteries can be found anywhere along the radial or brachial arteries. Its incidence rate is 3.8 % [1]. It is the twisting orbending of the artery. Patients with extremely tortuous arteries have a statically high procedural failure rate as it prevents the catheter wire from passing through the vessel smoothly and increases arterial spams (Fig. 3.8).

3.5 From Subclavian to Axillary Artery

The subclavian artery runs inferior to the clavicle and forms the axillary artery and this then forms the brachial artery, which further bifurcates under the elbow crease creating the radial and ulnar arteries (Fig. 3.9). Any traumatic injury to the branch along the route induced by wire advancement can cause artery perforation leading to uncontrolled bleeding and hematoma. There are several reports of mediastinal and neck hematoma that developed after transradial catheterization as results from injuring the small branch of innominate artery or aortic arch by either hydrophilic or J shape wire [7–9]. The main difficulties of transraidal approach in compare with transfemoral approach lie in the abnormal origin of subclavian/innominate artery from aortic arch, which we will deal it in detail in Chap. 10. Having patient take a deep breath to straighten subclavian/innominate arteries and subclavian/innominate-aortic junction will allow the direct catheter to ascending aorta in most cases.

Common radial anomalies are listed in Fig. 3.10. *The measures that deal with these anatomic difficulties will be explained further in the following chapters as a step to shorten the learning curve of the transradial intervention* [10].

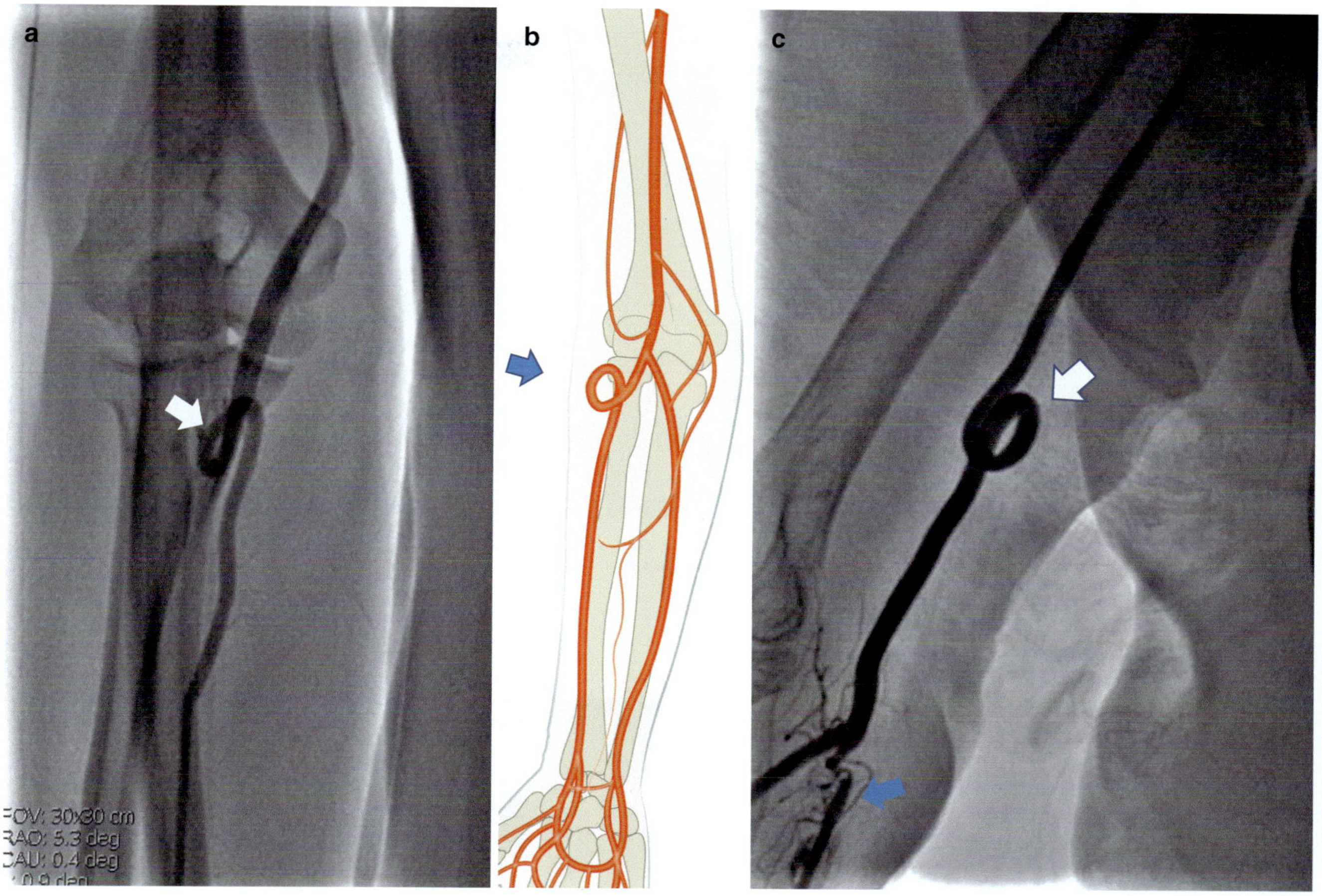

Fig. 3.6 (**a**, **b**) Radial loop (*arrows* indicate radial loop) (**c**) brachial loop (*white arrow*), tortuous radial artery (*white arrow*) and perforation induced by wire advancement (*blue arrow*)

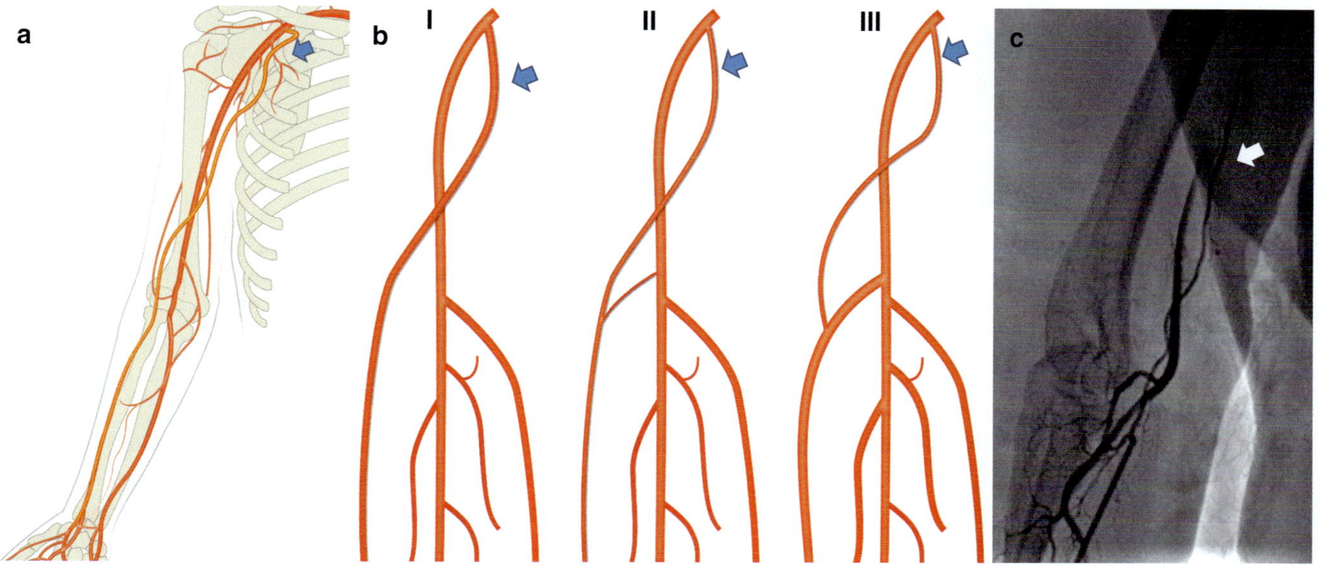

Fig. 3.7 (**a**, **b**) Variant form of high origin of radial artery (*blue arrow*) (**c**) An angiogram of high origin of radial artery (*white arrow*)

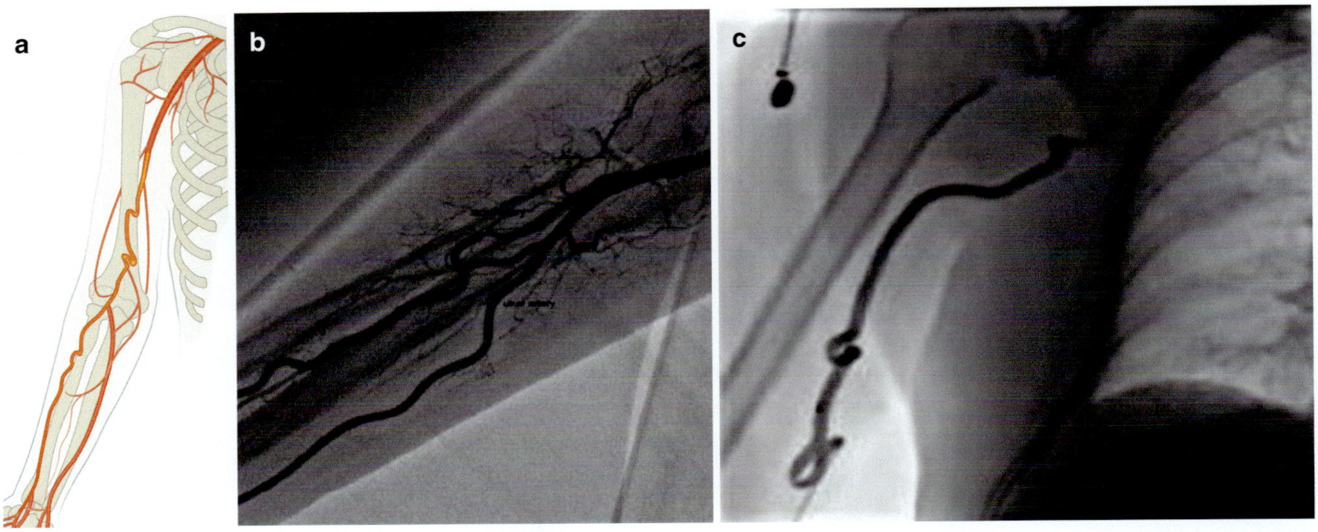

Fig. 3.8 Tortuous radial artery (**a**, **b**), ulnar artery (**b**), brachial artery (**a**, **c**)

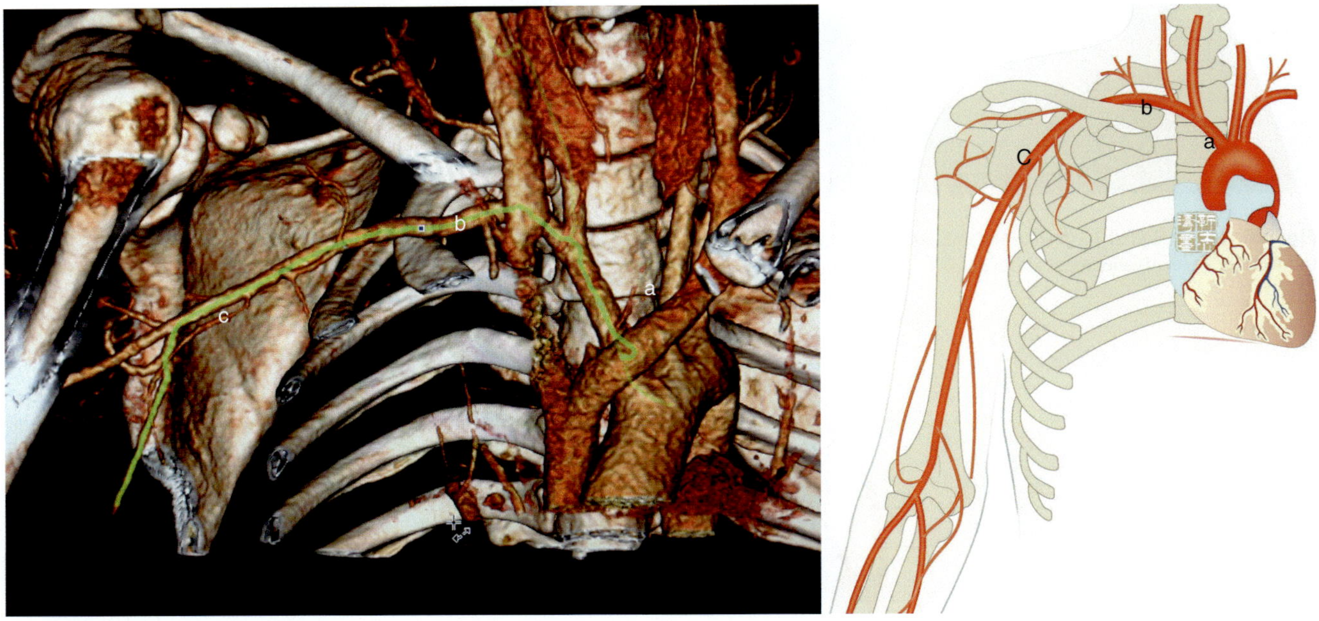

Fig. 3.9 Three dimensional rendered CT angiogram image (*left*) and artwork (*right*) of right subclavian/innominate artery showing branches of subclavian and axillary artery. Traumatic injury of these branches during transradial intervention could cause severe bleeding and hematoma such as mediastinal and neck hematoma (*a*) Innominate artery (*b*) subclavian artery (*c*) axillary artery

3.6 Common Reason for Transradial Failure

According to a previous study conducted in 2011, patients undergoing transradial percutaneous coronary intervention via low to intermediate transradial operators, there was 1 % occurrence of vascular complications, and 4.7 % observation of transradial-PCI failure. The mechanisms for failure were as following; inability to advance the guide catheter through the ascending aorta, insufficient guide catheter support, radial artery puncture failure as 51 %, 36 %, and 13 % respectively. On the multivariate analysis, with age more than 75 years, CABG history, and short stature were independent predictors of transradial percutaneous coronary interventions' lack of succession [11].

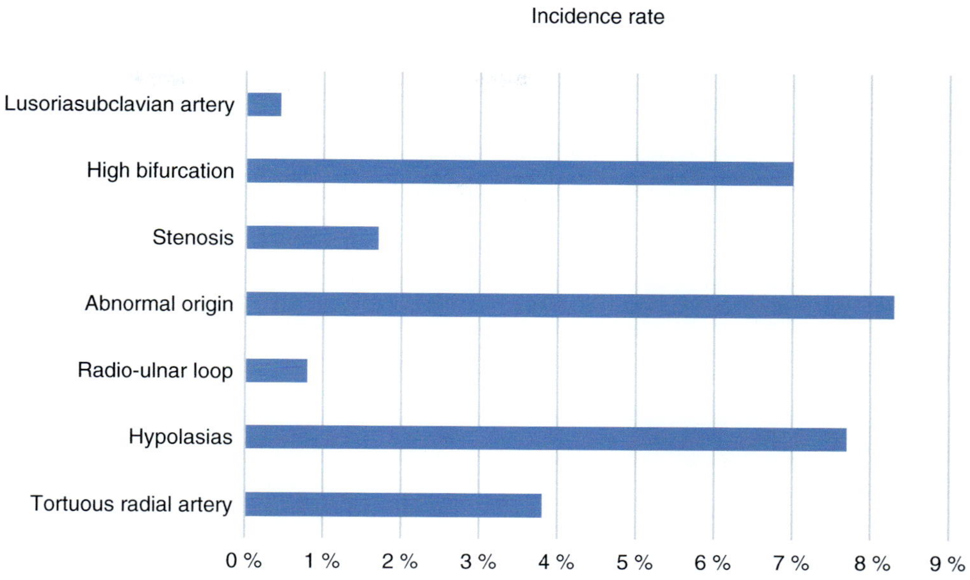

Fig. 3.10 Common radial annomalies and incidence rates [10]

3.7 Can Radial Artery Be a Bypass Graft Post Transradial Intervention ?

Although TRI has been shown to have less complication rate, be a safe and economic alternative to the femoral approach, there is an important limitation to this approach that RA injury could influence suitability of RA as a bypass conduit [12]. Previous study which directly assessed patency rates of RA's used as bypass grafts following RA-CA showing a significant adverse effect on graft patency (77 % patency in RA-CA, compared with 98 % in the control group) [13].

Using intravascular ultrasound (IVUS) to evaluate the radial injury demonstrated that the lumen diameters were smaller in repeat-TRI patients than in first-TRI patients due to intima-media thickening, especially in the distal radial artery [14]. Optical coherence tomography with much higher resolution clearly demonstrated significant acute injuries and chronic intimal thickening of RA after TRI. These changes may be due to an acute inflammatory reaction according to RA puncture and mechanical friction between the sheath and intima (Fig. 3.11). The frequency of intimal tears was greater in the RA distal (43.8 %) than proximal and the frequency of media dissections was significantly greater too (23 %) [15]. Early radial injury after transradial coronary intervention can also be assessed by high-resolution ultrasound biomicroscopy. Ultrasound biomicrosogy is an noninvasive ultrasound imaging system with a high-frequency transducer. The resolution is as high as 20–100 μm; The depth penetration may be limited depending on the frequency of imaging, which makes it suitable for precise imaging of the blood vessels under the skin surface 5–15 mm. This will be of great benefit to evaluate the patients with repeat cardiac catheterizations for availability of hemodialysis shunts and conduit in coronary bypass surgery [16] (Fig. 3.12).

3.8 Radial Ultrasound as a Pre-operative Evaluation Tool

Sufficient radial artery diameter and normal anatomy are important factors in getting a successful vascular puncture and completing the catheter cannulation. Thus measuring the radial artery diameter with radial ultrasound prior these procedures is helpful for the cardiologist to select suitable patients and prepare the difficulties in case of injuring the radial artery causing RAO (radial artery occlusion) and other complications [17] (Fig. 3.13). A prospective study performed by our team showed that the range of right radial artery diameters in Chinese adult patients is 1.3–3.6 mm (mean, 2.38 ± 0.56 mm) [18] which is similar to that in Japanese population (2.4 ± 0.4 mm) [19],and lower than that measured with US in Korean patients (2.60 ± 0.4 mm) [20]. The mean diameter of the left radial arty is similar to that of the right radial artery, the mean diameters of the ulnar artery is also similar to those of the radial artery. Radial artery ultrasound is also helpful in identifying radial and ulnar abnormalities (Fig. 3.14). In our study, the total incidence of anatomical abnormalities of the radial and ulnar artery was 15.4 %; largely due to high origin of the right radial artery or right ulnar artery (2.9 % vs 1.6 %), tortuosity (2.8 %), hypoplasia (1 %). Loops of the radial and ulnar were difficult to be detected by radial ultrasound. Radial diameter which is less than 2 mm and radial abnormalities are predicative for trans radial failure [18].

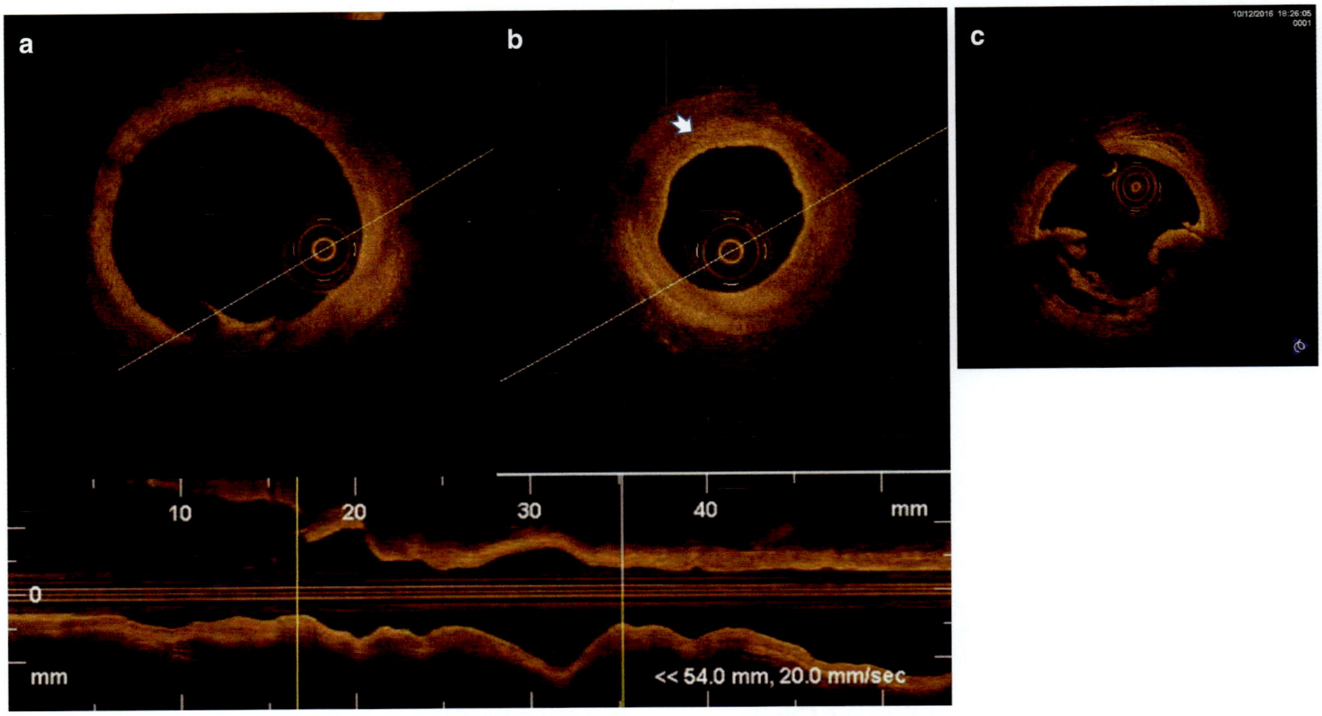

Fig. 3.11 Optical coherence tomography (OCT) of the radial artery post an elective left descending artery intervention. The patient had prior coronary angiogram via right transradial 2 weeks ago. OCT showed intimal tear and medial dissection (**a**) radial spasm (*White arrow* is the thickened media) (**b**) OCT of radial artery showed dissection and thrombus in a patient with previous PCI 7 times within a year, the latest PCI was 3 month ago (**c**)

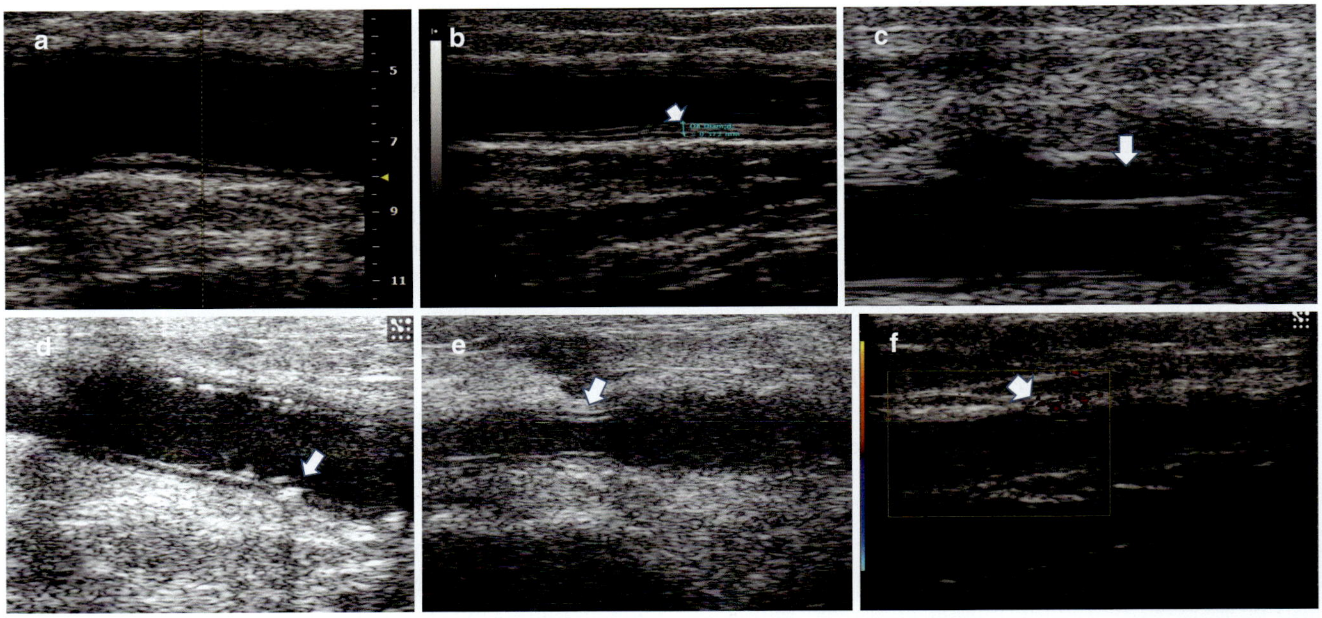

Fig. 3.12 Representative image of radial artery injury 1 day after procedure. (**a**) normal radial artery. (**b**) intima-media thickening of radial artery 1 day after procedure. (**c**) Intimal dissection of radial artery. (**d**) Intima tears of radial artery. (**e**) Radial artery stenosis 1 day after procedure. (**f**) Radial artery occlusion (RAO) 1 day after procedure. The intima-media thickening and intima dissection may be induced by an acute inflammatory reaction to radial artery puncture and mechanical friction between the sheath and intima. RAO may be due to acute radial artery thrombosis

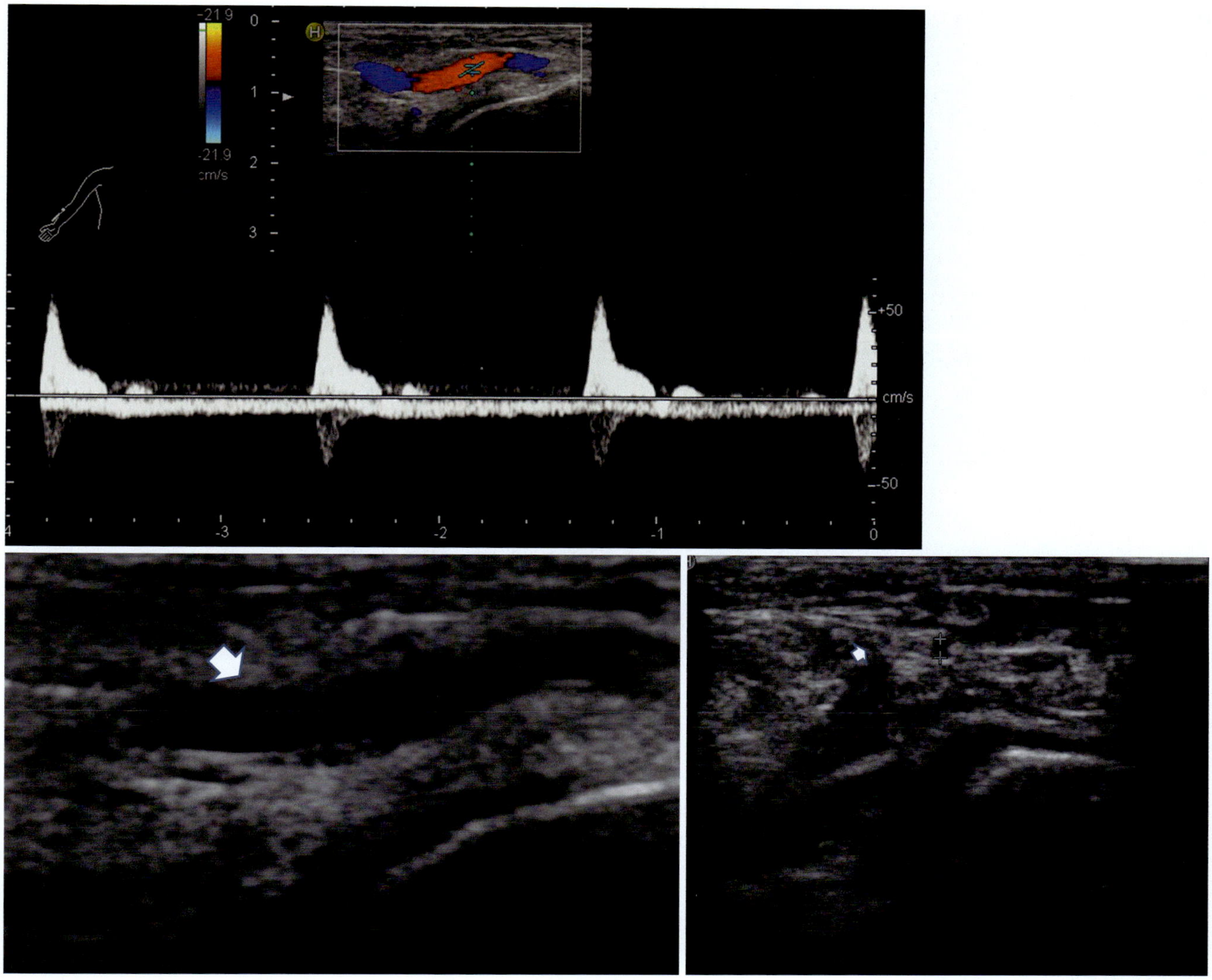

Fig. 3.13 Distal radial artery (PW Doppler) long axis view of radial artery, short axis view of radial artery

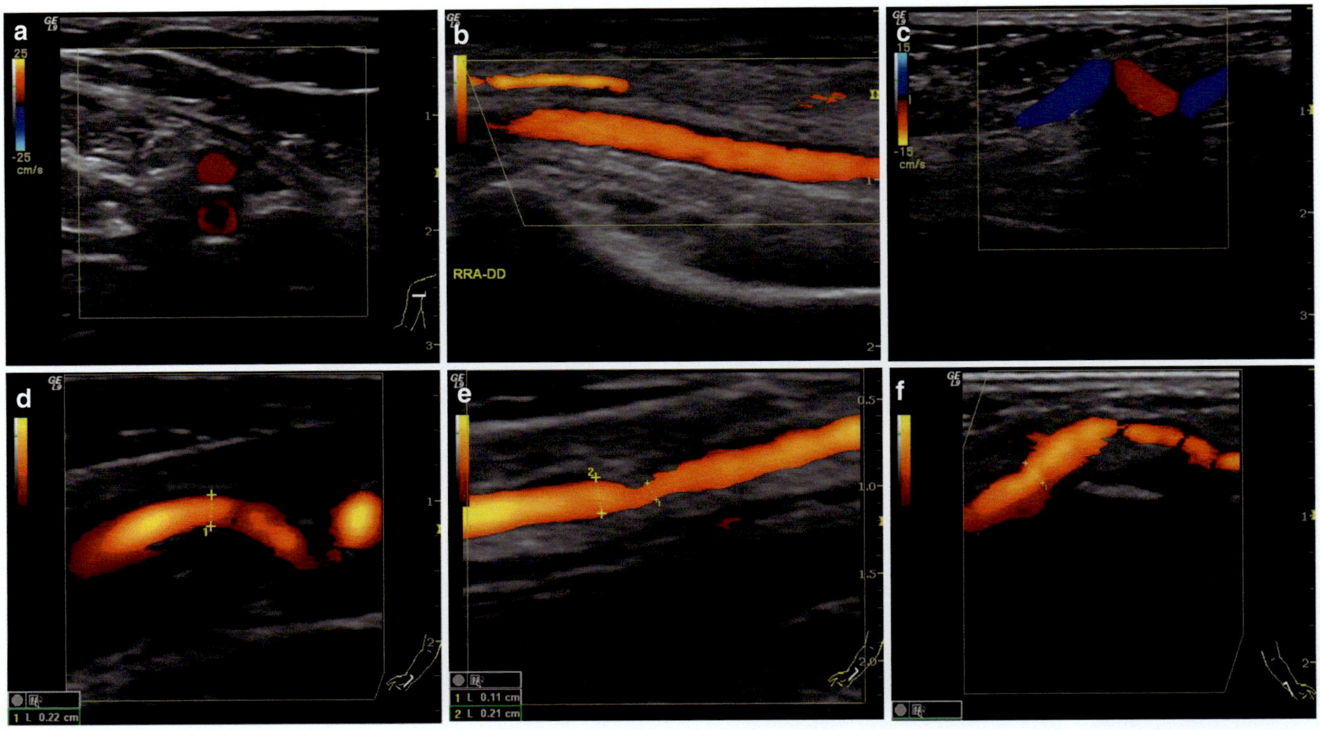

Fig. 3.14 (**a**) High bifurcation of right radial and ulnar artery. (**b**) Double radial arteries (axillary artery level). (**c**) Tortuosity of right radial artery. (**d**) Tortuosity of right ulnar artery. (**e**) Stenosis of right ulnar artery. (**f**) Maldevelopment of left ulnar artery

Some centres using live radial ultrasound in the cath lab as a guidance for transradial procedure which leads to more successful puncture rates [21, 22].

References

1. Joshi SB, Vatsalaswamy P, Bahetee BH. Variation in formation of superficial palmar arches with clinical implications. J Clin Diagn Res JCDR. 2014;8:AC06–9.
2. Ruengsakulrach P, Eizenberg N, Fahrer C, Fahrer M, Buxton BF. Surgical implications of variations in hand collateral circulation: anatomy revisited. J Thorac Cardiovasc Surg. 2001;122:682–6.
3. Asif M, Sarkar PK. Three-digit Allen's test. Ann Thorac Surg. 2007;84:686–7.
4. Barbeau GR, Arsenault F, Dugas L, Simard S, Lariviere MM. Evaluation of the ulnopalmar arterial arches with pulse oximetry and plethysmography: comparison with the Allen's test in 1010 patients. Am Heart J. 2004;147:489–93.
5. Greenwood MJ, Della-Siega AJ, Fretz EB, et al. Vascular communications of the hand in patients being considered for transradial coronary angiography: is the Allen's test accurate? J Am Coll Cardiol. 2005;46:2013–7.
6. Valgimigli M, Campo G, Penzo C, et al. Transradial coronary catheterization and intervention across the whole spectrum of Allen test results. J Am Coll Cardiol. 2014;63:1833–41.
7. Park KW, Chung JW, Chang SA, Kim KI, Chung WY, Chae IH. Two cases of mediastinal hematoma after cardiac catheterization: a rare but real complication of the transradial approach. Int J Cardiol. 2008;130:e89–92.
8. Jao YT, Chen Y, Fang CC, Wang SP. Mediastinal and neck hematoma after cardiac catheterization. Catheter Cardiovasc Interv Off J Soc Cardiac Angiography Interv. 2003;58:467–72.
9. Yang W, Qiao S, Liu R, et al. Clinical features and outcome of eight patients with mediastinal and neck hematoma after transradial cardiac catheterization approach. Zhonghua xin xue guan bing za zhi. 2014;42:406–12.
10. Valsecchi O, Vassileva A, Musumeci G, et al. Failure of transradial approach during coronary interventions: anatomic considerations. Catheter Cardiovasc Interv Off J Soc Cardiac Angiography Interv. 2006;67:870–8.
11. Lo TS, Nolan J, Fountzopoulos E, et al. Radial artery anomaly and its influence on transradial coronary procedural outcome. Heart. 2009;95:410–5.
12. Lim LM, Galvin SD, Javid M, Matalanis G. Should the radial artery be used as a bypass graft following radial access coronary angiography. Interact Cardiovasc Thorac Surg. 2014;18:219–24.
13. Kamiya H, Ushijima T, Kanamori T, et al. Use of the radial artery graft after transradial catheterization: is it suitable as a bypass conduit? Ann Thorac Surg. 2003;76:1505–9.
14. Wakeyama T, Ogawa H, Iida H, et al. Intima-media thickening of the radial artery after transradial intervention. An intravascular ultrasound study. J Am Coll Cardiol. 2003;41:1109–14.
15. Yonetsu T, Kakuta T, Lee T, et al. Assessment of acute injuries and chronic intimal thickening of the radial artery after transradial coronary intervention by optical coherence tomography. Eur Heart J. 2010;31:1608–15.
16. Shen H, Zhou YJ, Liu YY, et al. Assessment of early radial injury after transradial coronary intervention by high-resolution ultrasound biomicroscopy: innovative technology application. Chin Med J (Engl). 2012;125:3388–92.
17. Abazid RM, Smettei OA, Mohamed MZ, et al. Radial artery ultrasound predicts the success of transradial coronary angiography. Cardiol J. 2016. doi: 10.5603/CJ.a2016.0072. [Epub ahead of print].

18. Yan ZX, Zhou YJ, Zhao YX, Zhou ZM, Yang SW, Wang ZJ. Anatomical study of forearm arteries with ultrasound for percutaneous coronary procedures. Circ J Off J Jpn Circ Soc. 2010;74:686–92.
19. Nagai S, Abe S, Sato T, et al. Ultrasonic assessment of vascular complications in coronary angiography and angioplasty after transradial approach. Am J Cardiol. 1999;83:180–6.
20. Yoo BS, Yoon J, Ko JY, et al. Anatomical consideration of the radial artery for transradial coronary procedures: arterial diameter, branching anomaly and vessel tortuosity. Int J Cardiol. 2005;101:421–7.
21. Seto AH, Roberts JS, Abu-Fadel MS, et al. Real-time ultrasound guidance facilitates transradial access: RAUST (Radial Artery access with Ultrasound Trial). JACC Cardiovasc Interv. 2015;8:283–91.
22. Gao YB, Yan JH, Gao FQ, Pan L, Wang XZ, Lv CJ. Effects of ultrasound-guided radial artery catheterization: an updated meta-analysis. Am J Emerg Med. 2015;33:50–5.

4 Radial Access: Step by Step

Syed Gilani

Successful radial access starts with getting comfortable with arterial access especially in femoral artery. The basic principles of obtaining access are the same. Radial artery is smaller in size than femoral artery. Always have femoral access site also prepped and draped when using radial access first for coronary angiogram.

In a STEMI situation, radial access has an additional advantage that one can obtain access in radial artery while the cath lab nurse/tech is preparing the femoral access site and preparing the injector system or manifold.

4.1 Access Site Preparation

Once the patient is placed on cath lab table, place the radial board to support the right arm (or the left arm in case of left radial access), extent the elbow and wrist and place a small towel behind the wrist to support the wrist to provide mild hyperextension of the wrist (this helps make the radial artery access site more prominent and accessible). Wrap a tape softly around the palm or the fingers and attach the tape to the radial board to keep the right hand in stable position. Place a pulse oximeter on the right thumb for continuous oxygen saturation monitoring. Clean the distal forearm and wrist area with antiseptic solution. Place a drape (we use a sterile drape with a central hole) on the access site keeping the radial artery in the middle (Fig. 4.1a–c).

4.2 Two Puncture Techniques Can Be Used for Radial Artery Access

1. Single wall puncture technique using Micropuncture Access Set (Cook Medical, Bloomington, IN, USA) (Fig. 4.2). This provides the front wall single arterial puncture to radial artery using small 21-gage needle that comes in Micropuncture access set. The Micropuncture access set we use for radial access has a 21-gage 7 cm long needle, 0.018 in. 40 cm long guidewire and four or five French 10 cm long outer catheter with inner dilator.
2. Double wall puncture technique using Glidesheath Access Kit (Terumo Medical Corporation, Somerset, NJ, USA) (Fig. 4.3). The kit includes Glidesheath with dilator, Surflo IV catheter (1.25 in. long, 20 or 22 gage needle with plastic catheter) and a nitinol/plastic guidewire (0.021–0.025 in., 45 cm long).

Palpate the radial artery a few centimeters above the radial styloid process with the tips of the left hand index and middle fingers, separating the two by one centimeter or so. Palpate the radial pulse with both fingers and try to move both fingers side to side (medial to lateral or vice versa) over the radial artery so that you can correctly identify the location (site of the strongest pulse) and course of the radial artery under the fingers (avoid excess pressure as radial artery can be easily occluded by finger pressure). Once the location of the radial artery has been felt by both fingers of left hand, then you can place the artery at the tips of both fingers (radial artery coursing in straight line in-between the two points) (Fig. 4.4). Using the right hand, give small amount of local anesthetic to the skin in-between the fingers feeling the artery. Then for the single wall puncture technique, using the right hand hold micropuncture needle (Cook Medical, Bloomington, IN, USA) between the thumb and index finger at about 45–60° to the skin (Fig. 4.5) and advance the needle under the skin slowly until you have punctured the anterior wall of the artery and the blood is seen coming out from the hub. Due to smaller size of the micropuncture needle the pulsatile nature of the blood may be less prominent. At this point using your left hand thumb and index finger hold and stabilize the needle (thus freeing your right hand) (Fig. 4.6). With your right hand hold the micropuncture guide wire and slowly advance the wire into the radial artery (Fig. 4.7). Do not advance the guide wire against

S. Gilani, MD
Cardiology Department, University of Texas medical branch, Galveston, TX, USA
e-mail: sagilani@UTMB.EDU

Y. Zhou et al. (eds.), *Transradial Approach for Percutaneous Interventions*, DOI 10.1007/978-94-017-7350-8_4

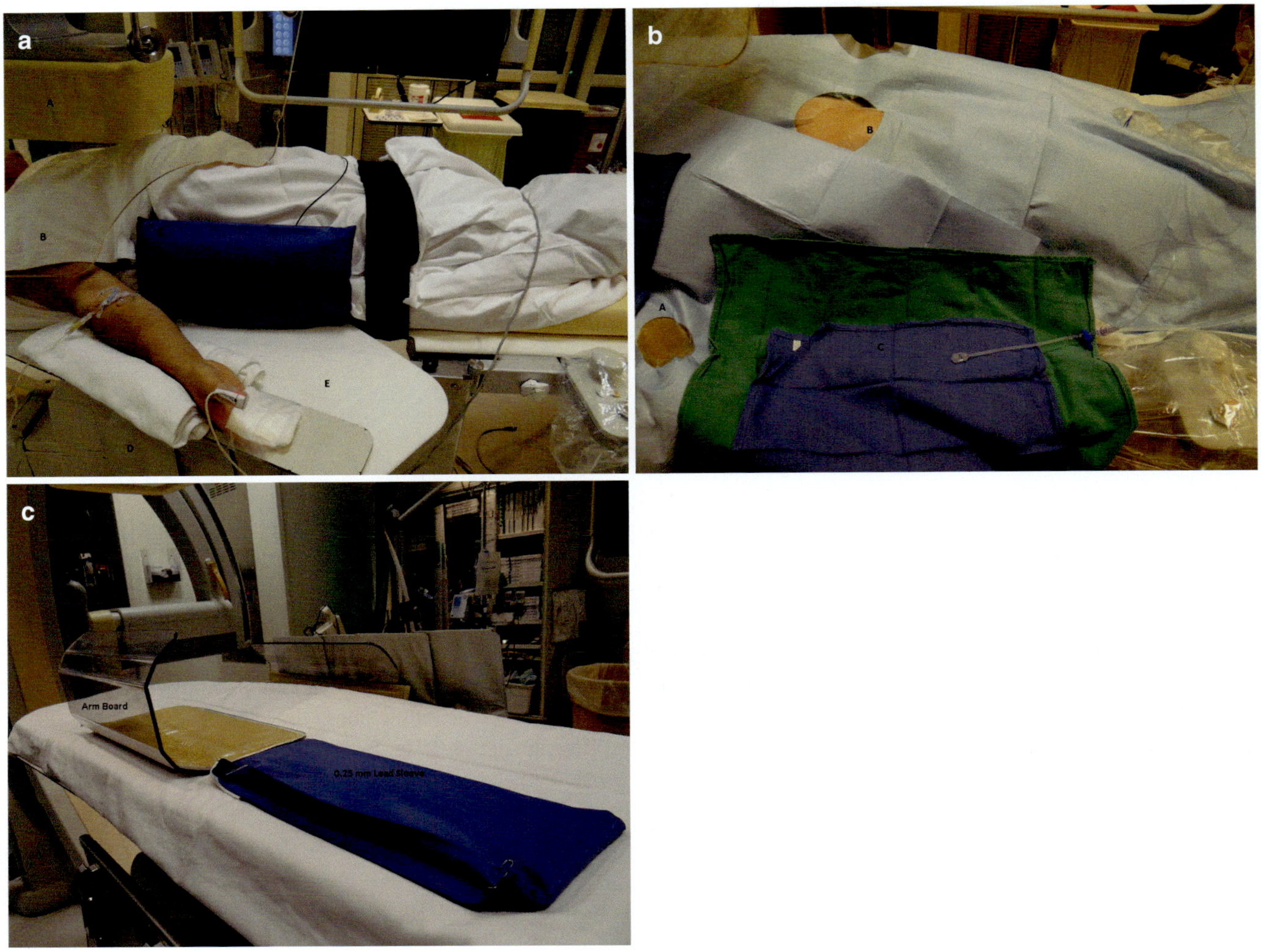

Fig. 4.1 (**a**) Right arm position prior to draping for right radial access. A-Image receptor. B-Ceiling mounted upper body radiation shield. C-Arm board draped with fitting Lead cover (reusable and kept under the sterile drape, also see **c**). D-Lower body radiation shield. E-a board placed half way under the patient to provide stable working area for the procedure. (**b**): Right radial access site draped and ready for the procedure. A-Right radial access site. B-Right femoral access site. C: Supported working area for procedure. (**c**): A-Arm board and B-0.25 mm Lead cover that is stitched to properly fit over the curved portion of the arm board. This arm board is placed between the pts arm and body (as shown in **a**) and helps reduce radiation exposure to the radial operator (Courtesy of Ajay Bhatia, RT, UTMB Cath Lab, Galveston, TX, USA)

resistance into the artery. If resistance is met then take these steps, (1) lower the needle hub slowly (thus changing the angle of entry of the needle into the artery) and try to advance the wire, (2) may turn the needle hub clock wise or counter clockwise (thus changing the bevel and direction of the wire entry into artery) and try advance the wire again,(3) slowly pull the needle back (thus making the position of the needle inside artery more central) while keeping the guide wire inside the needle and try to advance the wire into artery (using right hand) each time you pull the needle back a little (using left hand). This is a slow and controlled maneuver and if done properly, in author's opinion, will significantly increase the success rate of your radial artery access. Left hand palm could rest on the patient's arm to give stability and control in adjusting the needle position. If at any point you are not sure that needle is still inside the artery, then remove the guide wire and see if there is blood flow through the hub. If no blood is coming through the hub, you may still be able to salvage the access if the needle is through the back wall of the artery (double puncture) by pulling the needle back until you see blood again. After arterial puncture and placement of 0.018 in. guidewire the outer catheter is placed over the guidewire in the artery. Then inner dilator and guide wire is removed and 0.035 in. guidewire is introduced into the artery for placing the final sheath/catheter for the procedure. One can also directly place the final five or six French radial sheath over the 0.018 in. guidewire as long as the sheath has a narrow tip (0.018–0.021in.) dilator providing smooth transition for skin entry (Figs. 4.8, 4.9, 4.10, and 4.11).

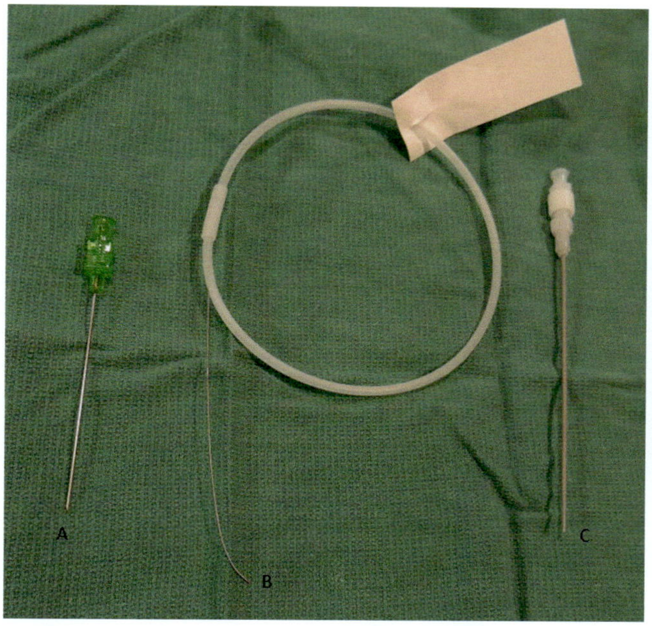

Fig. 4.2 Micropuncture Access set (Cook Medical, Bloomington, IN, USA). A-21 gage, 7 cm long needle. B-0.018 in., 40 cm long guidewire (Nitinol guidewire with Palladium tip). C-5 French 10 cm long outer catheter with inner dilator. *cm* centimeter

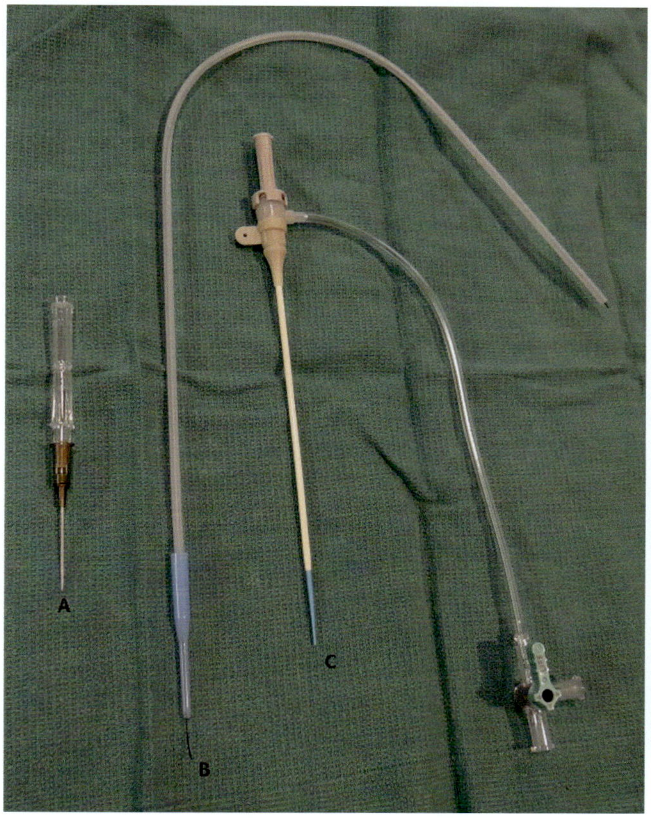

Fig. 4.3 Glidesheath Access Kit (Terumo Medical Corporation, Somerset, NJ, USA). A: Surflo IV catheter (1.25 in. long, 22 gage needle with plastic catheter). B- Nitinol/plastic guidewire (0.021 in., 45 cm long). C-5Fr Glidesheath with dilator. *cm* centimeter

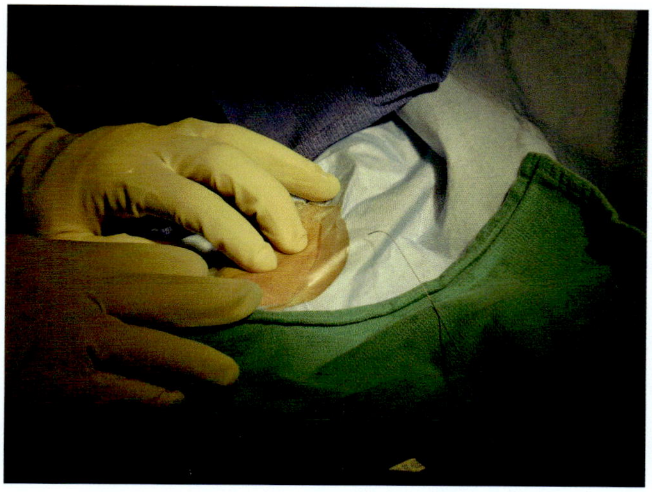

Fig. 4.4 Palpation of the radial artery a few centimeters above the radial styloid process

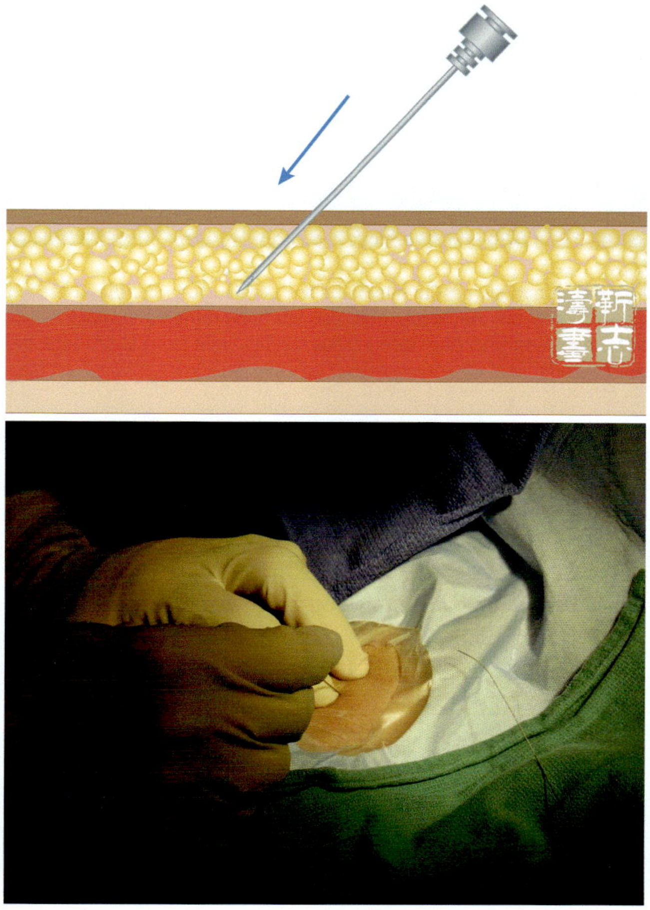

Fig. 4.5 Micropuncture needle insertion using right hand while palpating the radial artery with left hand

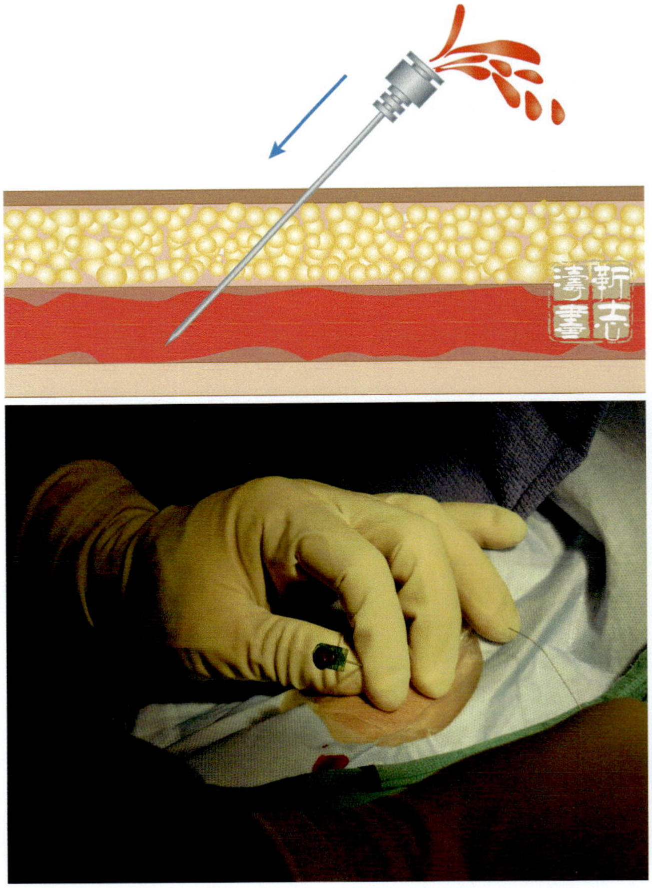

Fig. 4.6 Once the needle punctures the radial artery and blood is seen coming out from the needle hub, use left hand thumb and index finger to hold and stabilize the needle (thus freeing right hand to advance the guidewire)

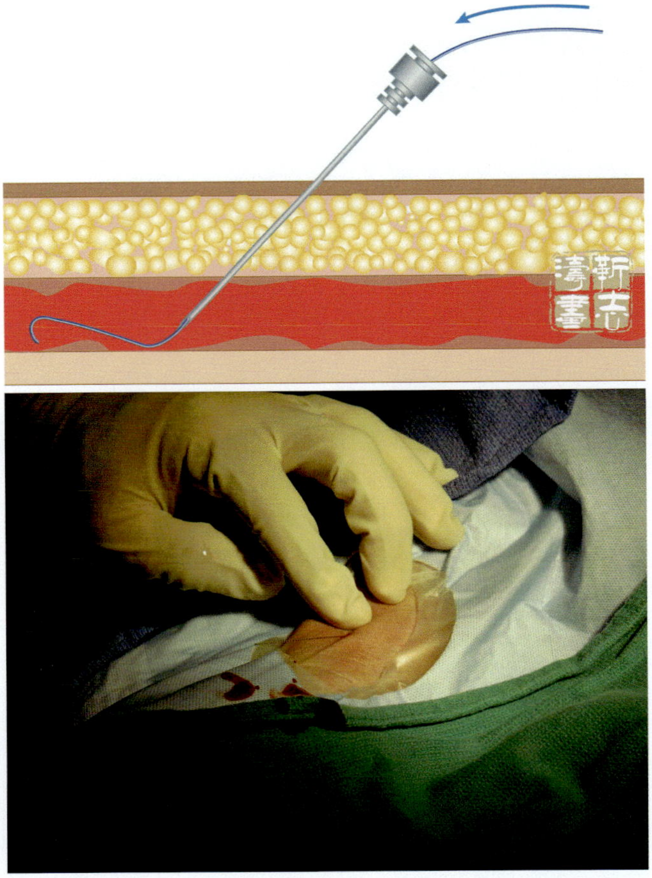

Fig. 4.7 Guidewire (0.018 in.) advanced into the radial artery and needle removed

For the double wall puncture technique, while palpating the radial artery with your left hand fingers, use the right hand to hold the Surflo IV catheter (1.25 in. long 20 gage needle and plastic catheter), (Fig. 4.3) between the thumb and index finger at about 45–60° to the skin and advance the needle under the skin slowly until you have punctured the anterior wall of the radial artery, a flush of blood is seen at the hub suggesting the needle is inside the radial artery, advance the Surflo IV catheter 2–3 mm further to puncture the posterior wall, then remove the needle and slowly pull back the plastic catheter until the pulsatile flow is seen coming through the hub of the plastic catheter (Figs. 4.12a, b, c, and d), then advance the guidewire that comes with the kit. Once the guidewire is sufficiently inside the radial artery, then remove the plastic tubing and advance the sheath over the guidewire. I usually advance the tip of the dilator into the radial artery and make a small skin nick with scalpel to help advance the radial sheath smoothly into the radial artery (Fig. 4.12e).

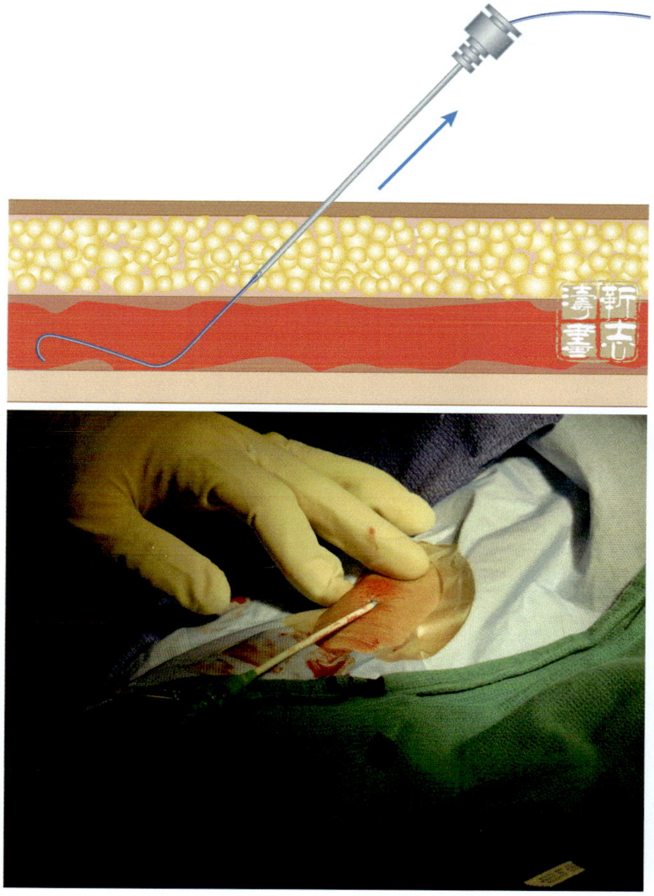

Fig. 4.8 6Fr Sheath with 0.021 dilator (GlideSheath, Terumo Medical Corporation, Somerset, NJ, USA) being advanced over the 0.018 in. guidewire

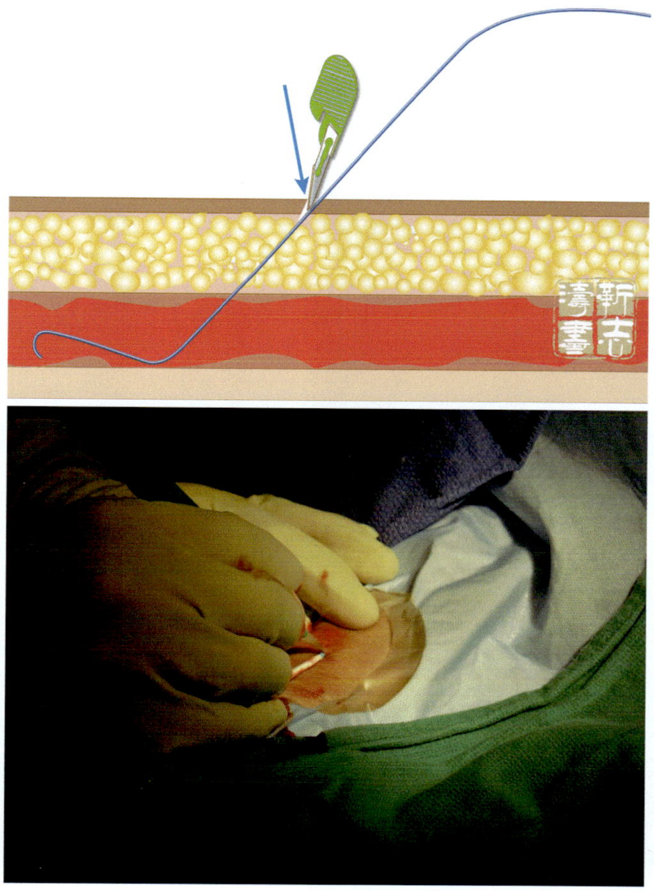

Fig. 4.9 Small skin nick using scalpel over the dilator or guidewire

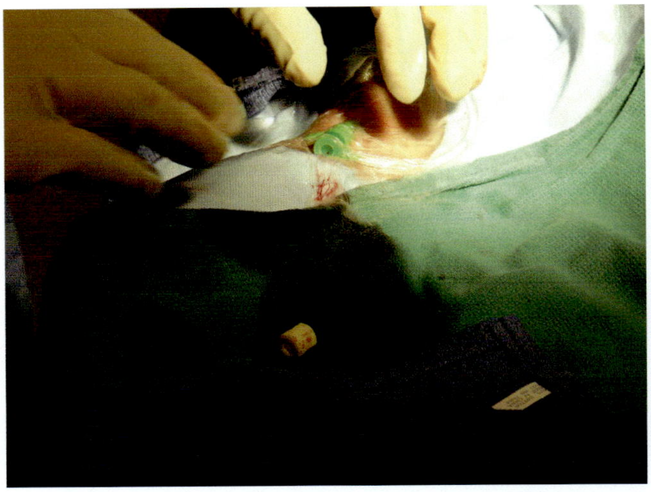

Fig. 4.10 Sheath advanced into the radial artery and secured in place

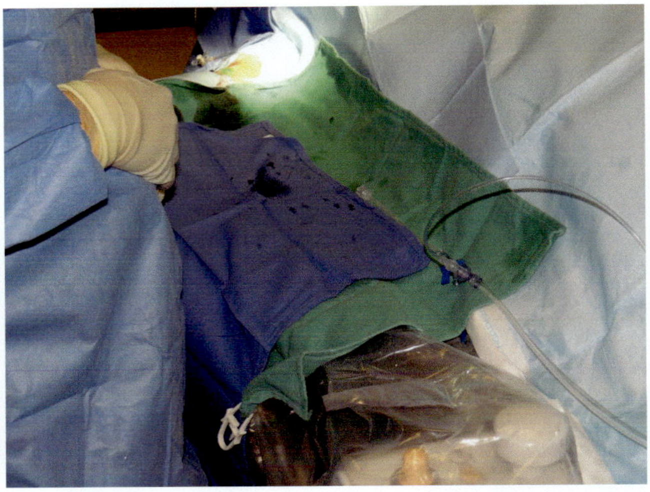

Fig. 4.11 Right radial access ready for the procedure

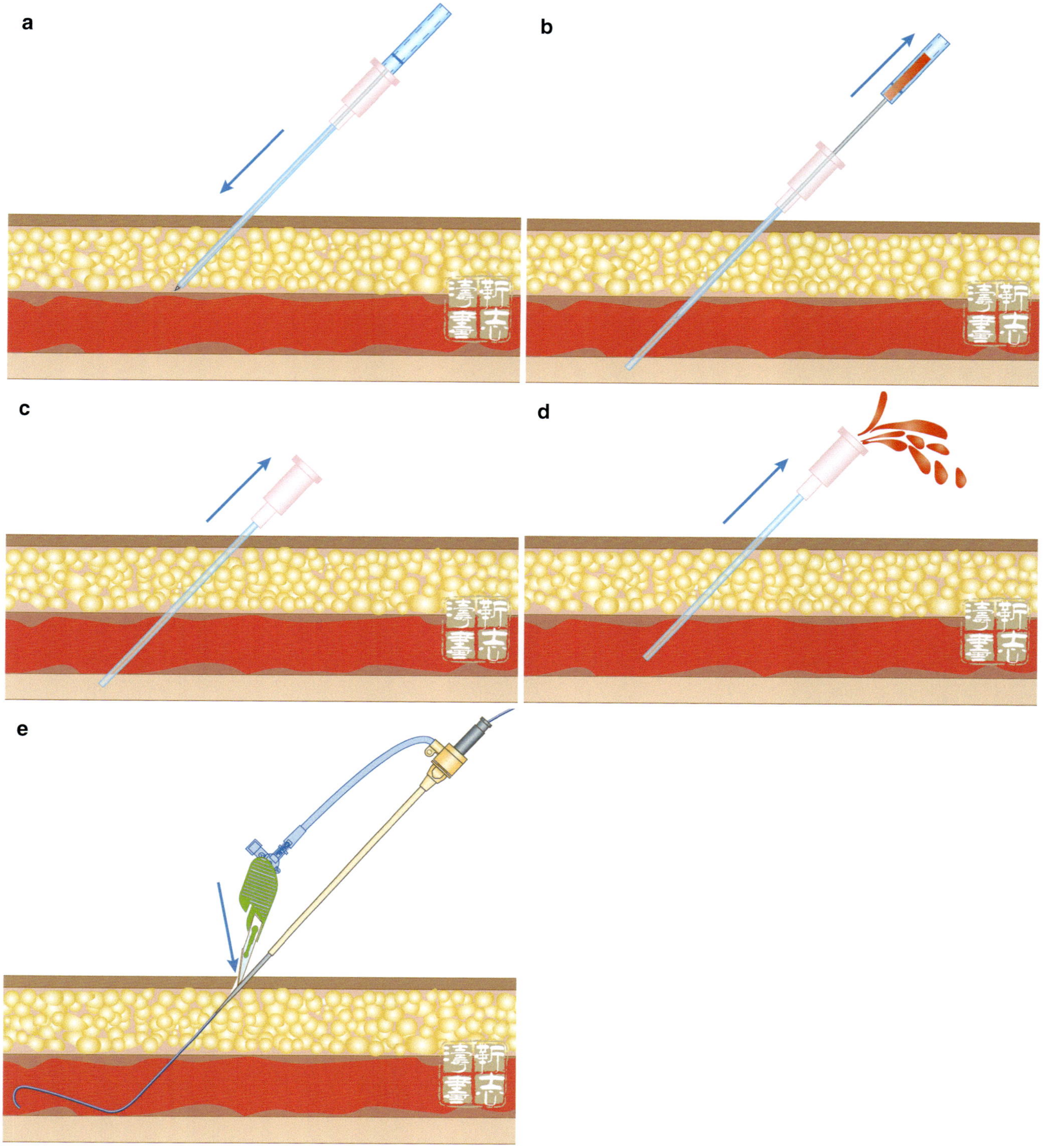

Fig. 4.12 Double wall puncture technique using Glidesheath Access Kit. (**a**): Arterial puncture using Surflo IV catheter. (**b**): Once the needle tip punctures the posterior wall of radial artery, remove the needle, leaving the plastic catheter in place. (**c**): slowly pull back the plastic catheter. (**d**): once the pulsatile blood flow is noticed coming out of catheter hub, advance the guidewire. (**e**): Advance the sheath over the guidewire. Small skin nick using scalpel over the dilator or guidewire will help advance the sheath smoothly

5 Prevention and Management of Complications in Transradial PCI

Weimin Li and Jianqiang Li

Abstract

Transradial approach for cardiac catheterization is associated with a reduced incidence of major access-related complications and has been adopted worldwide. As physicians become more comfortable with this approach, they start using it to perform complex procedures, leading to increased complications. There are common and rare complications with this approach which may lead to disastrous outcomes if they are not identified and treated immediately. Therefore, it is essential to be aware of these complications and to understand their prevention and management. In this chapter, we summarize the common and rare complications encountered in transradial intervention (TRI) and provide useful tips for their prevention and management.

5.1 Introduction

Routine use of transradial technique in percutaneous coronary intervention (PCI) has grown significantly over the past decade since its first introduction by Campeau in 1989 [1]. There are a number of advantages with transradial approach over transfemoral approach, including short recovery time, less bleeding complications, and better patient comfort, which gradually made radial artery the preferred access site in contemporary PCI [2]. As interventional cardiologists become more comfortable with this approach, they start using it to perform complex procedures, such as chronic total occlusion and bifurcation, leading to increased complications, particularly vascular complications. Therefore, it is vital importance to be aware of these complications and to deal with them immediately and properly.

Electronic supplementary material The online version of this chapter (doi:10.1007/978-94-017-7350-8_5) contains supplementary material, which is available to authorized users.

W. Li (✉) • J. Li
Department of Cardiology, The First Affiliated Hospital of Harbin Medical University, Harbin, China
e-mail: liweimin_2009@163.com; betterbetterman@126.com

5.2 Radial Artery Spasm

Radial artery spasm (RAS) remains one of the major challenges of TRI, which may result in difficult manipulation of devices and ultimately lead to procedural failure. RAS is defined as a temporary, sudden narrowing of the radial artery (Fig. 5.1) and the reported incidence varies dramatically from 4 to 20% [3]. Radial artery is usually small and contains abundant $\alpha 1$ adrenergic receptor, along with anatomical variation and tortuosity. Therefore, RAS is often caused by intensive anxiety of patients, insufficient local anesthesia, aggressive catheter manipulation, entrance of guidewire into side branch, and painful stimulus. Smaller artery diameter, female gender, lower body weight, advanced age, larger sheath size, and operator inexperience are considered risk factors for the occurrence of RAS [3]. If RAS is not relieved, pulling the sheath with force is extremely risky and may cause sheath fracture and artery injury. Thus, a number of measures have been applied to prevent or treat RAS, including the use of various vasodilatory cocktails, hydrophilic or small size sheaths, gentle catheter manipulation, adequate local anesthesia, and pre-operational sedation [4–6]. In terms of vasodilators, phentolamine, nicorandil, nitroprusside, nitroglycerin, and verapamil are commonly used in daily practice, either alone or in combination. In addition, brachial plexus block should be attempted if the above methods are not able to resolve the refractory RAS. Brachial plexus block

Y. Zhou et al. (eds.), *Transradial Approach for Percutaneous Interventions*, DOI 10.1007/978-94-017-7350-8_5

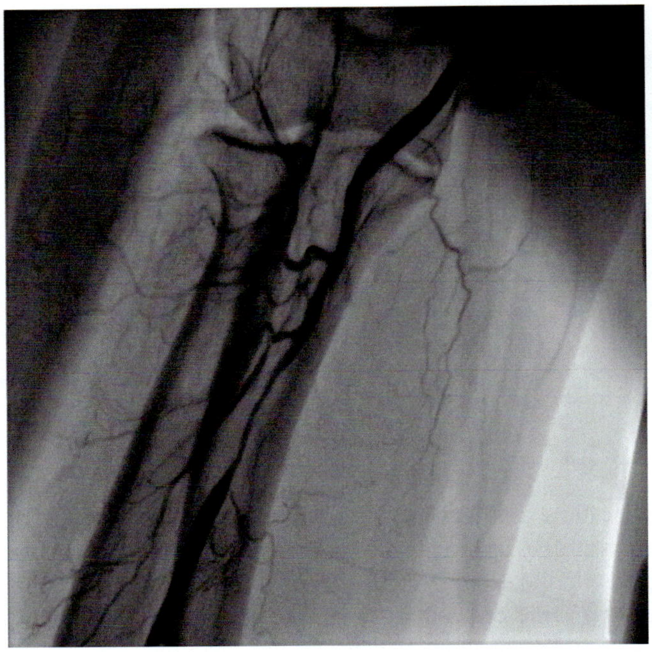

Fig. 5.1 Angiogram showing diffuse radial artery spasm

was initially used in orthopedic surgeries to relax muscles and vessels by blocking the dominant nerves. There are four kinds of pathways to perform brachial plexus block: interscalene, axilla, supraclavicular, and subclavicular. Needle insertion via interscalene can avoid pneumothorax and should be chosen for the treatment of RAS. A case of RAS is illustrated in Fig. 5.2.

5.3 Radial Artery Occlusion

Radial artery occlusion (RAO) (Fig. 5.3) is one of the most common complications in TRI with an incidence of 5–11% and is generally asymptomatic due to the dual blood supply of the hand [7–10]. Severe hand ischemia resulting from RAO is rare, except for the presence of some underlying pathology, such as defective palmar circulation and vascular dysfunction. Since simple pulse check at the radial artery is not reliable, ultrasound is recommended to assure the diagnosis. The occurrence of RAO has been found to be related to intimal hyperplasia, intima-media thickening, and thrombus formation mainly caused by artery injury and prolonged high-pressure compression. Although RAO usually requires no further treatment, measures should be taken to prevent it. Allen's test is critically important for selecting patients with patent palmar arch communications. Currently, the use of heparin is a standard procedure in TRI and adequate anticoagulation with heparin may reduce the incidence of RAO. Moreover, there are several commercially available radial compression devices with enough maintenance of perfusion during compression, which has been shown to decrease the rate of RAO [9–11]. Additionally, the use of a smaller size sheath or guide catheter may be potentially advantageous in the prevention of RAO. It's worth noting that reaccessing the occluded radial artery is a concern for future TRI. Although different techniques have been reported to recanalize a previously occluded radial artery [12, 13], none of them have been universally accepted and approved for clinical practice. Occasionally, a branch of radial artery can be occluded due to TRI. A special case of acute princeps pollicis artery occlusion is provided (Fig. 5.4).

5.4 Radial Artery Perforation

Radial artery perforation (RAP) is an uncommon complication (Fig. 5.5), which, if not identified promptly, can lead to severe forearm hematoma and compartment syndrome. The reported incidence of RAP is between 0.1 and 1% in different studies and it occurs more often in older and shorter women with tortuous arteries [14–16]. Risk factors of RAP have been related to artery spasm, small radial artery, excessive anti-coagulation, and over manipulation of guidewire. Generally, it is not easy to detect RAP during the procedure because of temporary tamponade provided by the catheter shaft. However, it can manifest as a forearm hematoma post-procedurally. Early detection of this complication can be achieved by angiography when the guidewire or catheter insertion meets resistance. If detected early, RAP can be treated simply with a pressure bandage; and if it progresses to a large hematoma to increase the risk of compartment syndrome, then surgical intervention is required. To carry on the procedure in patients with RAP, two strategies have been adopted: conversion to transfemoral approach or continuing the procedure either with the use of a long sheath, a guiding catheter, or a peripheral balloon to close the perforation [15, 17, 18]. A case of RAP is illustrated in Fig. 5.6.

5.5 Bleeding and Hematoma

Owing to the superficial location of the radial artery, hemostasis post-TRI can be achieved readily with a significant reduction of bleeding complications. However, this complication is not completely eliminated and it, if overlooked, can lead to forearm hematoma and even to compartment syndrome with disastrous outcomes. Hematoma is a subcutaneous collection of blood deriving from penetrating injury either on the vessel wall or its minor branches during the delivery of devices or from inadequate compression post-procedure. The factors

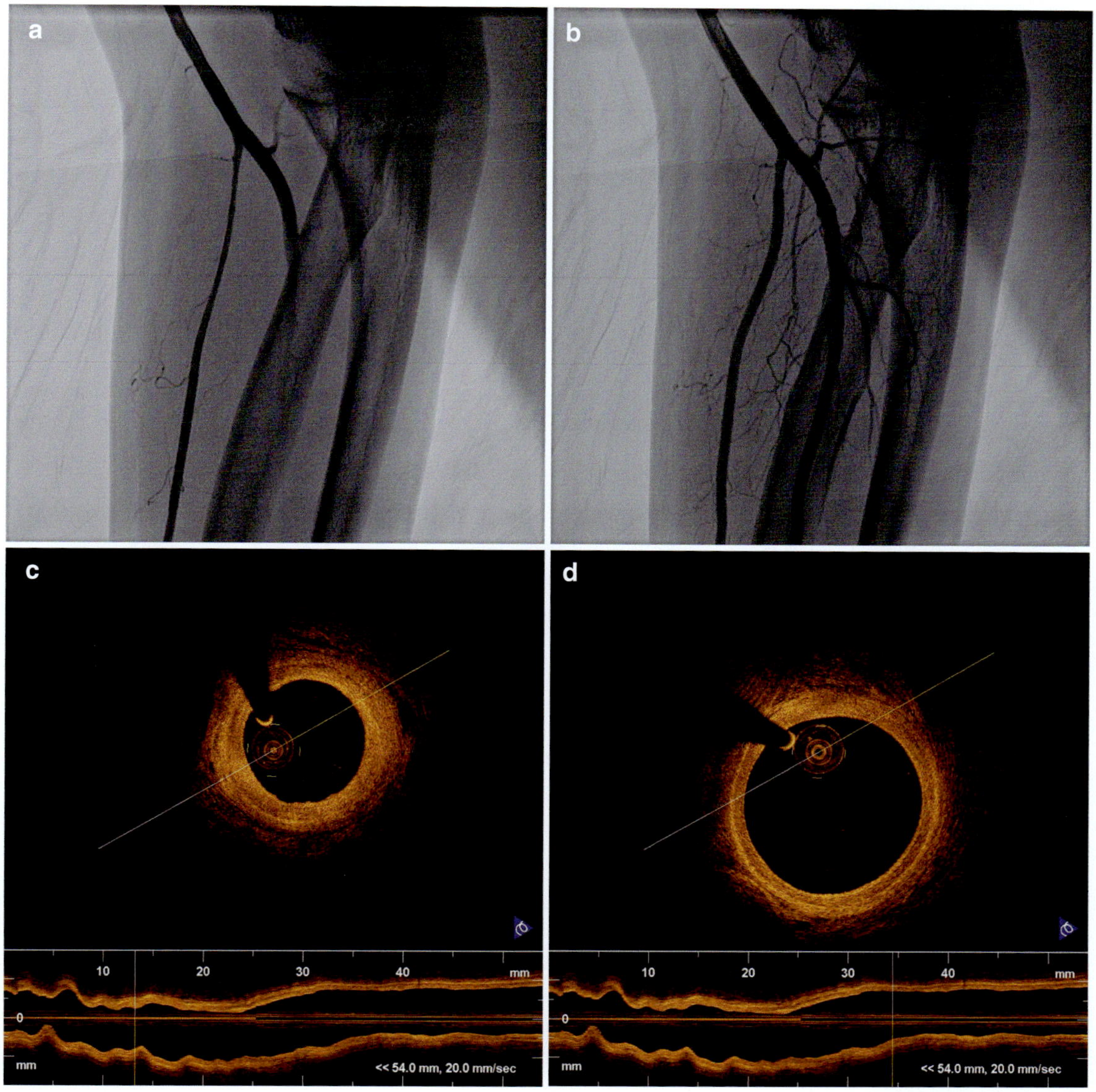

Fig. 5.2 A 40 years old male with a history of myocardial infarction underwent PCI for right coronary artery (*RCA*). The right radial artery was not palpable, and then left radial artery was chosen for access. Severe pain was noted when the catheter was pulled out. Angiogram showed severe spasm in left radial artery (**a**). Spasm was relieved after 200ug Nitroglycerin by iv (**b**). Optical coherence tomography (*OCT*) was performed in the left radial artery and spasm segment was characterized by thickened media and narrowed lumen (**c**). The normal reference vessel distal to the spasm segment showed clear structure with three layers (intima, media, and adventia) (**d**) (This case was provided by Dr. Jincheng Guo from Beijing Luhe Hospital)

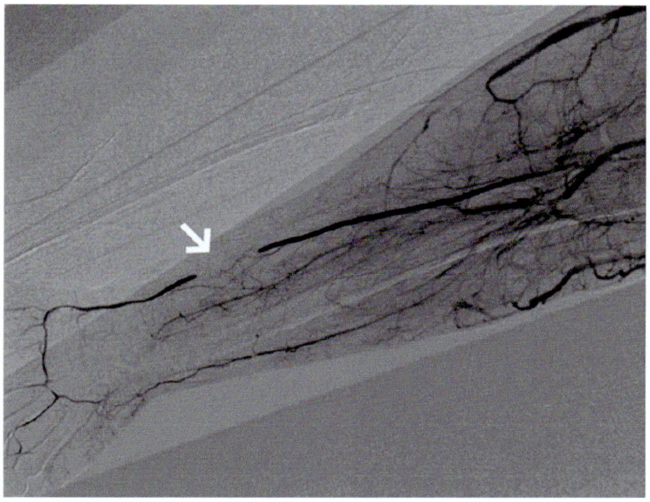

Fig. 5.3 Angiogram showing radial artery occlusion (*arrow*) and a small ulnar artery with diffuse spasm

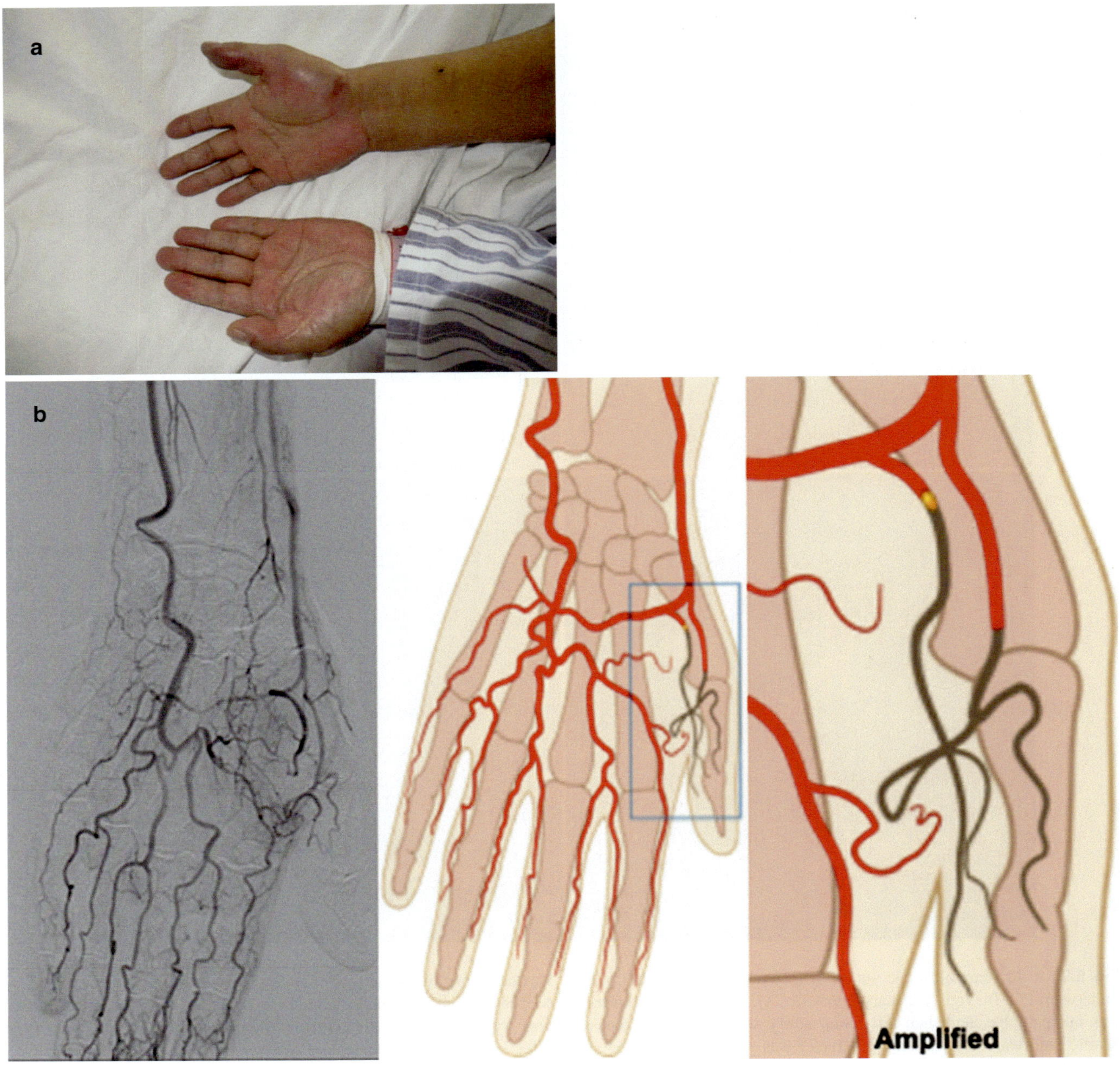

Fig. 5.4 A 53 years old male underwent PCI for a mid left anterior descending (*LAD*) lesion. One hour post hemostasis band removal, the patient complained of pain and pallor over right thumb and thenar muscle (**a**). The symptoms became worse on the 3rd day. An angiogram was performed via MPA catheter showing slow flow of princeps pollicis artery (also called primary artery of thumb, a branch of radial artery) (**b**). A 0.014 PT wire was crossed through the occlusion, then 10,0000U of urokinase was given via microcatheter (**c**) and the blood flow was recovered (**d**). The patient's symptom was relieved on the 4th day (**e**). Finally the patient was diagnosed as primary thrombocytosis, with platelet level of 514×10^9/L (This case was provided by Dr. Zhitao Jing from PLA Rocket General Hospital)

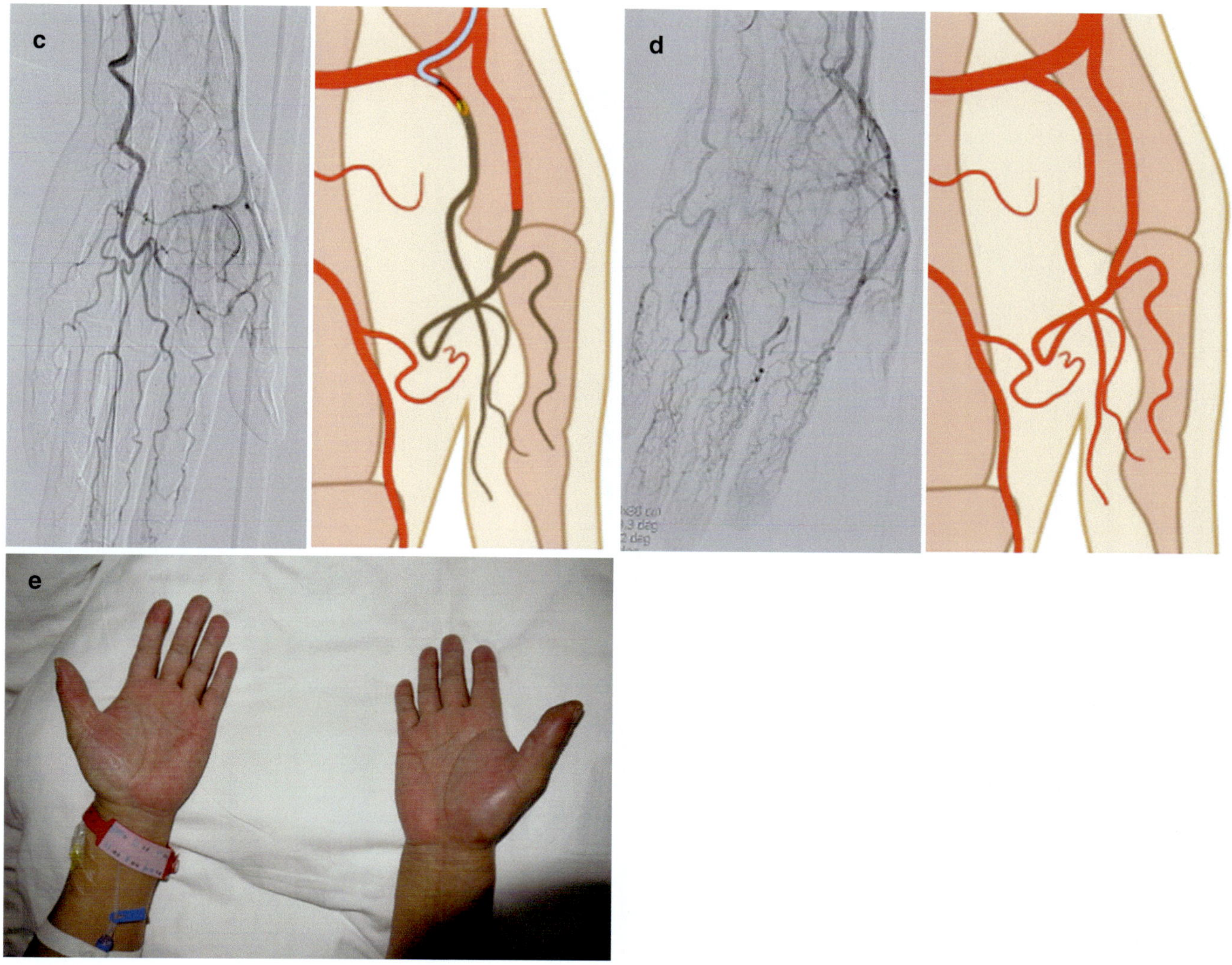

Fig. 5.4 (continued)

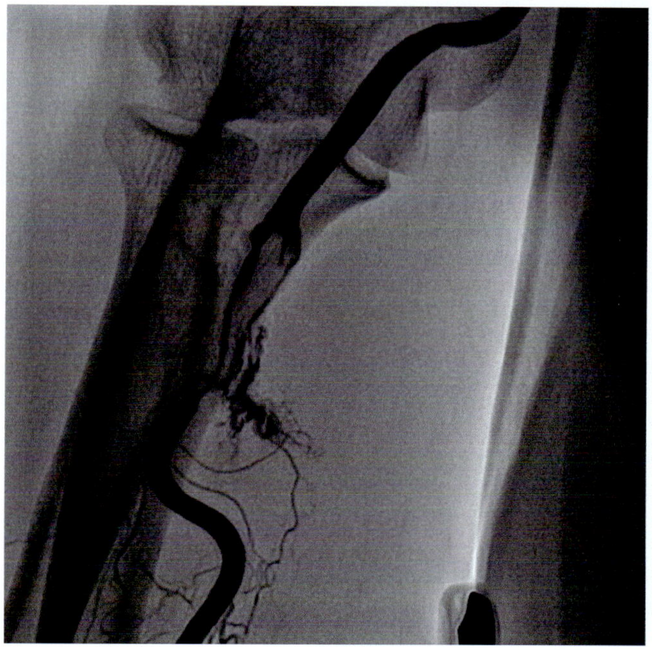

Fig. 5.5 Angiogram showing radial artery perforation with extravasation of contrast

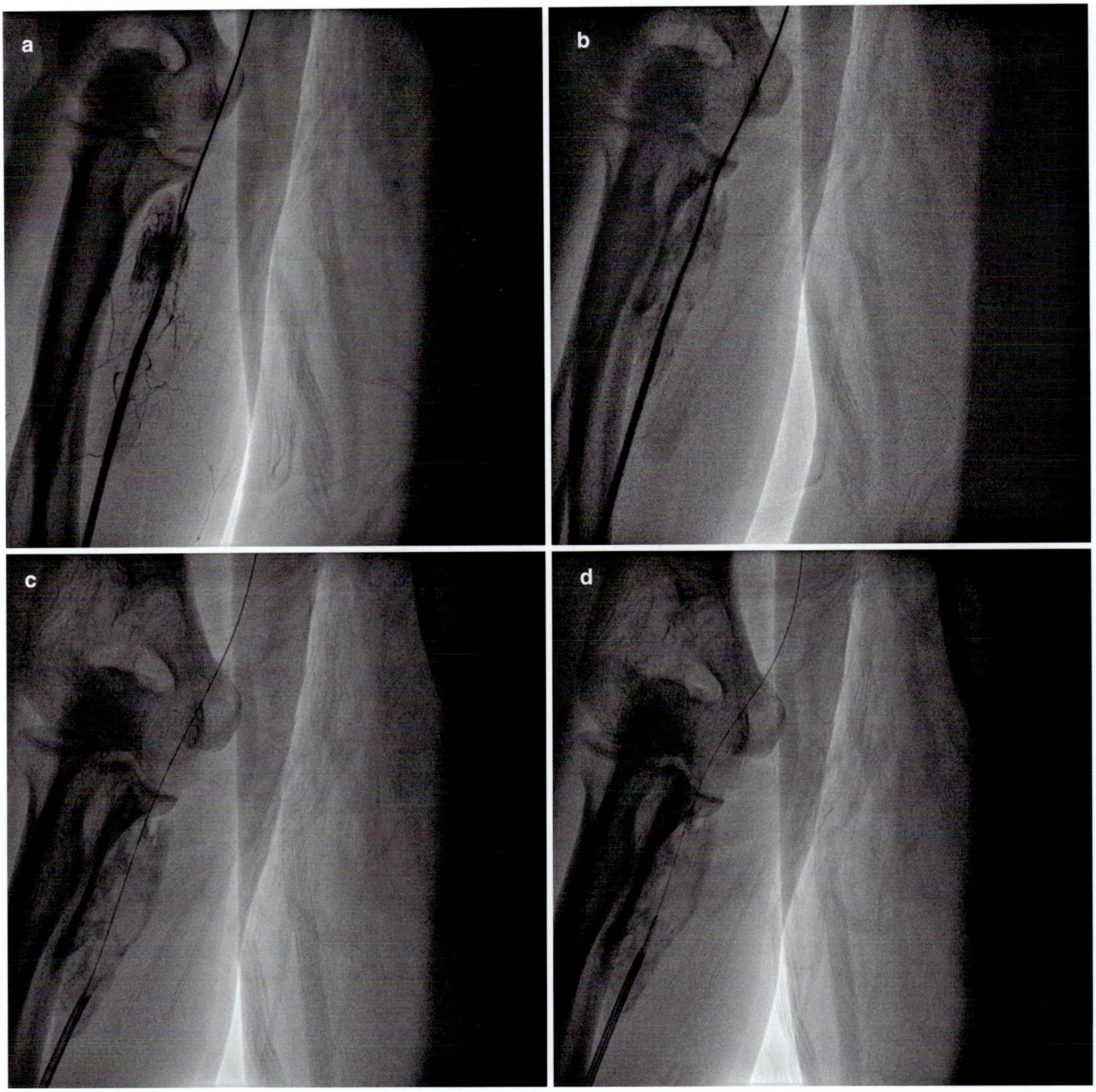

Fig. 5.6 A 52 years old male with a history of hypertension was admitted for chest pain. Angiogram was performed via right radial approach and a significant lesion at RCA was revealed. Arm pain was noted after advancing a MAC 3.5 catheter, and right radial artery perforation was found (**a**, **b**). A Tiger catheter was advanced over the perforation site to the level of elbow, and a BMW wire was exchanged. A MAC 3.5 catheter was successfully advanced with balloon assisting technique (**c**) and the intervention was completed (**d, e**). The radial angiogram showed narrowing and spasm in right radial artery after intervention (**f**). OCT revealed perforation of intima (**g**) (This case was provided by Dr. Jincheng Guo from Beijing Luhe Hospital)

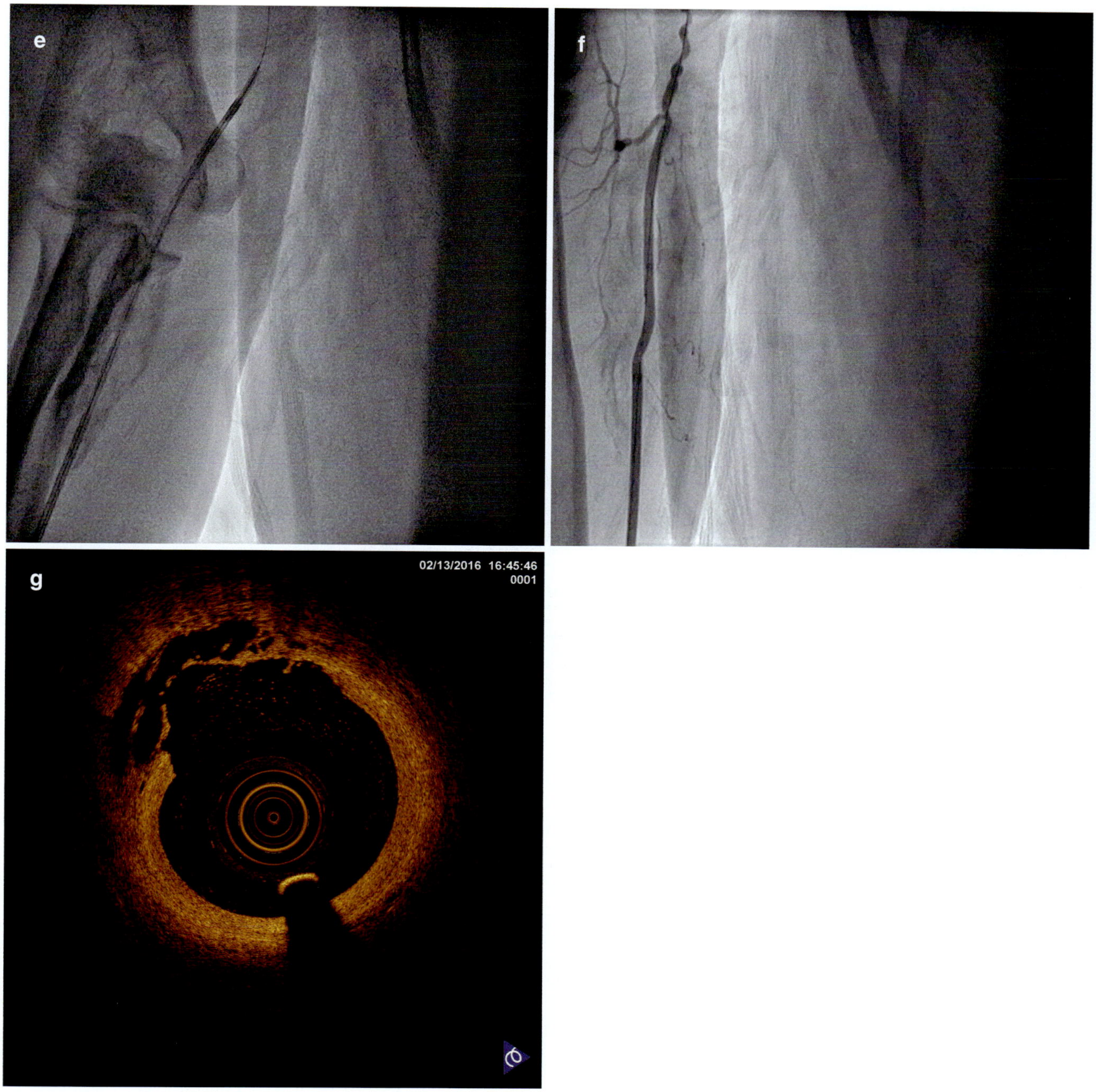

Fig. 5.6 (continued)

associated with bleeding after TRI include renal dysfunction, procedure duration, sheath size, female gender, advanced age, multiple puncture attempts, and aggressive use of anti-coagulation. Forearm hematoma is probably the most common bleeding complication of TRI and is described as the forearm swelling and pain, increased skin temperature and tension, and local skin bruising or blisters. Nevertheless, the exact incidence of forearm hematoma is not known because minor bleeding has no clinical implications. Conversely, more severe hematomas are noticed when swelling and pain of the puncture site are present. Usually prolonged compression may be enough to manage hematoma after ultrasound is used to exclude major injury of the artery. Forearm hematoma is caused by bleeding from the puncture site into the tissues of the forearm. A hematoma classification with different treatment strategies has been proposed by Bertrand, with Grade I and II being related to puncture site and Grade III and IV related to intramuscular bleeding (Fig. 5.7) [19]. In addition, major bleeding complications are markedly reduced with transradial approach over transfemoral approach.

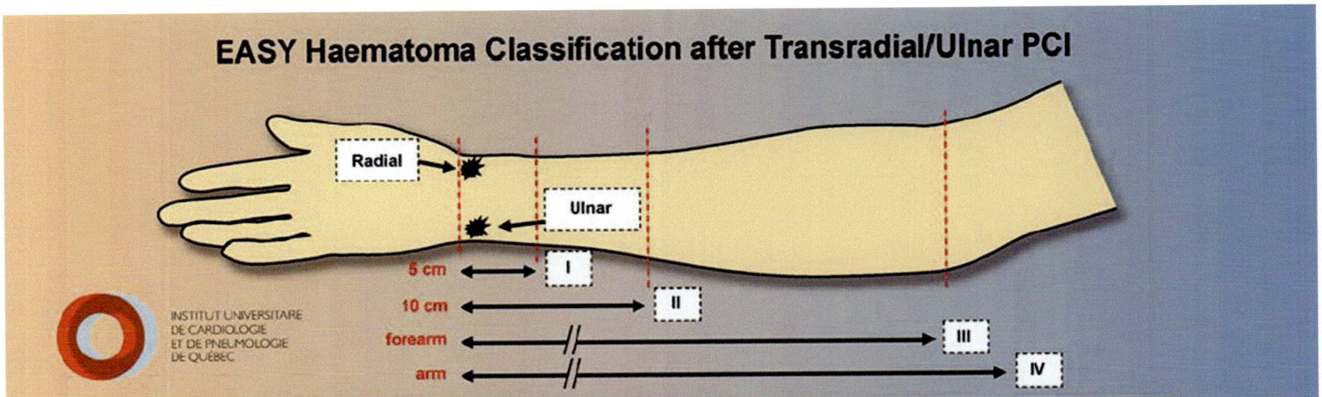

GRADE	I	II	III	IV	V
INCIDENCE	≤5%	<3%	<2%	≤0.1%	<0.01%
DEFINITION	Local hematoma, superficial	Hematoma with moderate muscular infiltration	Forearm hematoma and muscular infiltration, below the elbow	Hematoma and muscular infiltration extending above the elbow	Ischemic threat (compartment syndrome)
TREATMENT	Analgesia Additional bracelet Local ice	Analgesia Additional bracelet Local ice	Analgesia Additional bracelet Local ice Inflated BP cuff	Analgesia Additional bracelet, Local ice Inflated BP cuff	Consider surgery
NOTES		Inform physician	Inform physician	Inform physician	STAT call to physician
REMARKS	- Control blood pressure (BP) (importance of pain management) - Consider interruption of any anticoagulation and/or antiplatelet infusion - Follow forearm and arm diameters to evaluate requirement for additional bracelet and/or BP cuff inflation - Additional bracelet(s) can be placed alongside artery anatomy - Ice cubes in a plastic bag or washcloth are placed on the hematoma - Finger O_2 saturation can be monitored during inflated blood pressure cuff - To inflate blood pressure cuff, select a pressure of 20 mmHg < systolic pressure and deflate every 15 minutes - After bracelet removal, use "Velpeau bandage" around forearm/arm for a few hours to maintain mild positive pressure				

Fig. 5.7 EASY hematoma classification system after TRI

5.6 Compartment Syndrome

The forearm contains four inter-communicated compartments: superficial volar compartment, deep volar compartment, dorsal compartment, and Henry's mobile wad compartment, each of which consists of bone, interosseous membrane, intermuscular septa, and aponeurotic fascia, forming a closed chamber with tough and inflexible structure (Fig. 5.8). When there is a sharp increase in pressure of the chamber, the normal capillary flow and lymphatic drainage within the forearm is impeded, which progressively results in muscular and nervous damage. Compartment syndrome is a extremely rare complication of TRI. Possible causes can be unrecognized perforation at a distance from the puncture site, unsuccessful compression at the access site, or radial artery laceration induced by sheath insertion or removal because of severe spasm [20]. Typical symptoms of compartment syndrome are described as 5 "P" signs: pain, pallor, paresthesia, paralysis, and pulselessness. If compartment syndrome is not immediately identified and appropriately managed, patients may suffer amputation, acute renal failure, and even death. Given the catastrophic consequences of this complication, prevention is of vital importance. First, it is mandatory to check the patency of the hand collateral arteries during and after procedure. Second, radial tortuosities and anatomical variations should be managed properly during the procedure. If there is a severe spasm with the removal of the sheath, an anti-spasmolytic therapy should be given. The compression device should be placed accurately and periodically reviewed after procedure. Third, bleeding complications should be identified and treated promptly. Fourth, every complaint of the patient about pain or swelling of the arm should be taken into account. Treatment measures include dehydration and decompression. If pressure elevation caused by small hematoma is mild or modest and patients do not experience severe symptoms, conservative treatment should be applied, such as proper compression to stop the bleeding, dehydration with mannitol or furosemide to reduce the pressure, and discontinuation of anti-coagulation. If there is no symptomatic relief or the swelling aggravates, a surgical consultation is needed to perform fasciotomy. A case of compartment syndrome is illustrated in Fig. 5.9.

Fig. 5.8 Illustration of forearm compartments

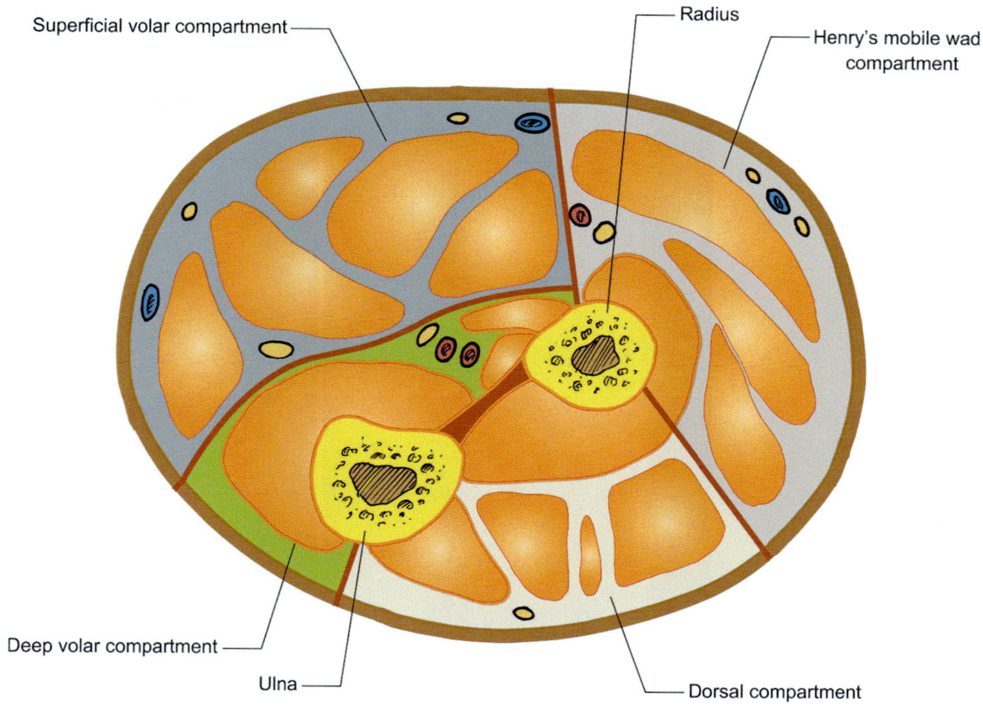

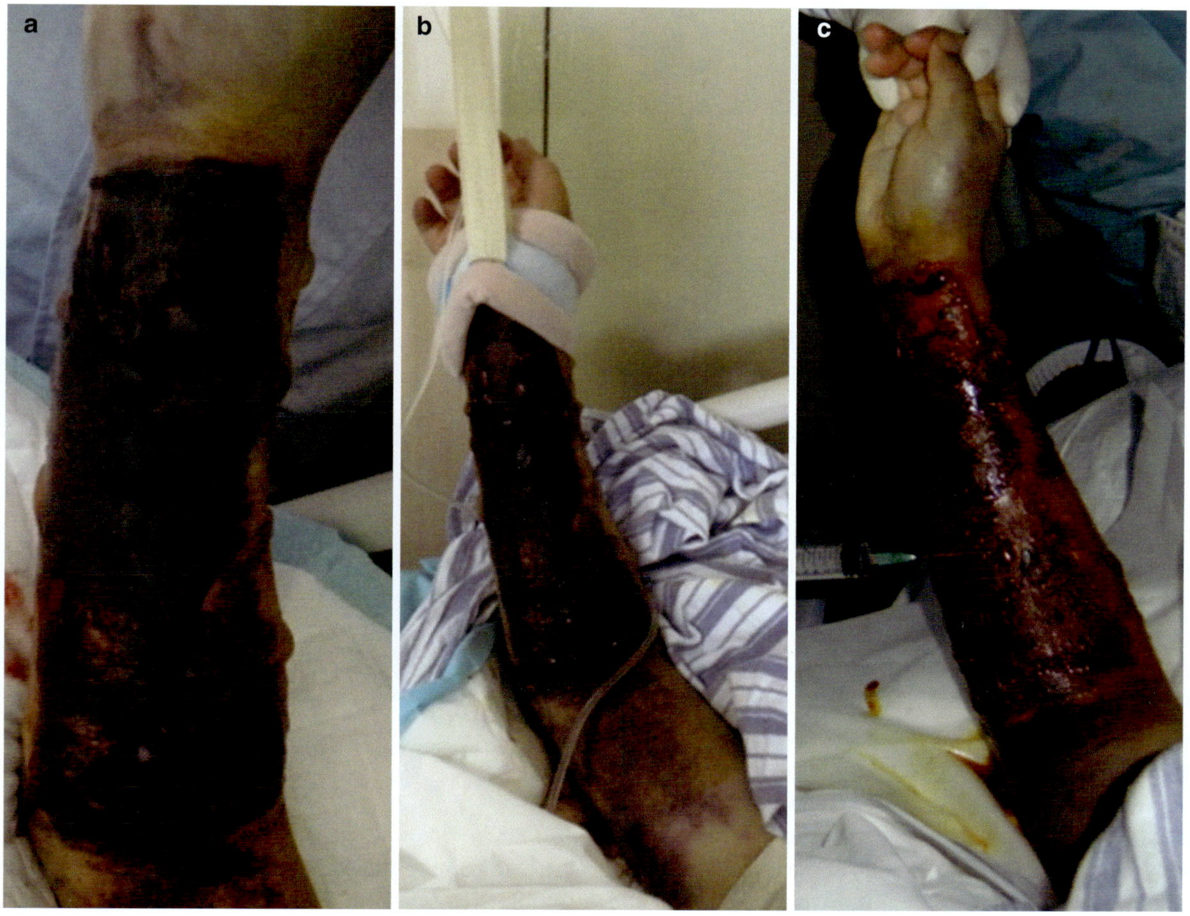

Fig. 5.9 A 79 years old male with acute myocardial infarction was admitted and an urgent PCI was performed via right radial approach. The patient was given tirofiban, low molecular weight heparin (*LMWH*), and double anti-platelet therapy (*DAPT*) after procedure. Radial sheath was removed 10 h after the procedure. TR band was released partially 1 h post sheath removal due to the patient's discomfort. Hematoma and blisters were developed the next day (**a**). Foasciotomy was advised by orthopedics, but it was not undertaken as discontinuation of anti-platelet and anti-coagulation is too risky after urgent PCI. A hanging position was applied to relieve the swelling by gravity (**b**). Blisters were aspirated with aseptic technique (**c**). The patient's forearm was partially recovered 1 week later (**d**) and completely recovered in 3 weeks (**e**) (This case was provided by Dr. Zhitao Jing from PLA Rocket General Hospital)

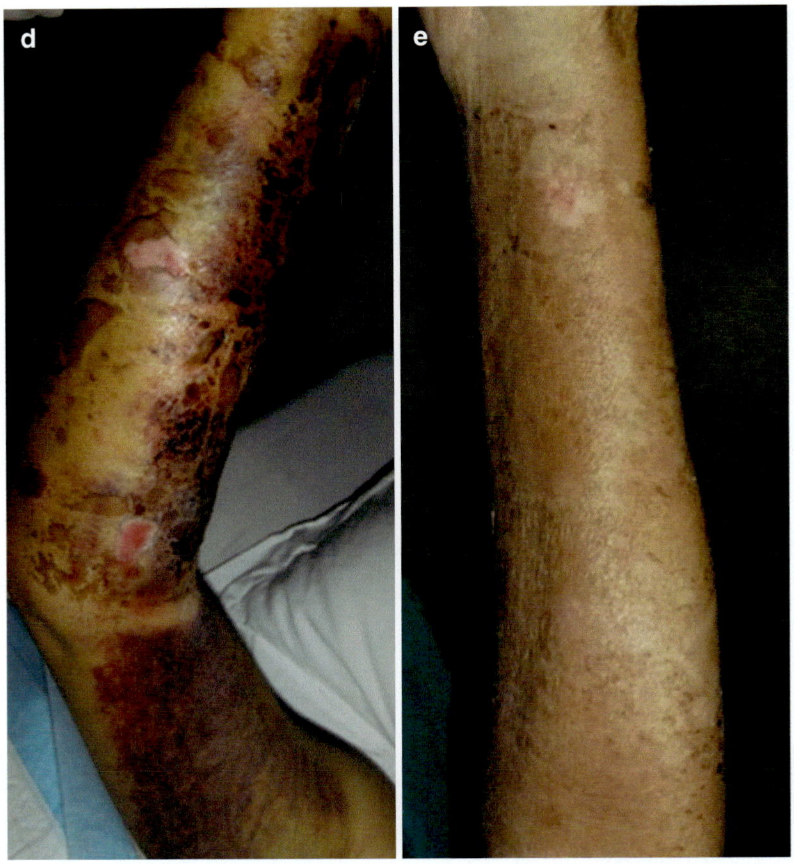

Fig. 5.9 (continued)

5.7 Pseudoaneurysm

Pseudoaneurysm is a very unusual complication after TRI with an incidence of <0.1% [21]. It results from penetrating injury of the arterial wall during procedure, leading to bleeding and pulsatile hematoma. A higher risk of pseudoaneurysm has been associated with multiple punctures, aggressive anti-coagulation, large size sheaths, and inadequate post-procedure compression. Radial artery pseudoaneurysm presents as the emergence of a local forearm pulsatile mass with systolic murmur and thrill which disappear by compressing the proximal part of radial artery. Large pseudoaneurysm may constrain the adjacent nerves and vessels, and subsequently cause forearm ischemia and upper limb dyskinesia. Ultrasound can confirm the diagnosis by demonstrating laminar flow entering and exiting through a neck region between the true vessel lumen and the pseudoaneurysm (Fig. 5.10) [2]. Early diagnosis and treatment of pseudoaneurysm are important to minimize further complications, such as spontaneous rupture or hand ischemia. Preventive measures include adequate compression, use of small size sheaths, and avoidance of strenuous upper extremity activities. Pseudoaneurysm can be treated with different approaches. Conservative strategy is to compress the neck region manually or by the use of Terumo TR Band™ (Terumo Medical Corporation) under ultrasound guidance [22]. Occasionally, surgical excision of the pseudoaneurysm and/or ligation of the radial artery may be necessary.

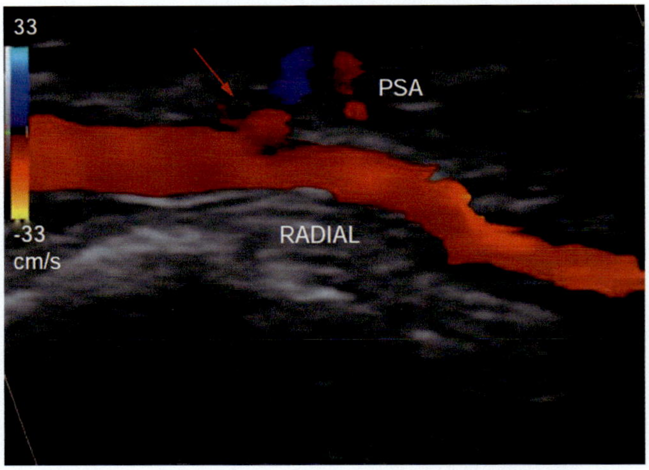

Fig. 5.10 Doppler ultrasound showing pseudoaneurysm (*arrow*) after TRI

5.8 Arteriovenous Fistula

Arteriovenous (AV) fistula is extremely uncommon with a reported incidence of $<0.03\%$ due to the fact that there are no major veins near the radial artery [23]. AV fistula often presents as persistent pain and swelling at the puncture site or an asymptomatic palpable thrill. About one third of iatrogenic AV fistula will close spontaneously within 1 year [24]. Therefore, conservative management is always attempted first. However, surgical or percutaneous approaches have been successfully performed to treat symptomatic AV fistula [25].

5.9 Nerve Damage

There is a paucity of significant neuronal structures around the radial artery and nerve damage is rarely encountered post TRI. Infrequently, median or radial nerves may be slightly injured owing to multiple punctures, which may result in digital numbness. This is usually a benign and minor complication that is self-limiting and can be relieved over time gradually. A more serious condition, the complex regional pain syndrome (CRPS), is a disorder of the involved limb characterized by pain, swelling, range of motion limitation, and vasomotor instability. There are two types of CRPS: type I with no demonstrable nerve damage and type II with obvious nerve damage [26]. The most common cause of type II CRPS is median nerve injury resulting from RAO, prolonged compression, and hematoma formation. CRPS is treated medically in most cases, such as sympathetic blockage, and the symptoms will eventually resolve.

5.10 Vasovagal Reflex

Vasovagal reflex, also called vasovagal response, is a malaise mediated by the vagus nerve. It is more frequent in patients with transfemoral approach, but can also be seen with transradial approach during pulling out the sheath, sometimes even shortly after the procedure. Patients are particularly predisposed to this complication when they suffer from great tension, insufficient local anesthesia, painful stimulus, and hypovolemia. Clinical manifestations of vasovagal reflex are related to decreased blood pressure and heart rate, including shortness of breath, nausea, vomiting, paleness, sweating, dizziness or sanity changes, and even syncope or death in worst cases. Prevention of vasovagal reflex is more important than treatment. Preoperative counseling and proper diet should be prepared to prevent emotional stress and hypovolemia. Once vasovagal reflex is identified, patients should be monitored and put on oxygen, and should be in the supine position without pillow with the head towards one side to avoid possible suffocation caused by vomiting. Meanwhile, vasodilators must be stopped and rapid infusion is given to maintain enough blood flow to important organs. If necessary, dopamine and atropine are used to increase the blood pressure and heart rate separately, and temporary pacing is considered in patients with severe bradycardia. If identified and treated early, the prognosis of vasovagal reflex is good.

5.11 Granuloma

Sterile granuloma formation is a rare self-limiting complication of TRI. It has been reported to be exclusively related with the use of a hydrophilic sheath and is considered as the consequence of a chronic inflammation [27]. Granuloma typically presents with swelling, redness, and tenderness 2 or 3 weeks after the procedure and is not responsive to antibiotics. Prior to confirming the diagnosis, ultrasound is recommended to exclude pseudoaneurysm. Usually, complete resolution of granuloma is expected to occur within several weeks without any sequela. In rare occasions, granulomas may need surgical excision, if it cannot resolve spontaneously. Thus, awareness of this complication is important to avoid unnecessary interventions.

5.12 Transradial Retrieval of Dislodged Stents

Stent dislodgement is a rare complication in interventional procedures and is associated with increased mortality. Coronary stent dislodgement can be secondary to severe angulation, calcified lesions, inadequate predilatation, and direct stenting. Retrieval of a dislodged stent should be performed either percutaneously or surgically. With the percutaneous method, femoral approach is commonly undertaken due to its larger diameter. A number of techniques via femoral approach have been attempted to successfully retrieve the dislodged stent, including low pressure balloon technique, small balloon technique, double wire technique, and loop snare technique [28]. The above stent retrieval methods can also be performed via transradial route if the dislodged stent is not inflated or deformed. However, transradial stent retrieval is slightly different from transfemoral approach and some modifications have to be made. First, the entire stent should be pulled into the guiding catheter before withdrawing the whole unit to prevent radial artery injury. Second, if the dislodged stent is partially inflated or deformed, it should be captured distally and then be pulled back into the guiding catheter. Third, if the dislodged stent cannot be pulled back into the guiding catheter, techniques described above may be used to pull the stent into the radial artery followed by the snare capture. Finally, if stent retrieval can not be achieved,

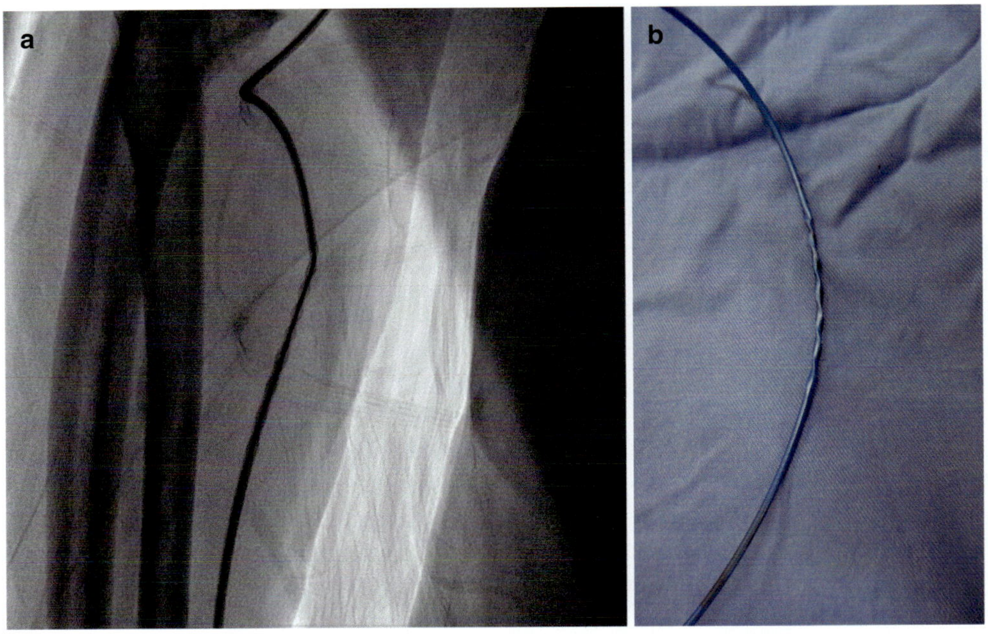

Fig 5.11 (**a**, **b**) Kinked catheter due to tortuous radial artery

the dislodged stent should be deployed directly in the radial artery, which causes no hand ischemia due to rich collateral circulation. A case of dislodged stent retrieval by forceps from right radial artery was recorded in Video 5.1.

5.13 Transradial Retrieval of Kinked Catheter

The occurrence of catheter kinking is not extremely exceptional during TRI, especially in patients with severe tortuosity (Fig. 5.11a, b). Manipulation of the entrapped catheter may harm the radial artery and lead to spasm, dissection, bleeding, and even occlusion. Prevention of this complication can be achieved by avoiding intense and repetitive rotation of the catheter. Usually, catheter kinking can be managed conservatively by gentle opposite rotation or straightening the catheter by crossing it with a regular or hydrophilic wire. Sometimes, an invasive approach for retrieval is required. So far, a few transradial techniques using long sheath or sheathless guiding catheter have been attempted successfully [29–32]. If all the transradial approaches to retrieve the entrapped catheter fail, then transfemoral or surgical approaches are considered.

As the use of transradial access becomes more common, cardiologists, particularly interventional practitioners, need to be aware of all minor and major complications related to this approach. The ability to recognize and manage complications unique to radial access is critical in decreasing their incidence and preventing serious long-term consequences. With better understanding of the cause and the appropriate management of these complications, transradial access will surely offer a terrific opportunity to deliver optimal care for patients with coronary heart disease.

References

1. Campeau L. Percutaneous radial artery approach for coronary angiography. Cathet Cardiovasc Diagn. 1989;16:3–7.
2. Bhat T, Teli S, Bhat H, et al. Access-site complications and their management during transradial cardiac catheterization. Expert Rev Cardiovasc Ther. 2012;10:627–34.
3. Ho HH, Jafary FH, Ong PJ. Radial artery spasm during transradial cardiac catheterization and percutaneous coronary intervention: incidence, predisposing factors, prevention, and management. Cardiovasc Revasc Med. 2012;13:193–5.
4. Rathore S, Stables RH, Pauriah M, et al. Impact of length and hydrophilic coating of the introducer sheath on radial artery spasm during transradial coronary intervention: a randomized study. JACC Cardiovasc Interv. 2010;3:475–83.
5. Kim SH, Kim EJ, Cheon WS, et al. Comparative study of nicorandil and a spasmolytic cocktail in preventing radial artery spasm during transradial coronary angiography. Int J Cardiol. 2007;120:325–30.
6. Ouadhour A, Sideris G, Smida W, et al. Usefulness of subcutaneous nitrate for radial access. Catheter Cariovasc Interv. 2008;72:343–6.
7. Kanei Y, Kwan T, Nakra NC, et al. Transradial cardiac catheterization: a review of access site complications. Catheter Cardiovasc Interv. 2011;78:840–6.
8. Stella PR, Kiemeneij F, Laarman GJ, et al. Incidence and outcome of radial artery occlusion following transradial artery coronary angioplasty. Cathet Cardiovasc Diagn. 1997;40:156–8.
9. Pancholy S, Coppola J, Patel T, et al. Prevention of radial artery occlusion-patent hemostasis evaluation trial (PROPHET Study): a randomized comparison of traditional versus patency documented hemostasis after transradial catheterization. Catheter Cardiovasc Interv. 2008;72:335–40.

10. Pancholy SB. Impact of two different hemostatic devices on radial artery outcomes after transradial catheterization. J Invasive Cardiol. 2009;21:101–4.
11. Cubero JM, Lombardo J, Pedrosa C, et al. Radial compression guided by mean artery pressure versus standard compression with a pneumatic device (RACOMAP). Catheter Cardiovasc Interv. 2009;73:467–72.
12. Patel T, Shah S, Sanghavi K, et al. Reaccessing an occluded radial artery: a 'proximal entry' technique. J Interv Cardiol. 2011;24: 378–81.
13. Babunashvili A, Dundua D. Recanalization and reuse of early occluded radial artery within 6 days after previous transradial diagnostic procedure. Catheter Cardiovasc Interv. 2011;77:530–6.
14. Patel T, Shah S, Sanghavi K, et al. Management of radial and brachial artery perforations during transradial procedures–a practical approach. J Invasive Cardiol. 2009;21:544–7.
15. Calvino-Santos RA, Vasquez-Rodriguez JM, Salgado-Fernandez J, et al. Management of iatrogenic radial artery perforation. Catheter Cardiovasc Interv. 2004;61:74–8.
16. Sanmartín M, Cuevas D, Goicolea J, et al. Vascular complications associated with radial artery access for cardiac catheterization. Rev Esp Cardiol. 2004;57:581–4.
17. Gunasekaran S, Cherukupalli R. Radial artery perforation and its management during PCI. J Invasive Cardiol. 2009;21:E24–6.
18. Rigatelli G, Dell'Avvocata F, Ronco F, et al. Successful coronary angioplasty via the radial approach after sealing a radial perforation. J Am Coll Cardiol Interv. 2009;2:1158–9.
19. Bertrand OF. Acute forearm muscle swelling post transradial catheterization and compartment syndrome: prevention is better than treatment! Catheter Cardiovasc Interv. 2010;75:366–8.
20. Tizón-Marcos H, Barbeau GR. Incidence of compartment syndrome of the arm in a large series of transradial approach for coronary procedures. J Interv Cardiol. 2008;21:380–4.
21. Collins N, Wainstein R, Ward M, et al. Pseudoaneurysm after transradial cardiac catheterization: case series and review of the literature. Catheter Cardiovasc Interv. 2012;80:283–7.
22. Liou M, Tung F, Kanei Y, et al. Treatment of radial artery pseudoaneurysm using a novel compression device. J Invasive Cardiol. 2010;22:293–5.
23. Eichhöfer J, Horlick E, Ivanov J, et al. Decreased complication rates using the transradial compared to the transfemoral approach in percutaneous coronary intervention in the era of routine stenting and glycoprotein platelet IIb/IIIa inhibitor use: a large single-center experience. Am Heart J. 2008;156:864–70.
24. Summaria F, Romagnoli E, Mustilli M. Arteriovenous fistula of the wrist after transradial coronary intervention. Heart Lung. 2012;41:410.
25. Summaria F, Romagnoli E, Preziosi P. Percutaneous antegrade transarterial treatment of iatrogenic radial arteriovenous fistula. J Cardiovasc Med. 2012;13:50–2.
26. Cho EJ, Yang JH, Song YB. Type II complex regional pain syndrome of the hand resulting from repeated arterial punctures during transradial coronary intervention. Catheter Cardiovasc Interv. 2013;82:E465–8.
27. Kozak M, Adams DR, Ioffreda MD, et al. Sterile inflammation associated with transradial catheterization and hydrophilic sheaths. Catheter Cardiovasc Interv. 2003;59:207–13.
28. Kwan TW, Chaudhry M, Huang Y, et al. Approaches for dislodged stent retrieval during transradial percutaneous coronary interventions. Catheter Cardiovasc Interv. 2013;81:E245–9.
29. Leibundgut G, Löffelhardt N, Neumann FJ. Percutaneous retrieval of a twisted guide catheter using a longer second radial sheath. Catheter Cardiovasc Interv. 2014;83:560–3.
30. Aminian A, Fraser DG, Dolatabadi D. Severe catheter kinking and entrapment during transradial coronary angiography: percutaneous retrieval using a sheathless guide catheter. Catheter Cardiovasc Interv. 2015;85:91–4.
31. Michael TT, Banerjee S, Brilakis ES. Percutaneous retrieval of a fractured guide catheter using contralateral snaring. J Invasive Cardiol. 2012;24:E176–8.
32. Waked A, Khoueiry G, Bhat T. Entrapment of a looped/kinked catheter in the brachial artery and its successful retrieval during transradial coronary catheterization. J Invasive Cardiol. 2012;24:471–2.

Common Anatomical Variants in Percutaneous Transradial Intervention and Trouble Shooting

6

HuayCheem Tan and XiaoFan Wu

Abstract

Transradial access has been advocated as the preferred vascular access because of its lower rate of vascular complications, improved patient comfort and satisfaction, and earlier ambulation. However transradial approach had its own limitations and challenges, including unique anomalous anatomies, small-calibred vessel, vasospasm etc. the We share some of the difficulties and offer possible solutions to commonly encountered problems.

6.1 Special Considerations in Transradial Intervention

The first obvious difference between the transfemoral and transradial approach is in the size of the arteries. Given the small size of the radial artery, devices will have to be modified and adapted for cannulation of the vessel as well as the coronary ostia. Radial access kits which provide progressive tapering tips and improved lubricated coating to ease insertion and decrease arterial spasm risk, at perhaps higher cost, are now commercially available. Most currently used femoral catheters are well-matched with radial access, however Judkins 3.5 shaped catheter is more suited to left coronary ostia from the right radial access in a normal aorta, unlike the standard Judkins 4.0 catheter chosen typically for femoral approach. The same standard Judkins Right 4.0 catheter is useful for cannulation of the right coronary ostium in a transradial approach. In difficult angle take-off situations, a Left Internal Mammary Artery (LIMA) catheter can be useful for horizontal take-off in an elongated aorta, and an Amplatz Left (AL) catheter can be used for superior take-off. Dedicated radial catheters such as Terumo Tiger catheter are available for cannulation of both coronary ostia and thus avoid the need for exchange of catheters during the procedures.

In addition to the challenges of pre-shaped guiding catheters that were designed initially not for the transradial route, anatomical variation in radial and brachial arteries may add further to the reduction in succession of the transradial cardiac procedures.

6.2 Radial and Brachial Artery Loop

Discrepancies among radial artery procedure are likely and occur in about 14% of patients [1]. These congenital anomalies have been attributed to differences in angiogenesis, selective hypertrophy and regression during early embryonic development, and alternative development around muscle and tendon bundles [2]. Navigating through tortuous radial artery, such as in the presence of vascular loops, may be challenging. Commonly the first sign of this is the difficulty in advancing the guidewire up the proximal arm [3]. It is important that one must not force the guidewire forward in the encounter of any resistance (Figs. 6.1 and 6.2; Videos 6.1 and 6.2.

Suggested techniques of negotiation (illustrated in Videos 6.3 and 6.4) would be to:

1. Do a radial artery angiogram with diluted contrast to outline the anatomy
2. When radial or brachial artery loop is confirmed, downside the guidewire to a 0.014 in. coronary angioplasty guidewire to negotiate through

Electronic supplementary material. The online version of this chapter (doi:10.1007/978-94-017-7350-8_6) contains supplementary material, which is available to authorized users.

H. Tan (✉) • X. Wu
National University Heart Centre, Singapore (NUHCS), Singapore, Singapore
e-mail: huay_cheem_tan@nuhs.edu.sg; drwuxf@163.com

Y. Zhou et al. (eds.), *Transradial Approach for Percutaneous Interventions*, DOI 10.1007/978-94-017-7350-8_6

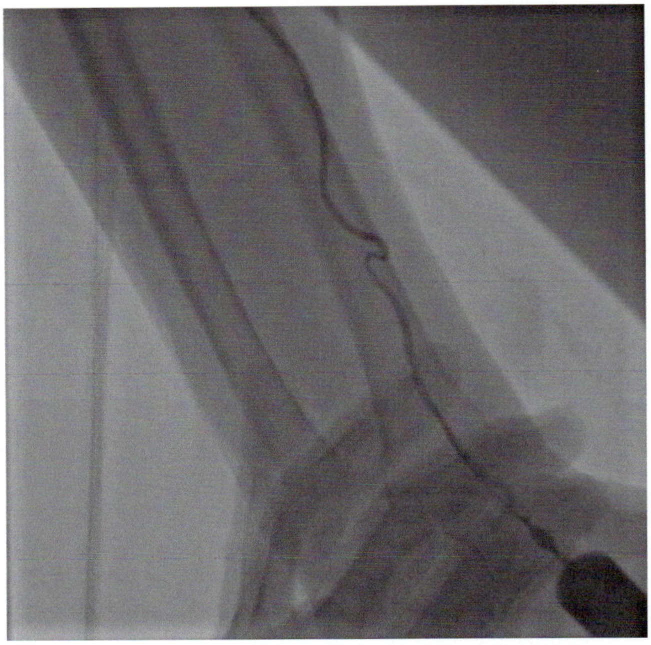

Fig. 6.1 Tortuous radial artery

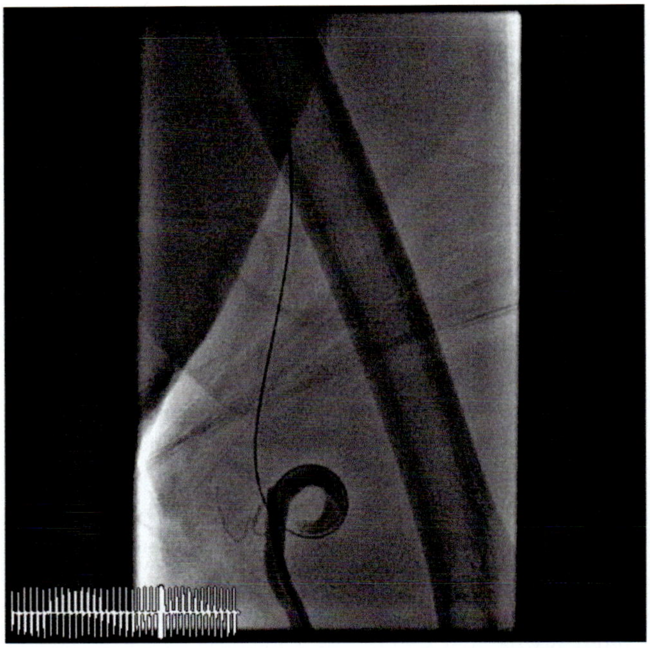

Fig. 6.2 Brachial artery loop

3. Once the diagnostic catheter has been advanced through the radial loop straightened by the coronary guidewire, one can switch to a polymer-jacket Terumo guidewire for further advancement

This technique of using coronary guidewire is not only safe and minimise the risk of radial artery perforation and trauma, it also facilitates the 'straightening' of the loop which allows for the subsequent passage of diagnostic or guiding catheters. Any change of the catheter is best done with the over-the-wire exchange technique (using a long 300 cm exchange guidewire) to prevent recurrent navigation of tortuosities of radial and brachial arteries.

Other techniques to consider include:

1. Use of second buddy guidewire in situations when a single coronary 0.014 in. guidewire delivers insufficient support to the catheter for crossing the loop
2. Upon difficulty in advancing into the loop: while keeping the tip of the catheter high, attempt to push as far as possible. And then pull back slightly (i.e., the catheter and the guidewire) which usually will be followed with straightening of the loop.
3. Balloon Assisted Tracking (BAT). This is a technique where an inflated PTCA balloon is slightly projected out of the distal end of the guide/diagnostic catheter and inflated at a pressure of 3–6 atmospheres. When 5 Fr diagnostic/guide catheters are used, balloon diameter of 1.5 mm is recommended. For 6 Fr guide catheters, balloon diameter of 2.0 mm is recommended. Balloon length of 15 mm or 20 mm will be sufficient. Once the partially protruded balloon is inflated in deployment, the entire structure is advanced over a soft-tipped 0.014 in. PTCA guidewire through the difficult vascular anatomy. This technique provides smooth and non traumatic passage and is useful not only in tortuous radial or brachial artery, complex radial artery loop, severe subclavian tortuosity, but also atherosclerotic lesions in the upper limb arteries (Fig. 6.3).

6.3 Tortuous Subclavian Artery

Tortuosity of the subclavian artery is commonly encountered in elderly patients while attempting the radial route. It may occur at the level of the subclavian or brachiocephalic trunk. Such tortuosities commonly result in difficulty in manipulating the catheter into the ostia or failure to advance the catheter to the aortic root. (Fig. 6.4).

One trick in negotiating the subclavian tortuosities is by asking the patient to take a deep breath to straighten the subclavian artery, to reach the ascending aorta and facilitate coronary ostia engagement and intubation. Another alternative is to exchange the diagnostic catheter for a guiding catheter for its enhanced stiffness. Some of the guiding catheters such as Cordis XB or Medtronic EBU guiding catheters may be used at times to interact with the left coronary ostium (Fig. 6.5).

6.4 Arteria Lusoria

The most common aortic arch anomaly is aberrant right subclavian arteries (ARSA), also called arteria lusoria which occurs in about 0.5–2 % in the population. Rather than

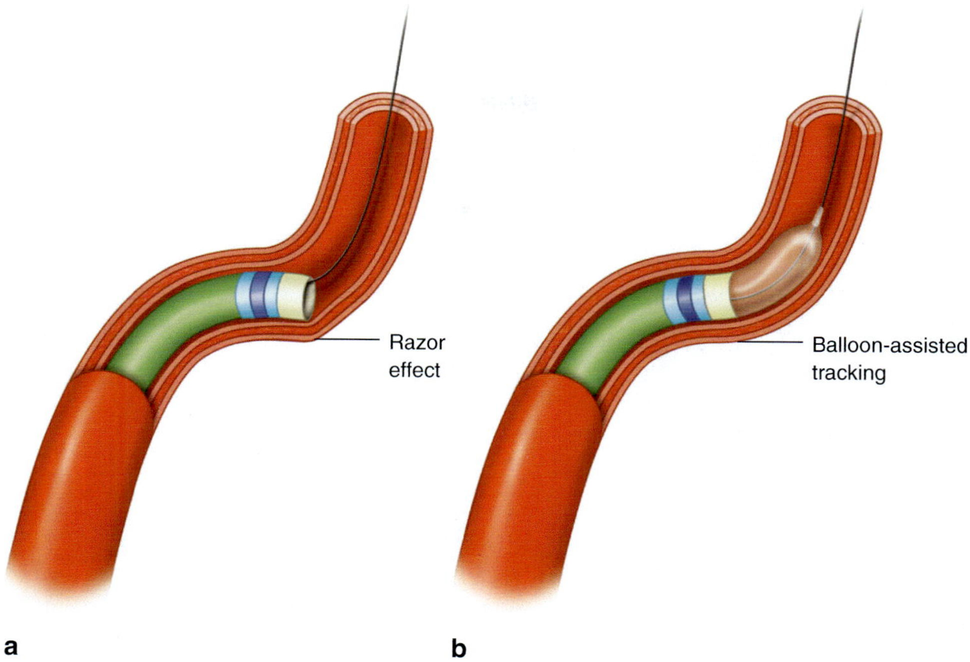

Fig. 6.3 Balloon assisted tracing Patel et al. CCI (2012) (**a**) Sharp edge of the guide catheter tip act like a "razor-blade" preventing the catheter navigation. (**b**) Balloon-assisted tracking in dealing with radial artery loop /radial artery spasm/ torturous radial artery by transradial approach

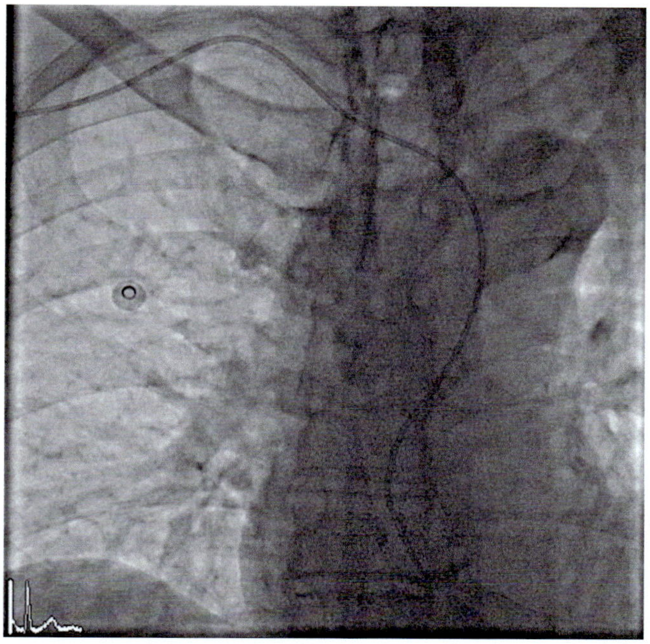

Fig. 6.4 Tortuous subclavian artery

forming with first branch (right common carotid as the brachiocephalic artery), it ascends independently on the fourth branch, post left subclavian artery and further hooks back to extend to the right. Its posterior to the esophagus between esophagus and trachea and anterior to trachea, 80 %, 15 %, 5 % respectively. In passing retro-esophageally in some cases, the artery may form vascular ring around and compress on the oesophagus to cause dysphagia. An upper GI contrast study will demonstrate displacement of the contrast-filled esophagus. This displacement by abnormal vessels results in the bayonet deformity of the abnormal right subclavian artery.

Arteria lusoria is one of the common causes of procedural failure during right transradial catheterisation. It makes the procedure challenging since the guidewire and catheters need to curve posteriorly towards the ascending aorta from the descending aorta, prior to arriving at the coronary sinus. If the guidewire re-enters the descending aorta, this promotes possibility of arteria lusoria. In such case it is viable to carry on the procedure, despite the technical challenges, rather than interchanging with the femoral artery. Techniques of engaging the coronary ostia is demonstrated in Videos 6.5, 6.6, and 6.7. A good alternative of transradial catheterisation will be to perform the procedure from the left radial route.

6.5 Radial Artery Spasm

Radial artery spasm should be suspected whenever patient mentions discomfort along the radial artery while passing the guidewire or catheter. In attempt of defining anatomy and distinguishing spasm, radial angiogram through the side-port of the introduce sheath or through the catheter should be performed (Fig. 6.6).

Radial artery (RA) spasm can present as spectrum of severity. Multiple attempts at radial artery puncture in beginner technicians is a common cause for encountering this scenario. The overall incidence is about 5.6 %, of which 0.5 % patients had severe spasm (3).

Initial steps to manage RA spasm would be to administer intraarterial spasmolytic such as glyceryl trinitrate (GTN) or

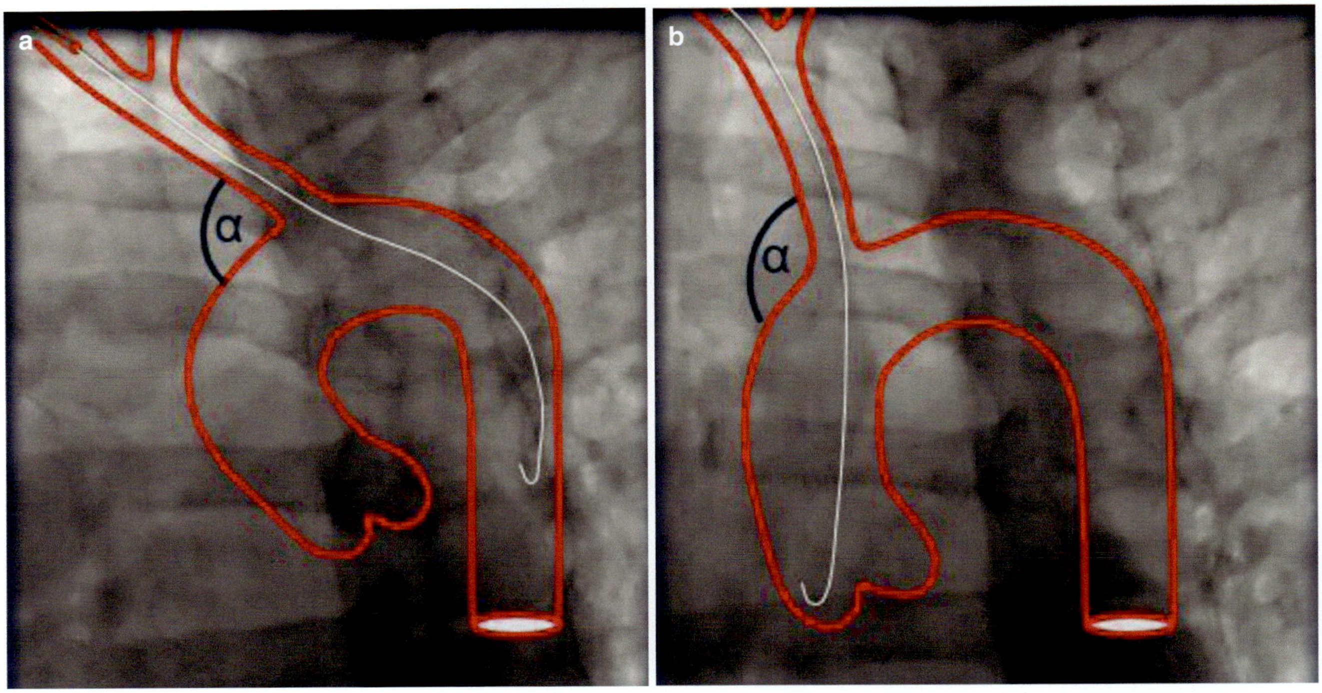

Fig. 6.5 (**a**) During expiration there is a more acute angle (α) between the brachiocephalic trunk and the ascending aorta, therefore the wire takes a more horizontal a more horizontal direction towards the descending aorta. (**b**) During deep inspiration, the diaphragm lowers the heart and straightens the angle (α) between the brachiocephalic trunk and the ascending aorta. The wire takes a more vertical direction towards the ascending aorta

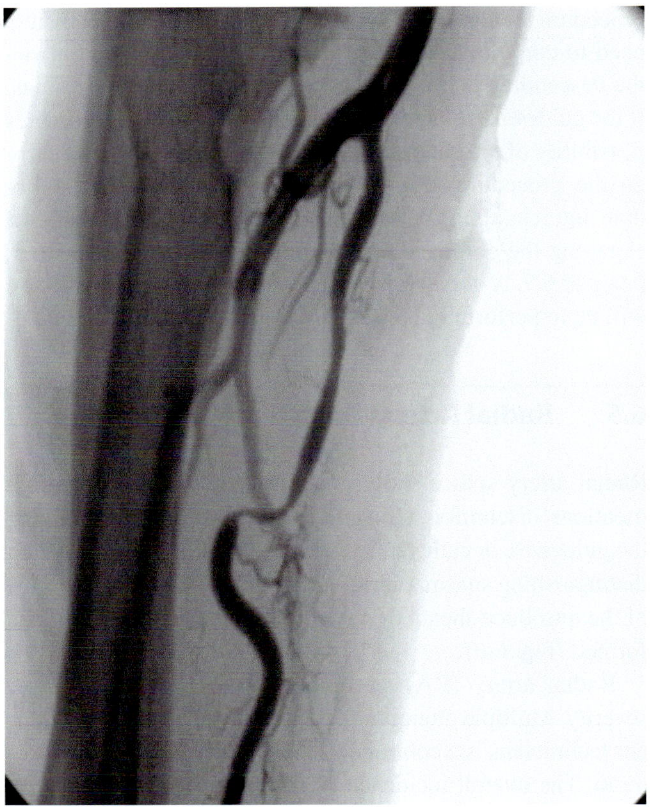

Fig. 6.6 Radial artery spasm

verapamil. A short wait time of between 30 and 60 s is recommended before attempting passage again. Analgesic and sedation are also helpful in reducing patients anxiety state and sympathetic tone, which is helpful in providing vascular relaxation.

Íf this is not successful, one can consider downsizing the guidewire to a 0.025" J shaped hydrophilic guidewire or a soft-tipped 0.014 in. PTCA guidewire. Upon successful completion of this, a diagnostic or guide catheter should be able to navigate over it. Rather than forcefully pushing the catheter, attempt at advancing in a manner of slow corkscrew movement. Sometimes, downsizing the guide catheter from 6 Fr to 5 Fr or diagnostic catheter from 5 Fr to 4 Fr may also be helpful. Balloon Assisted Tracking (BAT) technique may also be considered in the most difficult of situations. For catheter passage the semi-inflated balloon is used as a wedge to cause minimal trauma through the spastic segment.

Conclusions

Management of upper limb arterial anatomical variant is key to a successful transradial approach. Common vascular challenges may fortunately be managed through ensuing basic algorithm approach, and at the comfort and experience level of the operator. In the event that severe anatomical variant precludes a transradial approach, there should also be no hesitation in referring to the transfemoral route.

References

1. Lo TS, Nolan J, Fountzopoulos E, et al. Radial artery anomaly and its influence on transradial coronary procedural outcome. Heart. 2009;95:410–5.
2. Rodriguez-Niedenfuhr M, Vazquez T, Nearn L, Ferreira B, Parkin I, Sanudo JR. Variationsof the arterial pattern in the upper limb revisited: a morphological and statistical study, with a review of the literature. J Anat. 2001;199:547–66.
3. Caputo RP, Tremmel JA, Rap S, et al. Transradial arterial access for coronary and peripheral procedures: executive summary by the transradial committee of the SCAI. Catheter Cardiovasc Interv. 2011;15(78):823–30.

Single Catheter Usage for Both Left and Right Coronary Arteries

7

Seung-Woon Rha and Shaopeng Xu

Abstract

Transradial bilateral coronary angiography and angioplasty by single catheter is a useful technique but not a new one [1]. Since 1996, it has been reported that transradial percutaneous transluminal coronary angioplasty (PTCA) can be performed by single Kimny guiding catheter in single procedure [2]. Kiemeneij [3] reported several total coronary occlusion cases treated with single guiding catheter by simultaneous transradial coronary angioplasty and contralateral coronary angiography. The most remarkable characteristic is its ability of reducing the transradial intervention (TRI) related complications. Nowadays, transradial approach has been taken as the alternative of transfemoral access or the preferred access for percutaneous coronary intervention (PCI), given that transradial approach is known as being associated with lower vascular complication rates, improved patient comfort, and lower procedural costs than the femoral approach [4]. However the TRI related complications such as radial artery spasm is still worried by operators. Single catheter technique may amplify the priority of TRI buy reducing radial artery spasm because it does not need separate catheter for both left and right coronary arteries. Compared with conventional TRI, the advantages of single catheter for bilateral coronary artery intervention includes lower costs, reduction of vascular complications such as radial artery spasm, dissection, occlusion, perforation, reduction of radiation exposure, reduction of procedure time, and reduction of contrast volume.

7.1 Advantages of Transradial Single Catheter

7.1.1 Lower Costs

Compared with transfemoral intervention (TFI), the majority of cost saving in TRI comes from the post-procedural cost, due to early movement and discharge. The previous study demonstrated that TRI was associated with a total cost savings of $830, of which $130 were procedural savings and $705 were post-procedural savings for each patient [5]. Bilateral coronary angioplasty or angiography with single catheter can amplify the advantage by saving more cost due to less consumption of catheters [6, 7].

S.-W. Rha (✉) • S. Xu
Cardiovascular Center, Korea University Guro Hospital, Seoul, Korea
e-mail: swrha617@yahoo.co.kr; xsplzy@163.com

7.1.2 Reduction of Vascular Complications

Overall, transradial approach is safe and has advantages over femoral access, especially in patients with ST segment elevation myocardial infarction (STEMI) undergoing primary PCI, due to reduced bleeding and mortality [8]. However, there is hesitation which comes from the radial artery related complications. Radial artery spasm is one of the most common vascular complications induced by cannulation. The literature reported incidence of radial artery spasm during TRI ranged from 4 to 20 % [9]. Multiple catheters insertion by the radial approach might cause pain especially during catheter exchange [6], which may induce the radial spasm [10, 11]. Besides the anatomy factors such as smaller radial

Y. Zhou et al. (eds.), *Transradial Approach for Percutaneous Interventions*, DOI 10.1007/978-94-017-7350-8_7

artery diameter, the risk factors of radial artery spasm may include entrance of guidewires into side branches, larger arterial sheath diameters, longer procedure duration, number of catheters used and so on [9, 10]. The previous study demonstrated that more than three catheters during single procedure was related to three times higher risk of radial spasm [10]. Given the above evidences, reducing the catheter number is a helpful way to reduce the risk of radial spasm during procedure.

In addition to spasm, the passage and manipulations of catheters may induce dissections, and occlusion. Aseptic reactive inflammatory response in the arterial wall, intimal hyperplasia and thickening of intima–media due to proliferative mechanism [12], periarterial tissue or fat necrosis [13], medial dissections, and thrombi [14] which were observed in catheterized radial arteries ultimately lead to radial artery occlusion. In some cases, as previously reported,multiple cannulation or manipulation increase the risk of radial spasm, as well as the occlusion [12, 14]. The reported incidence of occlusion in the literature varies widely (0.8–30 %) [15] and so does the outcomes of occlusion, which range from asymptomatic occlusion of the lightest to finger amputation of the severest [16]. Single catheter technique can decrease the risk of radial artery occlusion induced by repeated catheter insertion.

7.1.3 Reduction of Procedure Time

Another hesitation in utilizing transradial approach is that procedure time is longer in TRI than that in TFI. For those patients undergoing primary PCI, the worry about needle to balloon time is more serious. Although the similar needle to balloon time was proven in previous study [17], the procedure time and x-ray times is considered slightly longer with the transradial than the transfemoral approach in the majority of reported or published studies [18, 19]. However, single catheter coronary intervention can attenuate the worry about the procedure time, needle to balloon time, or X-ray exposure. It has been demonstrated that single guiding TRI reduce the needle to balloon time compared with conditional TRI or TFI, and increased the proportion of patients achieving door to balloon time within 90 min [17] without increasing of major adverse cardiac events (MACE) rate [20]. Compared with conventional TRI intervention, single catheter intervention technique saves time required for exchange of catheter(s), shortens the procedure time, and also increases the possibility of no heparin procedure without increasing the risk of radial artery occlusion. It is more important for the patients who are not suitable to heparin [21]. Furthermore, using a single catheter may decrease fluoroscopy time that might be particularly important to high-volume operators doing multiple procedures [6, 7].

7.2 Choice of Single Transradial Catheter

Several catheters are selectable for single catheter transradial angiography (TRA) and TRI of both the right and left coronary artery. The diagnostic catheters include Tiger, multipurpose catheter, Amplatz left, RM or CR catheters (JSM, Korea). The Tiger II is manufactured by Terumo Corporation (Japan), and designed especially for right transradial or transbrachial approaches [6]. The shape of it is showed in the Table 7.1. The RM (Rha-Moon) and CR (Cheon-Rha) catheters are products of Jung Sung Medical (JSM), Korea. It was invented and entitled by Dr Rha SW. Those catheters have three side holes for enhanced image qualities thorough 4 F slender catheter and to prevent pulling out from the engagement position during forceful contrast injection. They are considered to be associated with a significantly shorter total procedure time and shorter total fluoroscopic time, compared with those with the conventional Judkins catheter (Figs. 7.1 and 7.2).

Many guiding catheters can be used for transradial bilateral coronary angioplasty. The choices are listed in Table 7.2.

In some of above catheters, such as kimny, Radial brachial and Radial Back-up, the shapes of these catheters are similar except the slight differences in the angle of second curve or distance between the first to the second curve. Kimny catheter (Boston Scientific) is the first multipurpose catheter designed for right radial approach TRI. The specific design of guiding catheters curves, such as Kimny, Ikari Left, can give optimum support besides the convenient engagement. Amplatz left guiding catheter is considered to provide the strongest support among them. Although Judkins left can be used in TRI, its curve is originally designed for TFI, which make the manipulation not as easy as it was in TFI, especially during engagement of

Table 7.1 Transradial diagnostic catheters for bilateral engagement

Catheter	Manufacturer	Illustration
Tiger	Terumo	
Multipurpose catheter		
Amplatz left		
CR	JSM Korea	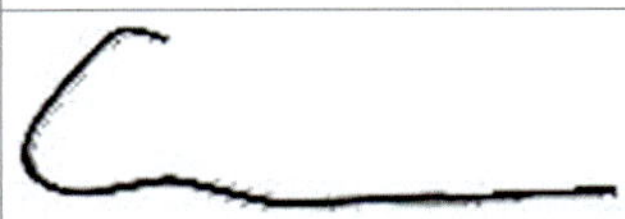
RM	JSM Korea	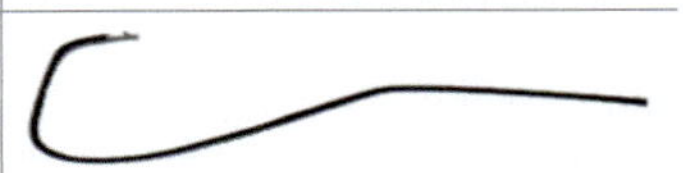

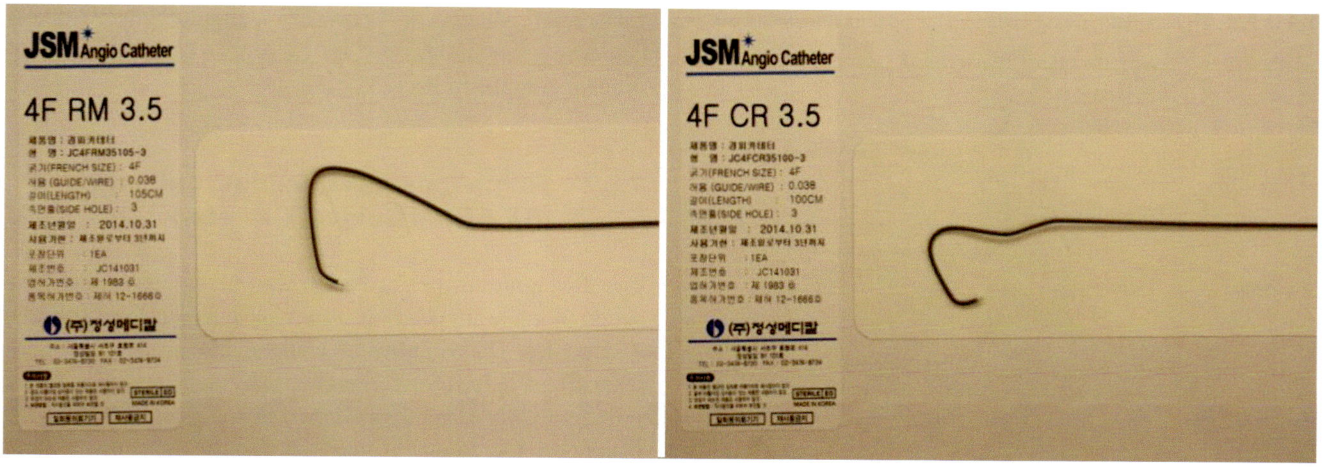

Fig. 7.1 RM & CR catheter (4 F, JSM Korea). Designed for 4 F transradial bilateral angiography with single catheter. Those catheters have three side holes to prevent pulling back during the contrast injection and to enhance more contrast delivery for better image quality through the slender 4 F catheter lumen

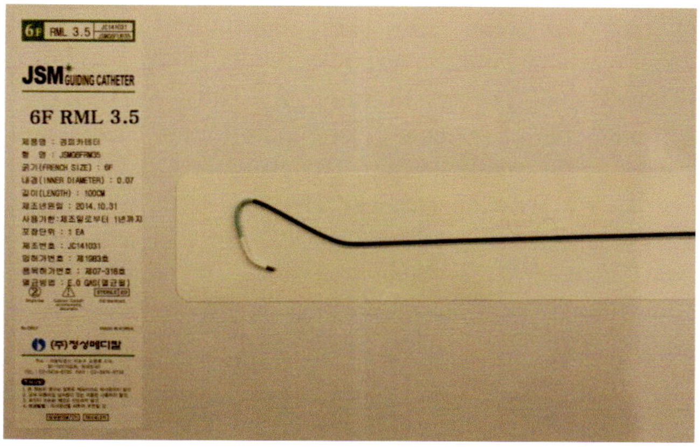

Fig. 7.2 RM Guiding catheter (5 F, 6 F) for transradial intervention

right coronary artery, and it is not as feasible as IL or Kimny during TRI procedure. However after its engagement, Judkins left can give excellent support. Just like Judkins catheter was named by Judkins, RM guiding catheter (5 F, 6 F, JSM Korea) was invented and entitled by Rha SW.

Overall, the use of single guiding catheter for transradial bilateral coronary intervention is safe, feasible and highly successful in most patients. The previous study reported 96.6 % of success rate as efficient at right and left of coronary arteries by single IL 3.5 transradial guiding, and 96.0 % by Kimny guiding catheter [2, 22]. In all cases, manipulating the catheter from one side to the other (especial from left to the right coronary artery) should be performed with care in order to prevent tip dissections or inadvertent and uncontrolled deep intubation [3]. Taking IL as an example, the overall incidence of right coronary artery (RCA) dissection is about 0.48 % according to previously reported study [22]. Compared to Judkins Right catheter, IL can provide stronger support, and also might engage into RCA deeply and forcefully (Fig. 7.3), however on the other side, it also may cause dissection, especially when the ostia are atherosclerotic.

7.2.1 Single Transradial Diagnostic Catheters (4 F RM & CR)

Transradial diagnostic coronary angiography is increasing and becoming popular because it can be safely performed at out-patient base with shorter procedure time without significant major procedure associated complications. Though, the use of an isolated diagnostic catheter can certainly cause severe spasm of the vessel, trauma and discomfort.

We developed and developed two new 4 F diagnostic catheters called RM and CR to be used with left and right coronary arteries through a single catheter. Judkins catheter and the new catheters were tested for 504 patients enduring TRA. Post LCA angiogram, upon failure to reach RCA, 035 Terumo wire was reintroduced for assistance. The safety and success rate of the two catheters, in comparison to the success rate for three variable diagnostic catheters were evaluated.

From the 504 patients, in comparison to JL catheter with 63.7 % success rate, the RM and CR presented with 95.1 %, 86.6 % success rate, respectively.

When we compare the success rate among three catheters, RM & CR catheters presented a superior succession irrespective of wire assistance in comparison to JL catheter. RM demonstrated itself superior to CR catheter (Table 7.3). Major complications including intractable radial artery spasm, perforation or procedure associated bleeding complications were not present. The recent 4 F RM and CR

Table 7.2 Transradial guiding catheters for bilateral engagement

Catheters	Manufacturer	Illustration
Kimny	Boston scientific	
TIGER	Boston scientific	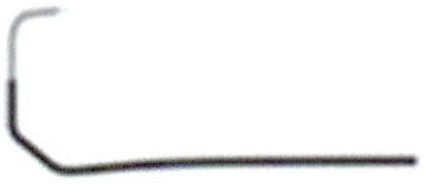
Barbeau	Cordis	
Radial brachial (RB)	Cordis	
Brachial left (Tilon)	Cordis	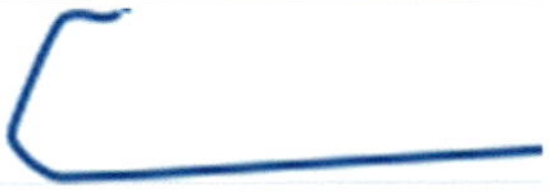
Radial Bi-lateral (RBL)	Cordis	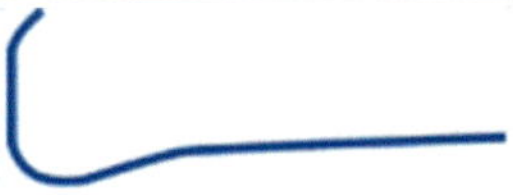
Ikari Left (IL)	Terumo	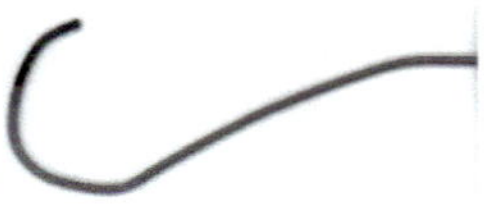
Radial curve	Boston scientific	
Radial Back-up	Boston scientific	
Amplatz left		
Multipurpose		
Judkins left		
Multi-Aortic curves (MAC)	Medtronic	
RM	JSM Korea	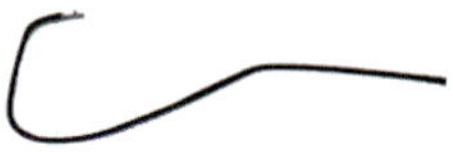

transradial diagnostic coronary angiography catheter achieved great success rate for LCA & RCA lacking of significant complications [23].

7.2.2 Single Transradial Guiding Catheter (5 F, 6 F RM Guiding Catheter)

The RM guiding performance was nicely evaluated in a series of acute myocardial infarction patients from a single TRI center. The viability of using guide catheter for non-culprit and culprit vessel angiography and intervention for primary PCI is currently unknown. A study with 242 STEMI patients undergoing primary PCI, 102 via trasfemoral approach and 109 via transradial approach by means of single guide catheter (6 F RMR_3.5).

Single guide catheter use present with 96.7 % success rate. The needle to balloon time were similar for conventional TFI and TRI groups (D28), while lower in single guiding TRI group (13.8 [TFI] and 14.1 [Conventional TRI] vs. 7.6 min, $P<0.001$; 89.5 [TFI] and 91.0 [Conventional TRI] vs.68.5 min, $P=0.008$, respectively), while amount of patients getting D28 time in 90 min was greater in the single guiding TRI group at 51.0 % for TFI and 49.5 % for Conventional TRI to 74.2 % ($P=0.023$). This concludes that primary trans radial PCI with single guide catheter is a viable and successful option which allows timely restoration of blood flow for infarct-related arteries [17].

Conclusion

TRA and TRI with single catheter was associated with lower costs, reduction of vascular complications such as radial artery spasm, dissection, occlusion, perforation, reduction of radiation exposure, reduction of procedure time, and reduction of contrast volume. TRA single guiding catheter such as RM guiding catheter and IL guiding catheter appears to be a preferred choice of guiding catheter for patients with multivessel diseases, particularly in the setting of primary PCI for STEMI patients with multivessel disease.

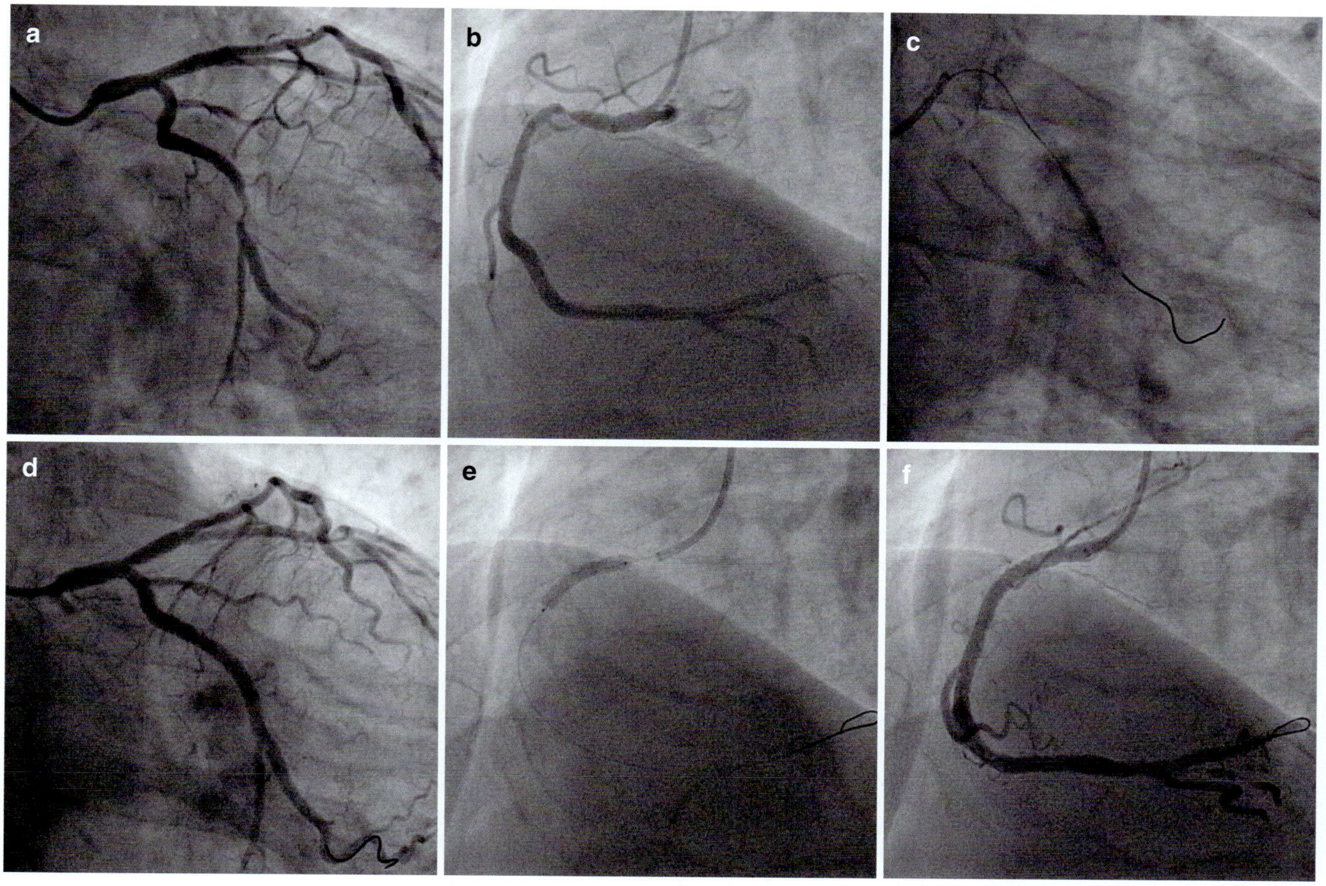

Fig. 7.3 The following figures illustrate the procedure of transradial bilateral coronary intervention with a single 6 F Ikari Left guiding catheter (Terumo). (**a**) angiogram of left coronary artery. (**b**) angiogram of right coronary artery. (**c**) stenting of circumflex lesion. (**d**) final angiogram of left coronary artery. (**e**) stenting of proximal right coronary lesion. (**f**) final angiogram of right coronary artery (Single transradial catheter performance from Korea University Guro Hospital)

Table 7.3 Independent and 035 Wire-Assisted Success Rate for engaging both LCA & RCA

	Overall success rate with/.ithout wire assist		
N (%)	No-wire assist	Wire assist	Total
RM catheter	121 (94.5)	14 (100)	135 (95.1)
CR catheter	94 (87.0)	3 (75.0)	97 (86.6)
JL catheter	149 (62.6)	7 (100)	156 (63.7)
RM vs JL	RM success rate compared with Judkins		
	RM	JL	p-value
	135 (95.1)	156 (63.7)	<0.001
CR vs JL	CR success rate compared with Judkins		
	CR	JL	p-value
	97 (86.6)	156 (63.7)	<0.001
RM vs CR	RM success rate compared with CR		
	RM	CR	p-value
	134 (95)	97 (86.6)	0.024

Rha et al. Presented at ACC 2010 meeting [23]

References

1. Sanmartin M, et al. Safety and efficacy of a multipurpose coronary angiography strategy using the transradial technique. J Invasive Cardiol. 2005;17(11):594–7.
2. Shibata Y, et al. New guiding catheter for transrad PTCA. Cathet Cardiovasc Diagn. 1998;43(3):344–51.
3. Kiemeneij F. Simultaneous transradial coronary angioplasty and contralateral coronary angiography with a single guide catheter for total coronary occlusions. J Invasive Cardiol. 2014;26(2):87–90.
4. Choussat R, et al. Vascular complications and clinical outcome after coronary angioplasty with platelet IIb/IIIa receptor blockade. Comparison of transradial vs transfemoral arterial access. Eur Heart J. 2000;21(8):662–7.
5. Amin AP, et al. Costs of transradial percutaneous coronary intervention. JACC Cardiovasc Interv. 2013;6(8):827–34.
6. Kim SM, et al. Novel diagnostic catheter specifically designed for both coronary arteries via the right transradial approach. A prospective, randomized trial of Tiger II vs. Judkins catheters. Int J Cardiovasc Imaging. 2006;22(3–4):295–303.
7. Mann 3rd JT, et al. Right radial access for PTCA: a prospective study demonstrates reduced complications and hospital charges. J Invasive Cardiol. 1996;8 Suppl D:40d–4.
8. Eleid MF, et al. Systematic use of transradial PCI in patients with ST-segment elevation myocardial infarction: a call to "arms". JACC Cardiovasc Interv. 2013;6(11):1145–8.
9. Ho HH, Jafary FH, Ong PJ. Radial artery spasm during transradial cardiac catheterization and percutaneous coronary intervention: incidence, predisposing factors, prevention, and management. Cardiovasc Revasc Med. 2012;13(3):193–5.
10. Ruiz-Salmeron RJ, et al. Radial artery spasm in transradial cardiac catheterization. Assessment of factors related to its occurrence, and of its consequences during follow-up. Rev Esp Cardiol (Engl Ed). 2005;58(5):504–11.
11. Saito S, et al. Influence of the ratio between radial artery inner diameter and sheath outer diameter on radial artery flow after transradial coronary intervention. Catheter Cardiovasc Interv. 1999; 46(2):173–8.
12. Brancati MF, et al. The occurrence of radial artery occlusion following catheterization. Expert Rev Cardiovasc Ther. 2012;10(10):1287–95.
13. Staniloae CS, et al. Histopathologic changes of the radial artery wall secondary to transradial catheterization. Vasc Health Risk Manag. 2009;5(3):527–32.
14. Yonetsu T, et al. Assessment of acute injuries and chronic intimal thickening of the radial artery after transradial coronary intervention by optical coherence tomography. Eur Heart J. 2010; 31(13):1608–15.
15. Uhlemann M, et al. The Leipzig prospective vascular ultrasound registry in radial artery catheterization: impact of sheath size on vascular complications. JACC Cardiovasc Interv. 2012;5(1): 36–43.
16. de Bucourt M, Teichgraber U. Digital ischemia and consecutive amputation after emergency transradial cardiac catheter examination. Cardiovasc Intervent Radiol. 2012;35(5):1242–4.
17. Moon KW, et al. Reducing needle-to-balloon time by using a single guiding catheter during transradial primary coronary intervention. J Interv Cardiol. 2012;25(4):330–6.
18. Louvard Y, et al. Coronary angiography through the radial or the femoral approach: the CARAFE study. Catheter Cardiovasc Interv. 2001;52(2):181–7.
19. Louvard Y, et al. Comparison of transradial and transfemoral approaches for coronary angiography and angioplasty in octogenarians (the OCTOPLUS study). Am J Cardiol. 2004;94(9): 1177–80.
20. Chow J, et al. Feasibility of transradial coronary angiography and intervention using a single Ikari left guiding catheter for ST elevation myocardial infarction. J Interv Cardiol. 2012;25(3): 235–44.
21. Pancholy SB, Bertrand OF, Patel T. Comparison of a priori versus provisional heparin therapy on radial artery occlusion after transradial coronary angiography and patent hemostasis (from the PHARAOH study). Am J Cardiol. 2012;110(2):173–6.
22. Youssef AA, et al. A single transradial guiding catheter for right and left coronary angiography and intervention. EuroIntervention. 2008;3(4):475–81.
23. Rha SW, Park JY, Poddar KL, Ramasamy S, Wang L, Choi BG, Kim JB, Shin SY, Choi CU, Lim HE, Kim JW, Kim EJ, Park CG, Seo HS, Oh DJ. Efficacy and safety of 4F new transradial diagnostic catheter; RM and CR catheter for engaging both left and right coronary arteries. ACC.10 59th Annual Scientific Session. USA. 14–16 Mar 2010. JACC p A214.

Selection and Manipulation of Guiding Catheter in Left Coronary Intervention via Radial Artery Approach

8

Qing Yang, Bin Nie, and Wei Liu

Abstract

Percutanous coronary intervention (PCI) via transradial approach could be more difficult in comparison to transfemoral approach due to frequently met anatomic route anomalies and limitations of Guiding Catheter GC size. Thus appropriate selection and skilful manipulation of GC is quintessential in increasing the operator's confidence to perform complex PCI procedures. The technique for manipulating GC via radial approach is different from that in femoral approach. In left coronary intervention, Extra Back up catheter (EBU) is the working catheter for most transradial interventionists. Mastering this catheter is important as it will shorten the procedure time, increase success rate and avoid complications. In this chapter, we outline the basic and advanced techniques of GCs in transradial left coronary intervention with a focus on EBU catheters.

8.1 The Advantages of EBU Catheter Over Judkins Catheter in Transradial Approach

Percutaneous coronary interventionists generally do not prefer using the Judkins left (JL) catheter for transradial intervention (TRI). The reason for this is that the JL catheter has a weak backup force when entering the left main coronary artery via the brachiocephalic artery as compared to entering the left main coronary artery directly from the aortic arch, as is the case for transfemoral intervention. For this reason, the extra backup catheter (EBU) is preferential when performing TRI. The EBU catheter has very strong backup force for TRI because it takes advantage of the reverse angle from the brachiocephalic artery, which was previously seen as a disadvantage of TRI, and uses it to create coaxial force against the aortic wall. The EBU also has a long, straight section just before the final curve and tip of the catheter to facilitate further coaxial force, as this section sits flat along the opposing side of the aortic wall allowing a greater surface area to be used for pushing against the force of the devices travelling though the catheter. In contrast, the JL catheter during transradial approach has a tendency not able to make a perfect coaxial aligment, as a result of 90 bend at its tip of the catheter to tap the ceiling of the left main artery instead of traveling through it. The JL catheter also comes to contact with a "point" instead of a "line" on contral lateral wall that is further up than the left coronary ostium, the passive back up force were restricted to second curve and further reduced at first curve, thus has a tendency to lose engagement when an interventional device is pushed through when doing TRI (Fig. 8.1).

Results of the first international transradial practice survey (Fig. 8.2) shows that standard extra back-up guiding

Q. Yang (✉) • B. Nie • W. Liu
Department of Cardiology, Beijing Anzhen Hospital, Capital Medical University, Beijing, China
e-mail: yq1963884@sina.com; Liuwei525@hotmail.com

Y. Zhou et al. (eds.), *Transradial Approach for Percutaneous Interventions*, DOI 10.1007/978-94-017-7350-8_8

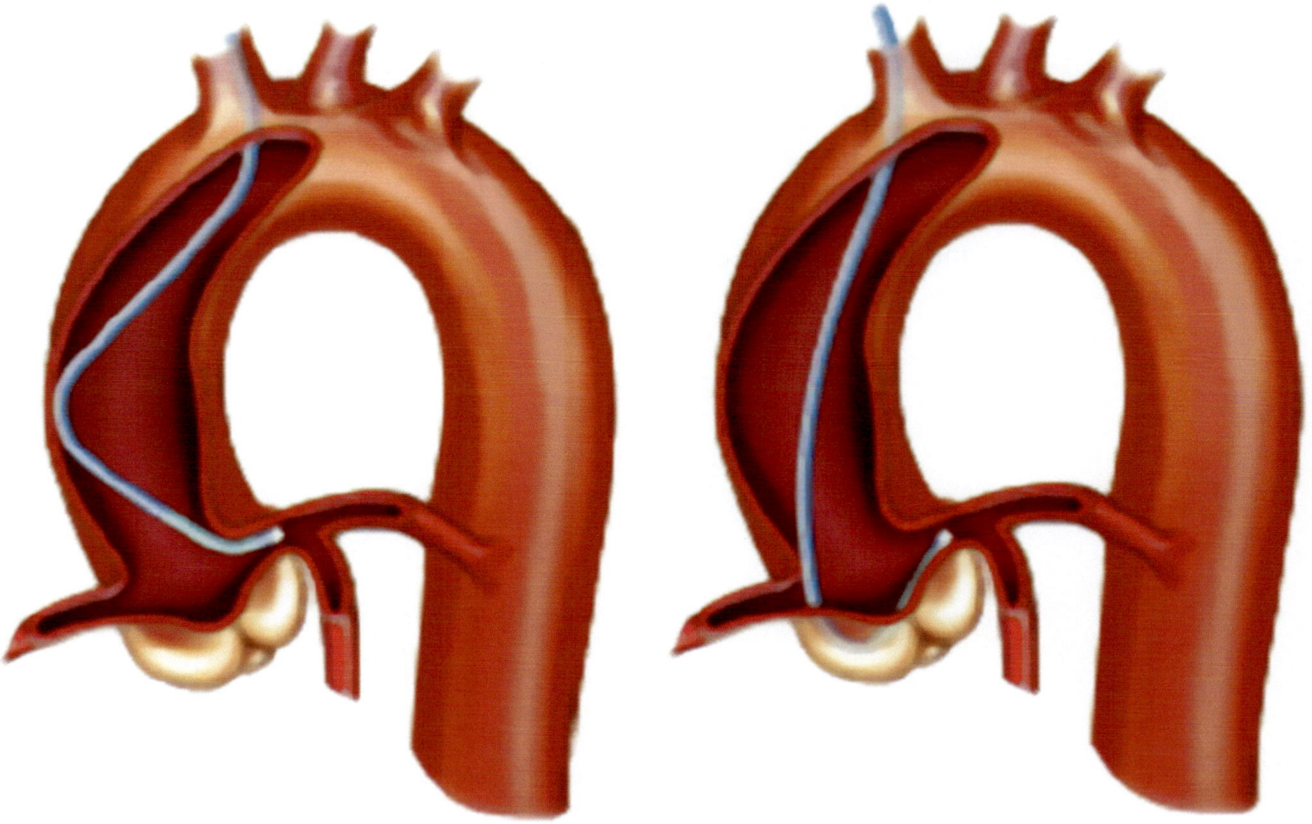

Fig. 8.1 Comparing the Judkin's catheter and EBU catheter in transradial intervention

catheters, especially EBU 3.5 (Medtronic, Minneapolis has been regarded as the first option in dealing with left coronary artery (LCA) intervenion compared to JL and other catheters [1].

The characteristics which make up an effective GC in TRI includes strong support, a large lumen, flexible manipulation and an atraumatic design. large majority of operators prefer to use 6-F catheter size. Adroit™ (Manufactured by Cordis comapany) has the largest inner lumen diameters among all the available 6Fr extra back-up shape GCs in the markets (Table 8.1). A large inner lumen design makes management of complex TRI possible including complex operations (Step balloon kissing, rotablator, etc) with a 6 F catheter, child in mother technique and better visibility especially when there are multiple devices within the GC. An ideal GC allows for a perfect balance between GC support and manoeuvrability allowing for easy engagement, easy adjustment, flexible changes of support mode, easy deep engagement, pressing against the contralateral aortic wall or aortic valve easily and a stable GC tip. The EBU catheter has these attributes which can be credited to the flexible manipulation of the primary curve yet strong coaxial support from the secondary curve.

8.2 The Size Selection of GC

Selection of the size of the GC is done according to the width of AO root (from the echocardiograph and coronary angiogram) and the orientation of the LCA. When the AO width is <3.0 cm, 3.0–3.5 cm and >3.5 cm the EBU size used is 3.0, 3.5 and ≥3.75 respectively. If the LM is oriented downwards, the EBU should be a half size larger (G1, blue). If the LM is oriented upwards the EBU should be half a size smaller G3, (yellow), in comparison to when the LM is horizontal (G2, green) (Fig. 8.3).

The other reason for using a catheter that is half a size larger is to increase back up for complex coronary lesions, including diffused lesions, Angulated lesions, left radial artery approach and LCX lesions.

8.3 Manipulation of EBU Catheter

8.3.1 Manipulation Method of EBU Catheter in Normal Conditions

The best view to engage an EBU catheter is LAO 45 or LAO caudal view. The basic methods to engage the EBU GC to LM ostium is the "rotating and pulling" or "Advancing and

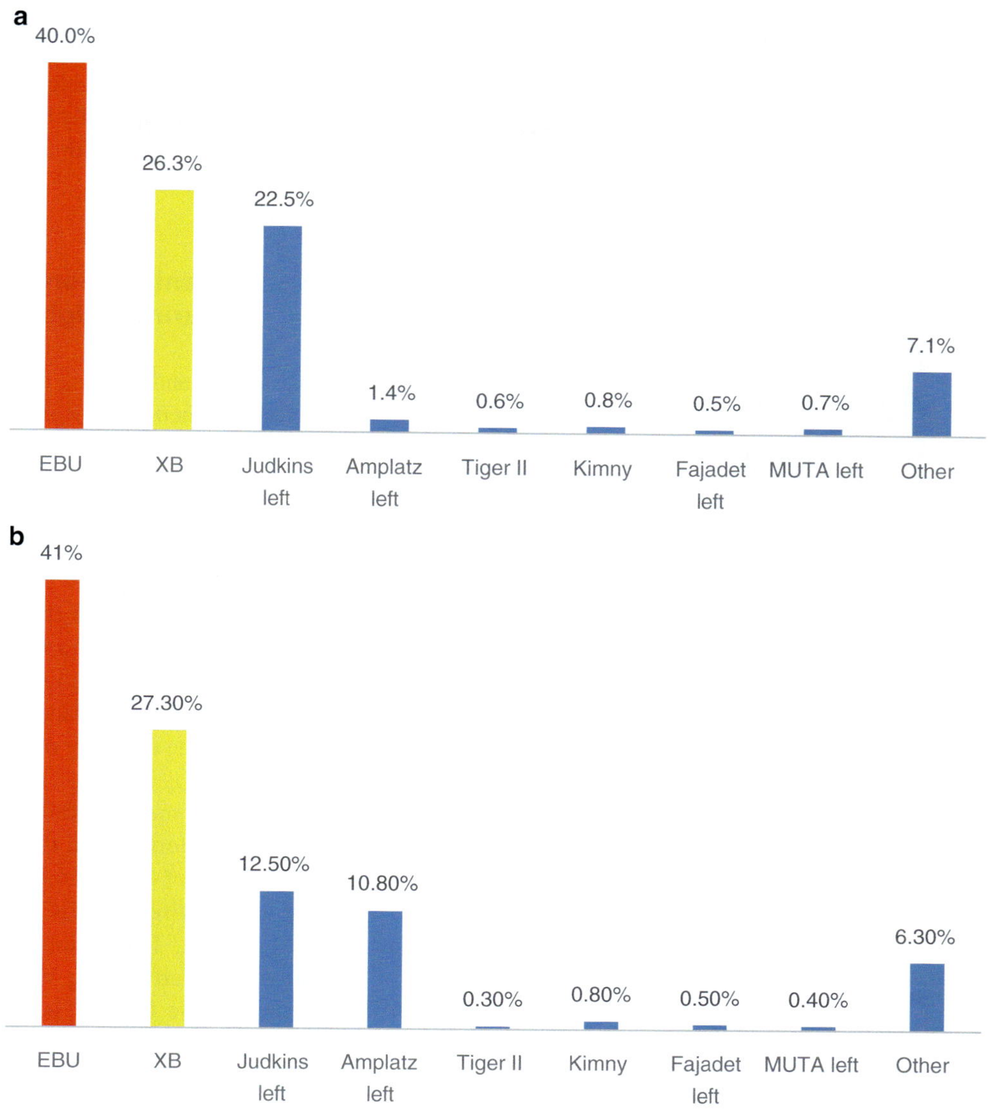

Fig. 8.2 (**a**) Preferred guiding catheter for left descending artery via transradial approach. (**b**) Preferred guiding catheter for left circumflex artery via transradial approach

Table 8.1 The inner lumen diameter of multiple EBU shape guiding catheter

	Vista brite tip Inner diameter	Launcer Inner diameter	Adroit Inner diameters
Manufacture	Cordis	Medtronic	Cordis
5 F	0.056″	0.058″	–
6 F	0.070″	0.071″	0.072″
7 F	0.078″	0.081″	–

forming U shape". However, due to a tortuous subclavian artery and widened AO root, a high take off or downward orientation of the LM ostium is not unfrequently met. Other methods of engaging the EBU catheter should be tried.

Rotating and pulling

This is the most common method to engage the EBU catheter to LM ostium. It involves the following steps. First step : Placing the guide wire into the aortic sinus under the fluoroscopy guidance. The wire should be curved just above the level of the sinotubular ridge so that it is located in the posterior sinus (Fig. 8.4a). Second step: While advancing the EBU catheter into the ascending aorta, manipulate it in a clockwise manoeuvre so that the tip of GC is directed to the left side (Fig. 8.4b). In the case of a tortuous brachiocephalic trunk, it is necessary to ask the patient to take a deep breath and hold it, which can facilitate the advancement of the EBU. After the EBU is shaped successfully in the posterior sinus, do not retract the wire from the GC until the air is removed.

Third step Pull it and rotate in a clockwise fashion if necessary. Generally, the GC jumps from posterior sinus to left sinus (Fig. 8.4b, c). Fourth step: Continue to withdraw the EBU to the level of the ostium of LCA, and rotate it with

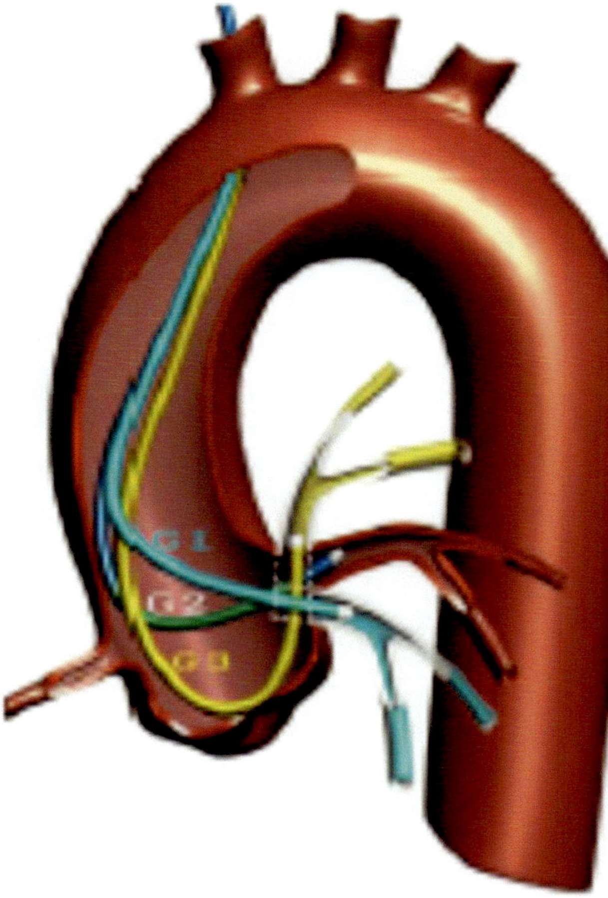

Fig. 8.3 Selection of size of the guiding catheter according to width of aortic root and orientation of left main

clockwise or anticlockwise torque until the catheter intubates the LM ostium (Fig. 8.4d).

Advancing and forming U shape

After the EBU is shaped in the posterior sinus, retract the wire till the secondary curve, then pull the GC softly and advance it into the left sinus (Fig. 8.5a). Instead of pulling the catheter up, aided by the force from the aortic sinus and opposite aortic wall, advance the GC until the tip reaches the level of the ostium of LCA. Ensure the GC maintains appropriate tension in case of it being bent backwards (Fig. 8.5b). When the tip of the EBU reaches the level of the ostium of LCA, rotate the catheter clockwise or anticlockwise to get close to the ostium of LCA (Fig. 8.5c). Once the GC tip is close to the ostium of LCA, do not remove the exchanged guidewire from GC until a PTCA guidewire is advanced into the LCA to keep the GC stabilized (Fig. 8.5d). The coaxial alignments of a GC to the LM ostium could be further obtained with the help of a PTCA guidewire or balloon catheter (Fig. 8.5d). While adjusting GC coaxiality, caution should be paid to avoid LM injury due to deep engagement (Fig. 8.5e). By siting in the aortic sinus, the guide can be kept stable without entering the LM ostium, which will be especially useful for left main ostial leiosns or LM body lesions with a short LM (see left main ostial lesions).

8.3.2 Manipulation Method of EBU Catheter During a High Takeoff

Advancing and forming a U shape of EBU catheter is most effective when deals with a high take off left main ostium (See Fig. 8.5).

For an unfolded aorta and high take off LM ostium, EBU catheter tends to being bent up by rotating and pulling maneuver and result in cannulation failure (Fig. 8.5a). A 0.035″ J type stiff wire can be used to effectively modulate the opening degrees of the GC tip (Fig. 8.5b) so that the tip of the catheter could go into the left sinus; The wire is then retracted back and kept in the GC ; by withdrawing and rotating the catheter, simultaneously accommodating the patient's breathing, the coronary ostium is finally engaged (Figs. 8.5c and 8.6).

If above methods fails, the horizontal rotation method could be attempted. In this method the tip of GC is at the same level of the LM ostium, while the EBU is kept open by a stiff wire. The GC is then rotated to search for the LM ostium. If coaxiality is not satisfactory, it can be solved by advancing a PTCA wire into the coronary artery, while the GC is manipulated to keep it co-axial (Fig. 8.7).

A tortuous brachiocephalic trunk with a wide aortic root and downward orientation of a high take-off coronary artery is the most difficult condition for GC engagement, especially when combined with lusoria. The operator should change the access route timely according to his or her own experience and the complexity of the coronary lesion.

8.3.3 Push Test to Confirm the Stability of Guiding Position

In PCI technique, experienced physicians test the stability and supporting force of the GC in the coronary ostia by using the push test (a). This is done by gently pushing the GC forward into the coronary ostia. If it further intubates the coronary artery, it means that the GC has good stability and supporting force (b) otherwise, if the GC prolapses into the aorta, poor stability and inadequate force is indicated (c) (Fig. 8.8).

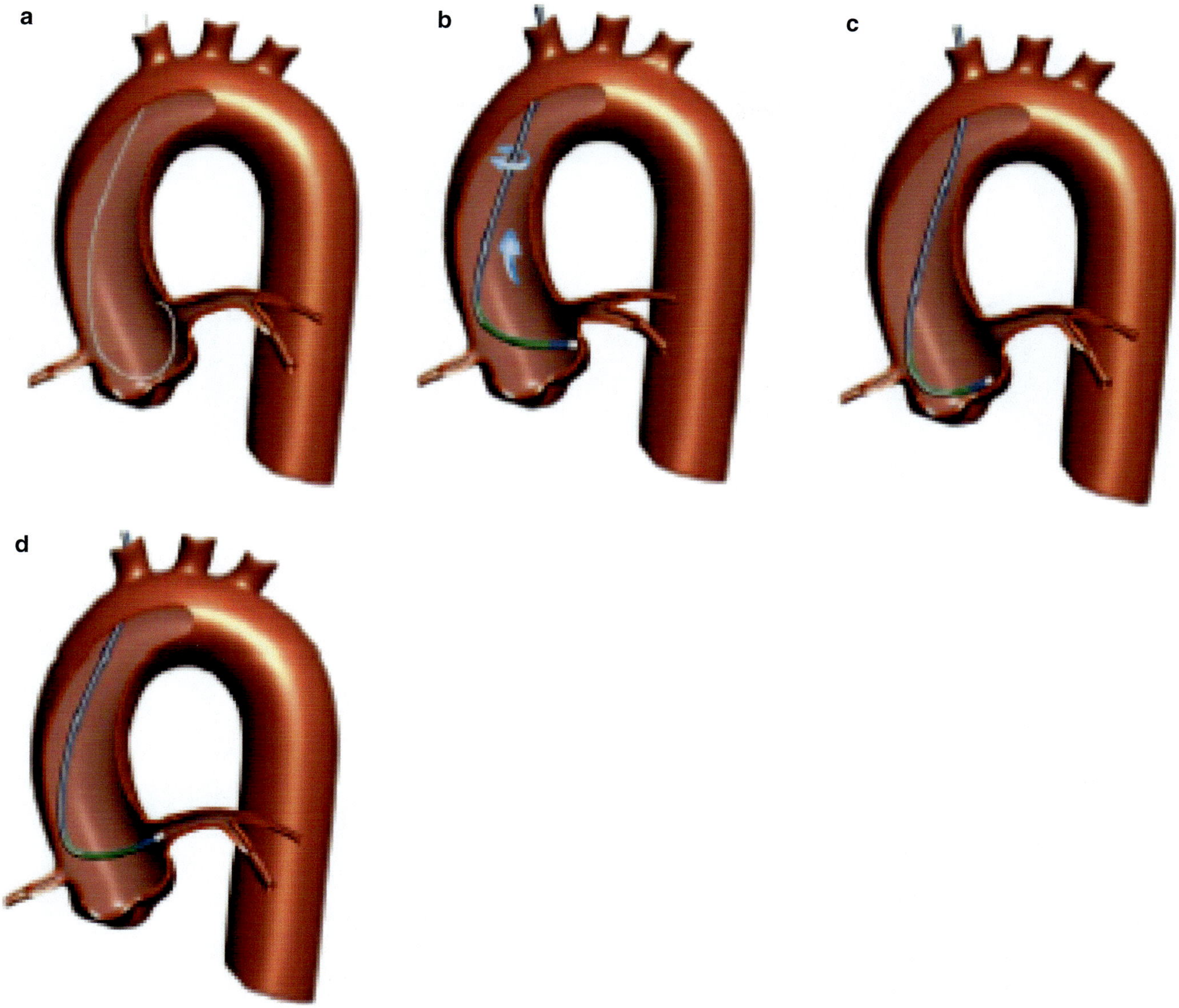

Fig. 8.4 Engaging the EBU by rotating and pulling (Image provided courtesy of Medtronic Inc. © Medtronic Inc. All rights reserved)

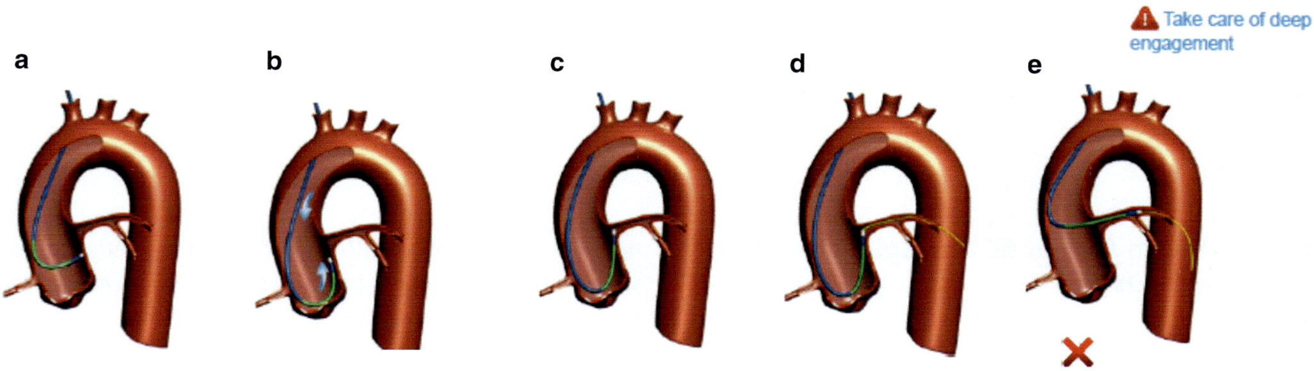

Fig. 8.5 Engaging EBU by advancing and forming U shape (Image provided courtesy of Medtronic Inc. © Medtronic Inc. All rights reserved)

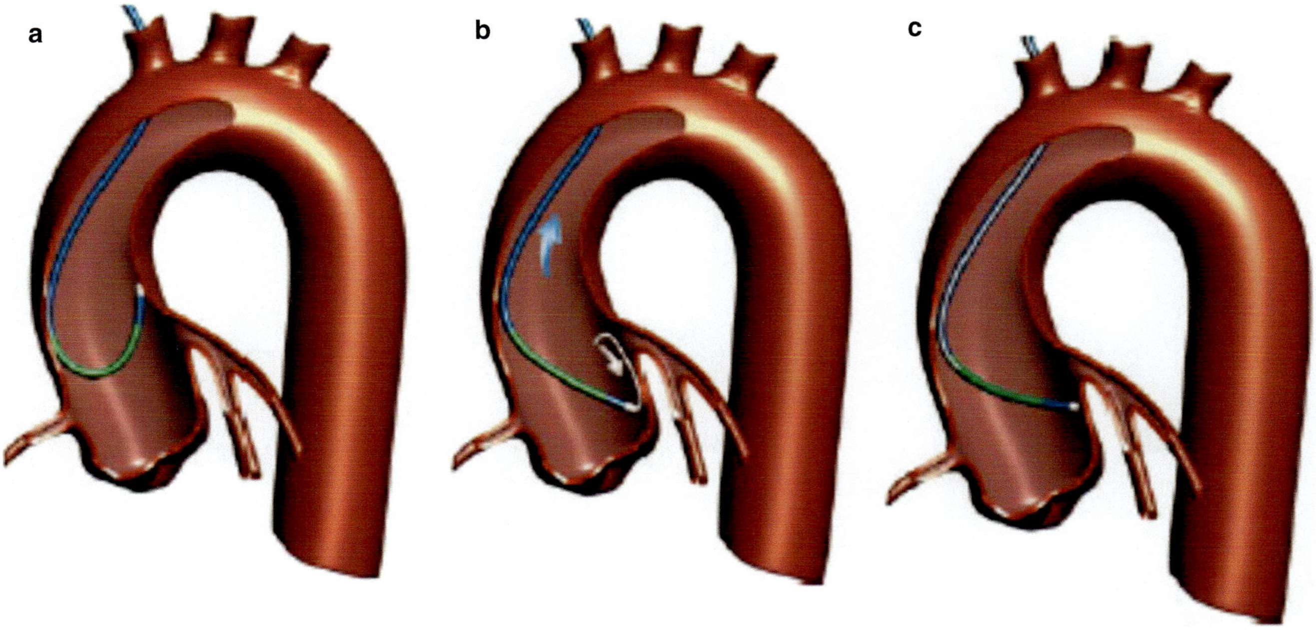

Fig. 8.6 Engaging EBU by rotating and pulling with the support of stiff wire for high take off LCA (Image provided courtesy of Medtronic Inc. © Medtronic Inc. All rights reserved)

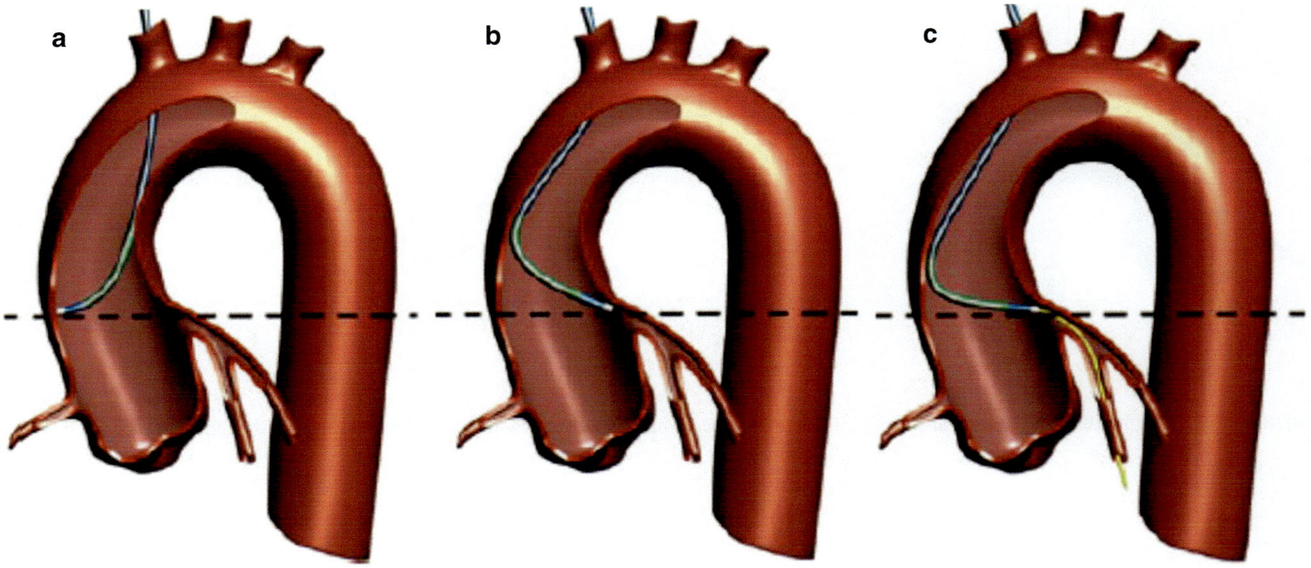

Fig. 8.7 Engaging EBU by horizontal rotation for high take off LCA (Image provided courtesy of Medtronic Inc. © Medtronic Inc. All rights reserved)

8.3.4 How to Advoid GC Damaging the Left Main Ostium

When perfoming transradial approach, it is not uncommon to see that the long tipped EBU GC deeply engages into the LCA and causes left main injury espically when the LM orients downwards. Furthermore, forceful injection of contrast tends to cause additional damage. Thus the pressure waves should be closely monitored (Fig. 8.7). Once coronary dissection has occurred, avoid GC disengagement from LCA too fast in order not to lose the positioning. The operator should advance the guidewire into the coronary artery distally and deal with the complication immediately (Fig. 8.9).

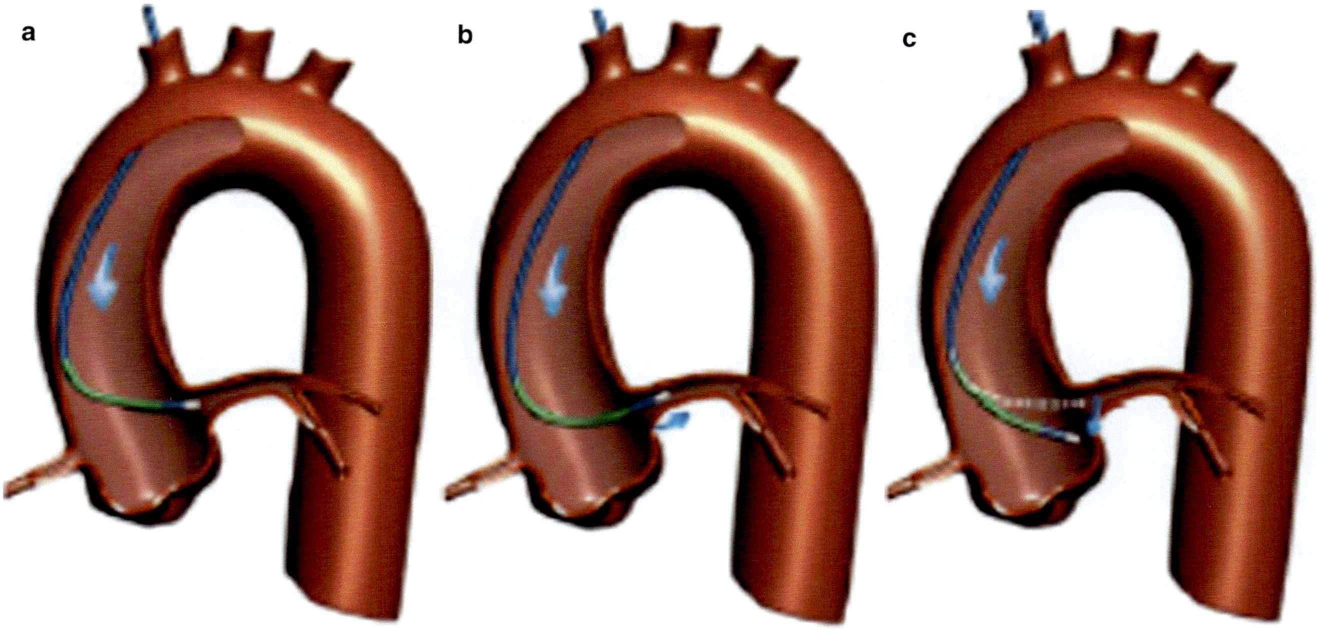

Fig. 8.8 Push test to confirm the stability of guiding position (Image provided courtesy of Medtronic Inc. © Medtronic Inc. All rights reserved)

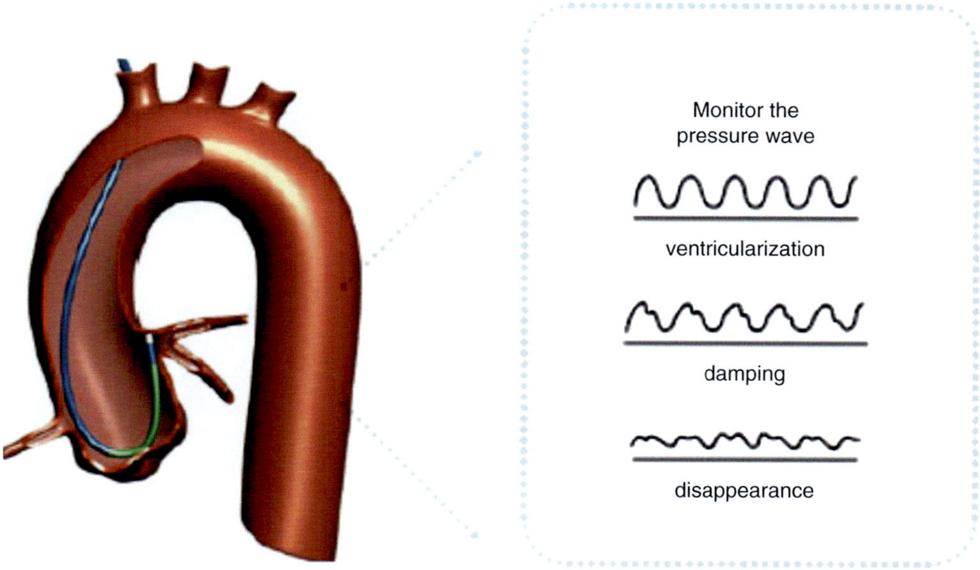

Fig. 8.9 Avoid GC damaging the left main ostium by closely monitoring the pressure wave ventricularization : fall of diastolic pressure; damping fall of both diastolic and systolic pressure (Image provided courtesy of Medtronic Inc. © Medtronic Inc. All rights reserved)

8.3.5 Avoid Deep Intubation of EBU Catheter

When adopting the U shape in AO left sinus, especially in the case of a tortuous brachiocephalic artery, the accumulated tension can be suddenly released while withdrawing the catheter hastily to improve the coaxial alignment. This could lead to the catheter deeply intubating into the LM and causing LM injury (Fig. 8.10a, b). While pulling out the PTCA instruments (balloon, stent), the GC tip can also be sucked into the coronary artery deeply. The operator should be especially cautious in these conditions. It is not necessary to pursue excessive coaxality when guiding support is enough.

8.3.6 Disengagement of GC From LCA

The disengagement of the catheter from the LCA can occur during the following conditions:

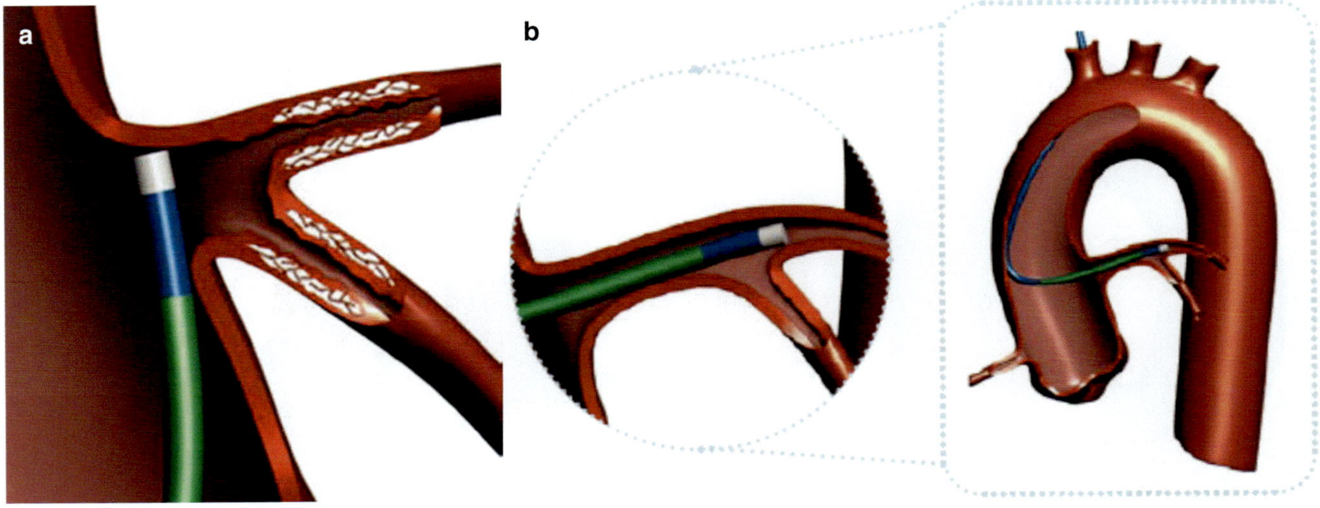

Fig. 8.10 Deep intubation of EBU catheter (Image provided courtesy of Medtronic Inc. © Medtronic Inc. All rights reserved)

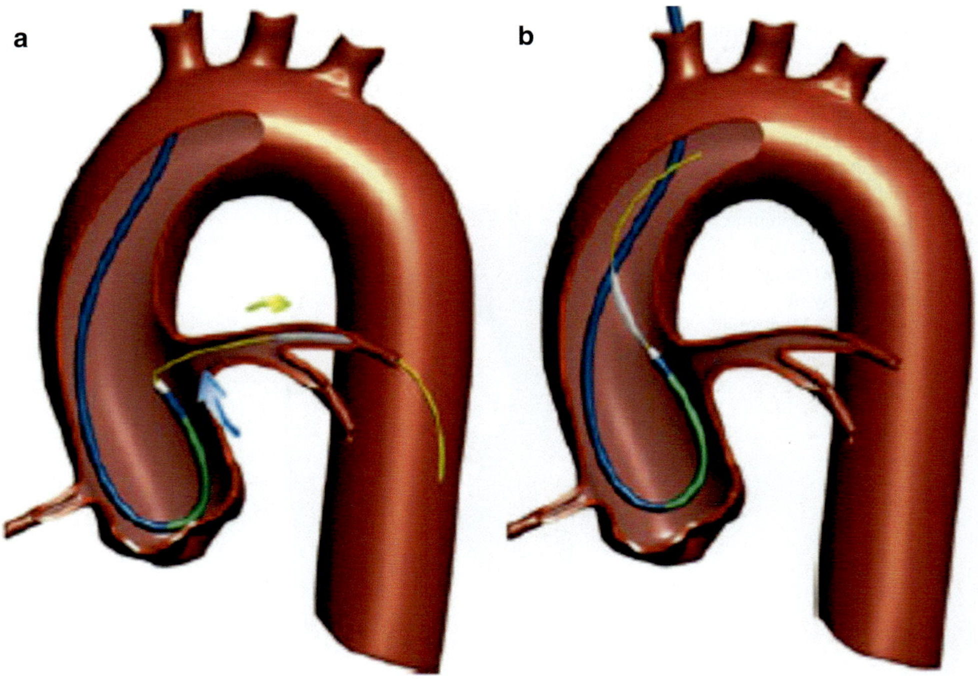

Fig. 8.11 EBC catheter disengaged from the LM when advancing the instruments (balloon, guidewire, stent) fast (Image provided courtesy of Medtronic Inc. © Medtronic Inc. All rights reserved)

1. Instruments (Balloon, Guide wire, stent, etc.) are advanced too fast, so the counterforce leads to catheter disengagement (Fig. 8.9).
2. GC might disengage in conditions when the GC is of small size, or due to poor backup, anatomic variations and a dilated aorta.
3. It is very necessary for the operator to balance the role of active and passive back-up of the GC in dealing with complex lesions, such as diffuse lesions, calcified lesions and bifurcation lesions in which the GC could dislodge from the coronary artery when instruments try to cross the struts in bifurcation lesions (Fig. 8.11).

8.4 Trouble Shooting and Advanced Techniques

Conventional interventional techniques and manoeuvers can sometimes literally lead to a dead end. These trouble shooting and advanced techniques allow for a greater range of manoeuvers in an interventionists arsenal.

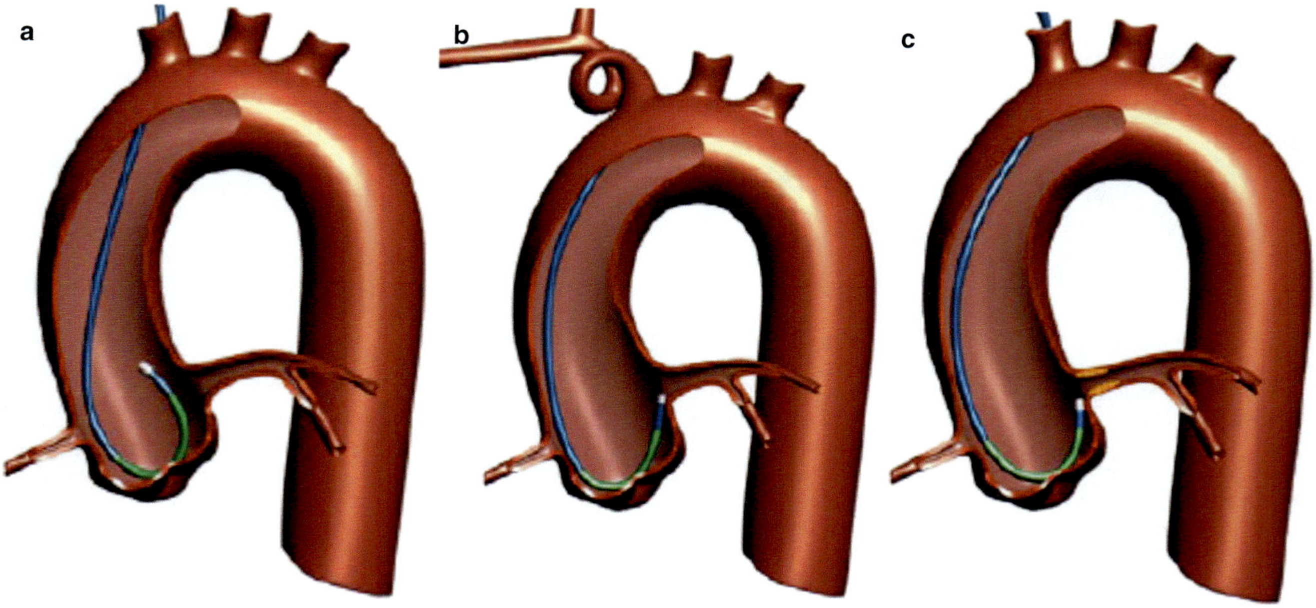

Fig. 8.12 Conditions while the wire shifting technique could be used to improve the EBU engagement (Image provided courtesy of Medtronic Inc. © Medtronic Inc. All rights reserved)

Wire shifting technique In the following circumstances, the wire shifting technique could be indicated

1. While a GC is smaller in size, the catheter tends to be bent up, resulting in the loss of engagement from the LM ostium (Fig. 8.12a),
2. During the case of an extremely tortuous aortic arch, if the support 0.035 angiographic wire is withdrawn too early, the torque force can be released and transmitted resulting in disengagement of the GC from the ostium (Fig. 8.12b).
3. While dealing with an ostial lesion, the GC needs to be stabilized without deep engagement into the LM (Fig. 8.12c).

The wire shifting technique can work around these problems. The GC is engaged into the LM ostium while keeping the stiff wire, such as a 0.035 J curve or glide wire in the guiding catheter, which allows an increase in the overall rigidity of the GC. The interventionist might advance a PTCA wire into either the LCX or LAD, then further adjust the stability of the GC by engaging the GC into the LM artery to improve coaxility or disengaging the GC to avoid deep intubation. Then the stiff 0.035 J curve wire being removed. This wire shift technique can prevent damage to the LM ostium, and allow for better coaxial force of the GC.

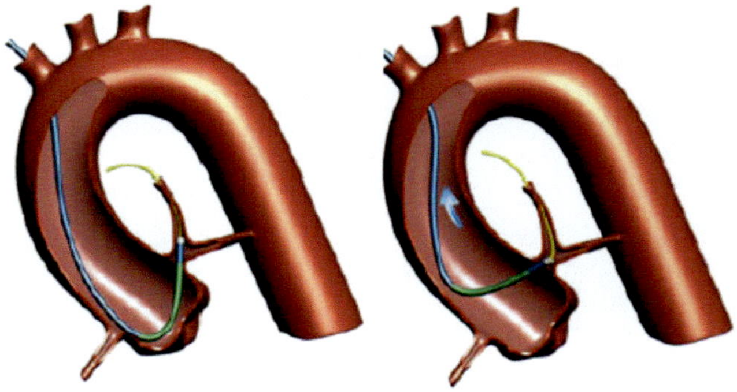

Fig. 8.13 Adjusting GC from LAD to LCX (Image provided courtesy of Medtronic Inc. © Medtronic Inc. All rights reserved)

Dealing with unwanted super-selection Sometimes, when the LM artery is shorter in length, the GC tends to enter the unwanted branches of the LM artery. A PTCA wire can be used to select a coronary artery first to stabilize the catheter. To select the LCX from LAD, a slide back movement and soft clockwise rotation of the GC is required (Fig. 8.13), while selection of the LAD from LCX requires an advance movement and soft counter-clock wise rotation.(Fig. 8.14) then the guidewire can be retracted and advanced into the intented artery.

The jailed wire and balloon anchor technique These are also useful manoeuvres when there is not adequate back up, despite the correct usage of the guiding catheter. In the jailed wire technique, after a stent is placed, the jailed wire under the stent retained temporarily, a second wire is then manoeuvred into the branch through the stent structs. This allows for an increase in back up force when advancing the balloon catheter through the 2nd guidewire (Fig. 8.15). The balloon anchor

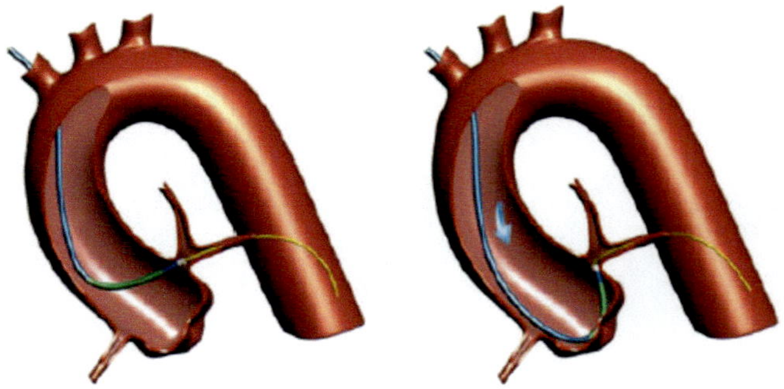

Fig. 8.14 Adjusting the GC from LCX to LAD (Image provided courtesy of Medtronic Inc. © Medtronic Inc. All rights reserved)

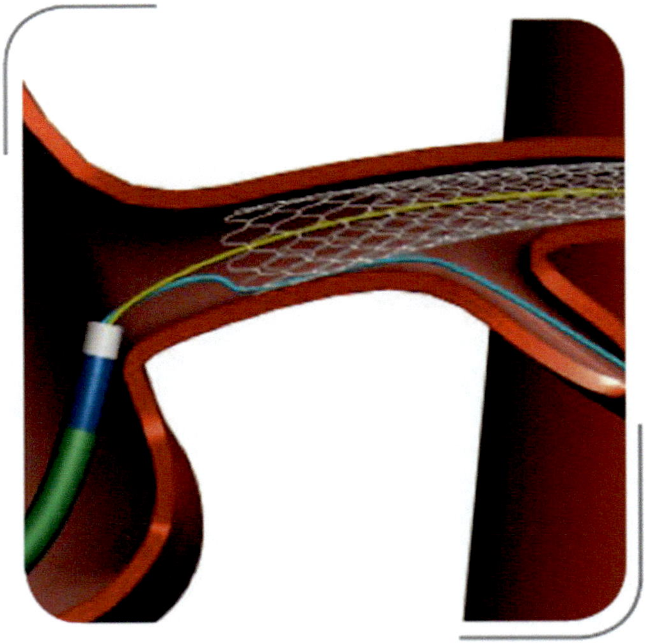

Fig. 8.15 Jailed wire technique (Image provided courtesy of Medtronic Inc. © Medtronic Inc. All rights reserved)

technique is very similar, in which by using a balloon inflated with low pressure at main branch, thus facilitates the balloon catheter crossing the structs with extra back up force (Fig. 8.16).

8.5 Tips for Managing the GC in LM Lesion

When dealing with LM ostial lesions, a short-tipped JL GC is usually used in clinical practice. However, when coupled with high take-off of the LCA and/or a dilated aorta, an EBU catheter would be more effective in engaging the target

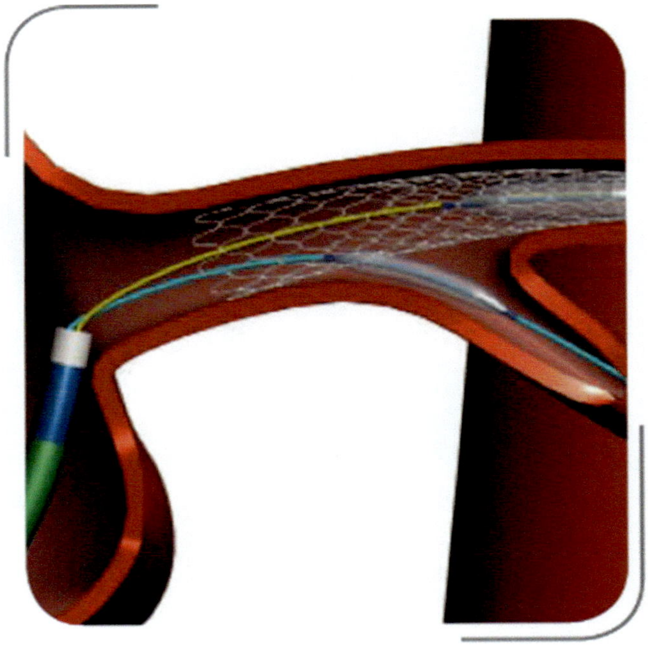

Fig. 8.16 Balloon anchor technique (Image provided courtesy of Medtronic Inc. © Medtronic Inc. All rights reserved)

artery. By using a long tipped GC, the interventionist runs the risk of damaging the ostium, obstructing LM blood flow, influencing the precise position of the stent and causing damage to the stent resulting in stent longitude deformation. So a special technique is required to disengage the GC readily.

8.5.1 Techniques in LM Ostial Lesions

Advancing and forming U shape method The operator should adjust the GC tension and torque force while advancing and forming EBU catheter to U shape in the left sinus. The wire shifting technique (mentioned earlier) could be used. These measures could maintain appropriate GC tension, prevent deep engagement and stabilize the guide catheter. After the guidewire has entered the coronary artery, loosen the Y valve connector and retreat the GC from LM ostium along the guidewire (Fig. 8.17). The balloon is then advanced to the ostium and pre-dilated fully. When implanting a stent, keep the tip of the GC stable and at this point ask the patient to hold their breath, which minimizes any respiratory interference. Using multiple angles to position the stent precisely, a LAO30 + CRA30 should be used. If difficulty is met in positioning the stent while dealing with ostial lesions, it is advisable to advance and retreat the GC and stent system in the whole system, or use an additional wire in the aorta (Fig. 8.16). While the stent is positioned well, keep the GC stabilized, inflate the stent at low pressure, then withdrawing the GC tip outside the ostium, the proximal stent is then dilated with stent

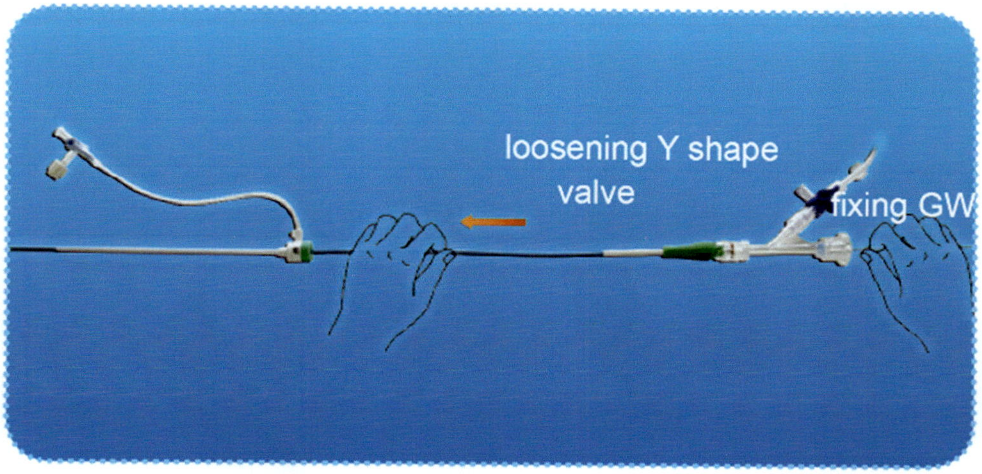

Fig. 8.17 Loosening the Y-shaped valve allows the guiding catheter manipulated while the guide wire being fixed (Image provided courtesy of Medtronic Inc. © Medtronic Inc. All rights reserved)

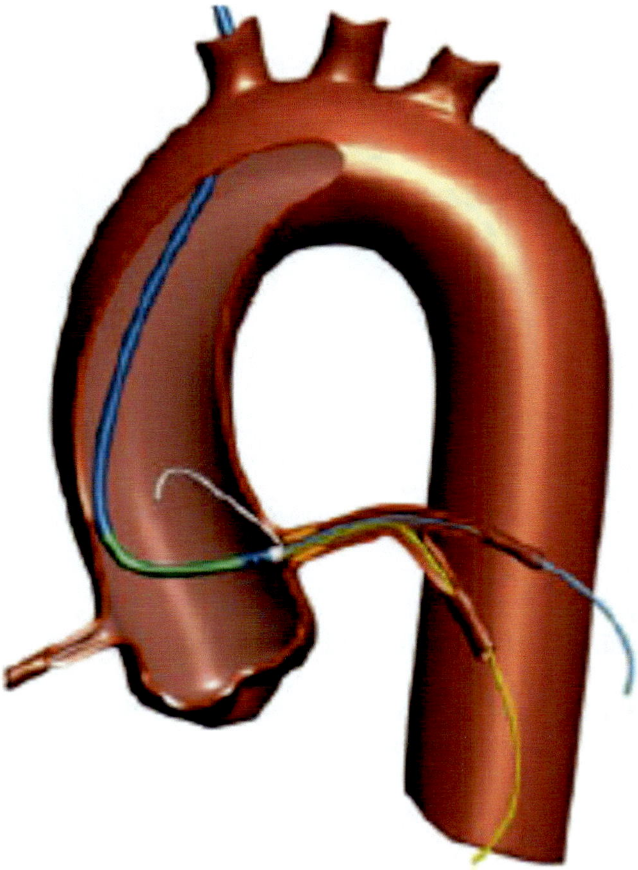

Fig. 8.18 Keep a wire in aorta to assist stent position (Image provided courtesy of Medtronic Inc. © Medtronic Inc. All rights reserved)

balloon at higher pressure. Following stent deployment and postdilation, it is suggested to slide the BC into the GC, which could assist GC coaxality with the LCA and prevent the damage and longitudinal deformation of the stent (Figs. 8.17, 8.18, 8.19, and 8.20).

8.5.2 LM Body Lesion

The GC is engaged in the LCA with the view from LAO 45 or spider view. The advancing and forming U shape method is then implemented as it is effective in stabilizing the GC tip. Find a workhorse view to expose the LM body lesion completely as it is important in GC tip stabilization. Occasionally the patient is asked to hold their breath, as it minimizes any respiratory interference. The GC tension is released by sliding it out along the BC after the stent is deployed and post-dilation is complete. As the balloon is retreated near the GC tip, the GC is advanced along the BC, obtaining perfect coaxial force with the LM.

8.5.3 LM Bifurcation Lesion

When dealing with LM bifurcation lesions with a normal length of the LM, operators should attempt to use the rotating and pulling method or the advancing and forming U shape method to place the GC in place. Following placement of the GC, the recommended projections include LAO45 + CAU30 or AP + CAU30. If the LM ostium needs to be covered, a stent could be positioned precisely under the view of LAO30 + CRA30. Increasing active back-up of the GC is often needed in complex conditions, such as two stent strategy, angulated lesion and diffused lesion. The common method to increase back-up is to advance the GC further, forming a U shape in the sinus bottom to add GC back-up force or advance the GC tip further into the vessel in order to obtain active-back force, moreover, an αloop shape can provide more support (Fig. 8.21).

When the LM is short in length, the EBU can easily super-select the LAD or the LCX. It would be more dangerous if the LM is too small or has serious ostial lesions. The procedure in the management of GC super-seletion of LCX is as

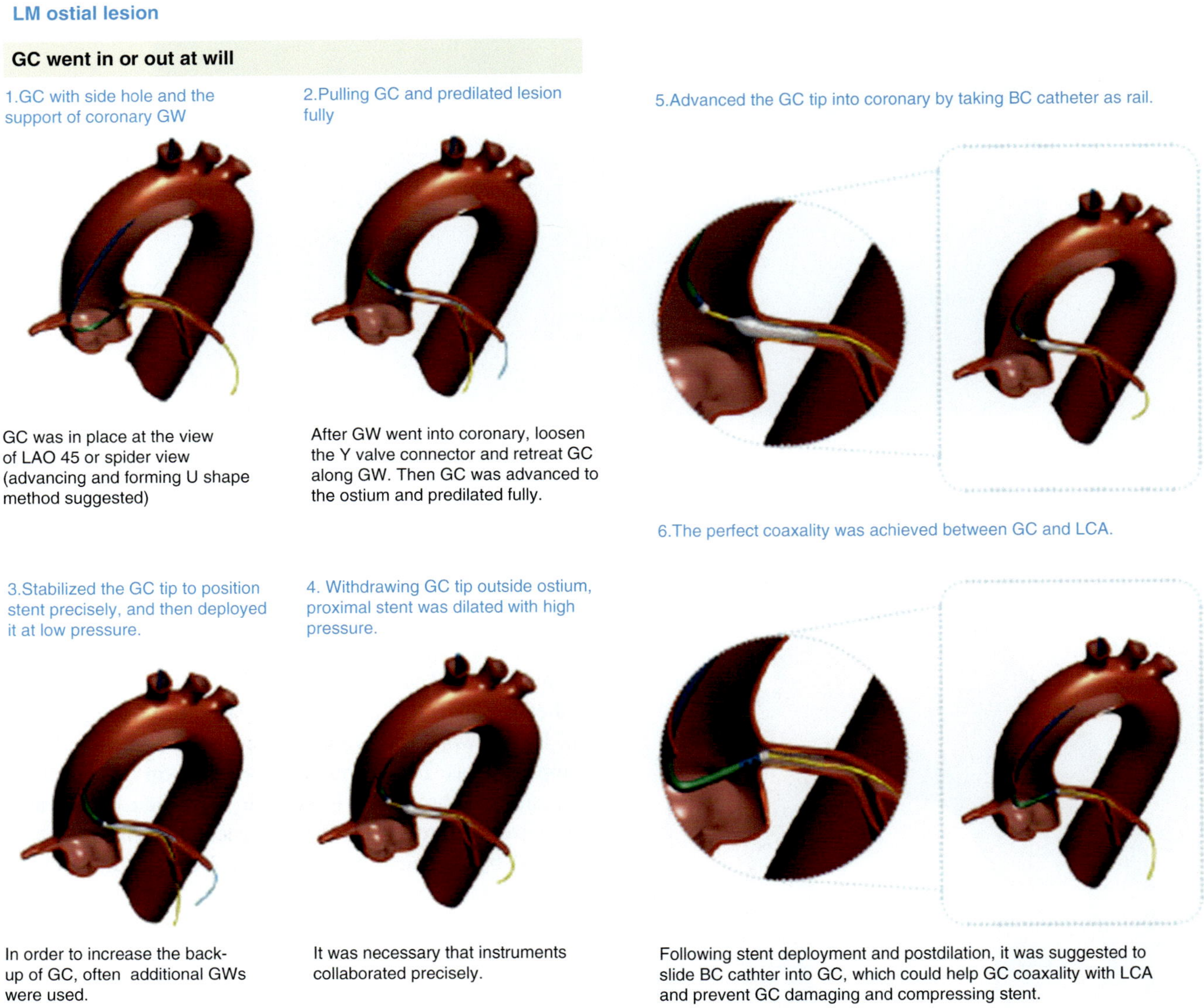

Fig. 8.19 Manipulating EBU catheter when dealing with LM ostial lesion (Image provided courtesy of Medtronic Inc. © Medtronic Inc. All rights reserved)

following method : First: Retreat the GC till its tip is positioned proximal to the LM bifurcation. Advance the GC slowly, gently adding an anti-clockwise rotation. Usually the GC can be redirected into the LAD smoothly (Fig. 8.22a). Second : Advance a PTCA guidewire into the LCX. In most cases, the GC can be redirected to LAD after advancing it slowly. When GC super-selection is too deep or the GC moves forward instead of being redirected to the LAD, the operator should pull the GC back and repeat the aforementioned technique and the operator must observe the tip movement (Fig. 8.22b).Third: Change an EBU catheter with smaller size (such as EBU 3.0).

8.6 Other Dedicated Transradial GC

8.6.1 Ikari Guiding Catheter: Especially Designed for TRI

Ikari is a new guide catheter for transradial intervention (TRI) that produces stronger back-up force by utilizing an unfavourable angle between the subclavian and brachiocephalic arteries. The Ikari left (L) GC was invented in 1995, first applied to PCI in 1996, and commercially available in 2002. The Ikari L catheter has three modifications from the Judkins L: (1) a shorter length between the third and the

Fig. 8.20 Manipulating EBU catheter when dealing with LM body lesion (Image provided courtesy of Medtronic Inc. © Medtronic Inc. All rights reserved)

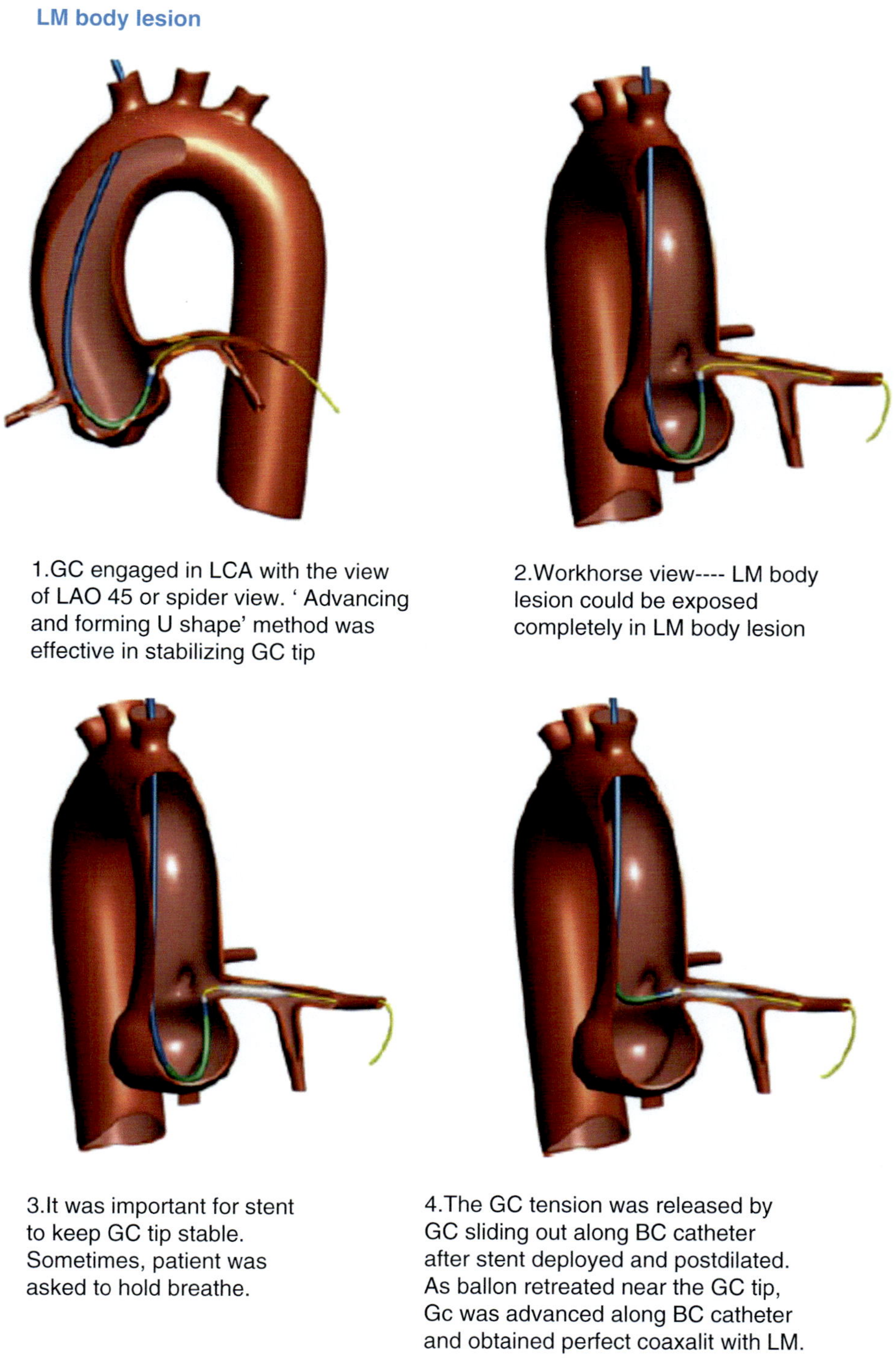

fourth angles, (2) longer length between the second and the first angles, and (3) the new first angle is added to fit the brachiocephalic artery [2].The Ikari L is essentially a modified version of the Judkins L catheter for TRI. Due to the modifications, the backup force of the Ikari L is stronger than the Judkins L in TRI, because the angle between the Ikari L catheter and the reverse side of the aorta is bigger than with the Judkins L. The Ikari L in TRI is actually stronger than the Judkins L in TFI.

Occasionally, a stronger backup force is necessary for an extremely complex lesion. There is an easy method of manipulation to increase backup force in the Ikari L. This technique is as easy as pushing the GC up to the reverse side angle of 90°. At this point, the backup force becomes much more significant. Deep engagement of the Judkins L also generates greater backup force; however, this can sometimes damage the left main. However, the power position with the Ikari L is safe, because the distal tip is never inserted deeply due to its differentiated design. To date, no left main dissections with Ikari L have been reported (Fig. 8.23).

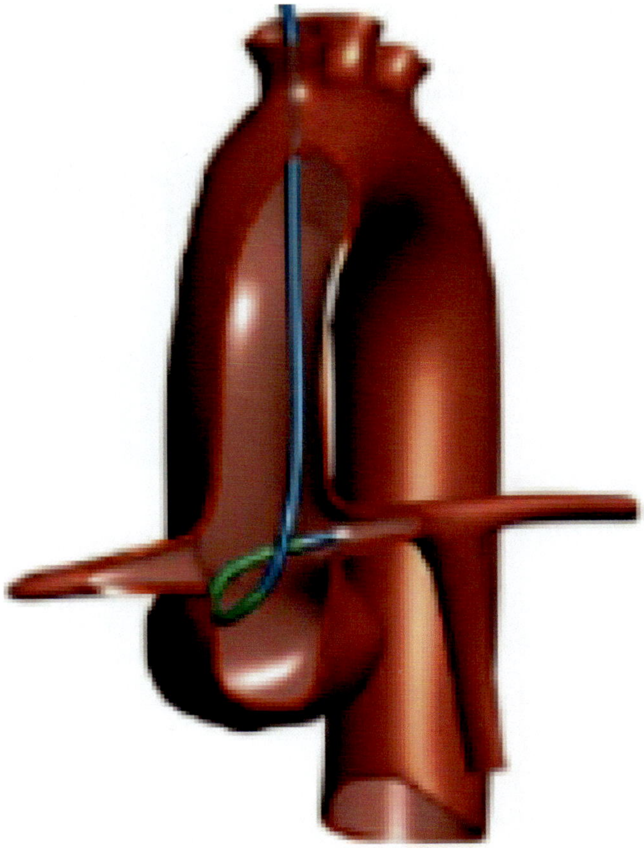

Fig. 8.21 EBU catheter can form an α loop to obtain active back up (Image provided courtesy of Medtronic Inc. © Medtronic Inc. All rights reserved)

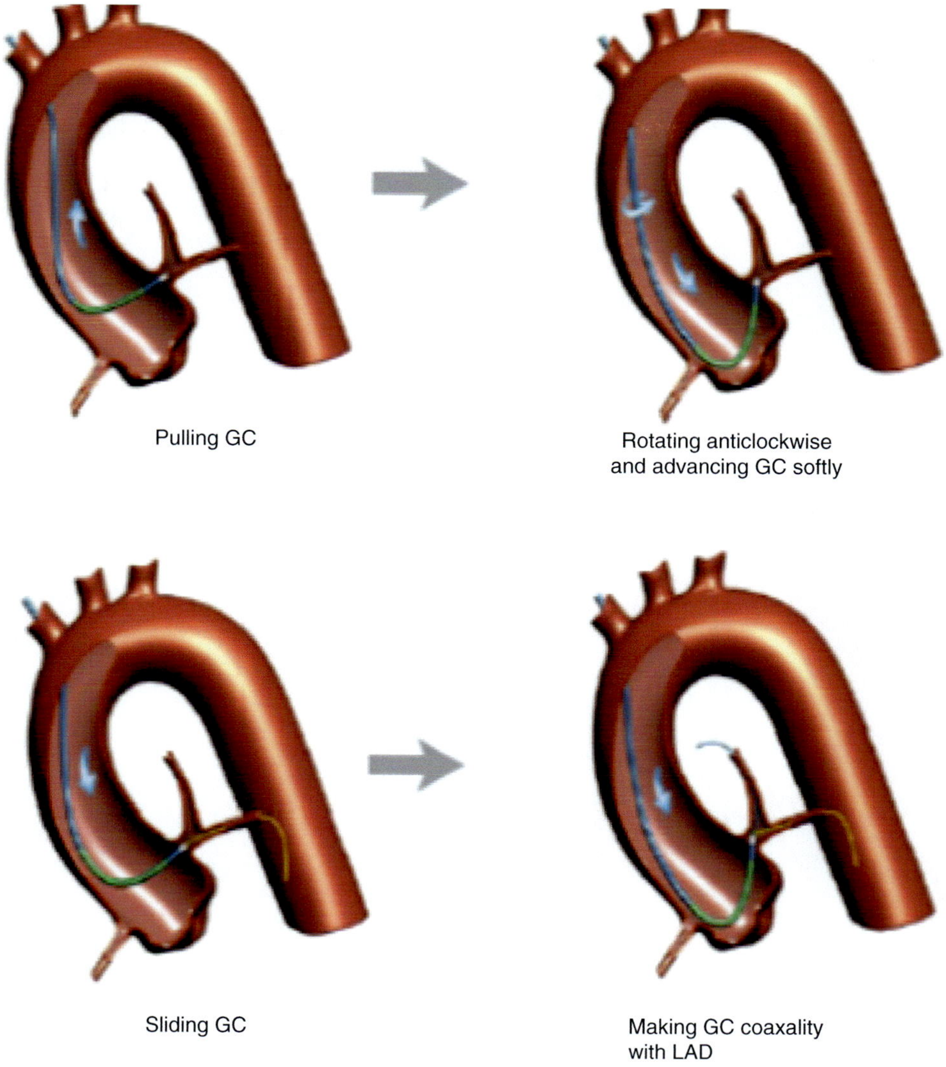

Fig. 8.22 Manipulating EBU catheter while GC superselected to LCX when dealing with LM bifurcation lesions (Image provided courtesy of Medtronic Inc. © Medtronic Inc. All rights reserved)

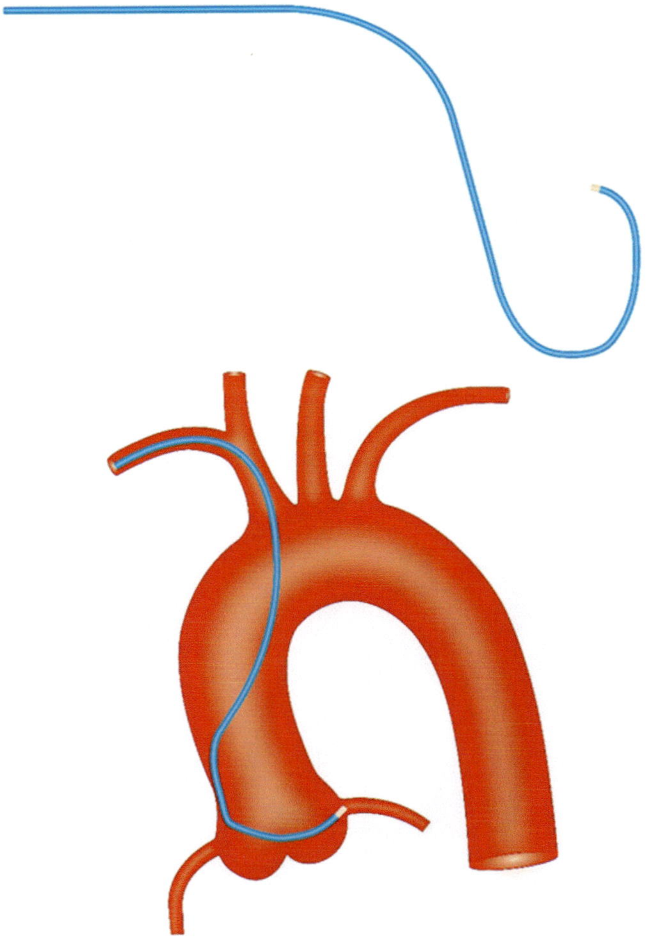

Fig. 8.23 Ikari catheter left

References

1. Bertrand OF, Rao SV, Pancholy S, et al. Transradial approach for coronary angiography and interventions: results of the first international transradial practice survey. JACC Cardiovasc Interv. 2010;3:1022–31.
2. Ikari Y, Nakajima H, Iijima R, et al. Initial characterization of Ikari Guide catheter for transradial coronary intervention. J Invasive Cardiol. 2004;16:65–8.

Intervention Through Transulnar Approach

9

Xianghua Fu

Since 1990s, transradial approach intervention has been gradually conducted in coronary angiography or angioplasty in China and now considered a preferable technique, which offers patients the greatest clinical benefit at the price of the minimal invasion. Compared with transfemoral approach, the main advantages of transradial approach are reduced risks of access site bleeding and major vascular complications, little influence on antithrombotic and anticoagulation treatment, short length of lying on bed, which significantly reduces psychological burden of operators and patients [1–3]. Therefore, not only the intervention access superiority, but the benefit of PCI and the overall treatment improvement can transradial approach achieved.

However, nearly 10–35 % patients are not suitable through transradial access because of factors like anatomic variation, dysplasia, vascular distortion, severe spasm, atherosclerosis and calcification of radial artery, subcutaneous induration, radial occlusion of secondary angiography and as a surgical bypass vessel of dialysis fistula [4, 5]. Transferring to transfemoral from transradial access, however, could increase the pain and mental stress of patients as well as the perioperative complications, deprive opportunity and benefit of transforearm minimal invasive intervention, what's worse, hindering the improvement of transiradial approach.

As we know, the radial artery and ulnar artery are two terminal branches of brachial artery. The ulnar artery normally originates at the bifurcation of the brachial artery near the elbow, and passes downward along the ulna in accompany with the ulnar nerve toward the wrist, where it crosses the transverse carpal ligament to enter the hand. In the forearm, the average diameter of the ulnar artery is comparable to that of the radial artery (Fig. 9.1). Besides, the ulnar artery is deeper than the radial artery. Transulnar coronary angiography was first reported by Terashima [6] et al in 2001, and the ulnar artery had been proposed for elective angiography in patients not suitable for the transradial approach. The first transulnar coronary angioplasty procedure was achieved in our cardiac center by Professor Fu Xianghua in 2001, and the safety and feasibility of coronary angioplasty via a transulnar approach in selective patients was reported by Fu et al in 2003 [7]. Recently, more reports have demonstrated that the transulnar approach may be both feasible and safe for coronary angiography and angioplasty in selective patients.

In clinical practice, we have summarized that the radial pulses of patients with radial puncture failure are more likely to be weak, while ulnar pulses at the same side are relatively strong. For those patients with wide diameters, strong beat and easy punctured ulnar artery, is it suitable for them to go through transulnar access? We referred to Chinese forearm arterial anatomic data and found that, just like dominance of left and right coronary artery, there also exists dominance between radial and ulnar artery. The diameter of ulnar artery in Chinese male is around 2.5–2.8 mm, and that of radial artery in female is 2.3–2.5 mm. Both sides are nearly the same and the right size of dextromanual patients is slightly wider than left. Therefore, no matter male or female, if a patient's ulnar artery diameters is above 2.3 mm, he can be operated with 6Fr guiding catheter (inner diameter 2 mm). Puncture needles, expanding sheath and operation equipment in transradial access operation are also suitable in transulnar intervention, which lays the foundation for transulnar access in anatomy and interventional equipment. Meanwhile, experts in hand surgery pointed out that since hand is supplied by bilateral blood circulation, puncturing ulnar artery and inserting sheath and catheter are safe, which do not affect hand function. However, since ulnar artery stretches closely to ulnar nerve, operators should pay attention to nerve damage.

Therefore, two main reasons have been considered for the choice of ulnar arterial approach. Firstly, when radial artery is contraindicated or unsuccessful as well as avoidance of the femoral arterial access, ulnar arterial access should be considered. Secondly, sometimes radial artery may be selected as the potential harvest for coronary bypass

X. Fu
Second Hospital of Hebei Medical University, Shijiazhuang, China
e-mail: fuxh999@163.com

Y. Zhou et al. (eds.), *Transradial Approach for Percutaneous Interventions*, DOI 10.1007/978-94-017-7350-8_9

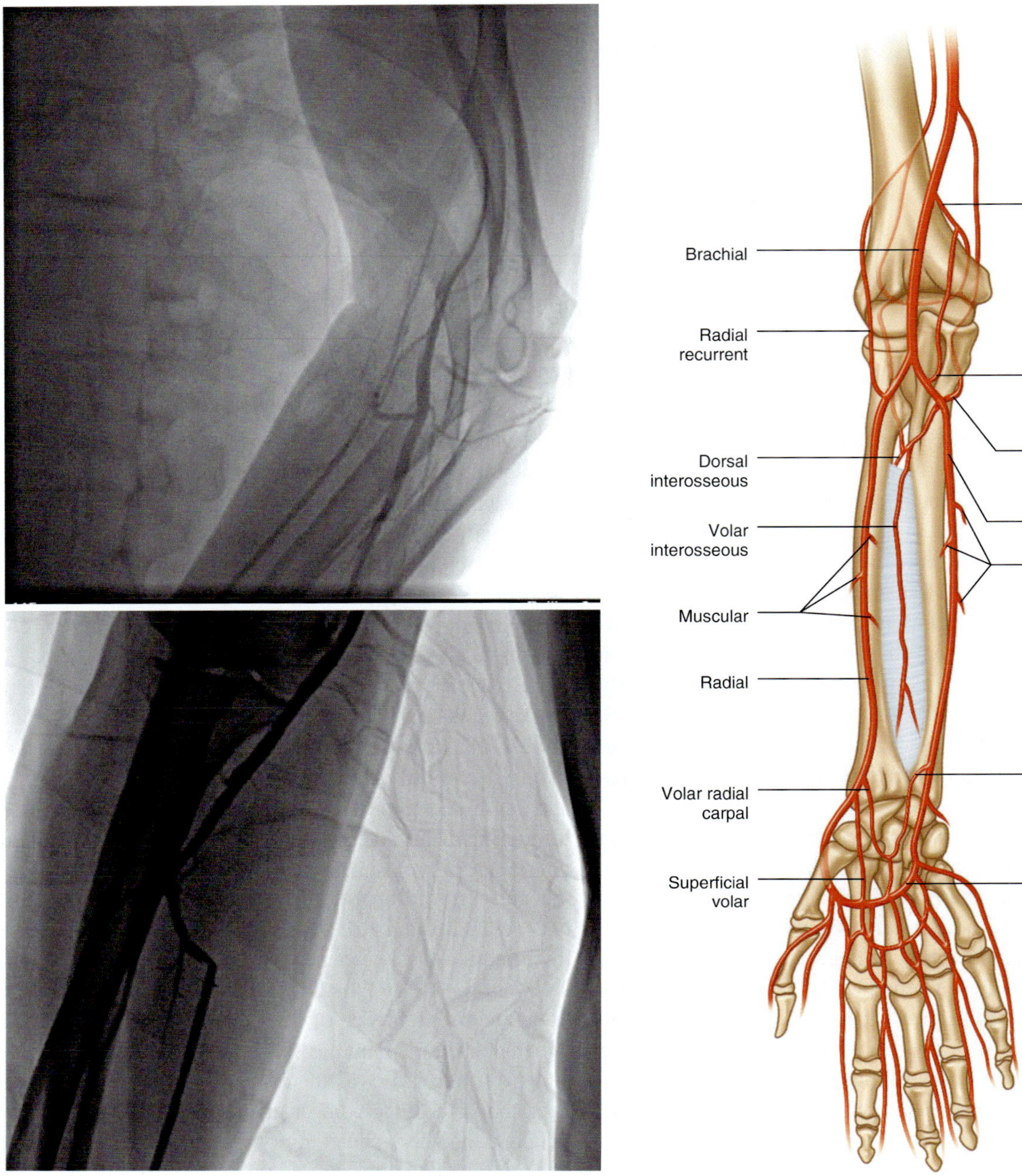

Fig. 9.1 Radial artery and ulnar artery anatomy

graft. For protection of the hand, safe ulnar arterial access remains predicated on the integrity of the palmar collaterals.

The ulnar artery puncture and cannulation is similar to the way of radial artery. The right forearm was abducted and placed on a rest attached to the catheterization table, with hyperextention of the wrist. After local subcutaneous anesthesia with 1 % lidocaine, the skin was infiltrated over the palpable artery at the site where the pulsation was the strongest, usually 1–5 cm proximal from the pisiform bone (ulnar artery), and 1–5 cm proximal from the styloid process (radial artery). The anterior wall of the artery was punctured using a 21 gauge needle. After the puncture, a 0.5334 mm (0.021 in.) guidewire was inserted (Cordis Corporation, Florida, USA). A short 4-French or 6-French tapering introducer (Cordis Corporation) was placed on the 0.5334 mm (0.021 in.) wire through a skin incision made by cutting gently with a surgical knife. A bolus of 3000 U unfractionated heparin and 200 μg of nitroglycerin were administrated to the access artery through the sheath catheter. In patients undergoing percutaneous coronary intervention (PCI), weight-adjusted unfractionated heparin (100 U/kg) was administrated through the sheath catheter to achieve and maintain an activated clotting time between 250 and 350 s. A 7-French introducer over a 0.038 in. wire was substituted for the 4-French or 6-French sheath catheter when a 7-French guiding catheter was needed in the procedure (Fig. 9.2). 4-French Judkins diagnostic catheters (Terumo, Tokyo, Japan) or 5-French TIG diagnostic catheters (Terumo) were used for diagnostic coronary angiography. Angioplasty was done with 6-French guiding catheters having an inner diameter of 1.8034 mm (0.071 in.) or 1.778 mm (0.070 in.) (Medtronic, Danvers, MA or Cordis Corporation) or 7-French guiding catheters having an inner diameter of 2.0574 mm (0.081 in.) (Medtronic). The catheters were advanced over a standard 0.035 in. spring guidewire. Commercially available guidewires for percutaneous transluminal coronary angioplasty (PTCA), rapid-exchange balloons, and balloon-expandable stents were used according to standard procedures. Forearm artery angiography was performed at the end of procedure before sheath removal, which was used to evaluate the anatomical variations of the forearm artery. The sheaths were immediately withdrawn after the procedure and a hemostasis strap over a gauze was applied to compress the puncture site for 4–6 h, followed by a non-occlusive pressure dressing.

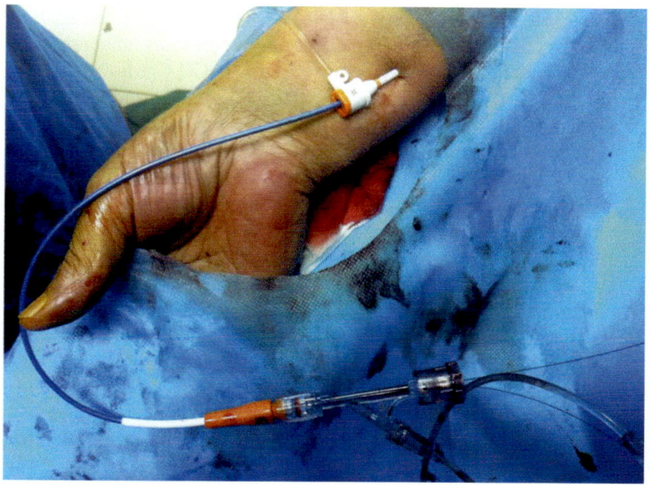

Fig. 9.2 Via right ulnar approach 7 Fr Guiding Catheter for left main bifurcation PCI

Subsequently, we started to propagandize and popularize TUI in many domestic conferences of cardiovascular disease, and gradually expanded its clinical PCI field including multivessel lesion, CTO lesion, in-stent restenosis, even AMI fit for TUI. It was found that TUI was similar to TRI in the door to balloon time and each procedural time, which suggested that for the patient with ulnar artery superiority, TUI could be not only used in common PCI, but in AMI-PCI as the superior or alternative vessel. Thus, almost all of AMI patients were fit for PCI via transforearm (radial/ulnar) artery, and the success rate of PCI was increased, while crossover to TFI was unnecessary. So far, many interventional cardiologists have tried to use ulnar artery as an alternative artery for PCI in lots of hospitals across the country. In 2004, I was invited to carry out TUI for over hundreds of German patients in St. Elizabeth Heart Center. We reported <Feasibility of percutaneous coronary intervention via transulnar artery approach in patients with

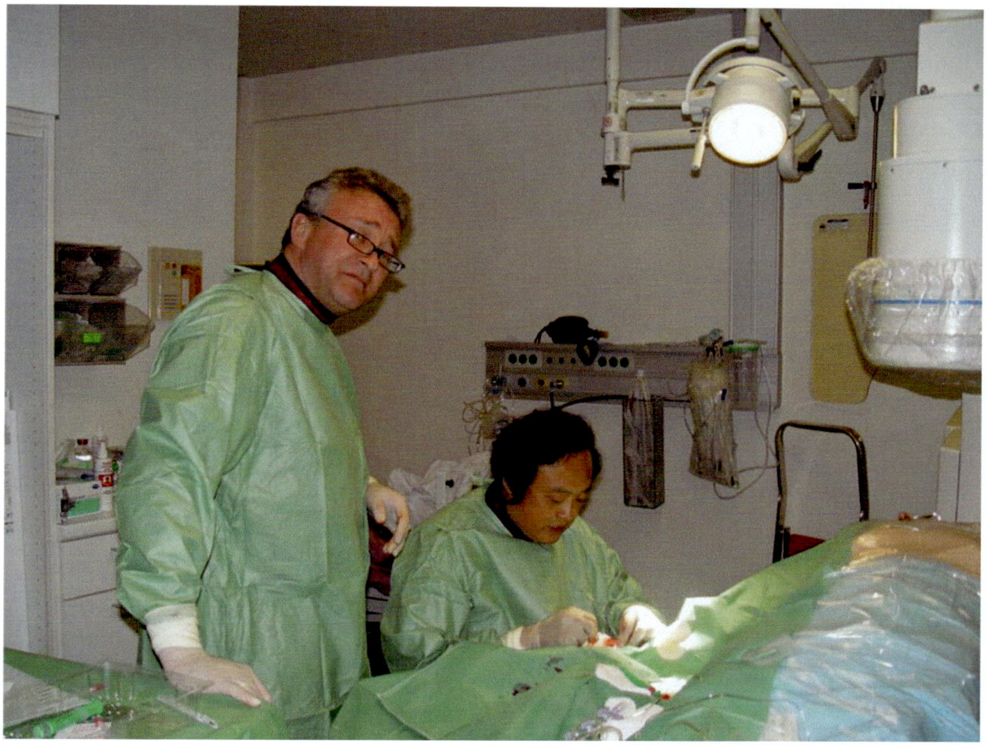

Fig. 9.3 Prof Xiang Hua Fu performed transulnar PCI in St. Elizabeth Germany (*Left Prof* Wende from Germany; *Right Prof* XiangHua Fu from China)

coronary heart disease>in the largest conference all over the world--TCT 2014, while the operation photo was published in <*American Journal of Cardiology*> (Fig. 9.3).

Several RCTs of transulnar compared with TRA in patients undergoing coronary procedures resulted in similar rates of major adverse cardiac events and access-related complications [7–10]. Higher access cross-over rates, and a small but significantly higher number of punctures were noted with the transulnar approach. No differences were found in procedure time, fluoroscopy time, or contrast volume between two approaches. A recent Meta-Analysis showed that TUA is safe and effective compared to TRA in patients undergoing coronary procedures [11]. However, large, multi-centers studies needed to be conducted in the further.

Presently, a consecutive randomized controlled trial concerning minimally invasive PCI via transforearm (radial/ulnar) artery is ongoing in our center, the existing results showing that TUI was also safe and effective compared with TRI in CAG and PCI. We try to prove that TUI is safe and effective as well as TRI in the selective cases of the real world; and TUI could be preferred for the patients with ulnar artery superiority. If puncture failure without sheath implantation in first TRI, you can instantly convert to ipsilateral TUI; if with sheath implantation, you can select contralateral TRI or TUI. Thus, the possibility and success rate of PCI via transforearm (radial/ulnar) artery are undoubtedly increased, which makes it more popular and in-depth development, and creates a new field of minimally invasive PCI.

References

1. Campeau L. Percutaneous radial artery approach for coronary angiography. Cathet Cardiovasc Diagn. 1989;16(1):3–7.
2. Karrowni W, Vyas A, Giacomino B, et al. Radial versus femoral access for primary percutaneous interventions in ST-segment elevation myocardial infarction patients: a meta-analysis of randomized controlled trials. JACC Cardiovasc Interv. 2013;6(8):814–23.
3. Valgimigli M, Gagnor A, Calabro P, et al. Radial versus femoral access in patients with acute coronary syndromes undergoing invasive management: a randomised multicentre trial. Lancet. 2015; 385(9986):2465–76.
4. Hamon M, Pristipino C, Di MC, et al. Consensus document on the radial approach in percutaneous cardiovascular interventions: position paper by the European Association of Percutaneous Cardiovascular Interventions and Working Groups on Acute Cardiac Care** and Thrombosis of the European Society of Cardiology. EuroIntervention. 2013;8(11):1242–51.
5. Abdelaal E, Brousseau-Provencher C, Montminy S, et al. Risk score, causes, and clinical impact of failure of transradial approach for percutaneous coronary interventions. JACC Cardiovasc Interv. 2013;6(11):1129–37.
6. Terashima M, Meguro T, Takeda H, et al. Percutaneous ulnar artery approach for coronary angiography: a preliminary report in nine patients. Catheter Cardiovasc Interv. 2001;53(3):410–4.
7. Aptecar E, Pernes JM, Chabane-Chaouch M, et al. Transulnar versus transradial artery approach for coronary angioplasty: the PCVI-CUBA study. Catheter Cardiovasc Interv. 2006; 67(5):711–20.
8. Gokhroo R, Bisht D, Padmanabhan D, Gupta S, Kishor K, Ranwa B. Feasibility of ulnar artery for cardiac catheterization: AJmer ULnar ARtery (AJULAR) catheterization study. Catheter Cardiovasc Interv. 2015;86(1):42–8.
9. Geng W, Fu X, Gu X, et al. Safety and feasibility of transulnar versus transradial artery approach for coronary catheterization in non-selective patients. Chin Med J (Engl). 2014;127(7): 1222–8.
10. Liu J, Fu XH, Xue L, Wu WL, Gu XS, Li SQ. A comparative study of transulnar and transradial artery access for percutaneous coronary intervention in patients with acute coronary syndrome. J Interv Cardiol. 2014;27(5):525–30.
11. Dahal K, Rijal J, Lee J, Korr KS, Azrin M. Transulnar versus transradial access for coronary angiography or percutaneous coronary intervention: a meta-analysis of randomized controlled trials. Catheter Cardiovasc Interv. 2016:87(5):857–65.

10 Tips and Tricks When Performing Transradial Intervention: A Supplement to Previous Chapters

Qing Yang, Bin Nie, and Wei Liu

Abstract

Percutaneous coronary intervention (PCI) via transradial approach (TRA) has been increased dramatically over the last 15 years and majority of operators adopt it as the default approach. Data from Chinese national PCI registry showed that 89.45 % of the PCI procedures were performed via TRA in China. Familiar with the tips and tricks when performing transradial intervention could shorten the learning curve and increase the successful rate. The tips and tricks of performing transradial intervention listed in this chapter are set as a supplement to the other chapters.

Question 1: What are the advantages and disadvantages of single wall versus double wall puncture technique? (Figs. 10.1 and 10.2a, b) Two puncture kits (Bare needle and plastic cannula) are most commonly used for TRA. Both puncture technique can obtain high rate of success at experienced hand, although majority of beginners prefer to use Terumo puncture kit due to its shorter learning curve. However, to some extent, one technique has advantage over the other, thus understanding both two puncture techniques are necessary.

	Bare needle	Plastic cannula
Components	21G needle 25 cm 0.021″wire 11 cm sheath (Cordis U.S)	20G needle 45 cm 0.025” wire 16 cm sheath (Terumo Japan)
Method	Single wall puncture Point to point	Counter wall puncture Point to line
Successful rate at 1st entry	Lower	Higher`
Need for skin incision	Yes	No
Penetrating the vessel wall	More frequent	Less frequent
Suitable for small/fine vessels	+++	+
Useful for multiple punctures	+++	+
Vessel spasm	More frequent	Less frequent

See also Chap. 4

Question 2: What should be done in case of first puncture failure? Attempt at a successful puncture at first hit. However, if the first puncture fails, do not completely remove the needle, keep the needle in situ. Next, feel the radial pulse

Q. Yang (✉) • B. Nie • W. Liu
Department of Cardiology, Beijing Anzhen Hospital, Capital Medical University, Beijing, China
e-mail: yq1963884@sina.com; 123nb@163.com; Liuwei525@hotmail.com

Y. Zhou et al. (eds.), *Transradial Approach for Percutaneous Interventions*, DOI 10.1007/978-94-017-7350-8_10

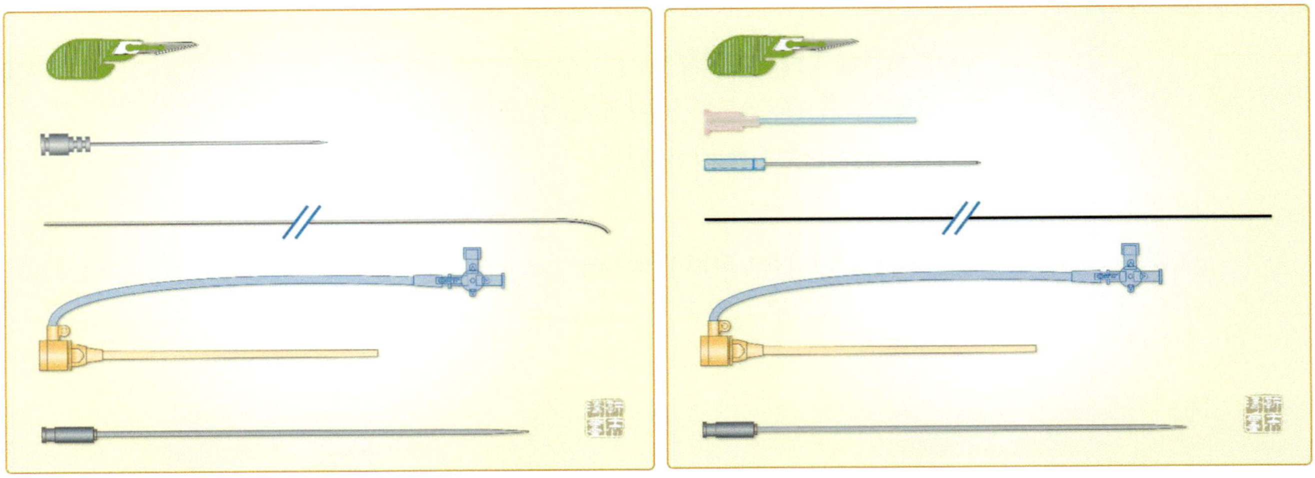

Fig. 10.1 Difference between two puncture kit. Bare needle (Cordis, co U.S), Plastic cannular (Terumo, Japan)

followed by reassessing the direction for re-inserting the needle. In case the current position of the needle is too far from the radial pulse, remove the needle completely and choose a more suitable position for re-inserting the needle. Sometimes, upon increased pressure of the left fingers on the radial artery while checking for pulse, the blood flow could be tampered and leads to the puncture failure. Then relieve the pressure slowly to re-instate the blood flow and repeat the puncture at the suitable site. In case of puncture failure by the plastic cannula (Terumo kit), switch to the bare needle to increase the likelihood of successful puncture, this is especially useful in case of small sized vessel and multiple punctures (Figs. 10.3 and 10.4).

Question 3: How to ensure higher success rate of first puncture? (1) Check radial pulse carefully; Perform a radial/ulnar ultrasound if the radial pulse is weak. (2) Positon the forearm flat to fully extend the wrist. (3) Analgesics or Lidocaine should be given to ensure patient's comfort and decrease the chance of vessel spasm. (4) Chose a proper site for puncture, Normally 1 cm above the radial styloid process. However, if the artery is tortuous or has puncture previously; puncture site should be slightly proximal to the tortuous segment to increase the success rate (Fig. 10.5). (5) The Angle of puncture is 30—45°. However, the angle should be adjusted according to the anatomical differences per patient. The angle should be smaller for thinner patients when the pulse is superficial and fine to increase the likelihood of successful puncture. The angle should be larger for obese patents when the pulse is deep (Fig. 10.6).

Question 4: Is the use of anti-spasm required routinely? Anti-spasm therapy includes lidocaine, nitroglycerin and verapamil, however, in a higher volume center with highly experienced interventionists and highly likelihood of first chance puncture, the cocktail administration may be neglected since administration of lidocaine can lead to patient discomfort.

Question 5: What should be done if the wire meets resistance after a successful puncture? Even in the presence of blood flow after a successful puncture, sometime the wire can encounter resistance. This could be due to the wire entering smaller branches or the vessel being tortuous and could also be due to vessel spasm. The wire may enter the medial layer causing dissection or penetrate the vessel wall, in this situation, do not further advance the sheath. Perform a fluoroscopy of the arm and adjust the wire. If the sheath is already inserted and blood flow is not present, withdraw the sheath slightly until the blood flow returns. If the blood flow does not return, remove the sheath and apply pressure to the puncture site.

Question 6: How to effectively treat forearm hematoma? The most effective way in treating forearm hematoma is not by surrounding the forearm with pressure bandages, elevation of the elbow or use of ice for decreasing the swelling but focus on identifying the bleeding site and performing manual compression on bleeding site for 30 min to 1 h until the tension is released, followed by covering with pressure bandages. Normally the accurate site of bleeding is where the patient feels the most pain (Figs. 10.7 and 10.8).

Question 7: What are the advantages and disadvantages of hydrophilic and J shape angiographic wire? J shape wire and hydrophilic wires can both be used to advance to the ascending aorta during angiogram, while they both present unique benefits and draw-backs.

Terumo hydrophilic guidewire with polyurethane radiopaque jacket provides smoother navigation (no friction) through the catheter and vessels with higher visibility (tungsten salts) and minimal blood adhesion to the wire. It's elastic

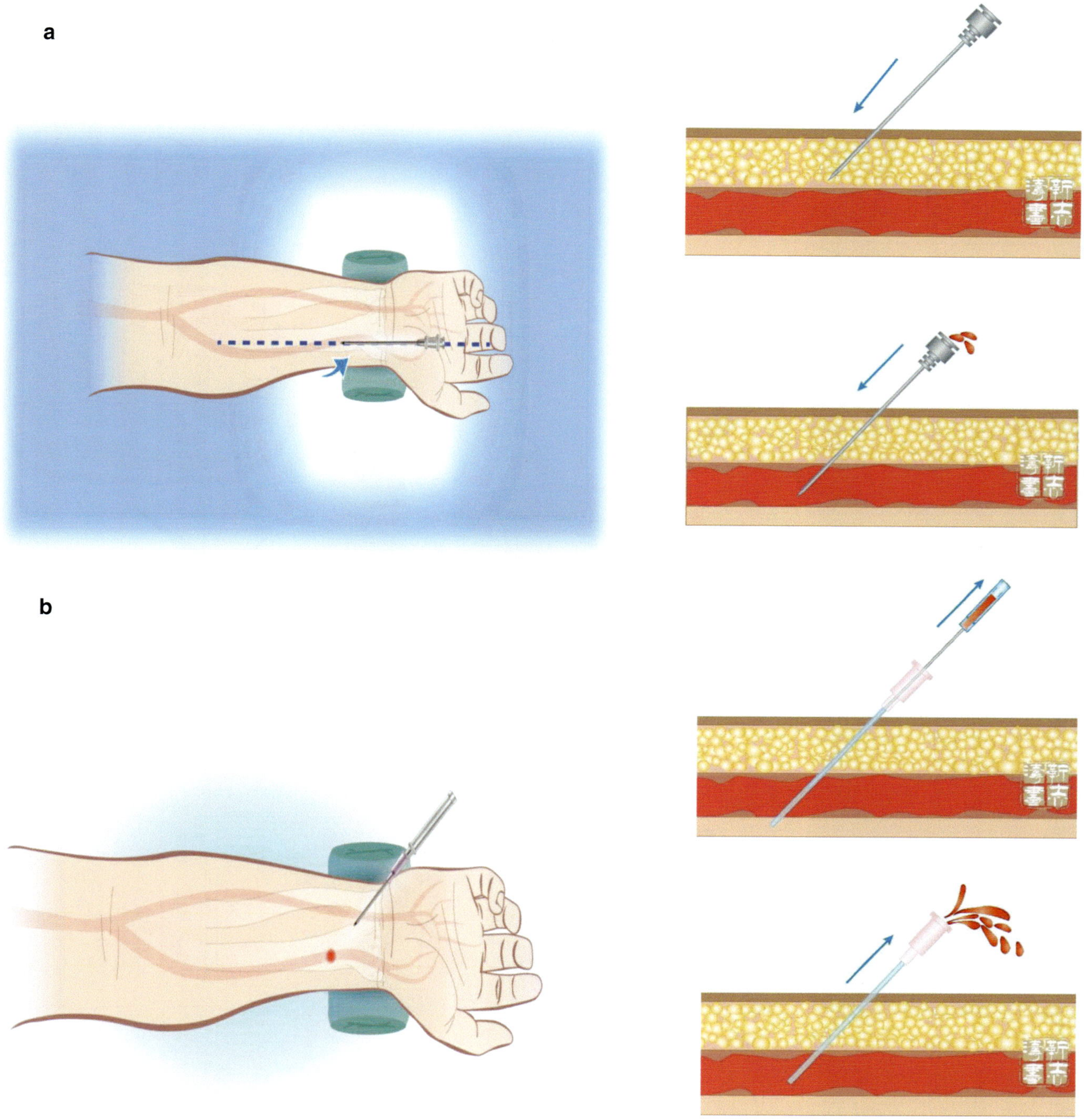

Fig. 10.2 (**a**) Characteristics of Single wall puncture: Only front wall being punctured, needle needs to be directed more coaxial to the vessel course (point to point), thus the successful rate at first attempt is less. There is Less pulsatile blood flow coming out after artery is punctured; The wire has diameters of 0.021 cm, non-coating with less support; The stiff tip is more easily to penetrate though the vessel wall to the surrounding tissue. Need make a skin incision with scalpel routinely before sheath insertion. (**b**) Characteristics of double wall puncture: Both front wall and counter wall being punctured (point to line), thus the successful rate at first attempt is higher. There is more prominent pulsatile blood flow coming out the hub after artery being punctured; Less chance of getting success while a hematoma formed after an unsuccessful attempt; The wire has diameters of 0.025 cm and coated, thus has chances of dissection by inadvertent advance; does not need make a skin incision with scalpel routinely for sheath insertion

nitinol core provides excellent shape memory, greater flexibility and increased control in difficult cases. The one-piece construction improves wire control through the vessel, true one-to-one torque transmission for an easier, faster and safer navigation through both the catheter and vessels. And the non-traumatic rounded edge decreased the likelihood of vessel trauma and smoother wire insertion. The hydrophilic wire's coating makes easier to cross the torturous artery.

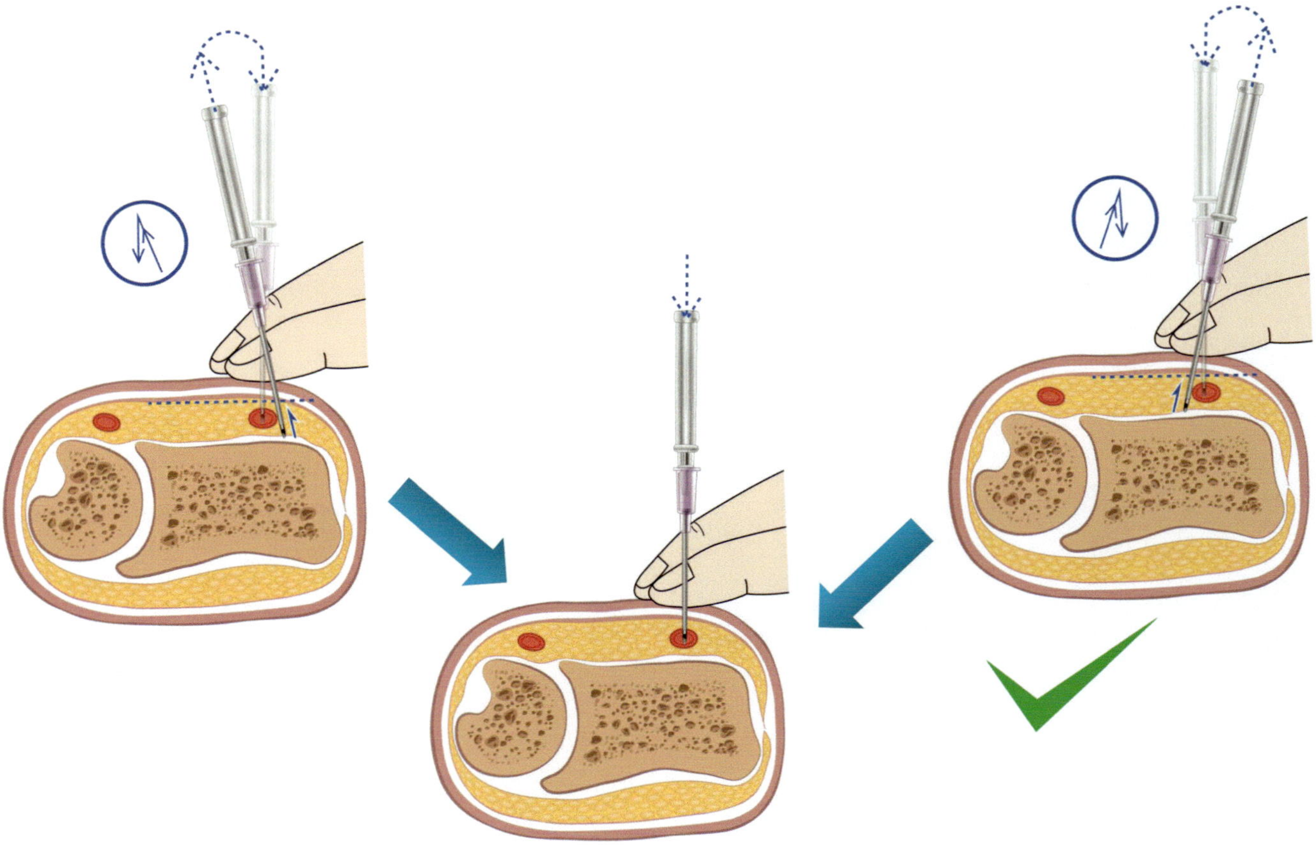

Fig. 10.3 Redirect the needle if the first attempt failed by defining the appropriate relationship between the position of needle and radial pulse

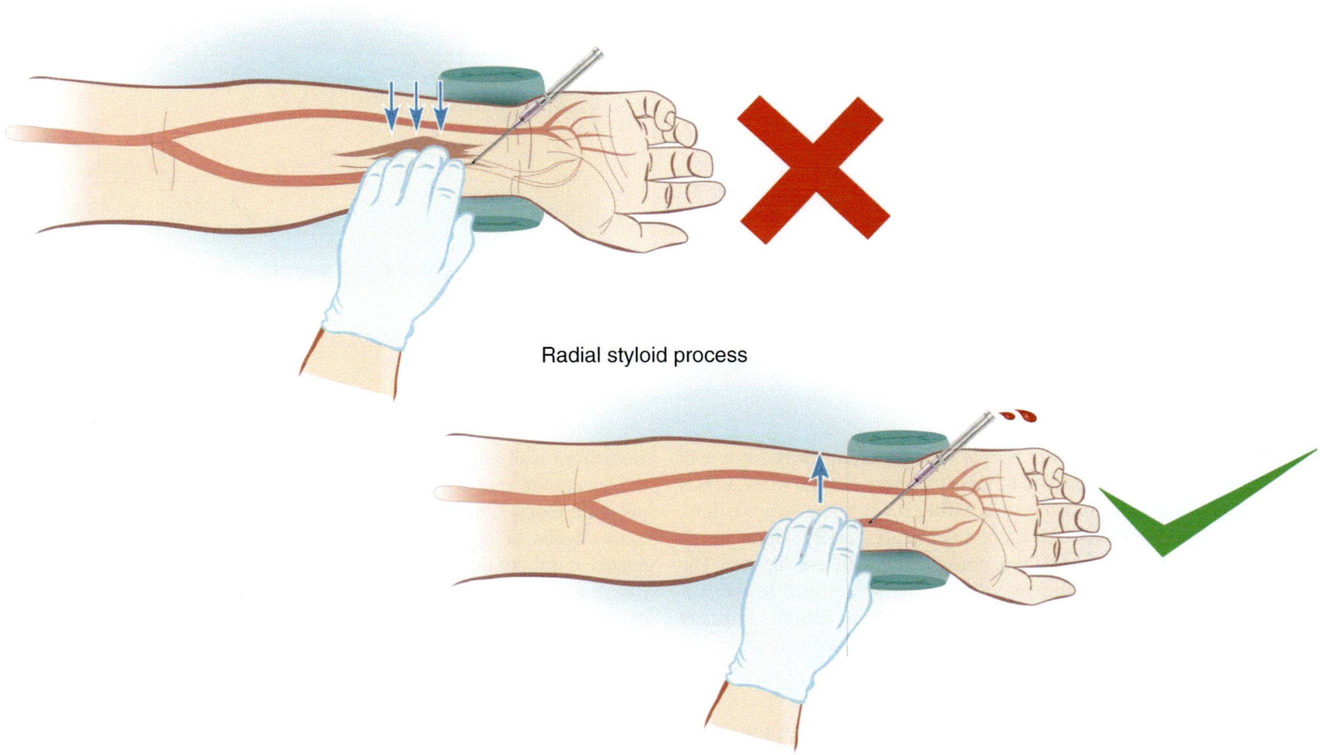

Fig. 10.4 Avoid excess pressure as radial artery can be easily occluded by finger pressure

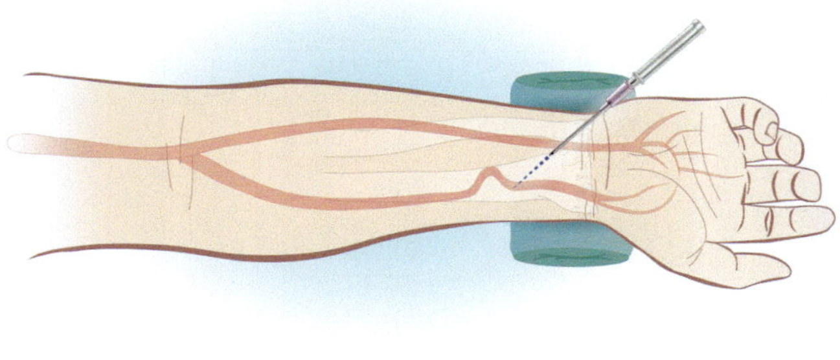

Fig. 10.5 Increase the successful rate for tortuous radial artery : choose more proximal puncture site, avoid access at radial styloid process, feel the relationship between the need and radial pulse properly, slowly advance

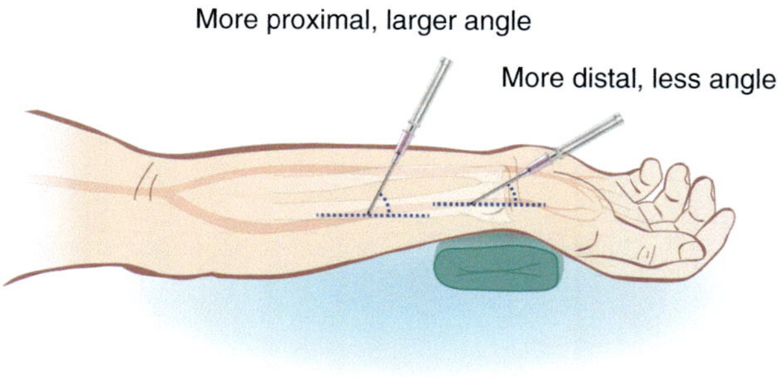

Fig. 10.6 Angle need to be adjusted according to variety of situation. The angle should be smaller for thinner patients when the pulse is superficial and fine. The angle should be larger for obese patents when the pulse is deeper

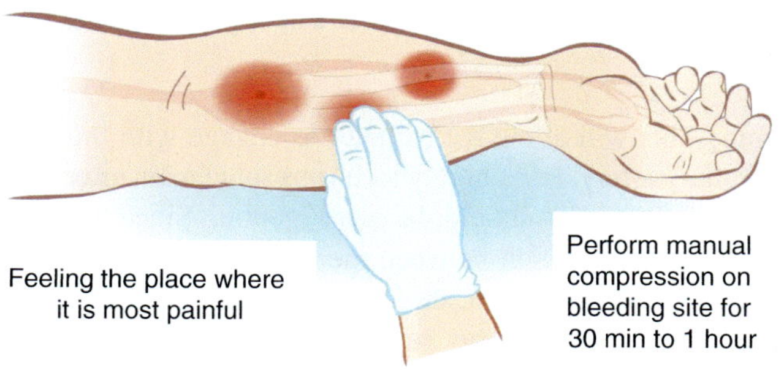

Fig. 10.7 The most effective thing to treat forearm hematoma: identifying the bleeding site within 10 min, manual compression until the tension is released,, then covering it with pressure bandage

However, there are higher chances of the wire to enter into the small branch and causing possible perforation. Close monitoring under fluoroscopy is required when advancing the wire.

On the other hand, the J shape wire is non- hydrophilic and has a 180°,3 cm curve at its tip. Resistance is easily to be felt when wire encountering small branches. It is not as likely as the hydrophilic wire to enter into the smaller branches and causes less complications. The J shape wire could be advanced with less fluoroscopy time. However, it presents with challenges when crossing extremely torturous radial or brachial arteries, Thus, requiring exchange to the hydrophilic wire.

Both hydrophilic wire and J shape wire can be used to cross torturous subclavian artery, while J. curve wire provides greater support for the guiding catheter when engaging with the coronary artery.

Question 8: How should the radial loop be dealt with? Refer to Chap. 6 (See picture 10.8)

Question 9: How to advance the catheter through torturous arteries? Refer to Chap. 6

Question 10: How to advance to catheter through torturous subclavian artery? Refer to Chap. 6

Upon reaching the cephalic arch and facing difficulty entering the ascending aorta; ask the patient to take a deep breath, allowing the angle between the cephalic arch and the ascending arota to decrease resulting in catheter advancing into the ascending aorta. In case this maneuver proves unsuccessful, advance the wire into the descending aorta Then progress the diagnostic catheter to the aortic arch, retract the wire to the catheter, and ask the patient to take a deep breath. Turn the catheter 45—90° counter clockwise facing the tip of the catheter towards the ascending aorta. This should allow the wire to advance into the ascending aorta. For an extreme torturous subclavian artery, a double wire technique could be used (Fig. 10.9).

Question 11: What is the basic technique for engaging left coronary artery by Tiger catheter via transradial approach? Advance the wire to sinus root until the wire bends upwards, then proceed with Tiger catheter along the wire into aortic root, simultaneously turning catheter clockwise to face the tip towards the left side, followed by pull-back of the catheter to the left sinus accompanied by clockwise or counterclockwise gentle movement at the level of the ostium, until the catheter pop into the left main ostium (Fig. 10.10).

If this maneuver fails due to torturous subclavian artery; ask the patient to take a deep breath causing the diaphragm to descend, then withdraw the catheter while gently turning the catheter counter clockwise, which will allow the catheter to pop into the left coronary artery.

Remember: For right radial approach, clockwise rotating the catheter will shorten the S band (caused by the torturous subclavian artery) and counter clockwise rotating the catheter will lengthen the S band. If the catheter is below the left main, gentle pull back with counter clock wise rotating will

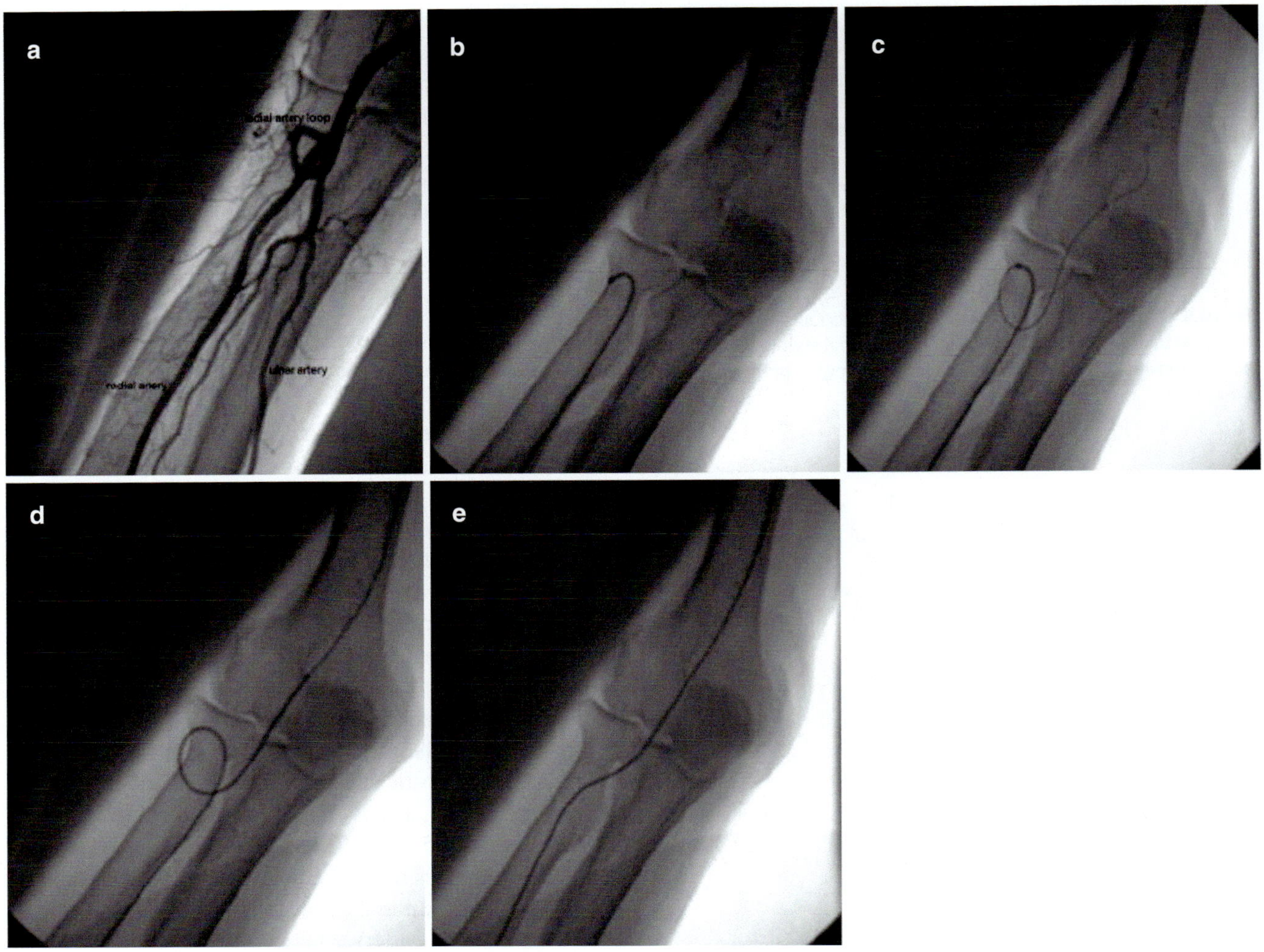

Fig. 10.8 Treatment of radial loop: (**a**) Wire encountered resistance, fluoroscopy showed radial loop. (**b**) Advanced a JR diagnostic catheter. (**c–e**) The tortuous artery was straightened by hydrophilic wire and diagnostic catheter

allow the catheter to pop into the left coronary artery. Alternatively, clockwise rotation from a higher sinus location and slightly withdraw the catheter will enable successful cannulation of LCA.

If the subclavian is severely tortuous, ask the patient to take a deep breath, while keeping 0.035 J shape wire inside the catheter to facilitate manipulation and to prevent the catheter from kinking.

Question 12: What is the basic technique for engaging the right coronary artery by Tiger catheter via transradial approach? Following the successful left angiogram, slightly withdraw the catheter away from the left coronary ostium while turning the catheter counter clockwise so that the primary and secondary curve come perpendicular to the screen until they are no longer discernible, and then push the catheter forward to direct the tip into the non-coronary sinus, while turning the catheter clockwise with gently withdraw. This will allow the catheter to engage with the right coronary artery. For a highly torturous subclavian artery, the toque movement should be very gentle. Since there is delayed transmission between the hand movement and the catheter tips movement, the trick is to anticipate the accurate amount of turning required to ensure best results (Fig. 10.11).

Question 13: What are the preventive measures for the catheter entering the cornus branches? The primary curve of the Tiger catheter is facing upwards, sometimes, the catheter stubbornly enters into the cornus branch. If the contrast medium is incidentally injected, it can lead to ventricular fibrillation. If the catheter is too deep causing obstruction of the coronary ostium, forceful injection can also lead to ventricular fibrillation (Fig. 10.12a).

The following methods could be used for prevention of the catheter from entering into the cornus branches?

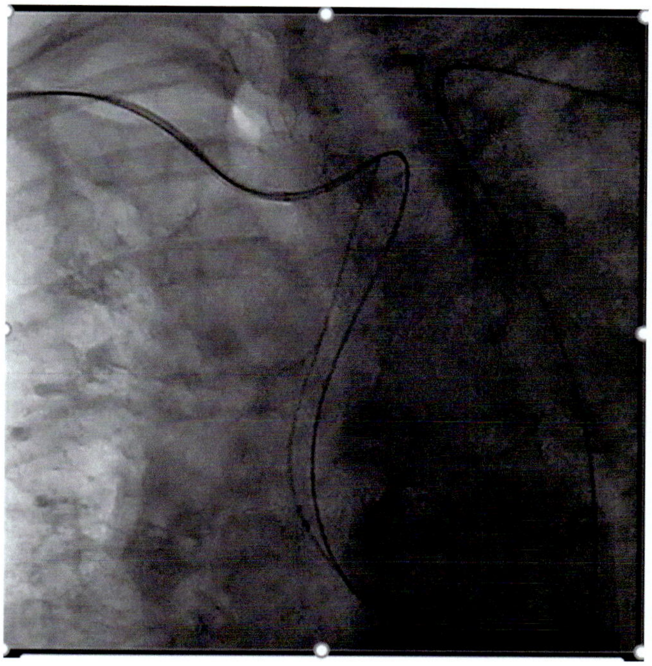

Fig. 10.9 Double wire technique: torque in the arm; Guide catheter manipulation with double 0.035 wire or 0.063 wire; May need to use supper stiff wires

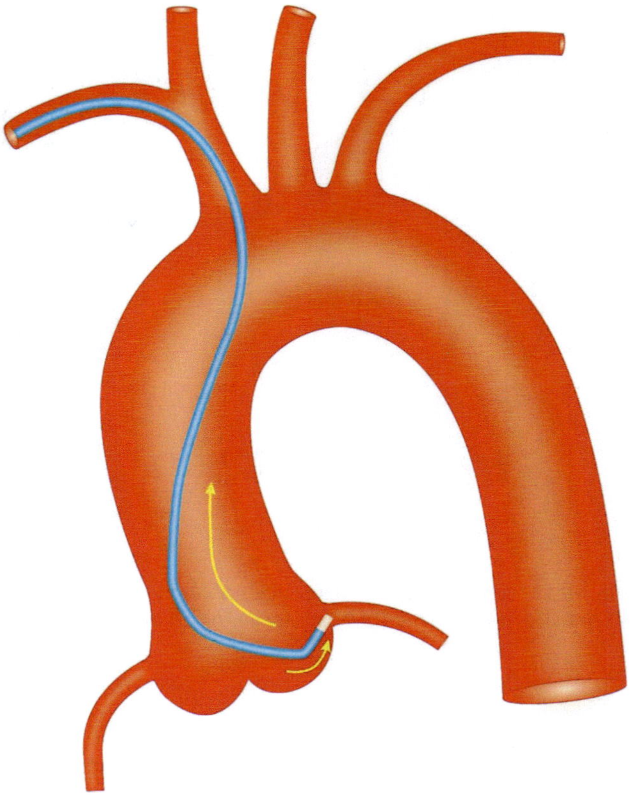

Fig. 10.10 Basic technique for engaging left coronary artery by tiger catheter via transradial approach

Fig. 10.11 Basic technique for engaging right coronary artery by tiger catheter via transradial approach

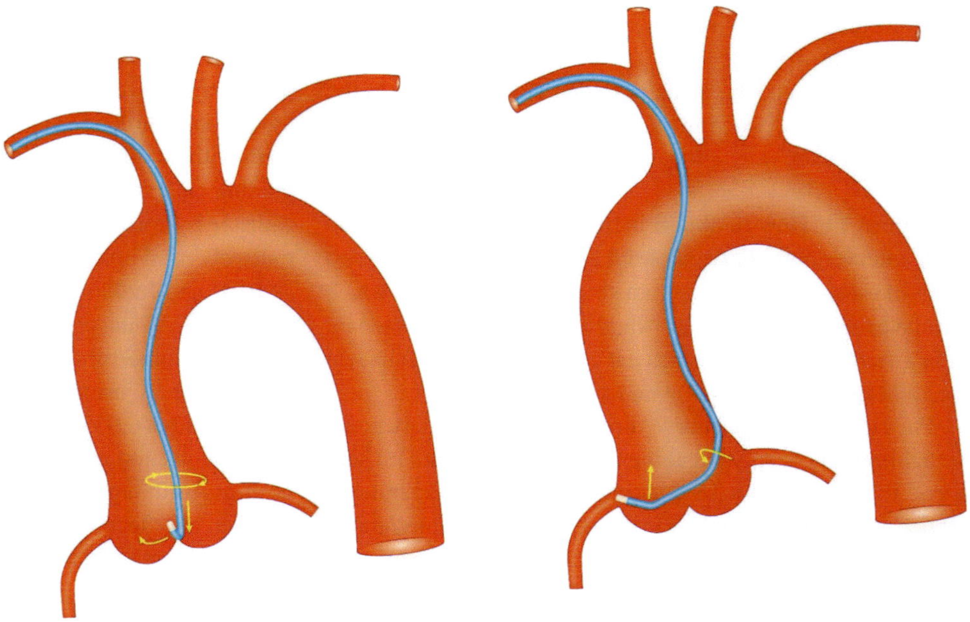

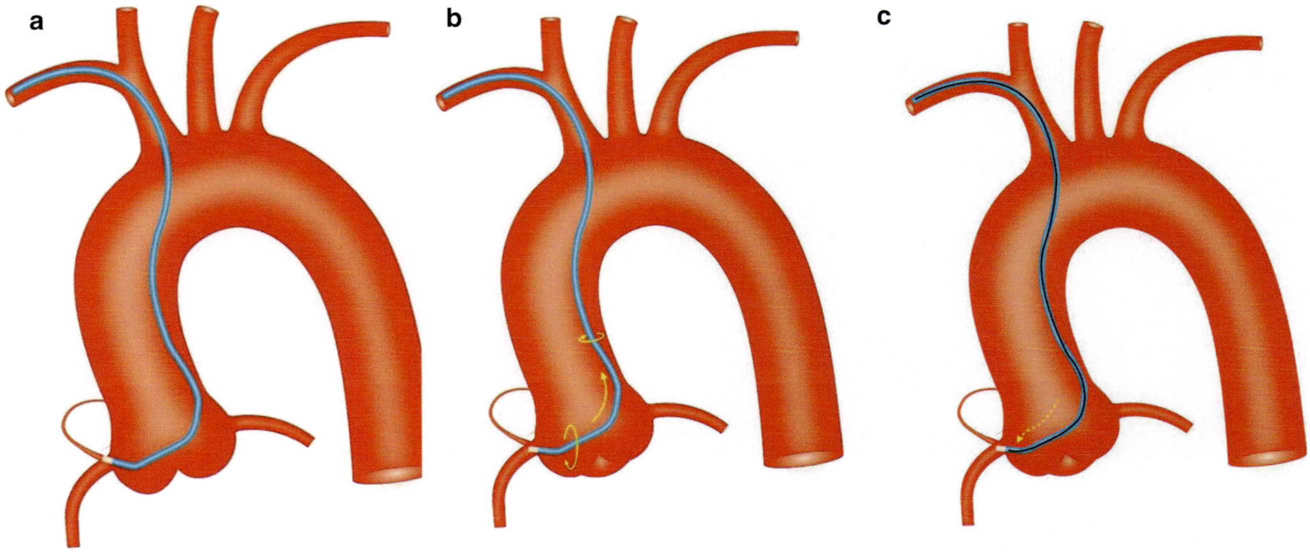

Fig. 10.12 (**a**) Tiger catheter stubbornly goes to the cornus branch. (**b**) Method 1: turning catheter towards right coronary artery. (**c**) Method 2: Keep 0.035″ J wire in the Tiger catheter and turn it as the same fashion as JR catheter

Method 1: Repeat the procedure with slowly withdrawing the catheter while turning less clockwise, consequently the catheter will enter the main branch. Sometimes, the problem can be solved by deep inspiration (Fig. 10.12b).

Method 2: Advanced the 0.035″ J wire into the first curve of the catheter to straighten the angle at its tip and make it more resembling the JR shape, while turning the catheter clockwise to promote the catheter to enter the right coronary ostium. Be cautious of the stiff part of J wire tip not protruding outside of the catheter and causing vessel injury (Fig. 10.12c).

Method 3: Reshape the catheter to decrease the angle of the first curve consequently matching the JR shape, or switch to JR catheter.

Questions 14: How to obtain better support for right coronary intervention via transradial approach? There are two types of backup for a guiding catheter, passive backup: in which a catheter will leave where it is when inserting in to the coronary artery, Active support: in which the operator should manipulate the catheter in some way to obtain a better support.

For right coronary intervention, an active support could be achieved by deeply engaging the JR catheter into 3rd segment through clockwise rotation along an interventional device (wire or balloon) to increase the coaxial alignment. Gentle counter clockwise pulling back will bring the guiding catheter to normal position.

Another power position could be achieved by JR guide is rotational amplatz maneuver, in which the JR guide is torqued counterclockwise and simultaneously push down gently to make a loop in the coronary sinus that it takes 90 band on its shaft and obtain direct support from the opposite aortic wall and coronary sinus. The position of the catheter tip should be closely monitored and the rotation maneuver should be adjusted accordingly. Excessive manipulation of JR catheter should be avoided to prevent the guide from being prolapsed into the ventricle and prevent it from kinking.

Amplatz left(0.75,1) catheter can provide a better passive support for RCA intervention and especially useful for shepherd crook configuration and will save more effort for calcified and tourous lesions when compared with JR. However, since the tip of Amplatz left is facing downward when inserting the right coronary artery, Amplaz left catheter will not be the optimal choice for ostial lesions. A better coaxial alignment without deep engaging should be achieved for Amplatz guiding catheter to avoid traumatic injury. Amplatz guiding catheter is prone to complications, therefore it should not be routinely used unless for an experienced operator.

EBU and Judkins left catheter may achieved a better support for RCA intervention than JR guide. Some interventionist prefers to perform the RCA intervention right after LCA intervention by using the same EBU or JL guide by keeping the stiff end of 0.035 J wire in the guide and rotating the guide the same fashion as that of the JR guide and obtain an active position. Although it works for most cases, cautions should be taken in order not to cause traumatic injury to the coronary ostium or cause other complications by deep engagement.

Some transrdial dedicated catheter such as Kimny, Barbeau, Fadajet are not introduced in this book since they are not frequently used. Multipurpose catheter for both left and right intervention and Wave 3 catheter for RCA intervention will be introduced in Chaps. 14 and 20 respectively.

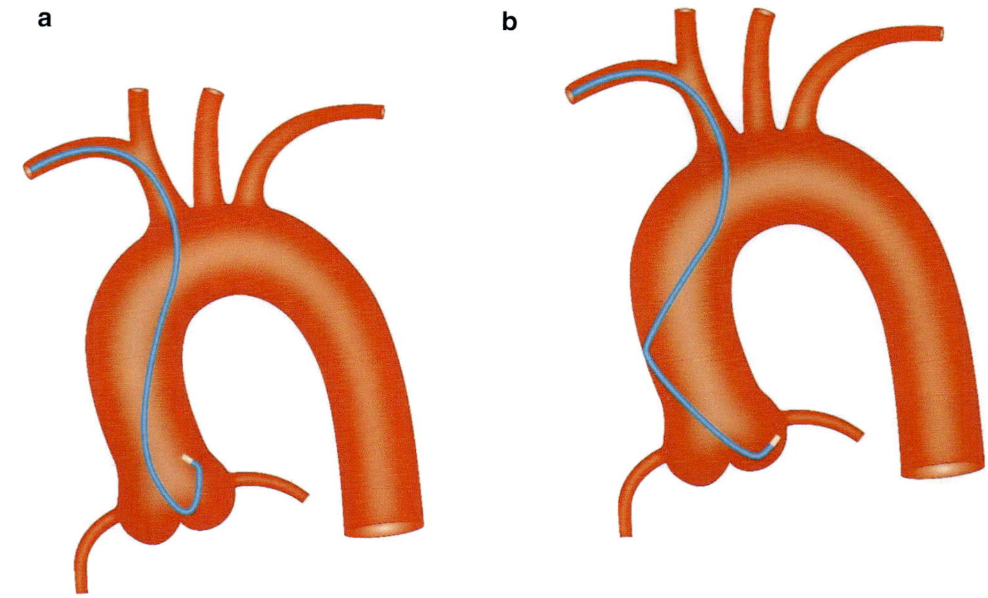

Fig. 10.13 (**a**) Catheter is too small for the aortic root, tip is facing upwards and catheter is bent up. (**b**) Catheter is too big for the aortic root. Tip is facing downwards

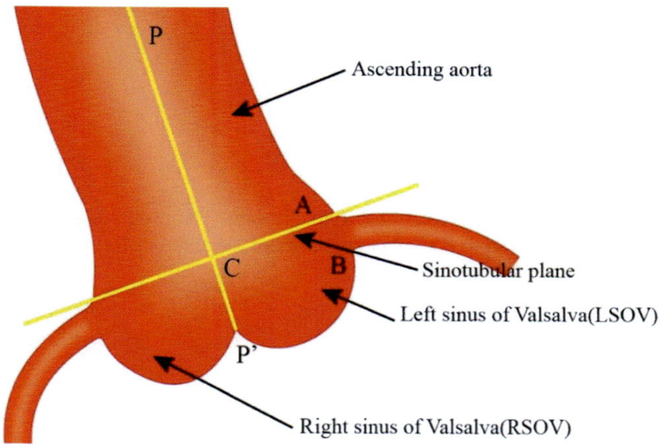

Fig 10.14 Origin of anomalous RCA from left sinus. Representative diagram of aortic root and sinuses in LAO projection. P–P′ indicates a hypothetical plane running through the midline. Sites A through C represents common sites for the origin of the anomalous artery. *A*. Origin just above the ostium of the left coronary artery (*LCA*) *B*. Origin just below the ostium of the left coronary artery *C*. Origin along the midline

Question 15: How to cannulate RCA which arising from left coronary cusp abnormally When the RCA arises from the left cusp, usually it is anterior and cephalad to the LM (type A), a JL guide with the secondary curve one size smaller than the one used for the patient for LM could be used (usually Judkins left 3.0) from right radial approach. In this case, the back up support of this catheter is from ipsilateral aortic wall instead of the contra lateral aortic wall. For Type B, which take off below the origin of LCA and type C which originating in or near the midline (type C), a AL or JL 4 guide could be used (Fig. 10.14) [1].

Question 16: How to select the appropriate sized guiding catheter for the left coronary artery intervention? The standard choice for TRI is to use a catheter half the size smaller than that of Transfemoral intervention. JL 3.5 catheter EBU 3.5 catheter are most common for patients with standard sized aortic root (Asian patients 3.5–4.0 cm). Performing an angiograph prior to procedure is the main method to provide relevant information in selection of catheter size. If the Tiger catheter is too large; select EBU 3.0. On the other hand if it is too small; choose EBU3.75 or above. If the position of the left ostium is found superiorly, EBU 3.0 would be the most appropriate. For circumflex lesions; larger sized catheter provides better support (Fig 10.13).

Question 17: What are the different types of aortic arches, and their relationships with catheter choice? Distal origin of the brachiocephalic trunk from aortic arch and subclavian-brachiocephalic tortuosities are frequently encountered in the elderly and hypertensive patients. Thus understanding the different anatomy of aortic arch then selecting the appropriate Guiding catheter are key elements for successful transradial PCI (Fig. 10.15).

For the left coronary artery, when the distal cephalic arch origin becoming more distally to the ascending aorta, the greater sized catheter is needed for sufficient support (Fig. 10.16).

Likewise, For the right coronary artery, when the distal cephalic arch origin becoming more distally to the ascending aorta, the larger sized catheter should be chosen for engaging RCA to ensure a better backup (Fig. 10.17).

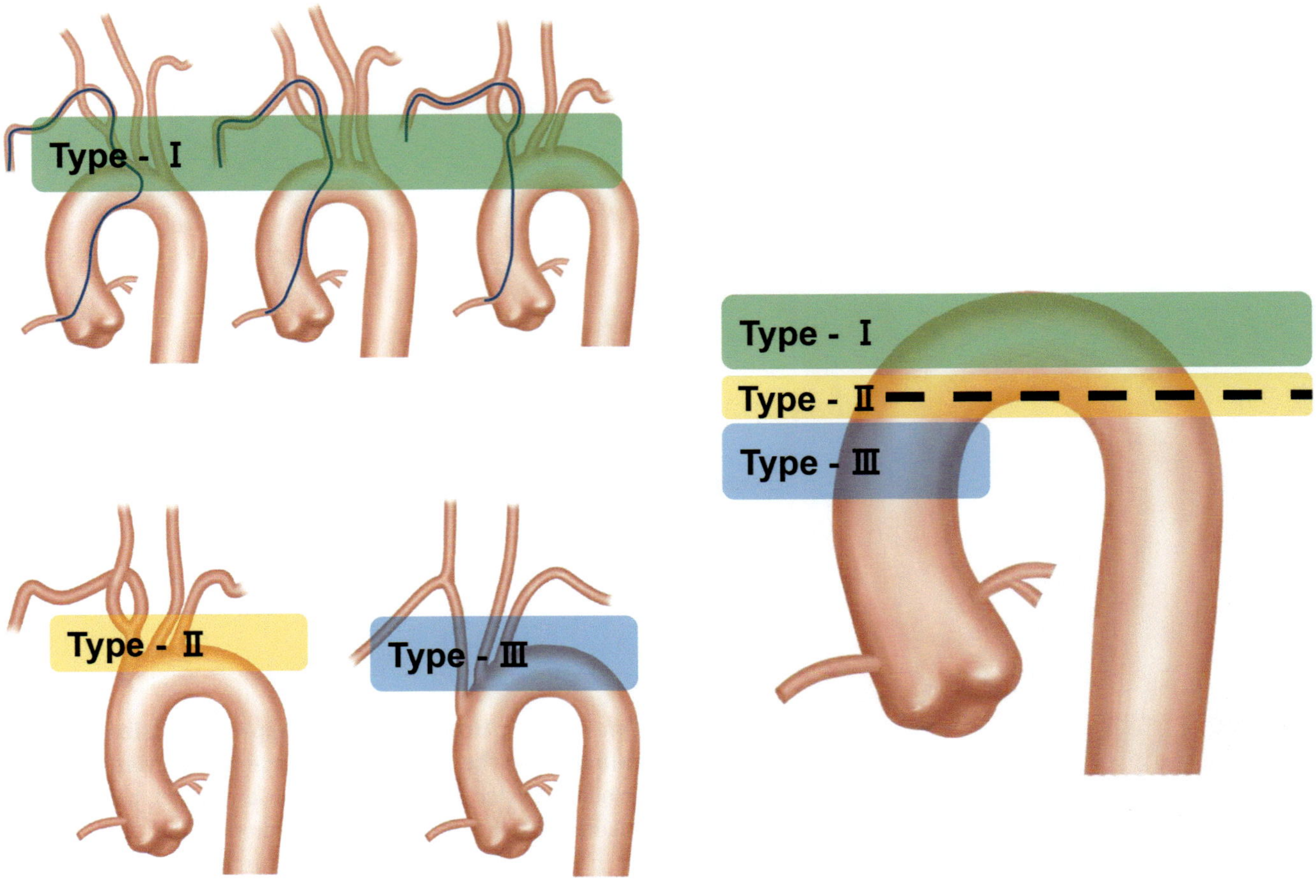

Fig. 10.15 Three different types of cephalic arch. Type I arch. The arch vessels arise from the outer curvature of the arch in the same horizontal plane (no angulation). Type II arch. The arch vessels arise between the parallel planes delineated by the outer and inner curves of the arch (moderate angulation). Type III arch. The arch vessels arise proximal or caudal to the lesser curvature of the arch or off the ascending aorta (severe angulation)

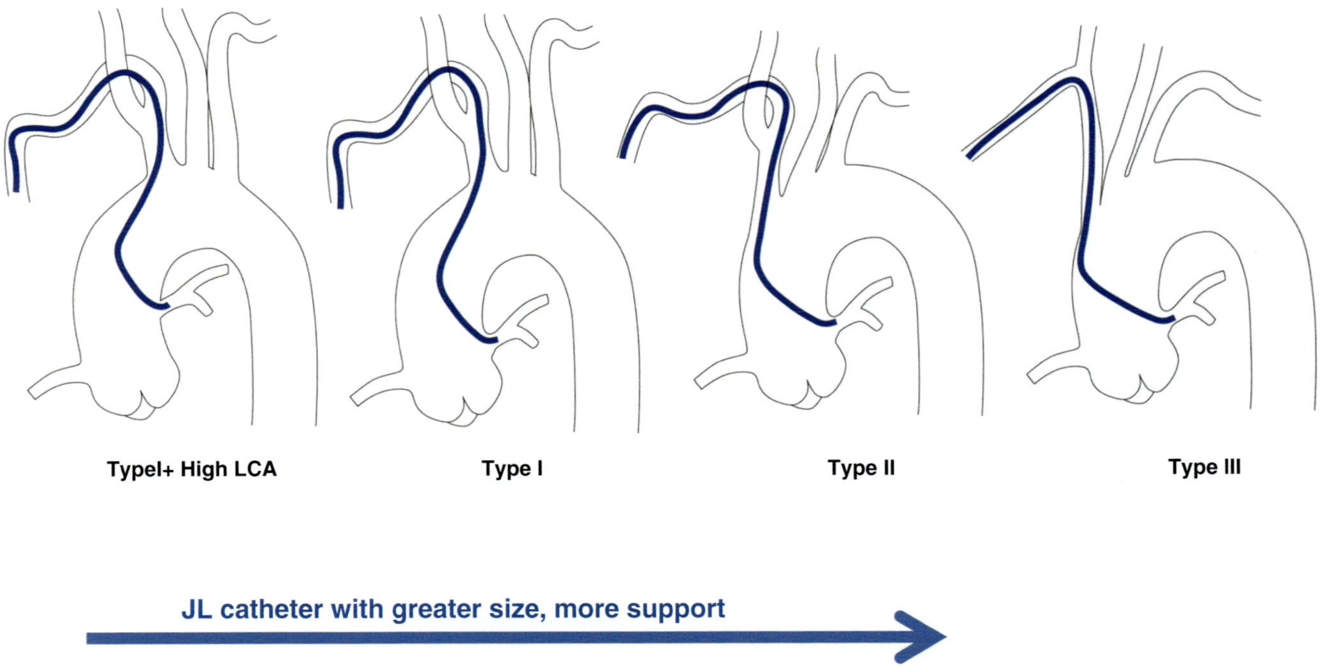

Fig. 10.16 Choose of JL catheter according to different types of cephalic arch

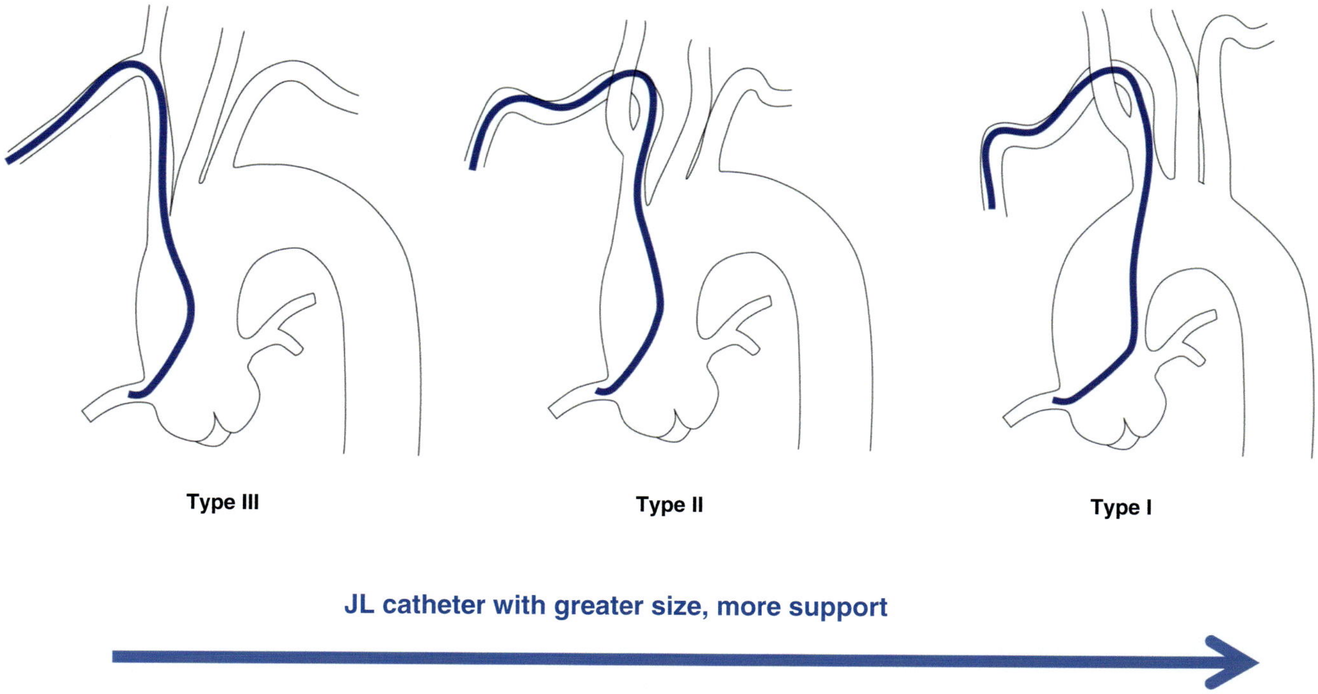

Fig. 10.17 Choose of JR catheter according to different types of cephalic arch

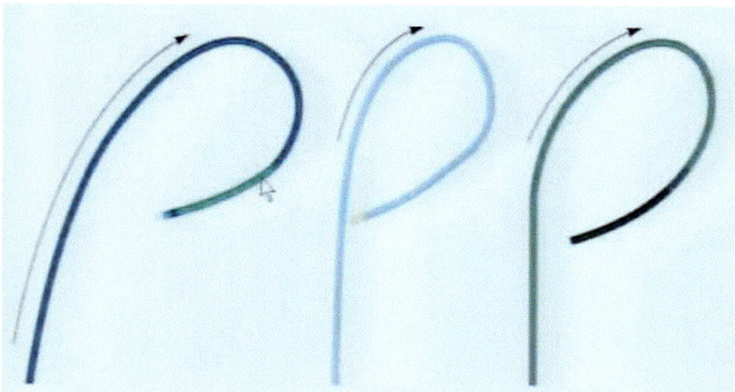

Fig. 10.18 The differences among various extra back guiding catheter from different manufacturers? EBU (Laucher, Medtronic U.S), XB (Vista brite tip, Cordis U.S) BL (Heartrail Terumo Japan)

Question 18: Are there any differences among various guiding catheter from different manufacturers? In our institution, the most commonly used guiding catheter are made by the 3 manufacturers Fig. 10.18:

1. CORDIS (Vista Brite tip)
2. MEDTRONIC (Launcher)
3. TERUMO (heartrail)

The stiffness and formability are the main differences found between the catheters. The stiffness decreases as we go down the list while the formability increases. This concludes that the latter manufacturers' guiding catheter can conform better with severely torturous arteries at the sacrifice of back-up support. The heartrail guiding catheter (from Terumo Jp) present superior tractability to cross even spastic radial and brachial artery or severely tortuous subclavian artery when other guides fail. The soft tip made this catheter less traumatic. However, since the support of BL catheter (Back up left) is relatively weak, most operators do not chose it as the default guiding catheter but EBU (Launcher) is regarded as most widely used guiding catheter for left coronary artery cannulation. The new generation of Vista brite tip, "Adroit" by CORDIS, provides larger lumen diameter as well as improved conformability function.

Reference

1. Sarkar K, Sharma SK, Kini AS. Catheter selection for coronary angiography and intervention in anomalous right coronary arteries. J Interv Cardiol. 2009;22:234–9.

Part III

Transradial Approach for Complex Intervention

11 Transradial PCI for Complex PCI: An Overview

Sunil V. Rao

Abstract

As outlined in this textbook, radial approach for angiography and coronary intervention is rapidly growing worldwide. This adoption is being driven by improved safety over the traditional femoral approach and by studies demonstrating lower costs and patient preference for radial access. Details of these studies are reviewed elsewhere in this text and strongly support the use of radial approach to achieve the best outcomes, in terms of bleeding or vascular complications, at the lowest cost. An equally important issue is whether radial access can achieve similar *efficacy* to femoral approach – namely, can complex PCI be performed successfully via radial approach? In order to examine this issue appropriately, it is important to review the existing data comparing radial with femoral approach for procedure success, determine whether ad hoc PCI can be performed after transradial diagnostic angiography, and whether a "radial first" approach can be used for all lesion subset.

11.1 PCI Success

The traditional definition of PCI success in coronary intervention varied according to whether a stent was placed. Since the vast majority of PCIs involve the placement of a stent, the angioplasty definition is less relevant. In the stent era, procedure success is generally defined as at least a 50 % reduction in diameter stenosis and ≤20 % residual stenosis [1]. This definition pre-supposes that the lesion has been crossed with a guidewire, guide support has been sufficient to deliver devices to dilate the lesion, and that the stent has been successfully deployed across it. For a transradial PCI, all of this requires that radial access was successfully achieved, the arm and chest arterial vasculature was negotiated, diagnostic catheters were advanced into the ascending aorta and cannulated the coronary arteries to provide adequate opacification during angiography, and the guide catheter successfully intubated the coronary artery ostium.

Many observational studies have compared radial approach with femoral approach, but selection bias and confounding hamper the validity of these data. In order to determine which of the two approaches are superior, randomization is key. The largest randomized trial comparing radial and femoral is the RIVAL trial, which randomized over 7000 patients with acute coronary syndrome (with or without ST-segment elevation) undergoing angiography or intervention to either radial access or femoral access [2]. PCI success, a secondary endpoint, was defined as partial or full, with full success defined as successful dilation of all attempted lesions with <50 % residual stenosis and TIMI 3 flow. There was no significant difference between the two approaches (radial 95.4 % vs. femoral 95.2 %, p=0.83). While angiographic details of the PCI procedures are not available, 65.9–66.8 % of patients underwent PCI, which is consistent with the proportions seen in national registries [3]. This suggests that PCI was not likely deferred due to the access site chosen.

11.2 Access Site Crossover

An important dimension to the concept of PCI success is that the definition does not take into account whether the procedure was ultimately completed using the initial arterial access site. Therefore, the issue of *procedure success* versus *PCI*

S.V. Rao
Duke University Medical Center, Durham, NC, USA
e-mail: sunil.rao@duke.edu

Y. Zhou et al. (eds.), *Transradial Approach for Percutaneous Interventions*, DOI 10.1007/978-94-017-7350-8_11

success must take into account access site crossover from radial to another arterial site (most commonly the femoral artery). In this context, proficiency with transradial procedures is of paramount importance. The RIVAL Trial investigators were required to have some experience with transradial procedures in order to participate. The requirement was for at least 50 transradial procedures within the prior year, although many operators had significant proficiency, performing > 142 procedures annually [2]. Access site crossover occurred in 7.6 % of patients assigned to radial access and 2.0 % of patients assigned to femoral access [hazard ratio 3.82 (2.93–4.97); $p < 0.0001$]. At centers with the highest volumes, access site crossover was much lower (4.4 %), but still higher in the radial arm. These data demonstrate that transradial procedure success (as opposed to PCI success) exceeds 90 % when performed by experienced operators.

11.3 Ad hoc PCI

Ad hoc PCI is a PCI procedure performed subsequent to a diagnostic catheterization during the same cath lab visit. The incidence of ad hoc PCI in the large US-based National Cardiovascular Data Registry CathPCI registry is > 50 %, but this likely varies across different countries. The performance of transradial ad hoc PCI assumes that the diagnostic portion of the procedure was performed via radial access. Transradial ad hoc PCI is feasible for several reasons. First, the diagnostic catheterization will provide detail on arm and subclavian arterial anatomy, which may allow for easier seating of the guide catheter. Studies examining procedure times and radiation exposure have shown that increases associated with radial approach are generally limited to the diagnostic cath with no significant difference for PCI [1]. Second, as stated above, data from the RIVAL trial indicate no difference in the proportion of patients undergoing PCI between radial and femoral access, thus indicating that PCI was not deferred based on the initial access site. Finally, the learning curve for becoming proficient at transradial procedures is not steep – approximately 30–50 cases [4] – and is easily overcome by performing ad hoc PCI.

11.4 "Radial First" Approach for All Lesions

The term "radial first" means that every procedure is approached with intent to start and end the case with radial access. While this may seem straightforward for Type A lesions, the issue is whether this can be applied to more complex lesions like heavily calcified stenoses, bifurcation lesions, unprotected left main stenosis, or chronic total occlusions. Technical aspects of transradial PCI of each of these lesion subsets are described in detail in the following chapters. In summary, the radial approach offers few limitations since almost all lesions can be successfully treated through 6-French systems, which are readily accommodated by the radial artery in most patients. Larger bore guide catheters can be used with or without a sheath, if appropriate, to minimize radial artery trauma. Dedicated transradial 7.5-French sheathless guide catheters are commercially available [5]. These guides have outer diameters of 2.49 mm (compared with an outer diameter of 2.52 mm for 6-French sheaths), and their inner luminal diameter easily accommodates two stents simultaneously. They are introduced into the ascending aorta over a 0.035″ standard guidewire. A long tapered dilator facilitates entry through the skin. Procedure success for complex PCI is excellent with these guides, but radial artery occlusion rates may not be lower compared with the use of arterial sheaths [5]. From and colleagues have described a sheathless approach using standard 7-French and 8-French guide catheters [6]. A long (125 cm) 5 or 6-French diagnostic angiographic catheter is placed through a standard length 7 or 8-French guide to facilitate entry through the skin into the radial artery.

Calcified lesions present a challenge for stent delivery and lesion dilation (i.e., procedure success). Adjunctive devices like rotational atherectomy and orbital atherectomy can ablate plaque to facilitate stent placement and expansion. Rotational atherectomy burrs up to 1.75 mm can be placed through 6-French guide catheters. Larger burrs require bigger guide catheters and commercially available sheathless guides can be used, or a system can be set up using the mother-in-child technique [6]. Alternatively, a 7-French sheath can be used in patients with radial arteries large enough to accommodate it. The orbital atherectomy device from CSI has a crown that is 6-French compatible and operates at 2 speeds, 80,000 RPM and 120,000 RPM, to ablate calcification and create different size lumens.

Most bifurcation stenting techniques can be performed through 6-French guide catheters. Techniques such as the "sequential mini-crush," "balloon crush," and "culotte stenting," as well as provisional stenting using the "T," "V", or "Y" approaches are all feasible via 6-French radial access and have been previously described [7–10]. In addition, Yang and colleagues have retrospectively compared radial and femoral approaches to unprotected Left Main PCI showing similar rates of procedure success [9]. The majority of the radial cases in this series were performed using 6-French systems and the balloon crush technique. Kissing balloon inflation with two rapid exchange non-compliant balloons can also be accomplished through 6-French guides.

Simultaneous two-stent techniques such as "simultaneous kissing stents" or variations of the two-stent crush technique require 7-French or larger guide catheters. Although the optimal two-stent approach has not been identified, operators wishing to use simultaneous two-stent techniques via the radial approach are faced with a challenge due to the relatively small caliber of the radial artery in many patients. Again, larger bore guide catheters can be used either with or without a sheath depending on the size of the radial artery.

Advanced techniques for recanalization of chronic total occlusions (CTOs) include procedures requiring access to collaterals for retrograde approaches. In addition, deliberate subintimal tracking of wires often necessitates supportive guide catheters and occasionally large bore guides. The feasibility of a "bi-radial" approach for complex CTOs has been described with the limitation that procedure and fluoroscopy times may be longer than with a bi-femoral approach [11].

Conclusion

The technique and technology of transradial procedures has evolved significantly over the past decade. This evolution has led to increased feasibility of radial approach for all patients while preserving its safety. Most lesions are addressable with 6-French guide catheters that are readily accommodated by most radial arteries. For procedures that require larger bore guides, sheathless techniques can be used. The published literature demonstrates no difference in PCI success between radial and femoral access when experienced operators perform the procedures. In addition, proficiency increases overall procedure success by reducing the rate of femoral crossover. Once the shallow learning curve is overcome, a "radial first" approach for all lesions is not only possible, but preferred.

References

1. Rao SV, Ou FS, Wang TY, Roe MT, Brindis R, Rumsfeld JS, Peterson ED. Trends in the prevalence and outcomes of radial and femoral approaches to percutaneous coronary intervention: a report from the national cardiovascular data registry. JACC Cardiovasc Interv. 2008;1:379–86.
2. Jolly SS, Yusuf S, Cairns J, Niemela K, Xavier D, Widimsky P, Budaj A, Niemela M, Valentin V, Lewis BS, Avezum A, Steg PG, Rao SV, Gao P, Afzal R, Joyner CD, Chrolavicius S, Mehta SR. Radial versus femoral access for coronary angiography and intervention in patients with acute coronary syndromes (RIVAL): a randomised, parallel group, multicentre trial. Lancet. 2011;377: 1409–20.
3. Dehmer GJ, Weaver D, Roe MT, Milford-Beland S, Fitzgerald S, Hermann A, Messenger J, Moussa I, Garratt K, Rumsfeld J, Brindis RG. A contemporary view of diagnostic cardiac catheterization and percutaneous coronary intervention in the United States: a report from the CathPCI Registry of the National Cardiovascular Data Registry, 2010 through June 2011. J Am Coll Cardiol. 2012;60: 2017–31.
4. Hess CN, Peterson ED, Neely ML, Dai D, Hillegass WB, Krucoff MW, Kutcher MA, Messenger JC, Pancholy S, Piana RN, Rao SV. The Learning Curve for Transradial Percutaneous Coronary Intervention among Operators in the United States: A Study from the National Cardiovascular Data Registry(R). Circulation. 2014;129:2277–86.
5. Mamas M, D'Souza S, Hendry C, Ali R, Iles-Smith H, Palmer K, El-Omar M, Fath-Ordoubadi F, Neyses L, Fraser DG. Use of the sheathless guide catheter during routine transradial percutaneous coronary intervention: a feasibility study. Catheter Cardiovasc Interv. 2010;75:596–602.
6. From AM, Gulati R, Prasad A, Rihal CS. Sheathless transradial intervention using standard guide catheters. Catheter Cardiovasc Interv. 2010;76:911–6.
7. Lim PO, Dzavik V. Balloon crush: treatment of bifurcation lesions using the crush stenting technique as adapted for transradial approach of percutaneous coronary intervention. Catheter Cardiovasc Interv. 2004;63:412–6.
8. Mamas MA, Fath-Ordoubadi F, Fraser DG. Atraumatic complex transradial intervention using large bore sheathless guide catheter. Catheter Cardiovasc Interv. 2008;72:357–64.
9. Yang YJ, Kandzari DE, Gao Z, Xu B, Chen JL, Qiao SB, Li JJ, Qin XW, Yao M, Wu YJ, Yuan JQ, Chen J, Liu HB, Dai J, Chen T, Wang Y, Li W, Gao RL. Transradial versus transfemoral method of percutaneous coronary revascularization for unprotected left main coronary artery disease: comparison of procedural and late-term outcomes. JACC Cardiovasc Interv. 2010;3:1035–42.
10. Liang M, Puri A, Linder R. Transradial simultaneous kissing stenting (SKS) with SheathLess access. Catheter Cardiovasc Interv. 2010;75:222–4.
11. Rinfret S, Joyal D, Nguyen CM, Bagur R, Hui W, Leung R, Larose E, Love MP, Mansour S. Retrograde recanalization of chronic total occlusions from the transradial approach; early Canadian experience. Catheter Cardiovasc Interv. 2011;78:366–74.

Transradial Approach for STEMI: A General View

12

Josef Ludwig

Abstract

The PAMI trials Stone et al. [1] suggested that angioplasty provides clinical advantage over thrombolytic therapy with t-PA.in patients presenting with acute ST-elevation myocardial infarction. Significant advantages for primary stenting were found for death (2.7 % vs. 0.6 %, p=*0.03),* re-infarction or infarct-related artery (IRA) closure (5.1 % vs. 1.3 %, p=0.002) Stone et al. [1]. Since then, primary angioplasty combined with stent deployment is considered the default method for myocardial reperfusion in STEMI patients. According to ESC and ACC/AHA guidelines the **placement of a stent (bare-metal stent [BMS] or drug-eluting stent [DES]) is useful in primary PCI for patients with STEMI (*Level of Evidence: A*).** However, bleeding complications still represent the Achilles's heel of primary PCI (PPCI). When the femoral artery is used as the approaching vessel, local hemorrhagic complications, especially in the era of potent antithrombotics, are not rare. The relevance of such bleeding complications must not be underestimated [2, 3]. In fact, recent studies have suggested that peri-procedural bleeding complications after PCI are associated with increased short- and long-term morbidity and mortality. Therefore, reducing the number of bleeding events is an area of major importance in the modern treatment of acute coronary syndromes.

Radial angioplasty was introduced by Kiemeneij et al. [4] more than 20 years ago. He and his colleagues clearly demonstrated thar the radial access reduces bleeding events, increased patient comfort and decreased the duration of hospital stay for elective coronary interventions. Following Dr. Kiemeneij's work, small scale randomized observational studies as well as meta-analysis were performed to compare radial versus femoral access regarding the outcome of primary PCI [5–7].

12.1 Evidence of Transradial Versus Transfemoral Approach in Primary PCI

Recently, De Luca et al. [8] performed a comprehensive meta-analysis of randomized and non-randomized trials comparing transradial versus transfemoral approach in primary angioplasty for STEMI. The literature was scanned by searching electronic databases (MEDLINE, Pubmed) for relevant publications between January 1990 and October 2012. A total of 27 publications were included, of which 11 reported on randomized trials. The analysis comprised a total of 29,194 patients of whom radial PCI had been performed in 10,052 patients (34.5 %). The authors used 30-day mortality as the primary endpoint of data analysis and further evaluated long-term mortality (range 2–6 years) after the index PCI. A total of 2069 patients (8.75) died at 30 day follow-up. Of note, radial access was associated with a significant reduction in mortality (5.2 % vs. 10.3 %; $p<0.001$). The benefits in mortality were also seen at long-term follow-up (6.6 % vs. 10 %; $p<0.001$). Major bleeding complications were observed in 808 patients (2.8 %). Bleedings were significantly less frequent in the radial group (1.9 % vs.

J. Ludwig
Beijing, China
e-mail: josef.ludwig@web.de

Y. Zhou et al. (eds.), *Transradial Approach for Percutaneous Interventions*, DOI 10.1007/978-94-017-7350-8_12

4.7 %; $p < 0.001$). Both benefits in death and major bleeding complications were not related to baseline risk profile. The profound importance of this meta-analysis by De Luca et al. is the inclusion of observational studies in addition to randomized trials, because randomized trials have strict inclusion and exclusion criteria and, thus, may not fully represent clinical practice. De Luca et al, however, found significant reductions in mortality in both types of publications. Interestingly, they observed a greater reduction in major bleedings in the observational study group when compared to the randomized group. A potential publication bias could be excluded as depicted as funnel plot. A funnel plot is a useful graph designed to check the existence of publication bias in systematic reviews and meta-analysis.

The British Cardiovascular Intervention Society found that the use of radial access for PPCI (primary PCI) has steadily increased over time from 7.6 % in 2008 to 32.7 % procedures in 2011. As it became evident that patients with acute coronary syndromes (ACS) have higher rates of bleeding complications than those without ACS, and, that bleedings result in higher morbidity and mortality, a debate has emerged as to whether radial access could have better clinical outcomes compared to femoral access PPCI. Nine studies were included in the analysis by The National Institute for Health and Care Excellence on Myocardial Infarction with ST segment elevation and their findings are given as Forest plots. The results which exactly mirror those of De Luca et al. [8] are not depicted. Taken together, this randomized trials included in this review provide evidence that radial arterial access for PPCI is associated with lower short-term all-cause mortality and reduce bleeding when compared with femoral arterial access. In addition, radial arterial access is associated with fewer vascular access site complications and shorter hospital stay, but more access site crossover. There was no evidence of benefit of radial arterial access PPCI versus femoral arterial access for the outcome of stroke (Fig. 12.1a, b).

The association between access and non-access site bleeding and mortality in people with acute coronary syndrome has been the subject of intense research over the last decade [9]. Hypothetical mechanisms link bleeding and mortality in acute coronary syndrome include the hemodynamic consequences of blood loss, complications related to blood transfusion, and the need to modify antithrombotic medication. Nevertheless, a clear causal relationship between bleeding and mortality has not been confirmed and it is possible that major bleeding simply identifies people with an underlying mortality risk. According to data analysis by The National Institute for Health and Care Excellence on Myocardial Infarction with ST segment elevation the following statement was given.

In all-cause mortality Radial access PPCI has a clinically effective association when compared to femoral access PPCI with reduced all-cause mortality rates at ≤ 30 days [8 studies, $n = 3825$]. Radial access PPCI potentially has a clinically effective association when compared to femoral access PPCI with reduced all-cause mortality in the longer term, but the direction of the estimate of effect could favor either intervention [2 studies, $n = 306$].

Regarding reinfarction Radial access PPCI potentially has a clinically effective association when compared to femoral access PPCI at reducing reinfarction rates at ≤ 30 days, but the direction of the estimate of the effect could favor either intervention [7 studies, $n = 3661$]. However, femoral access PPCI potentially has a clinically effective association when compared to radial access PPCI with reduced reinfarction rates in the longer term, but the direction of the estimate of effect could favor either intervention [2 studies, $n = 306$].

In major bleeding incidence and repeat revascularization rates Radial access PPCI potentially has a clinically effective association when compared to femoral access PPCI with reduced major bleeding incidence at ≤ 30 days [10] [8 studies, $n = 3825$]. Evidence suggested that there may be no clinical difference between radial access PPCI and femoral access PPCI with an association with repeat revascularization rates at ≤ 30 days, but the direction of the estimate of effect could favor either intervention [5 studies, $n = 1558$]. Very low quality evidence also suggested that there may be no clinical difference between radial access PPCI and femoral access PPCI with repeat revascularization rates in the longer term, but the direction of the estimate of effect could favor either intervention [2 studies, $n = 308$].

In stroke incidence No clinical difference between the association of radial access PPCI and femoral access PPCI with reduced stroke incidence at ≤ 30 day [3 studies, $n = 3059$].

In access site crossover Low quality evidence showed that femoral access PPCI was more clinically effective when compared radial access PPCI at reducing rate of access site crossover during PPCI [9 studies, $n = 4195$].

In fluoroscopy time The analysis showed that there is no clinical difference between radial access PPCI and femoral access PPCI and PPCI procedural success [9 studies, $n = 3903$]. Fluoroscopy time of PPCI showed that there was no clinical difference between radial access PPCI and femoral access PPCI at fluoroscopy time [5 studies, $n = 671$].

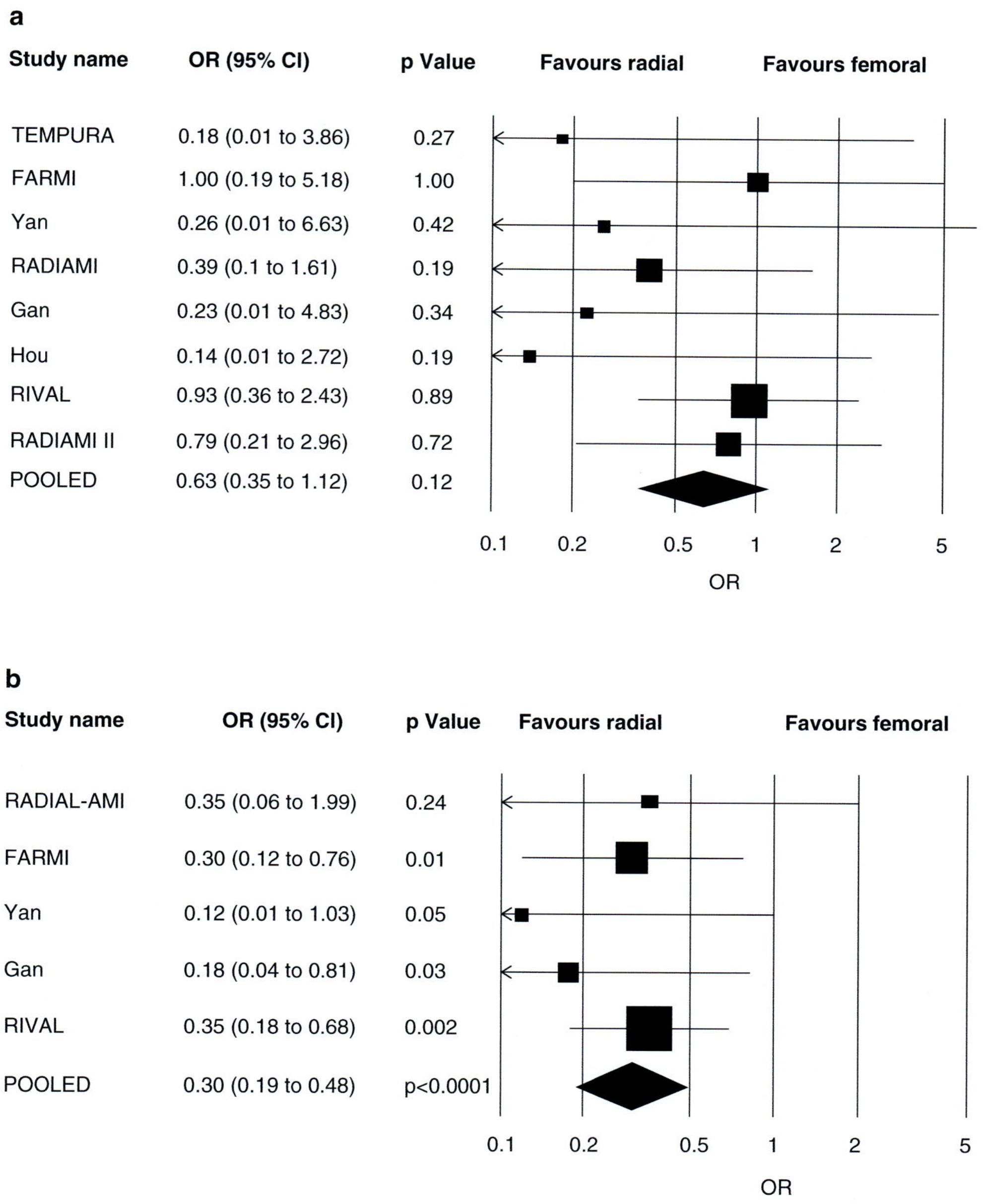

Fig. 12.1 (**a**, **b**) It assumes that the largest studies will be near the average, and small studies will be evenly spread on both sides of the average. Deviation from this assumption can indicate publication bias. Of note, similar to confidence interval plots, funnel plots are conventionally drawn with the treatment effect measure on the horizontal axis, so that study size appears on the vertical axis (Reprint with permission from Ref. [8])

In total radiographic contrast media use Total radiographic contrast media used during PPCI procedure suggested that there may be no clinical difference between radial access PPCI and femoral access PPCI at reducing total radiographic contrast media use, but the direction of the estimate of effect could favor either intervention [4 studies, n = 471].

In reducing vascular access site complications Radial access PPCI is more clinically effective when compared to femoral access PPCI at reducing vascular access site complications at ≤30 days [4 studies, n = 2416].

In reducing hospital stay Additional evidence showed that radial access PPCI was more clinically effective when compared with femoral access PPCI at reducing hospital stay [4 studies, n = 644].

In procedure length Very low quality evidence showed that femoral access PPCI is more clinically effective when compared with radial access at reducing procedure length [7 studies, n=1235].

In cost analysis One original comparative cost analysis found that PPCI carried out by femoral access was more costly than PPCI carried out by radial access. There was insufficient evidence to reliably predict the size of the cost difference. This analysis was assessed as directly applicable with minor limitations.

Cardiogenic shock Cardiogenic shock remains the leading cause of mortality in patients hospitalized with AMI. Even though TRA has become increasingly adopted as a default PCI; however, even in experienced centers that favor the radial artery as the primary access site during PCI, patients presenting in CS are often treated via the transfemoral access site (TFA); and commentators have suggested that CS remains the final frontier even for experienced radial operators. However, even in cardiogenic shock, recent studies showed that the transradial access site was independently associated with a lower 30-day mortality, in-hospital major adverse cardiac and cerebrovascular events and major bleeding [11, 12]. In addition to lower bleeding rates, transradial PCI in patients with cardiogenic shock has the advantage of preserving bilateral femoral access for hemodynamic support devices such as IABP, impeller, ECMO and others.

12.2 Strategy of Anticoagulant and Antiplatelet Therapy During Primary PCI

Recently, Lee MS et al. stated that the benefits of radial over femoral PPCI were strongly influenced by suboptimal antithrombotic regimens as well as liberal use of potent parenteral antiplatelet agents [13]. Thus, the influence of access site alone on outcomes could be accurately measured. Radial access and bivalirudin usage. In the National Cardiovascular Data Registry it was found that the combination of radial access and bivalirudin anticoagulation is associated with a significant reduction in post-PCI bleeding compared with either radial access alone or the combination of femoral access, bivalirudin, and a vascular closure device. The overall bleeding rate was 2.59 %: 2.71 % in the femoral group, 2.5 % in the radial group, and 1.8 % in radial access-bivalirudin group ($P<0.001$) The authors calculated the relative risk of bleeding events for radial combination therapy to be 0.79 (0.72–0.86), as compared to 0.96 (0.88–1.05) for radial only. The numbers are given as adjusted OR (95 % CI). However, the limitation of the reported data is that they are observational. Moreover, the data of the US National Cardiovascular Data Registry are contrasted by, the report by the European Ambulance Acute Coronary Syndrome Angiography (EUROMAX) trial. This trial had been designed to test whether bivalirudin given already during transport for STEMI is superior to heparins with regards to major bleedings. The results showed that radial access was not associated with major bleedings or patients' outcomes at 30 days. This trial, however, was not conducted and powered to show superiority or non-inferiority of one access site over the other. In addition, it should be mentioned, that in EUROMAX acute stent thrombosis was more frequent with bivalirudin (1.1 % vs. 0.2 %; $p=0.07$) compared to heparin.

In summary, there are still some controversies regarding the access site in PPCI. Indeed, a large randomized trial designed to evaluate bleeding outcomes in patients referred for primary PCI assigned to either TRA or TFA has yet to be published and no trial has been designed which includes bivalirudin as the routine anticoagulant used for PPCI. Consequently, the SAFARI-STEMI trial was designed, a trial to specifically address the bleeding differences between TRA and TFA using the direct thrombin inhibitor bivalirudin in the two groups. If TRA is shown to be equally safe or safer than TFA, this may influence interventional cardiologists to change their practice for primary PCI in favor of TRI. In addition to all objective data, TRI also provides better patient comfort, cost-effectiveness and, last not least, usually constitutes patient preference especially amongst elderly patients. Never investigated, but commonly accepted, is the discreteness of the puncture site at the wrist far from the pubic area. Thus, The Task Force on the Management of ST-Segment Elevation Acute Myocardial Infarction of the European Society of Cardiology (ESC) recommended TRI as a Class II A-Level B indication for PPCI as long as performed by experienced radial operators. (Published in European Heart Journal, 2012) [14].

Therefore operator and volume center activity will strongly influence successful development of a radial PPCI program. As recently outlined by Hamon et al. [15] 2013. The recommendations are printed in italic letters (see below).

12.3 Learning Curve for Primary PCI

The radial approach is a demanding technique, requiring expertise in both the operator and his/her team. Inability to puncture or cannulate the radial artery, inability to select the coronary artery and insufficient support to perform PCI is minimised by experience. An operator's annual procedure volume of more than 80 transradial cases correlates with a significant reduction in access failure, sheath insertion time and procedure time [17].

To achieve the best results in TRI, individual operators and institutional teams should aim at maintaining the highest feasible rate of TRI. However, a reasonable objective for achieving an average satisfactory proficiency is aiming, after

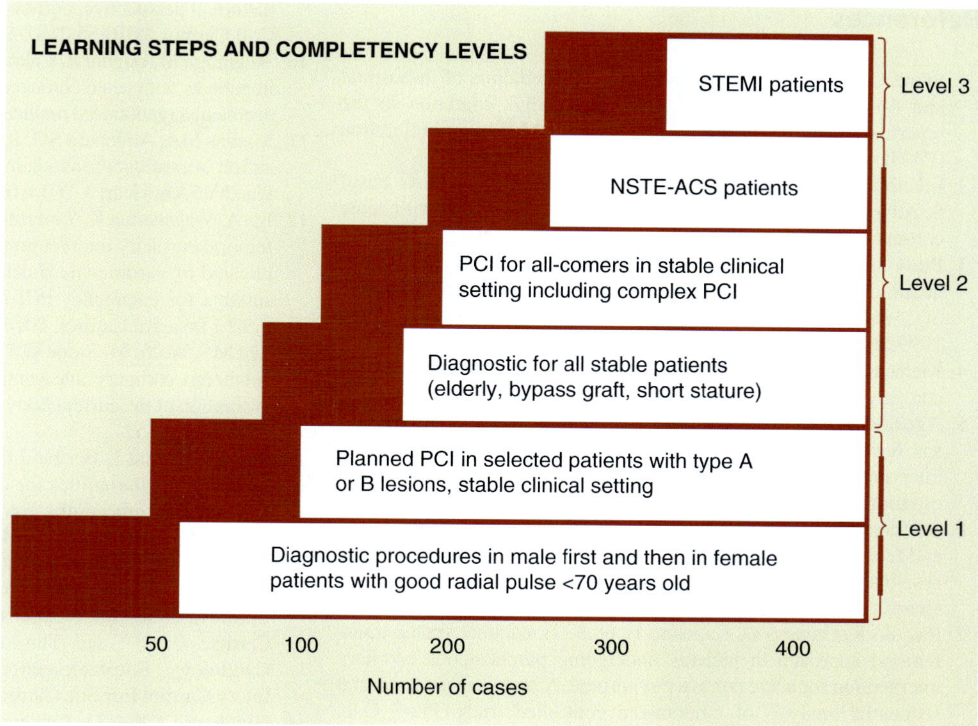

Fig. 12.2 Proposed framework for learning steps and competency levels for TRI. ACS-PCI is proposed as the last step (NSTEMI and STEMI patients), due to expected anatomical variations and to less suitable clinical settings, where time constraints and/or complex pharmacological and clinical management are often required during the procedure [15]

the learning curve has been completed, for over 50 % radial access in routine practice with a minimum of 80 procedures/year per operator (including diagnostic and interventional procedures).

Figure 12.2 *shows the proposed framework for the required learning steps to finally achieve the necessary skills for doing PPCI by radial access (Hamon et al. 2013). Such a step by step learning will reduce cross-over rates to TFI, facilitate immediate radial arterial access and quickly overcome anatomic variations due to the radial route.*

Finally, it has been suggested that thrombectomy prior to stenting could be a new option to better treat STEMI prior to stenting. Theoretically this could limit radial access as of larger size catheters needed for this procedure. However, most of the available thrombectomy devices are now 6 F compatible and, thus, there is no real restriction to perform "thrombus aspiration- PPCI" through the radial. But, as of now, thrombus aspiration during primary PCI for people with acute STEMI is not generally recommended (National Clinical Guideline Centre, 2013).

12.4 In Conclusion

For all those familiar with transradial access, the available body of evidence should be an encouragement to use it in these patients who need it most, namely, the patients at highest risk for bleeding complication like STEMI patients. Especially if co-morbid, elderly and frail Table 12.1.

Table 12.1 Summarize the advantage and disadvantage of TR approach for STEMI patients [16]

	TR approach
Advantage	Reduce access bleeding
	Reduce cost and hospital stay
	Reduce access complications
	Safety after higher dose of antiplatelet and anticoagulation or thrombolytic therapy
	Improved survival
	No limitations of thrombectomy aspiration
	Save femoral routes for hemodynamic support
Disadvantage	Procedural metrics and outcomes[a] are dependent on transradial case volume
	Potential for femoral crossover
	Lack of standardized transradial training programs
	Inability to use same entry site to insert hemodynamic support systems like intra-aortic balloon pump
	Catheter size is limited by radial artery caliber
	Longer D2B time for beginners
	Longer procedure time for anatomy difficulties patients; tortuous subclavian etc

[a]Includes radiation exposure, procedure time, D2BT, procedure success rate

Key points Transradial approach, transfemoral approach, anticoagulant and antiplatelet therapy

References

1. Stone GW, Grines CL, Browne KF, et al. Predictors of in-hospital and 6-month outcome after acute myocardial infarction in the reperfusion era: the Primary Angioplasty in Myocardial Infarction (PAMI) trail. J Am Coll Cardiol. 1995;25:370–7.
2. Eikelboom JW, Mehta SR, Anand SS, Xie C, Fox KA, Yusuf S. Adverse impact of bleeding on prognosis in patients with acute coronary syndromes. Circulation. 2006;114:774–82.
3. Psaty BM, Weiss NS, Furberg CD, et al. Surrogate end points, health outcomes, and the drug-approval process for the treatment of risk factors for cardiovascular disease. JAMA. 1999;282:786–90.
4. Kiemeneij F, Laarman GJ. Percutaneous transradial artery approach for coronary stent implantation. Cathet Cardiovasc Diagn. 1993;30:173–8.
5. Agostoni P, Biondi-Zoccai GG, de Benedictis ML, et al. Radial versus femoral approach for percutaneous coronary diagnostic and interventional procedures; systematic overview and meta-analysis of randomized trials. J Am Coll Cardiol. 2004;44:349–56.
6. Bertrand OF, Belisle P, Joyal D, et al. Comparison of transradial and femoral approaches for percutaneous coronary interventions: a systematic review and hierarchical Bayesian meta-analysis. Am Heart J. 2012;163:632–48.
7. Piccolo R, Galasso G, Capuano E, et al. Transradial versus transfemoral approach in patients undergoing percutaneous coronary intervention for acute coronary syndrome. A meta-analysis and trial sequential analysis of randomized controlled trials. PLoS One. 2014;9:e96127.
8. De Luca G, Schaffer A, Wirianta J, Suryapranata H. Comprehensive meta-analysis of radial vs femoral approach in primary angioplasty for STEMI. Int J Cardiol. 2013;168:2070–81.
9. Rao SV, Cohen MG, Kandzari DE, Bertrand OF, Gilchrist IC. The transradial approach to percutaneous coronary intervention: historical perspective, current concepts, and future directions. J Am Coll Cardiol. 2010;55:2187–95.
10. Valgimigli M, Gagnor A, Calabro P, et al. Radial versus femoral access in patients with acute coronary syndromes undergoing invasive management: a randomised multicentre trial. Lancet. 2015;385:2465–76.
11. Mamas MA, Anderson SG, Ratib K, et al. Arterial access site utilization in cardiogenic shock in the United Kingdom: is radial access feasible? Am Heart J. 2014;167:900–8.e1.
12. Iga A, Wagatsuma K, Yamazaki J, Ikeda T. Transradial versus transfemoral coronary intervention for acute myocardial infarction complicated by cardiogenic shock: is transradial coronary intervention suitable for emergency PCI in high-risk acute myocardial infarction? J Invasive Cardiol. 2014;26:196–202.
13. Lee MS, Wolfe M, Stone GW. Transradial versus transfemoral percutaneous coronary intervention in acute coronary syndromes: re-evaluation of the current body of evidence. JACC Cardiovasc Interv. 2013;6:1149–52.
14. Rao SV, Bernat I, Bertrand OF. Clinical update: Remaining challenges and opportunities for improvement in percutaneous transradial coronary procedures. Eur Heart J. 2012;33:2521–6.
15. Hamon M, Pristipino C, Di Mario C, et al. Consensus document on the radial approach in percutaneous cardiovascular interventions: position paper by the European Association of Percutaneous Cardiovascular Interventions and Working Groups on Acute Cardiac Care** and Thrombosis of the European Society of Cardiology. EuroIntervention J EuroPCR Collab Work Group Interv Cardiol Eur Soc Cardiol. 2013;8:1242–51.
16. Hinohara TT, Rao SV. Current State of Radial Artery Catheterization in ST-Elevation Myocardial Infarction. Prog Cardiovasc Dis. 2015;58:241–6.
17. Ball WT, Sharieff W, Jolly SS, et al. Characterization of operator learning curve for transradial coronary interventions. Circ Cardiovasc Interv. 2011;4:336–41.

Transradial Approach for STEMI: From US Perspective

13

Syed Gilani

Abstract

Despite a significant interest in transradial percutaneous coronary intervention (PCI) in the United States (US), transradial primary percutaneous coronary intervention (PPCI) lags behind. Femoral approach continues to be the preferred approach for PPCI among most US interventional cardiologists.

13.1 Radial Versus Femoral Access for Primary Percutaneous Coronary Intervention (PPCI) in ST-Segment Elevation Myocardial Infarction in the United States (US)

Adoption of transradial PPCI has been slow in the US. Menees DS et al. [1] reviewed data on 96,738 admissions for patients undergoing PPCI for ST-segment elevation myocardial infarction (STEMI) from July 2005 through June 2009 at 515 hospitals across the US, participating in the CathPCI Registry of the National Cardiovascular Data Registry (NCDR). They found that femoral access was used for 98 % of all cases in 2005–2006 (vs. 0.7 % radial), and 98.5 % of all cases in 2008–2009 (vs. 1.0 % radial) suggesting no significant increase in radial approach for PPCI in STEMI during the period from 2005 to 2009.

Another NCDR data review from 2007 to 2011 found gradual but slow increase in use of radial access for PPCI in STEMI from just 0.9 % in 2007 to 6.4 % in 2011 [2]. Somewhat similar trend was reported by Nallamothu et al. in a contemporary analysis of patients undergoing PPCI using the NCDR CathPCI data [3]. Data showed gradual increase in transradial PPCI from 0.7 % in 2005 to 4.7 % in 2011 in the reported US STEMI patient population. The NCDR for fiscal year 2012–2013 reports only 18 % of all PCIs used radial access.

S. Gilani
Cardiology Department, University of Texas Medical Branch, Galveston, TX, USA
e-mail: sagilani@UTMB.EDU

Limiting, In a review of 2009–2010 STEMI patient data obtained from New York State's PCI Reporting System, only 7.6 % of the patients had radial access and 92.4 % of patients had femoral access for immediate primary or rescue PCI. Is this study, radial access increased from 4.9 % in the first quarter of 2009 to 11.9 % in the last quarter of 2010 suggesting slow increase in uptake of radial access for PCI in STEMI patients [4].

In an electronic survey of US interventional cardiologists (conducted by SCAI among its members, one of the survery question was, What is your preferred access approach for STEMI PCI? Femoral vs. Radial), only 17 % of the respondents preferred radial artery access (vs. 83 % femoral artery) for STEMI PCI [5].

Several factors as listed below are limiting the adoption of Radial access for PPCI in the US.

13.2 Learning Curve for Transradial PCI and Volume of PCI Among US Interventional Cardiologists

In the US, most interventional cardiologists are unfamiliar with transradial PPCI because they have been trained in programs using femoral access for PPCI [1]. These operators will require overcoming a significant learning curve before they become comfortable in performing transradial PPCIs. Trials comparing radial versus femoral access for PPCI using high volume operators showed no increase in reperfusion times when radial PPCI is performed by experienced radial operators. In the US, there is a large increase

Y. Zhou et al. (eds.), *Transradial Approach for Percutaneous Interventions*, DOI 10.1007/978-94-017-7350-8_13

in number of hospitals capable of performing PCI from 2001 to 2006 (1176 of 4609 in 2001, to 1695 of 4673 in 2006, a 44 % relative increase) without a significant increase (a mere 0.9 %) in the proportion of population with access to the procedure. Data from 2006 shows that 1695 of 4673 US hospitals (36 %) have a primary PCI program [6]. Meanwhile, the PCI volumes have been steadily declining within the Medicare population (data from 2001 to 2009) from the peak in 2004 [7]. According to the 2015 update of the heart disease and stroke statistics in the US, an estimated 954 000 inpatient PCI procedures were performed in the US in 2010, compared to 1 313 000 inpatient PCI procedures in 2006, thus showing declining PCI numbers over past several years [8]. Together, declining PCI volumes and the increasing number of the PCI centers has led to a decrease in the volume of PCI procedures at both the center and the operator level [9]. Thereby making it difficult for interventional cardiologists experienced in transfemoral approach to switch to transradial approach for PPCI.

In the US, PCI centers of excellence are not as developed as in Europe or Canada. Most US interventional cardiologists in practice are relatively low volume operators [10]. The 2011 ACCF/AHA/SCAI PCI guidelines recommended that PCIs be performed by operators with an annual volume of >75 procedures at hospitals with an annual volume of >400 procedures [11]. In the face of declining PCI volumes, the 2013 ACCF/AHA/SCAI update of the clinical competence statement on coronary artery interventional procedures now recommends that PCIs should be performed by operators with an annual volume of ≥50 coronary interventions (averaged over a 2 year period) and a hospital minimum of 200 PCI/year to maintain competency [10, 12]. Due to a significant learning curve for the transradial approach, interventional cardiologists not having a high volume exposure to transradial PCI in elective cases cannot be expected to prefer this approach in PPCI. Therefore experienced radial PCI operators are limited but gradually increasing. Centers that have reported their experience with adoption of transradial PCI for elective and STEMI cases that it was a relatively easy transition and not difficult mounting the learning curve [13, 14].

13.3 Higher Crossover (From Radial to Femoral) Rates

Transradial catheterization/PCI is associated with higher cross over rate compared to transfemoral catheterization/PCI. A meta-analysis of randomized controlled trials of radial versus femoral access for STEMI PPCI found crossover rates were 4.6 % with the radial and 1.1 % with femoral approach [15]. In the randomized trial of radial vs. femoral approach for primary PCI in STEMI patients by experienced operators (the STEMI-RADIAL trial) in both access sites, the cross over from radial to femoral approach was 3.7 % [16]. Cross over from radial to femoral artery may lead to longer door to balloon times [17]. This cross over could be related to radial access site issues, radial artery spasm/small size, radial artery loop, subclavian artery tortuosity and catheter/guide manipulation for coronary engagement. Each one of these can be overcome with experience/special techniques that require knowledge and experience. We recommend following SCAI transradial working group best practices recommending significant transradial PCI experience demonstrating low cross over rate prior to starting PPCI in STEMI cases [18].

13.4 Door-to-Balloon Times

In STEMI patients, timely reperfusion is the primary goal. Studies show minimal or no increase in DTB time with radial access vs. femoral access [2, 19]. In a review of five year data (from 2007 to 2011) of CathPCI Registry of the NCDR including 90,879 patients undergoing primary or rescue PCI for STEMI (6.8 % transradial, 93.2 % transfemoral) at 541 US sites, transradial PCI was associated with a median 4 min increase in DTB time (radial 78 vs. femoral 74 min; $p = < 0.0001$). Despite longer DTB times, the radial approach was associated with lower risk of bleeding and risk of in-hospital mortality [2]. The data regarding the relationship between DTB time and mortality are inconsistent. This variation in DTB and mortality could be due to the fact that the DTB is a limited measure of the processes of care in STEMI care and is just one component of the total ischemic time. There is need for comprehensive efforts to improve all aspects of acute MI care to improve survival rates. Measures of other time delays i.e. reducing symptom onset to reperfusion time, peri-procedural and post-procedural management including access site (radial vs. femoral) are also important components in improving outcomes and need to be focused upon. Studies examining effects of symptoms onset to door time and DTB time on longer term mortality have suggested that short DTB times (90 min or less) are associated with a lower mortality rate in patients with early presentation but have less impact on the mortality rate in patients presenting later [20].

Gibson et al., in an analysis of data from the National Registry of Myocardial Infarction (NRMI), reported a significant reduction in in-hospital mortality among patients undergoing PPCI for STEMI, from 8.6 to 3.1 % ($p < 0.001$), associated with a decline in DTB times from 111 min in 1994 to 79 min in 2006 [21].

Flynn et al. [22] published data from Blue Cross Blue Shield of Michigan Cardiovascular Consortium, a multi-hospital regional quality improvement collaborative in Michigan, USA on effect of improvement in DTB time on in-hospital mortality outcome in patients undergoing PPCI for STEMI. This study included 8771 patients with STEMI who were undergoing PPCI from January 2003 to December 2008. They found no change in the in-hospital mortality between 2003 and 2008 (in hospital mortality 4.1 % in 2003 and 3.62 % in 2008, p = 0.69, this continued to be insignificant after adjustment for baseline risks) despite a decrease in median DTB time from 113 min in 2003 to 76 min in 2008.

Menees DS et al. [1] reviewed data on 96,738 admissions for patients undergoing PPCI for STEMI from July 2005 through June 2009 at 515 hospitals across the United States participating in the CathPCI Registry of the NCDR. Their data suggests that despite the decrease in median DTB times (from 83 min in 2005–2006 to 67 min in 2008–2009) the adjusted and unadjusted in hospital mortality among the pts undergoing PPCI for STEMI has not changed (unadjusted 4.8 % in 2005–2006 vs. 4.7 % in 2008–2009 p = 0.43, adjusted 5.0 % in 2005–2006 vs. 4.7 % in 2008–2009 p = 0.34).

In a recent analysis of the NCDR CathPCI data performed by Nallamothu et al. [3], authors reexamined the association between DTB time and mortality at both individual level and population levels using rigorous statistical approaches. Authors tried to unravel the relation between the patient-specific DTB time and morality from the secular trends in outcomes for the PPCI population over the study period. Authors reviewed data on 150116 patients undergoing PPCI for STEMI from Jan 2005 to December 2011 at 423 hospitals across the United States participating in the CathPCI Registry of the NCDR. Annual DTB times decreased significantly from median of 86 min in 2005 to 63 min in 2011 with a concurrent rise in risk adjusted in hospital mortality (from 4.7 to 5.3 %;p = 0.06) and risk adjusted 6 month mortality (from 12.9 to 14.4 %;p = 0.001). The adjusted population level mortality increased overtime, suggesting temporal increase in use of PPCI in high risk patient subgroups. However, shorter patient specific DTB times were associated at the individual level with lower in hospital mortality and lower 6 month mortality.

Achieving a DTB time (first medical contact to device time) of 90 min or less is a Class I (LOE:A) guideline recommendation for STEMI care and should be the goal as recommended in the 2013 ACCF/AHA clinical practice guidelines for STEMI [23]. The slight increase in DTB times with radial access are unlikely to adversely affect the patient outcomes and should not prevent the operators from adopting transradial PPCI.

13.5 Radiation Exposure

Most but not all studies show higher radiation exposure to the patient and the operator with radial access compared to femoral access [19, 24]. Operator volume of transradial cases and experience help reduce the amount of excess radiation exposure. Measures that can be taken to reduce radiation exposure include appropriate shielding, minimizing scatter by keeping the camera as close to the patient, avoiding excess angulation, use of collimation, less magnification when possible, use of fluoro save when possible, use of low energy fluoro/low frame rate etc. Current imaging systems have helped reduce radiation exposure so much that overall exposure, even with radial access has dropped significantly compared to past. In our lab we use various maneuvers to reduce radiation exposure during transradial procedures (Figs. 13.1 and 13.2).

13.6 Technical Difficulties with Catheter Placement and Guide Catheter Support

Transradial access may be met with greater anatomic variability in the course of radial/subclavian artery as well as challenges in cannulation of the coronary arteries. These Factors may increase the procedure time and account for higher rate of cross over to the femoral access. Starting initially with elective PCIs will help improve the confidence in quickly overcoming anatomic challenges and successful manipulation of the guide catheters for transradial PPCIs. We routinely use standard femoral guides for transradial

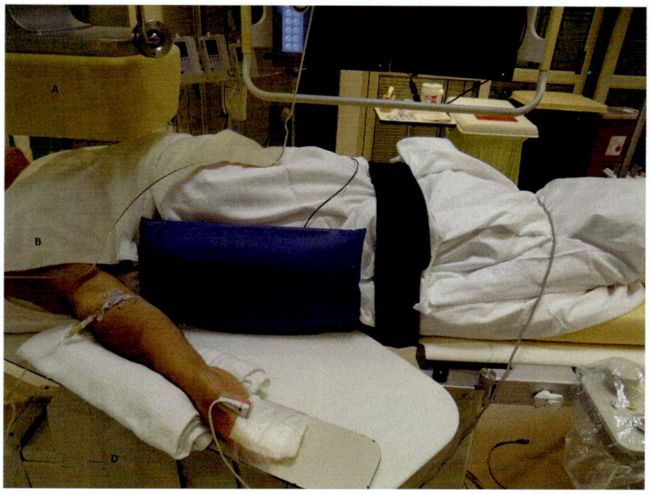

Fig. 13.1 Some methods to reduce radiation exposure to the operator in radial access. *A*-Image receptor being close to the patient's chest. *B*-Ceiling mounted upper body radiation shield. *C*-An arm board draped with fitting Lead cover (reusable and kept under the sterile drape, also see Fig. 13.2). *D*-Lower body radiation shield

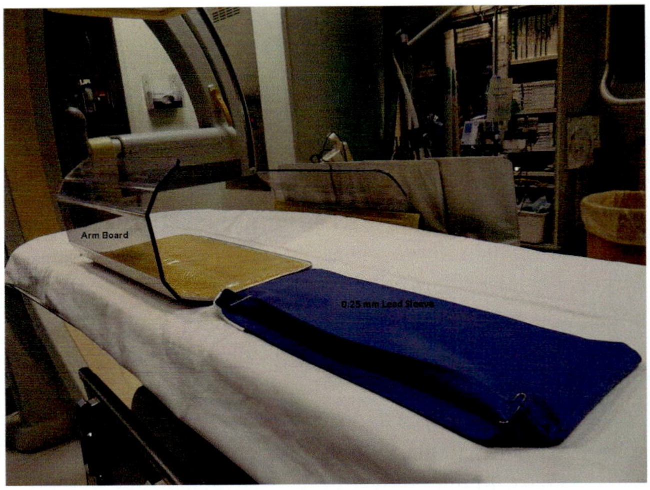

Fig. 13.2 *A*-Arm board and *B*-0.25 mm Lead cover that is stitched to properly fit over the curved portion of the arm board. This arm board is placed between the pts arm and body (as shown in Fig. 13.1) and helps reduce radiation exposure to the radial operator (Courtesy of Ajay Bhatia, RT, UTMB Cath lab, Galveston TX, USA)

PPCI JR-4 for right coronary and Launcher EBU-3.0 (Medtronic, Inc., Minneapolis, MN, USA) guide for LM cannulation from right radial access. From left radial access, we use Launcher EBu 3.5 guide for UN and JR-4 guide for reight coronary artery cannulation. We use buddy wire in same artery or adjacent branch to stabilize the guide catheter if needed. Especially taken using right radial access.

13.7 Procedure Time

Radial primary PCI procedure in STEMI patients may be associated with significantly longer procedure time especially if performed in low volume radial PCI centers [25]. A recent meta-analysis of 12 randomized controlled trials of radial versus femoral access for STEMI PPCI found a mean of 1.52 min increase in procedure time ($p=0.01$) with radial access versus femoral access. Despite slightly longer procedure times the data suggests significant reduction in mortality, major bleeding and access site bleeding [15]. Most of the studies included in this meta-analysis are either single center or include only a few centers, with high concentration of experienced radial operators. Therefore, the minimal increase in procedure time for PPCI when performed by experienced radial operators, may not be generalizable to the practice in the US.

13.8 Contrast Use

The subgroup analysis of the STEMI cohort from the RIVAL (Radial versus Femoral access for Coronary Intervention Trial) showed that with considerably experienced radial operators (median 400 radial cath or PCI procedures/year), transradial PPCI is associated with similar contrast use (median 180 ml contrast use for both access sites, $p=0.2223$) and longer fluoroscopy time (radial 9.3 min vs. femoral 8.0 min, $p=<0.0001$) [26]. In the randomized trial of radial vs. femoral approach for primary PCI in STEMI patients by experienced operators (the STEMI-RADIAL trial) in both access sites, the contrast utilization was actually lower (mean 12 ml lower in radial vs. femoral approach) [16]. A review of five year data (from 2007 to 2011) of CathPCI Registry of the NCDR, including 90,879 patients undergoing primary or rescue PCI for STEMI (6.8 % transradial, 93.2 % transfemoral) at 541 US sites, suggested that transradial access was associated with longer fluoroscopic time (median 1.4 min longer for transradial) and less contrast use (median 5 ml less for transradial) [2]. Therefore, transradial PPCI performed by an experienced operator is not associated with increase contrast use compared to femoral access.

13.9 Data from the Trials Comparing Radial Versus Femoral Access for PPCI

In the subgroup analysis of the STEMI cohort from the RIVAL (Radial versus Femoral access for Coronary Intervention Trial) showed that with considerably experienced radial operators (median 400 radial cath or PCI procedures/year), transradial PPCI is associated with reduced major vascular access site complications and mortality [26]. The RIFLE-STEACS (Radial versus femoral randomized investigation in ST-elevation acute coronary syndrome) trial showed that radial access was associated with decrease in the rate of major adverse cardiac events driven by reduction in mortality and bleeding. The operators in RIFLE-STEACS performed >150 PCIs per year (of which >50 % radial PCIs) [27]. By contrast, the STEMI-RADIAL (A Prospective randomized trial data of radial vs. femoral access in patients with ST-segment elevation myocardial infarction) trial conducted at 4 high volume radial centers, showed a significant reduction in bleeding and access site complications with radial access, but did not demonstrate a mortality benefit for radial access over femoral access for PPCI [16]. A meta-analysis of randomized controlled trials of radial versus femoral access for STEMI PPCI found a 45 % decrease in mortality ($p<0.001$) associated with radial access [15]. An analysis of the NCDR data from 2007 to 2011, including 90,879 patients undergoing primary or rescue PCI for STEMI (6.8 % transradial, 93.2 % transfemoral) at 541 US sites, found a 24 % reduction in mortality ($p=0.0455$) associated with radial access [2].

The MATRIX trial (Minimizing Adverse Hemorrhagic Events by Transradial Access Site and Systemic Implementation of angioX) randomized 8404 patients with

ACS (52 % NSTEMI/48 % STEMI) to coronary angiography and PCI using radial vs. femoral access, demonstrated significant reduction in BARC major bleeding unrelated to CABG (33 % relative risk reduction) and all-cause mortality (28 % relative risk reduction) with radial access compared to femoral access. In the MATRIX trial, the operators performed at least 75 PCIs and at least 50 % of interventions in ACS via the radial route during the previous year. Despite including the skilled operators, in the MATRIX trial, there was a significant interaction of proportion of PCIs undertaken transradially by each center to the outcome of each co-primary endpoints and mortality, but not for major bleeding. The greatest benefit of radial access was seen in highest volume radial centers (ie, those doing at least 80 % of their procedures via radial access). This suggests that although the bleeding benefit accrues at an earlier stage of the learning curve of transradial intervention, but superior efficacy compared with femoral access needs substantial expertise that can be met only by high-volume radial operators [28, 29]. This data is also supported by the prespecified subgroup analysis of the RIVAL trail suggesting that primary outcome (death, MI, stroke, non CABG major bleeding) was reduced with radial versus femoral access in high volume radial centers (>146 radial PCI/year/operator) but not in intermediate (61–146 radial PCI/year/operator) or low volume (≤60 radial PCI/year/operator) radial centers. Low-volume radial centers performed 20 % of PCI procedures per year via radial access, whereas high-volume centers performed 75 % of PCIs per year via radial access. Therefore suggesting that procedural volume and expertise of the radial centers are important, particularly for radial PCIs [25].

Radial artery access for PPCI is also appealing in patients with coagulopathy, elevated international normalized ratio due to warfarin, novel anticoagulants, or morbid obesity. Therefore in STEMI patients undergoing primary PCI, the radial approach is associated with favorable outcomes and should be the preferred approach for experienced radial operators.

Most recent STEMI guidelines by ACCF/AHA, give radial access for STEMI Class IIa designation [23]. 2011 ACCF/AHA/SCAI Guideline for PCI recommends patients to be evaluated for risk of bleeding before PCI and measures considered to minimize the risks of bleeding complications that include among others radial artery access site [11].

13.10 Right Versus Left Radial Access in PPCI in STEMI

Transradial PPCI through either arm is a feasible and safe approach. The use of left radial approach for PPCI in STEMI patients is associated with comparable success rates and reperfusion times when compared with right radial approach [30]. Left radial approach for PPCI may be considered in patients with features associated with failure of right radial approach i.e. history of prior CABG, right subclavian tortuosity, age >75 years and short stature [31].

13.11 Applying This to Practice

PPCI in STEMI is a stressful situation with patients that are acutely sick, having acute symptoms and possibly hemodynamic compromise. Obtaining quick angiogram followed by timely revascularization of the culprit coronary artery using the access site that is to provide the best clinical outcome for that specific patient is the primary goal. Radial access for PPCI for STEMI patients is associated with better clinical outcomes and reduced duration and cost of hospitalization. The data supporting transradial PPCI is derived mostly from studies involving operators highly skilled in transradial PCIs. Therefore, in order to replicate these findings in clinical practice, PPCI for STEMI using radial access requires experienced operators at high volume radial catheterization laboratories. Data from a large unselected patient population derived from the British Cardiovascular Intervention Society database suggests that the benefits of adoption of transradial PPCI can be achieved in real world practice [32]. This led to a bold editorial comment by Di Mario C and Secco G "Radial Primary Angioplasty- The Gold Standard Treatment for STEMI patients" [33]. Adoption of transradial PPCI is becoming essential but needs training and physicians will have to go through the discomfort of a learning curve. In order to avoid losing precious time overcoming the transradial access related technical/learning curve issues, it is important to initially start with transradial catheterization/PCI in elective cases and gradually ease into the ACS/NSTEMI cases followed by PPCI in STEMI. The SCAI's Transradial Working Group recommends best practices for transradial interventions and recommends operators and sites not to start performing transradial PPCI until they have performed at least 100 elective PCI cases with a "radial first" approach and their femoral cross over rate is ≤4 % [18]. This gradual transition is very important to obtain the best outcomes of transradial approach for PPCI in STEMI patients.

Conclusion

Transradial PPCI is associated with reduced non CABG major bleeding (especially access site related bleeding), all-cause mortality, hospital length of stay and cost of hospitalization. In a health care era in which patient-centered outcomes are being recognized to be increasingly important, hospitals should strive to maximize their volumes of radial procedures (rather than reserving for patients in whom femoral access is not possible) in order to derive the maximum benefit from transradial PPCI [34]. These benefits are especially relevant for the countries such as the USA where use of the radial approach in currently uncommon. As the adoption of transradial PCI and PPCI increases in the US, this will help reduce the cost of health care and improve the quality of patient care and help bring it to the level of other industrialized nations [35].

References

1. Menees DS, Peterson ED, Wang Y, Curtis JP, Messenger JC, Rumsfeld JS, et al. Door-to-balloon time and mortality among patients undergoing primary PCI. N Engl J Med. 2013;369(10):901–9.
2. Baklanov DV, Kaltenbach LA, Marso SP, Subherwal SS, Feldman DN, Garratt KN, et al. The prevalence and outcomes of transradial percutaneous coronary intervention for ST-segment elevation myocardial infarction: analysis from the National Cardiovascular Data Registry (2007 to 2011). J Am Coll Cardiol. 2013;61(4):420–6.
3. Nallamothu BK, Normand SL, Wang Y, Hofer TP, Brush Jr JE, Messenger JC, et al. Relation between door-to-balloon times and mortality after primary percutaneous coronary intervention over time: a retrospective study. Lancet. 2015;385(9973):1114–22.
4. Hannan EL, Farrell LS, Walford G, Berger PB, Stamato NJ, Venditti FJ, et al. Utilization of radial artery access for percutaneous coronary intervention for ST-segment elevation myocardial infarction in New York. JACC Cardiovasc Interv. 2014;7(3):276–83.
5. Chiang A, Gada H, Kodali SK, Lee MS, Jeremias A, Pinto DS, et al. Procedural variation in the performance of primary percutaneous coronary intervention for ST-elevation myocardial infarction: a SCAI-based survey study of US interventional cardiologists. Catheter Cardiovasc Interv. 2014;83(5):721–6.
6. Concannon TW, Nelson J, Goetz J, Griffith JL. A percutaneous coronary intervention lab in every hospital? Circ Cardiovasc Qual Outcomes. 2012;5(1):14–20.
7. Riley RF, Don CW, Powell W, Maynard C, Dean LS. Trends in coronary revascularization in the United States from 2001 to 2009: recent declines in percutaneous coronary intervention volumes. Circ Cardiovasc Qual Outcomes. 2011;4(2):193–7.
8. Mozaffarian D, Benjamin EJ, Go AS, Arnett DK, Blaha MJ, Cushman M, et al. Heart disease and stroke statistics – 2015 update: a report from the American Heart Association. Circulation. 2015;131(4):e29–322.
9. Langabeer JR, Henry TD, Kereiakes DJ, Dellifraine J, Emert J, Wang Z, et al. Growth in percutaneous coronary intervention capacity relative to population and disease prevalence. J Am Heart Assoc. 2013;2(6):e000370.
10. Badheka AO, Patel NJ, Grover P, Singh V, Patel N, Arora S, et al. Impact of annual operator and institutional volume on percutaneous coronary intervention outcomes: a 5-year United States experience (2005–2009). Circulation. 2014;130(16):1392–406.
11. Levine GN, Bates ER, Blankenship JC, Bailey SR, Bittl JA, Cercek B, et al. 2011 ACCF/AHA/SCAI Guideline for Percutaneous Coronary Intervention. A report of the American College of Cardiology Foundation/American Heart Association Task Force on Practice Guidelines and the Society for Cardiovascular Angiography and Interventions. J Am Coll Cardiol. 2011;58(24):e44–122.
12. Harold JG, Bass TA, Bashore TM, Brindis RG, Brush JE, Jr., Burke JA, et al. ACCF/AHA/SCAI 2013 update of the clinical competence statement on coronary artery interventional procedures: a report of the American College of Cardiology Foundation/American Heart Association/American College of Physicians Task Force on Clinical Competence and Training (Writing Committee to Revise the 2007 Clinical Competence Statement on Cardiac Interventional Procedures). J Am Coll Cardiol. 2013;62(4):357–96.
13. Bheemarasetti MK, Shawar S, Chithri S, Khalife WI, Rangasetty UM, Fujise K, et al. Influence of access, anticoagulant, and bleeding definition on outcomes of primary percutaneous coronary intervention: early experience of an US Academic Center. Int J Angiol. 2015;24(1):11–8.
14. Blankenship JC, Scott TD. What matters and what does not: variations in STEMI PCI techniques. Catheter Cardiovasc Interv. 2014;83(5):727–8.
15. Karrowni W, Vyas A, Giacomino B, Schweizer M, Blevins A, Girotra S, et al. Radial versus femoral access for primary percutaneous interventions in ST-segment elevation myocardial infarction patients: a meta-analysis of randomized controlled trials. JACC Cardiovasc Interv. 2013;6(8):814–23.
16. Bernat I, Horak D, Stasek J, Mates M, Pesek J, Ostadal P, et al. ST-segment elevation myocardial infarction treated by radial or femoral approach in a multicenter randomized clinical trial: the STEMI-RADIAL trial. J Am Coll Cardiol. 2014;63(10):964–72.
17. Rubartelli P, Crimi G, Bartolini D, Bellotti S, Iannone A, Fontana V. Switching from femoral to routine radial access site for ST-elevation myocardial infarction: a single center experience. J Interv Cardiol. 2014;27(6):591–9.
18. Rao SV, Tremmel JA, Gilchrist IC, Shah PB, Gulati R, Shroff AR, et al. Best practices for transradial angiography and intervention: a consensus statement from the society for cardiovascular angiography and intervention's transradial working group. Catheter Cardiovasc Interv. 2014;83(2):228–36.
19. Jang JS, Jin HY, Seo JS, Yang TH, Kim DK, Kim DK, et al. The transradial versus the transfemoral approach for primary percutaneous coronary intervention in patients with acute myocardial infarction: a systematic review and meta-analysis. EuroIntervention. 2012;8(4):501–10.
20. Hannan EL, Zhong Y, Jacobs AK, Holmes DR, Walford G, Venditti FJ, et al. Effect of onset-to-door time and door-to-balloon time on mortality in patients undergoing percutaneous coronary interventions for st-segment elevation myocardial infarction. Am J Cardiol. 2010;106(2):143–7.
21. Gibson CM, Pride YB, Frederick PD, Pollack Jr CV, Canto JG, Tiefenbrunn AJ, et al. Trends in reperfusion strategies, door-to-needle and door-to-balloon times, and in-hospital mortality among patients with ST-segment elevation myocardial infarction enrolled in the National Registry of Myocardial Infarction from 1990 to 2006. Am Heart J. 2008;156(6):1035–44.
22. Flynn A, Moscucci M, Share D, Smith D, LaLonde T, Changezi H, et al. Trends in door-to-balloon time and mortality in patients with ST-elevation myocardial infarction undergoing primary percutaneous coronary intervention. Arch Intern Med. 2010;170(20):1842–9.
23. American College of Emergency P, Society for Cardiovascular A, Interventions, O'Gara PT, Kushner FG, Ascheim DD, et al. 2013 ACCF/AHA guideline for the management of ST-elevation myocardial infarction: a report of the American College of Cardiology Foundation/American Heart Association Task Force on Practice Guidelines. J Am Coll Cardiol. 2013;61(4):e78–140.
24. Shah B, Bangalore S, Feit F, Fernandez G, Coppola J, Attubato MJ, et al. Radiation exposure during coronary angiography via transradial or transfemoral approaches when performed by experienced operators. Am Heart J. 2013;165(3):286–92.
25. Jolly SS, Cairns J, Yusuf S, Niemela K, Steg PG, Worthley M, et al. Procedural volume and outcomes with radial or femoral access for coronary angiography and intervention. J Am Coll Cardiol. 2014;63(10):954–63.
26. Mehta SR, Jolly SS, Cairns J, Niemela K, Rao SV, Cheema AN, et al. Effects of radial versus femoral artery access in patients with acute coronary syndromes with or without ST-segment elevation. J Am Coll Cardiol. 2012;60(24):2490–9.

27. Romagnoli E, Biondi-Zoccai G, Sciahbasi A, Politi L, Rigattieri S, Pendenza G, et al. Radial versus femoral randomized investigation in ST-segment elevation acute coronary syndrome: the RIFLE-STEACS (Radial Versus Femoral Randomized Investigation in ST-Elevation Acute Coronary Syndrome) study. J Am Coll Cardiol. 2012;60(24):2481–9.
28. Valgimigli M, Gagnor A, Calabro P, Frigoli E, Leonardi S, Zaro T, et al. Radial versus femoral access in patients with acute coronary syndromes undergoing invasive management: a randomised multicentre trial. Lancet. 2015;385(9986):2465–76.
29. Le May MR, Singh K, Wells GA. Efficacy of radial versus femoral access in the acute coronary syndrome: is it the operator or the operation that matters? JACC Cardiovasc Interv. 2015;8(11): 1405–9.
30. Larsen P, Shah S, Waxman S, Freilich M, Riskalla N, Piemonte T, et al. Comparison of procedural times, success rates, and safety between left versus right radial arterial access in primary percutaneous coronary intervention for acute ST-segment elevation myocardial infarction. Catheter Cardiovasc Interv. 2011;78(1):38–44.
31. Dehghani P, Mohammad A, Bajaj R, Hong T, Suen CM, Sharieff W, et al. Mechanism and predictors of failed transradial approach for percutaneous coronary interventions. JACC Cardiovasc Interv. 2009;2(11):1057–64.
32. Mamas MA, Ratib K, Routledge H, Neyses L, Fraser DG, de Belder M, et al. Influence of arterial access site selection on outcomes in primary percutaneous coronary intervention: are the results of randomized trials achievable in clinical practice? JACC Cardiovasc Interv. 2013;6(7):698–706.
33. Di Mario C, Secco G. Radial primary angioplasty: the gold standard treatment for STEMI patients. JACC Cardiovasc Interv. 2013;6(7):707–8.
34. Jolly SS, Mehta SR. Coronary intervention: radial artery access comes of age. Lancet. 2015;385(9986):2437–9.
35. Laslett L, Anderson HV, Clark 3rd B, Dewhurst TA, Waits TF, Wilson S, et al. American College of Cardiology: environmental scanning report update 2015. J Am Coll Cardiol. 2015;66(19 Suppl):D1–44.

14 Transradial Approach for STEMI: Focus on Technique Using a Single MAC Guiding Catheter for Transradial Primary PCI

Jincheng Guo

14.1 Introduction

Radial angioplasty was introduced 20 years ago by Kiemeneij et al. [1], and immediately showed advantages in terms of reduction in bleeding, patient discomfort, and hospital stay. Transradial approach (TRA) in percutaneous coronary interventions (PCI) today becomes widely accepted and practiced procedure worldwide. Available evidence indicates that TRA is the optimal treatment approach for patients presenting with ST-segment elevation myocardial infarction (STEMI) due to reduced bleeding and mortality [2]. Mamas et al. [3] showed a highly significant 29 % reduction in 30-day mortality in 46,128 STEMI patients using the radial access site compared with transfemoral approach. The 2014 European Society of Cardiology myocardial revascularization guidelines give a strong Class IIa Level A recommendation for transradial primary PCI [4]. Achieving door-to-balloon (DTB) time in less than 60 min is an important quality metric in the setting of primary PCI [4].

Although radial approach for percutaneous coronary artery catheterization and intervention has been previously demonstrated to be as effective as the femoral approach [3, 5, 6], and to be associated with a reduction in vascular complications [3, 6]. The longer procedural and fluoroscopic time is the disadvantage of tansradial over transfemoral access [6, 7]. To avoid the disadvantages of a multi-catheter strategy, using a dedicated radial guiding catheter for both the diagnostic and interventional procedures is the "one-pass" technique, with potentially less procedure and fluoroscopic time, lower costs, and diminished radial artery spasm.

J. Guo
Department of Cardiology, Luhe Hospital,
Capital Medical University, Beijing, China
e-mail: guojcmd@126.com

14.2 Catheters for Coronary Angiography and Intervention

In general, there are two types of radial guiding catheters (1) dedicated left and right coronary catheters and (2) universal catheters, intended to cannulate both the left and right coronaries with a single instrument.

In an international transradial practice Survey [8], Judkins left (JL) catheters are the most popular for left coronary artery (LCA) angiographies (66.5 %) and right coronary artery (RCA) angiographies (58.8 %). For PCI, 6 F standard extra back-up guiding catheters (>65 %) such as EBU3.5 (Medtronic, Minneapolis, MN) or XB 3.5 (Cordis, Bridgewater, NJ) were preferred for LCA. For RCA, 70.4 % use Judkins right (JR) catheters. Although TRA pioneers designed several catheter shapes to cannulate LCA and RCA with a single catheter, these catheters are rarely used.

14.3 Procedural Variation and Catheters Selection for Primary PCI

An important issue to consider in the context of transradial primary PCI is sequence of catheters and coronary angiography. No consensus exists about which coronary artery should be firstly catheterized in primary PCIs. There is a significant variability in the way of performing primary PCI by different interventional cardiologists [9]. Some of this variability (e.g., sequence of catheters) is not addressed by current guidelines/consensus documents. According to the sequence of catheters and coronary angiography, five types of method for primary PCI were divided (Fig. 14.1).

Y. Zhou et al. (eds.), *Transradial Approach for Percutaneous Interventions*, DOI 10.1007/978-94-017-7350-8_14

Type 1: Start with multiple diagnostic catheters (for example: JR for RCA or JL for LCA) or one single diagnostic catheter (Tiger or Kimny) for complete coronary angiography followed by using a guiding catheter to perform PCI of the culprit artery [9].

Type 2: Start with a diagnostic catheter for the presumed non-culprit artery based on the Electrocardiogram (ECG) identification followed by guiding catheter selection to treat the culprit artery [9].

Type 3: Start with diagnostic catheter for angiography of the presumed culprit artery followed by guiding catheter selection for primary PCI or start with guiding catheter for angiography and intervention of the presumed culprit artery and then performed contralateral diagnostic angiogarphy [10].

Type 4: start with a guiding catheter for the angiography and PCI of the "culprit artery" followed by contralateral diagnostic angiography [11].

Type 5: Start with a single guiding catheter for the non-culprit artery coronary angiography and then performed primary PCI for the culprit artery.

Simply, three types of method were also applied in clinical practice, The definition, advantage and disadvantages of different approaches regarding coronary angiography before primary PCI seen Table 14.1.

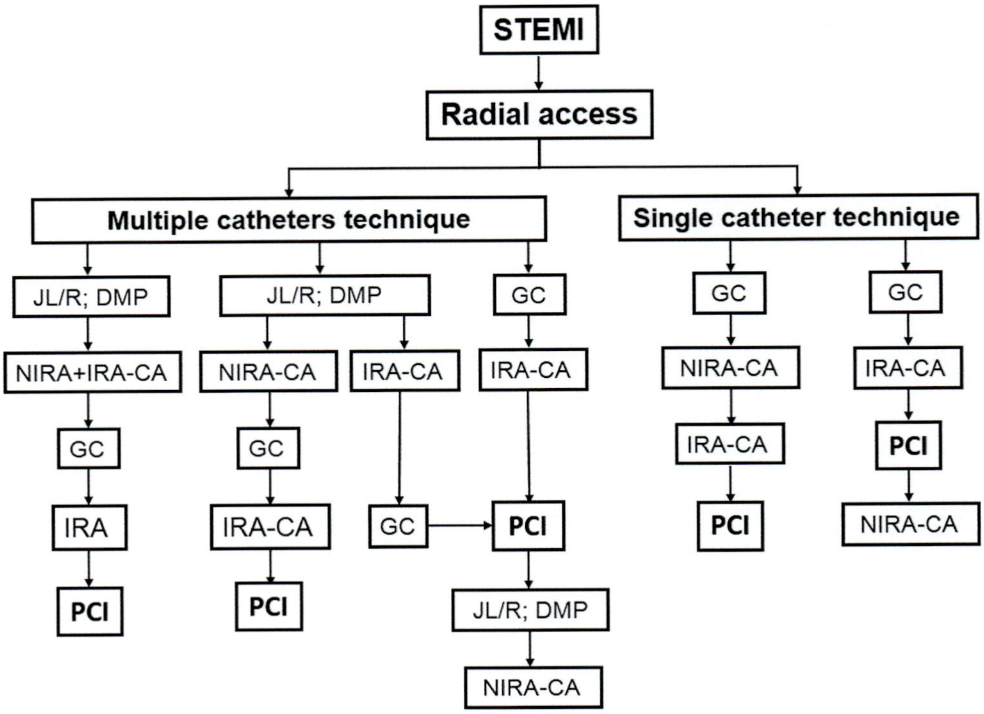

Fig. 14.1 Different sequence of catheters in performing primary PCI including multiple catheters technique and single catheter technique. *STEMI* ST-segment elevation myocardial infarction, *JL/R* judkins left or right catheter, *DMP* diagnostic multipurpose catheter, *IRA* infarct-related artery, *NIRA* non infarct-related artery, *GC* guiding catheter, *PCI* percutaneous coronary intervention,*CA* coronary angiography

Table 14.1 Different approaches regarding coronary angiography before primary PCI

Method	Definition	Reperfusion time	Revascularization strategy
Ipsilateral approach	Start the procedure with a guiding or diagnostic catheter for the angiography followed by PCI of the "culprit artery" (based on ECG)	Reduced	No change
Contralateral approach	Start with a diagnostic or guiding catheter for the "non-culprit artery" (based on ECG) followed by angiography and PCI of the culprit vessel	Increase	May be modified after get the knowledge of multivessel or left main disease before Primary PCI
Full diagnostic catheterization	Completing the angiography of left and right coronary arteries with diagnostic catheters before primary PCI	Increase	May change

Table 14.2 Recent studies demonstrating single guiding catheter for transradial primary PCI

First author (Ref. #)	Year	Study type	Default access	Sample size	Guide catheter	Median procedure time (min)	Success rate % (CA) LCA	RCA	Success rate %(PCI)
Roberts et al. [12]	2011	Observational	Right	42	Q	47	100	85	85
CHOW et al. [13]	2012	Retrospective	Right	162	Ikari left (IL) 3.5	34	100	95	98.8
Malaiapan et al. [14]	2013	Observational	Right	39	6 F Kimny	50	100	100	100
Moon et al. [15]	2012	Observational	NA	31	6 Fr RM 3.5	NA	96.7		96.7

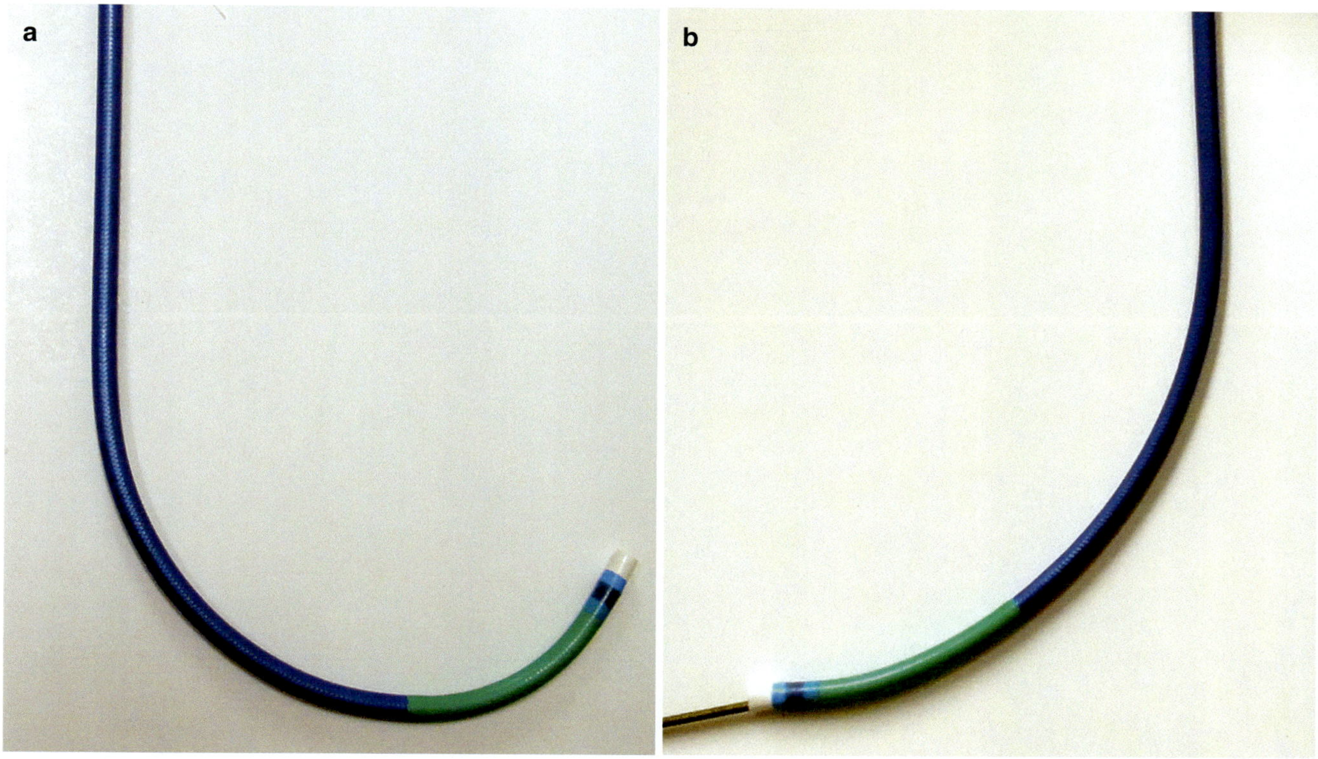

Fig. 14.2 MAC 3.5 guiding catheter designed by Medtronic INC., (**a**) natural shape, (**b**) the wire modifies the MAC catheter to simulate a Judkins Right conformation

A few studies have examined the effect of a single universal guide catheter such as Ikari or Kimny catheter on reducing catheterization laboratory door to balloon (CTB) times and DTB times and showed using that a single guiding catheter can reduced CTB time (Table 14.2).

14.4 Manipulation of the MAC Guiding Catheter

The Multi-aortic Curve (MAC) guiding catheter (Fig. 14.2 Medtronic, Inc.) is a long-tip guide that provides backup from the contralateral aortic wall. MAC guiding catheter was advanced over a 0.035-in. wire, the catheter tip will typically end up in the left coronary sinus. Withdrawing the wire but keeping the guidewire in the catheter prevents kinking of the catheter. Cannulation of the RCA using a MAC guiding catheter is performed in left anterior oblique (LAO) projection. Maneuver is basically same as with the JR catheter if failed, formed a smaller U-shaped curve in the right sinus with its tip directed to the left coronary orifice. Rotate the catheter clockwise until its tip engage the RCA (Fig. 14.3a–d).

Cannulation of the LCA is also performed in the LAO projection. For selective engagement of the left coronary ostium after finishing coronary angiography of RCA, MAC require more manipulation while it is gently pull the catheter toward the contralateral aortic wall (Fig. 14.4a–c), push the catheter at the moment until it looks like a U-shape (Fig. 14.4d–f), slightly rotate the catheter tip clockwise toward the left sinus Valsalva (Fig. 14.4g–i) while pushing it with counterclockwise or slightly pulling it to enter the left coronary artery ostium (Fig. 14.4j).

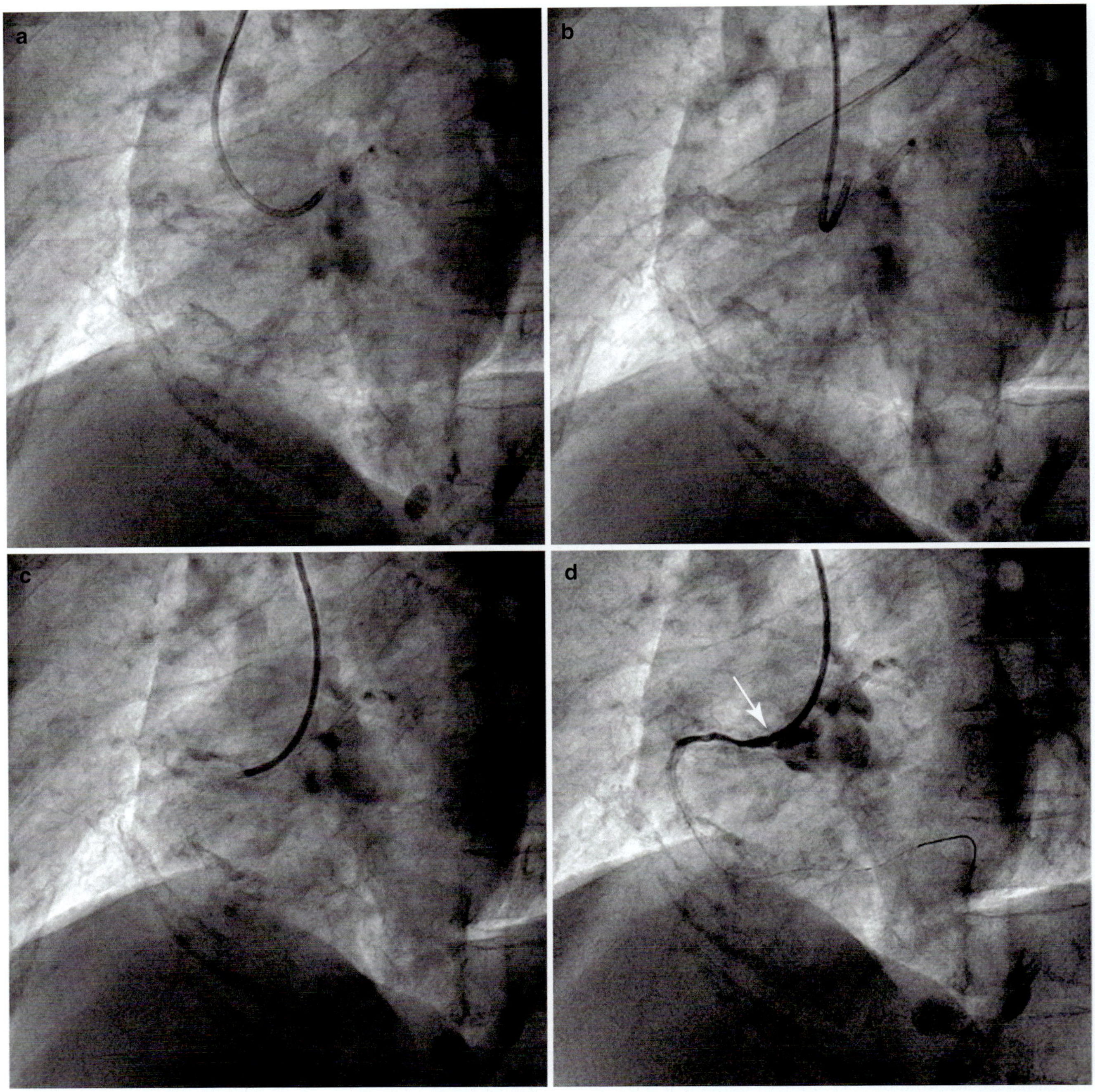

Fig. 14.3 Catheterization of Right coronary artery (*RCA*) in the left anterior oblique projection using MAC3.5 guiding catheter, (**a**) formed a small u shape curve in right cusp with it tip directed to left; (**b**) rotate the catheter clockwisely; (**c**) its tip points toward RCA; (**d**) slightly pull or push the catheter and engage RCA (*white arrow*)

14.5 Primay PCI Procedures in Luhe Hosptial

Algorithm routinely used for primary PCI in Luhe hospital see Fig. 14.5. For patients who are going to be performed primary PCI,after being given loading dose aspirin 300 mg and clopidogrel 600 mg or ticagrelor 180 mg,the patient was transferred to catheterization laboratory. Right radial artery with papable pulse was default access, if failed, switching to right or left femoral artery or left radial access. Heparin was the first choice for anticoagulation. In our catheterization laboratory, we routinely start with a 6 F MAC3.5 guiding catheter for coronary angiography and intervention. MAC 3.5 guide catheter is advanced into the aortic root over a standard 0.035-in., 1-mm, J-tipped guide wire. If any resistance is encountered during passage, dilute contrast should be injected via the guiding catheter to identify the problem (e.g., loop, spasm, cannulation of side-branch). If 0.035-in. wire fails then 0.035-in. hydrophilic wire or 0.14-in. guide wire can be used. An angiography of the non-infarcted artery should be performed first to allow identification of multivessel disease and collateral flow into the infarct zone with multiple projections. Angiography of the infarcted artery is performed with only limited projections to visualized the culprit lesion followed by using adjunctive techniques: non hydrophilic wire, aspiration catheter, balloon or stent.

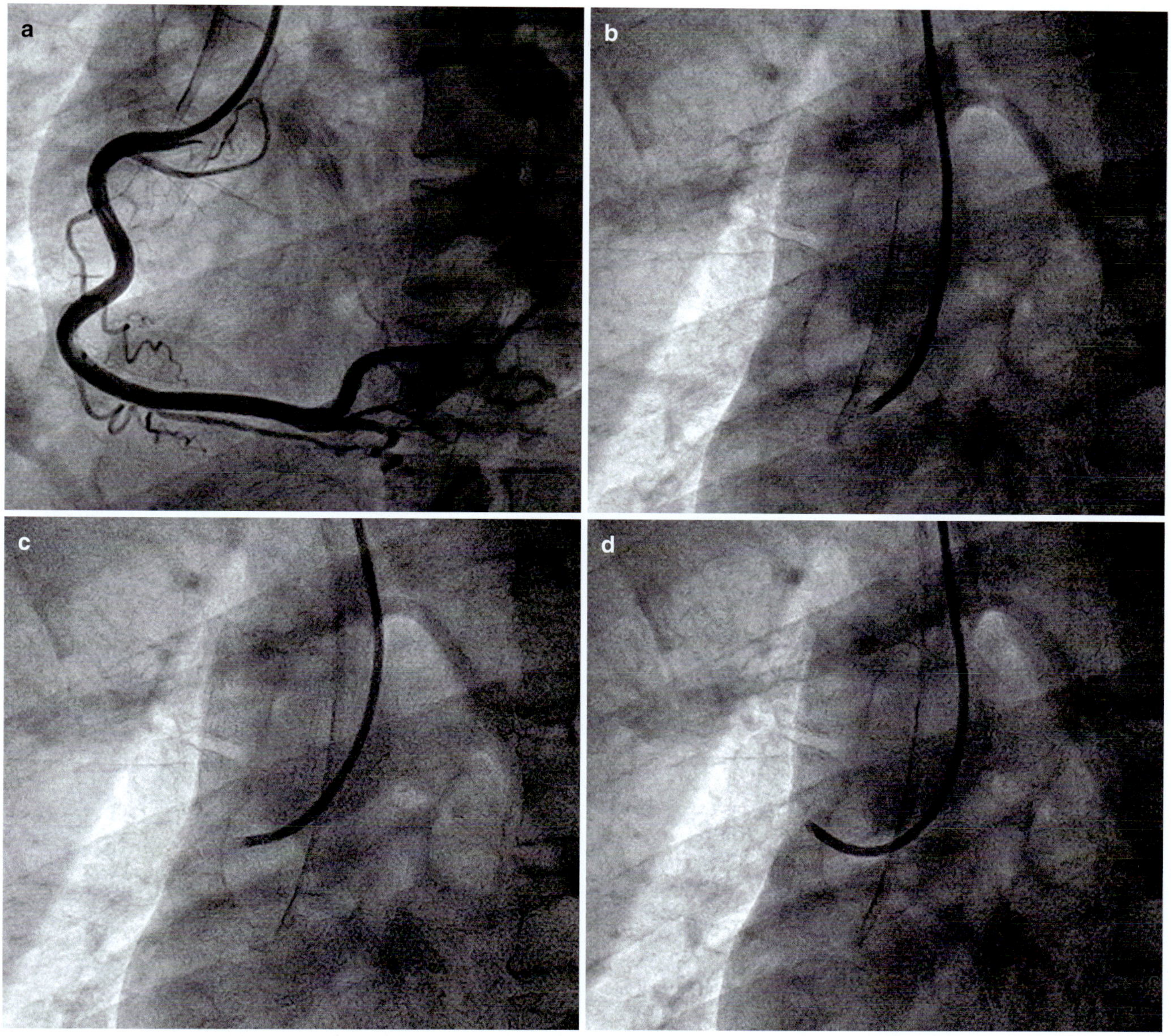

Fig. 14.4 Coronary angiography of RCA was performed by MAC3.5 guiding catheter (**a**);slightly pull the catheter and let the MAC3.5 guiding catheter left ostium of RCA (**b**, **c**); push the catheter to form a big U shape (**d–f**); rotate the catheter clockwisely until its tip toward the left (**g–i**); push while counterclockwise or slightly withdraw the catheter to engage LCA with test injection (*white arrow*) (**j**)

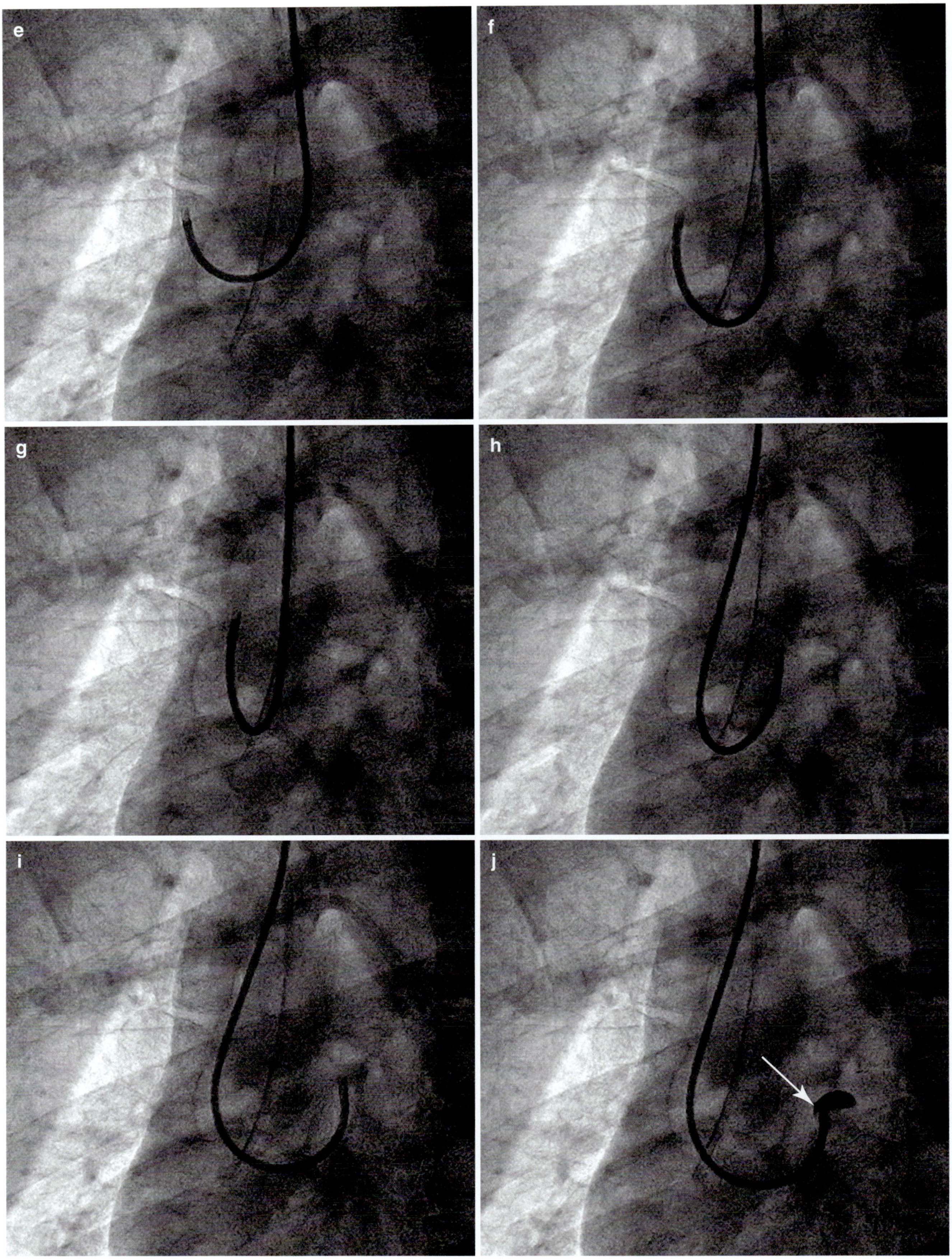

Fig. 14.4 (continued)

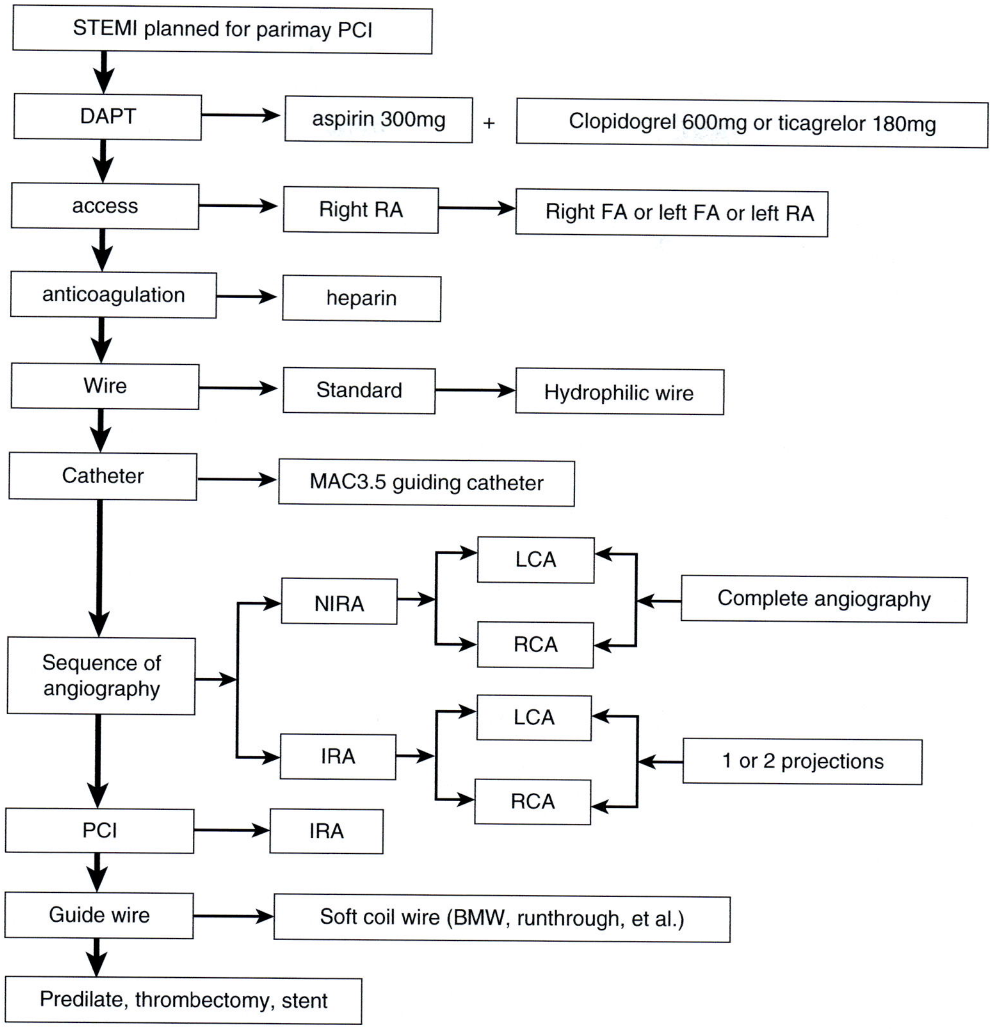

Fig. 14.5 Suggested management algorithm for primary PCI in Luhe hospital. *STEMI* ST segment elevation myocardial infarction, *DAPT* dual antiplatelet therapy, *RA* radial artery, *FA* femoral artery, *NIRA* non infarct-related artery, *IRA* infarct-related artery, *LCA* left coronary artery, *RCA* right coronary artery, *PCI* percutaneous coronary intervention

14.6 Typical Cases Using a Single MAC Guiding Catheter for Primary PCI

Case 1

A 43-year-old male collapsed while walking on the way, around 8:00 am. When an ambulance arrived, the patient was unresponsive, pulseless, and not breathing. Cardiopulmonary resuscitation was started, and ventricular fibrillation was the initial rhythm recorded. Ventricular defibrillation (VF) was applied twice to terminate VF during resuscitation. After intubation, intravenous access was obtained, He was transferred to the Emergency Department for further resuscitation. Subsequent ECG revealed ST-segment elevation in leads I, II, V_{2-6} (Fig. 14.6). After administration of aspirin (300 mg) and ticagrelor (180 mg) *via* a nasogastric tube, he was transferred to the catheterization laboratory. Hemodynamic support was provided with dopamine and norepinephrine *via* the intravenous route. Coronary angiography was performed via the right radial artery using a 6 F single MAC3.5 guiding catheter (Medtronic, Inc., Minneapolis, MN, USA), based on the ECG, the RCA was the non-culprit vessel and firstly engaged, coronary angiography demonstrated normal RCA was dominant and normal. Left circumflex (LCx) was also normal as well as total occlusion of the mid-segment of the left anterior descending artery (LAD) (Fig. 14.7a). Two drug-eluting stents (3.5×30 mm and 3.5×15 mm) were implanted into the LAD (Fig. 14.7b), resulting in Thrombolysis in Myocardial Infarction (TIMI) grade 3 flow. Intra-aortic balloon pump (IABP) was inserted during the procedure. Consciousness was restored 3 days later. Impairment of short term memory was restored by hyperbaric oxygen therapy. The IABP was removed on day-2 and he underwent extubation on day-7. On day-21, he was discharged from hospital with prescriptions of aspirin, ticagrelor, a beta-blocker, a lipid-lowering drug, and an angiotensin-converting-enzyme inhibitor.

Comment: This case showed using a single guiding catheter MAC3.5 for RCA angiography and LAD intervention to avoid catheter exchange and save time in such a comatose patient after cardiac arrest out of hospital.

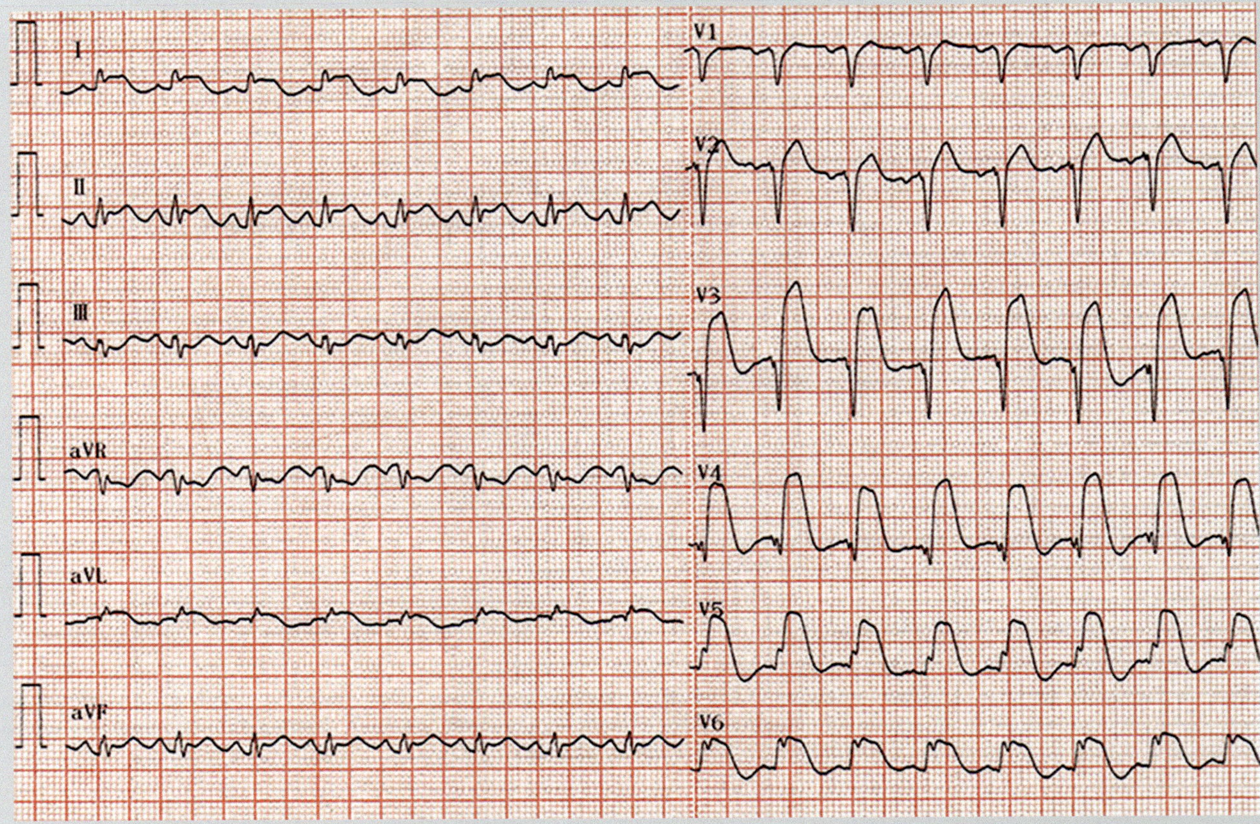

Fig. 14.6 Twelve-lead electrocardiogram (ECG) in the emergency department reveals ST elevation in leads I, II, V2–6

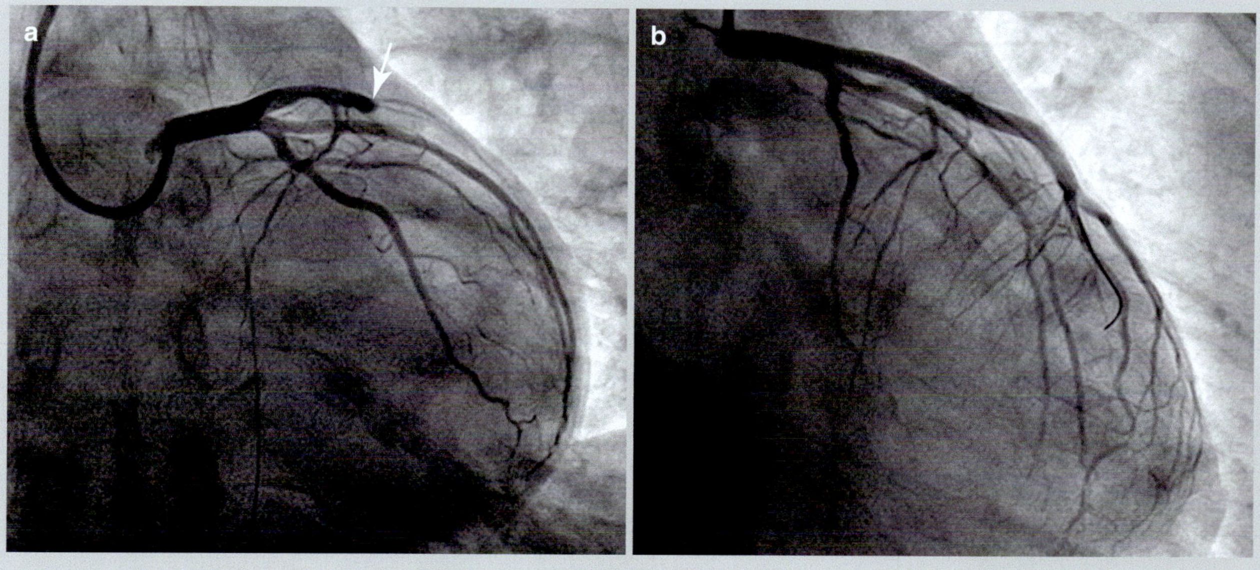

Fig. 14.7 (**a**) Mid-segment LAD is totally occluded (*white arrow*). (**b**) Results after 2 stents deployment

Case 2

A 64-year-old man with heavy smoking presented to the emergency department after experiencing left-sided anterior chest pain for 45min. Two years prior to presentation, he underwent PCI with placement of a 2.5 mm diameter by 36 mm long sirolimus-eluting stent in the LCx and a 3.5 mm diameter by 30 mm long sirolimus-eluting stent in the mid-RCA. The initial 12-lead ECG revealed inferior ST-segment elevation and severe ST depression in leads V_{1-4} (Fig. 14.8). He was promptly treated with aspirin,clopidogrel and was referred to the cardiac catheterization laboratory.

LCx considered as a culprit vessel based on ECG identification, the patient was catheterized via the right radial artery using a standard 6F arterial sheath. A 6F-MAC 3.5 guiding catheter was then introduced and positioned in the aortic root. After u shape formed (Fig. 14.9a) and rotate the catheter clockwisely, the right ostium is easily cannulated (Fig. 14.9b–d). After coronary angiography of RCA, slightly pull the MAC3.5 guiding catheter, the catheter tip will deflect to the right coronary cusp, push the catheter to form a big U shape and rotate clockwisely to engage LCA (Fig. 14.10a–j)

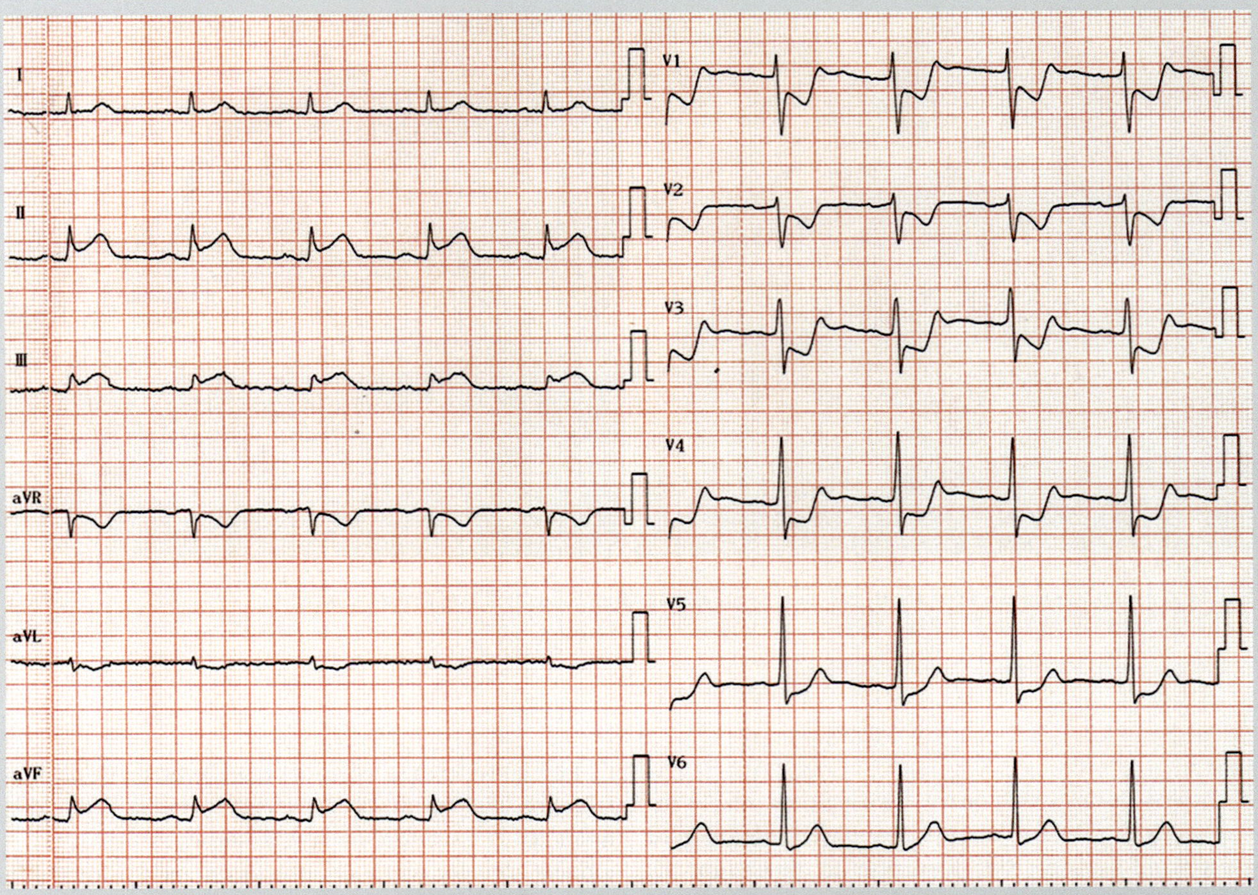

Fig. 14.8 Twelve-lead ECG in the emergency department shows ST-segment elevation in inferior leads (II,III and aVF) and ST-segment depression in leads aVR, aVL and V_{1-4}

Case 3

A healthy 33-year-old man with no prior cardiac history developed acute onset of midsternal chest pain radiating to back associated with sweat. He presented to the emergency department after experiencing symptoms for 45 min. His medical history is notable for smoking. A 12-lead ECG showed sinus rhythm of 95 beats per minute, with pathologic Q-waves in leads III,aVF and ST-elevation in leads II, III, aVF (Fig. 14.11). After 300 mg aspirin and 180 mg ticagrelor was given, he was transferred to the catheterization laboratory.

According to ECG, RCA was identified culprit vessel, a MAC3.5 guiding catheter was advanced into ascending artery via right radial artery, after U shape was formed against contralateral wall (Fig. 14.12a), rotate the catheter clockwisely (Fig. 14.12b), when the catheter was directed to left (Fig. 14.12c), slightly pull the catheter and engage LCA (Fig. 14.12d). Coronary angiography revealed a right dominant coronary artery with 80 % stenosis LCx after it gives rise obtuse marginal (Fig. 14.13a). Collateral circulation to the distal RCA from LAD was noted (Fig. 14.13b). After RCA was engaged with MAC3.5 guiding catheter, Coronary angiography showed RCA was totally occluded with huge thrombus burden at proximal segment (Fig. 14.13c). An Export aspiration catheter (Medtronic) was used to extract a large amount of thrombus after making multiple passes (Fig. 14.13d–g), severe stenosis in mid-RCA (Fig. 14.13h) was predilated (Fig. 14.13i) with a 2.0 mm balloon, a 3.5 mm×24 mm stent was implanted into mid-RCA with good angiographic result (Fig. 14.13j).

Comment: MAC guide catheter is designed for RCA, the key point of MAC3.5 engaging LCA is to form a U shape and rotate clockwise with upward movement of the tip the left main aortic trunk.

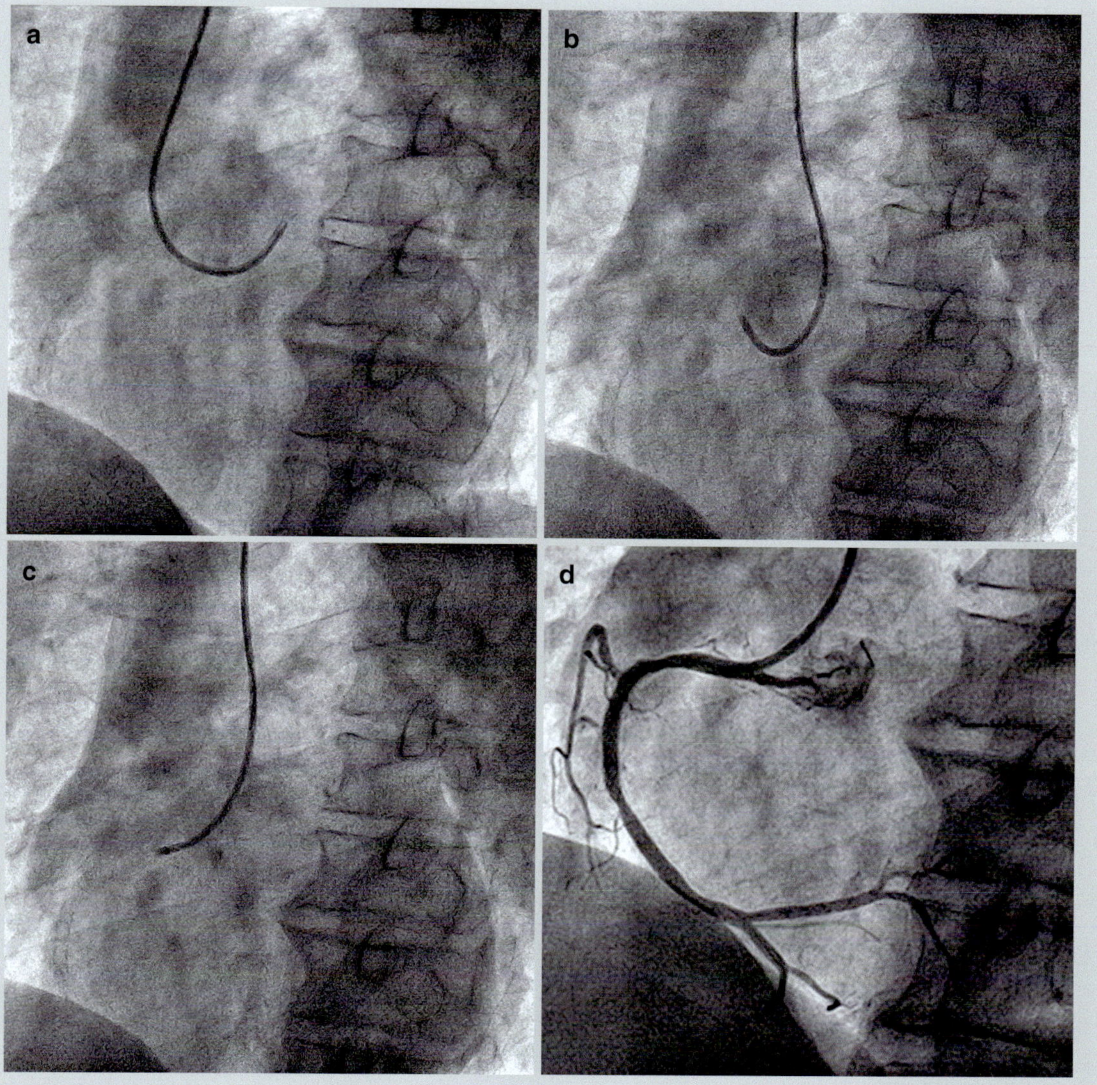

Fig. 14.9 Catheterization of RCA using a single MAC3.5 guiding catheter. Push the catheter to form a small u-shape (**a**); rotate the catheter clockwisely with it tip toward the RCA (**b**, **c**); RCA was engaged with mild stenosis in proximal segment and 50 % stenosis in mid-RCA (**d**)

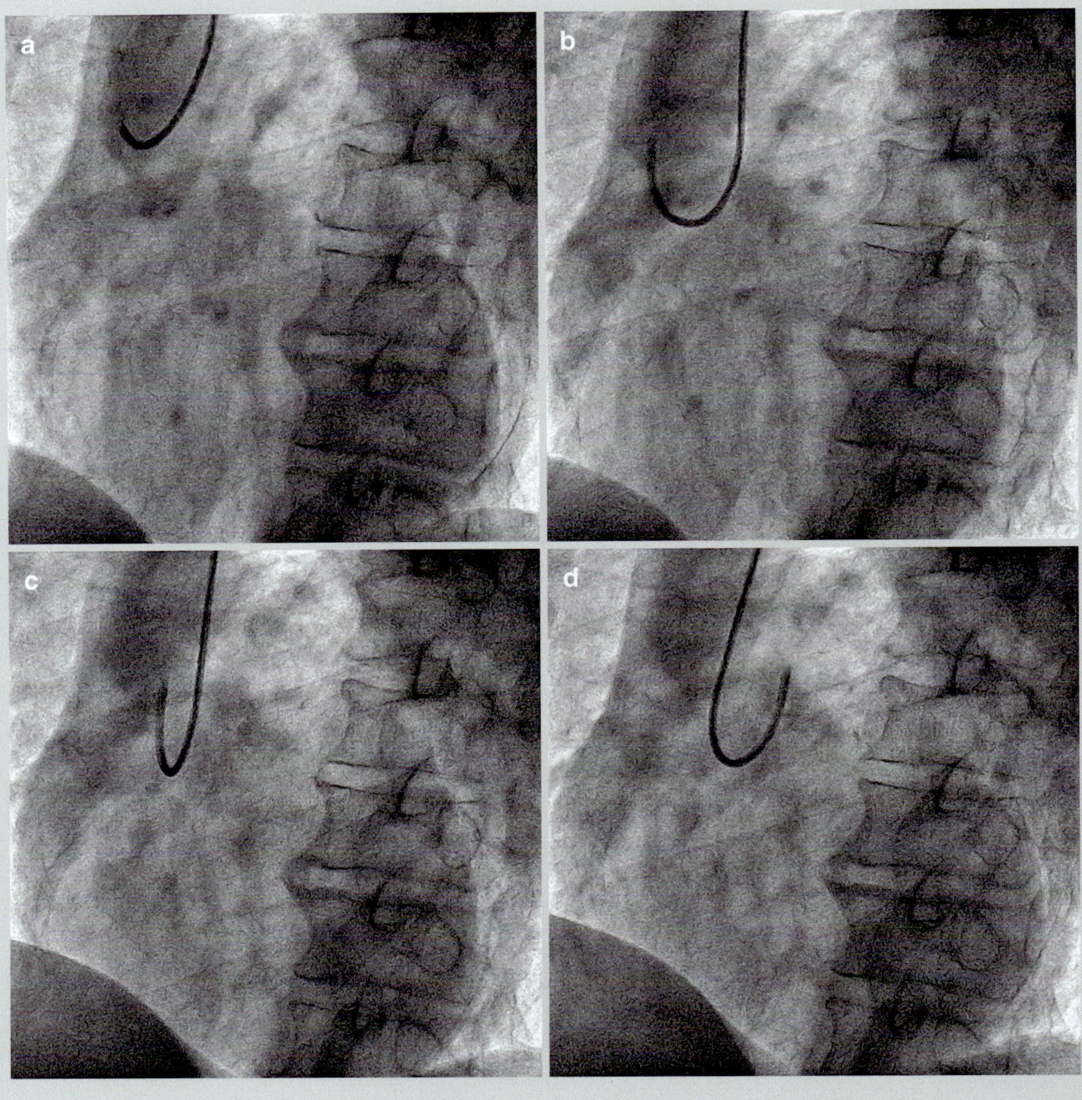

Fig. 14.10 After finished angiography of RCA, pull the MAC3.5 guiding catheter against the contralateral wall of LCA (**a**); push the catheter to formed a U shape (**b**); apply clockwise torque (**c**, **d**) until its tip facing LCA (**e**); the tip position below the left main ostium was verified with small contrast media injections (**f**); slightly pull the catheter (**g**) and engage the ostium of LCA with test injection (white arrow) (**h**). The LCx was totally occluded after give rise to a branch (**i**); aspirate the thrombus after a wire passes the lesion to distal of LCx, the lesion was stented with good result (**j**)

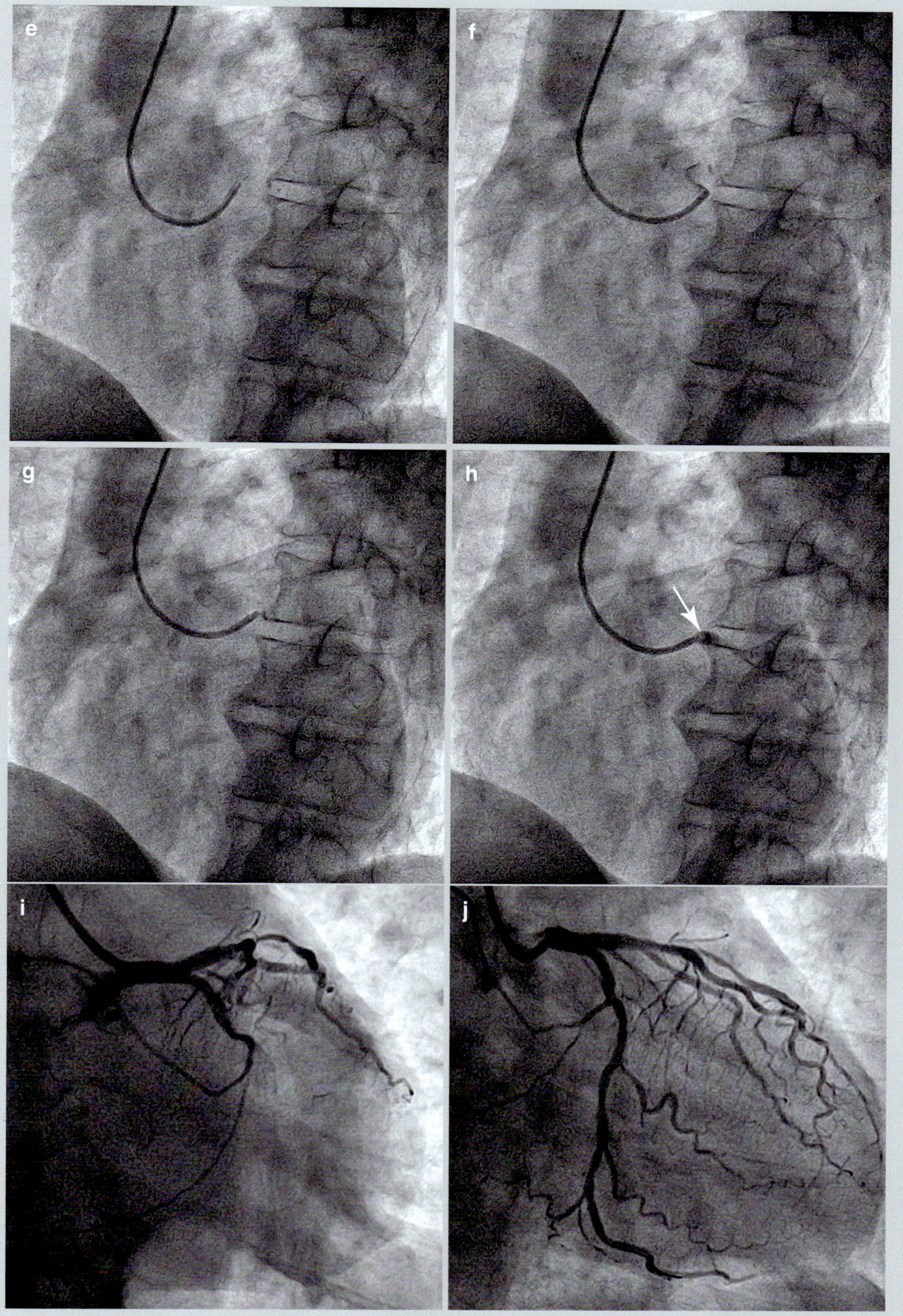

Fig. 14.10 (continued)

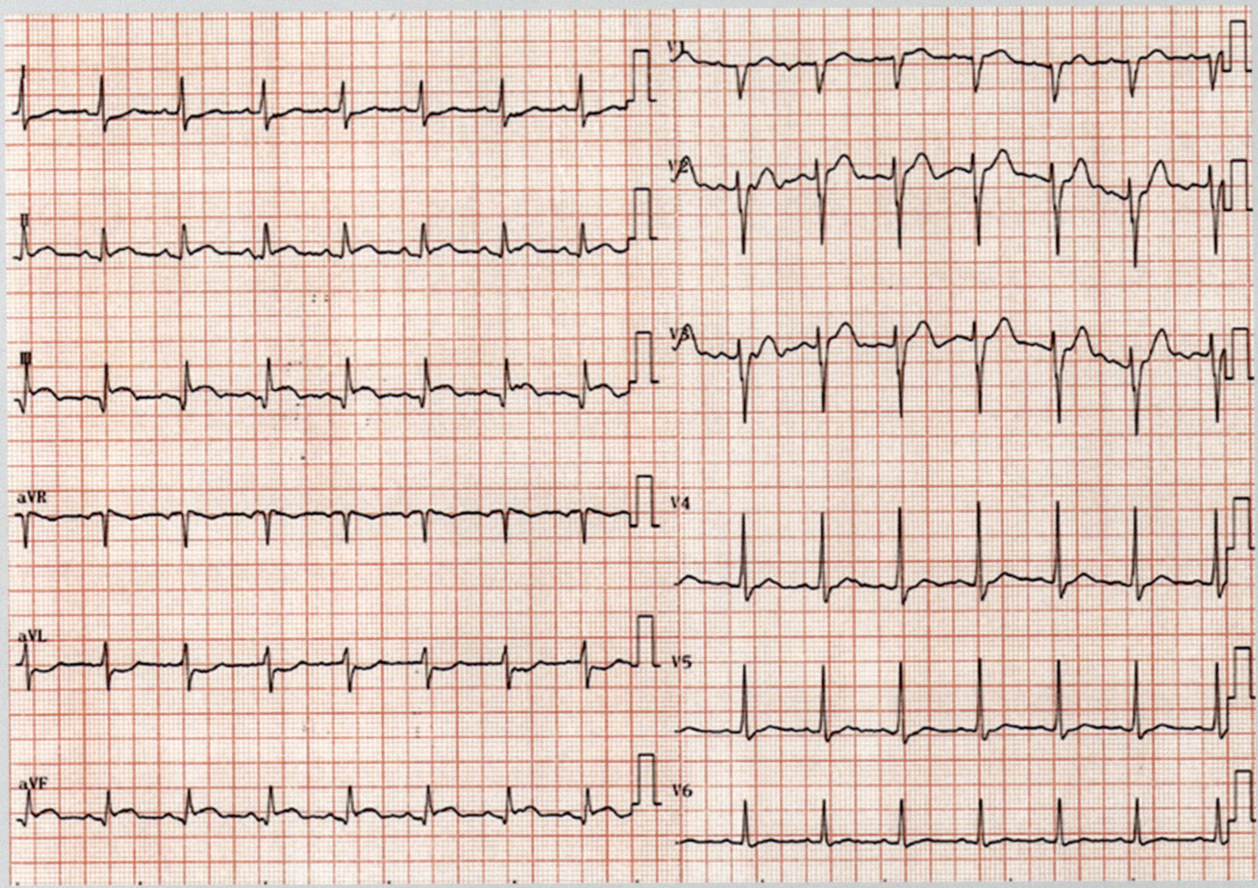

Fig. 14.11 Twelve-lead ECG demonstrate a sinus rhythm and ST-segment elevation in inferior leads (II,III and aVF) with pathologic Q-waves (III and aVF)

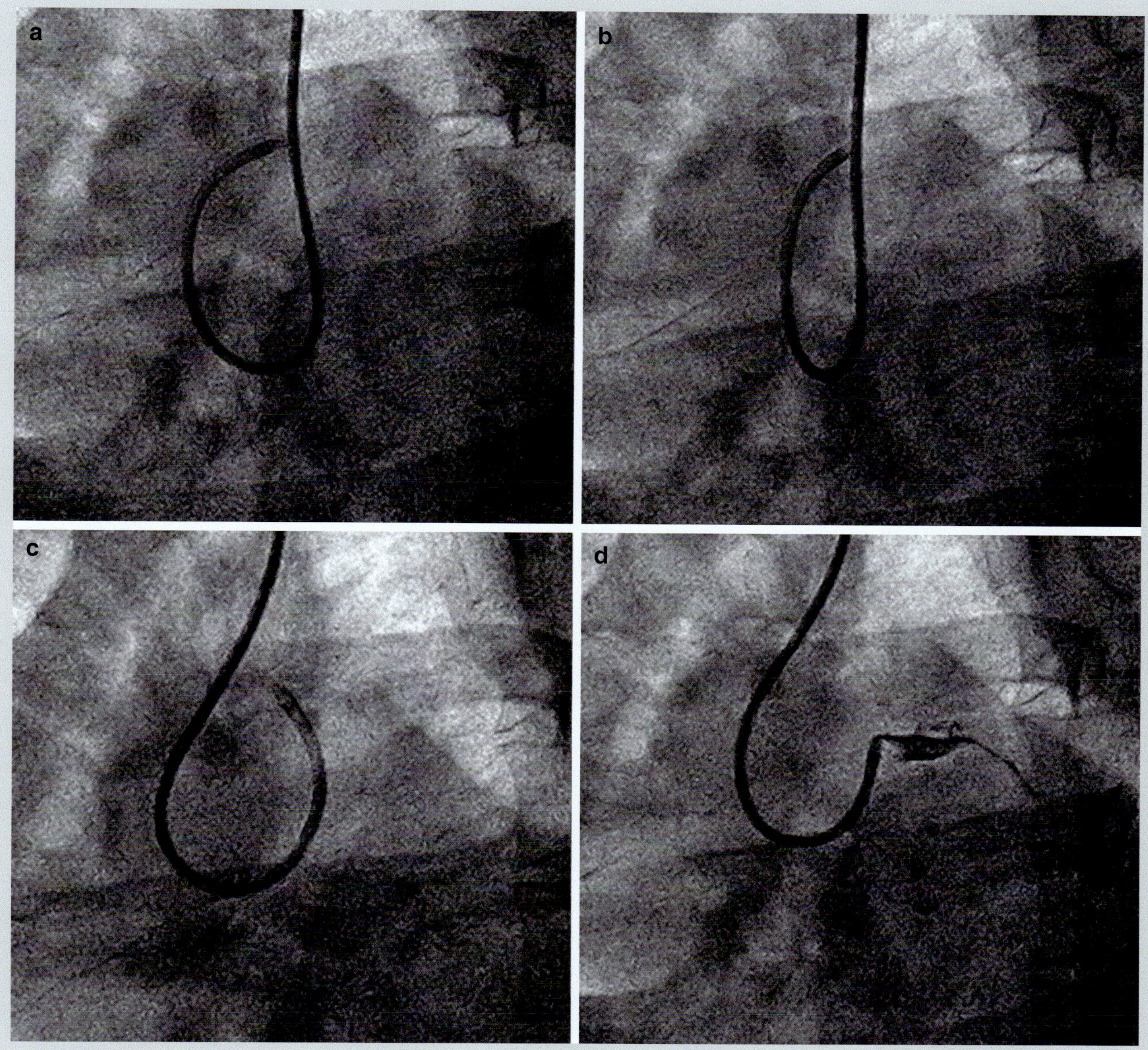

Fig. 14.12 Manipulation of MAC3.5 guiding catheter for coronary angiography of left coronary artery. A big U shape was formed (**a**); clockwise catheter rotation with its tip upward (**b**); when the catheter is in left cusp (**c**); pullback is required to carefully engage the artery (**d**)

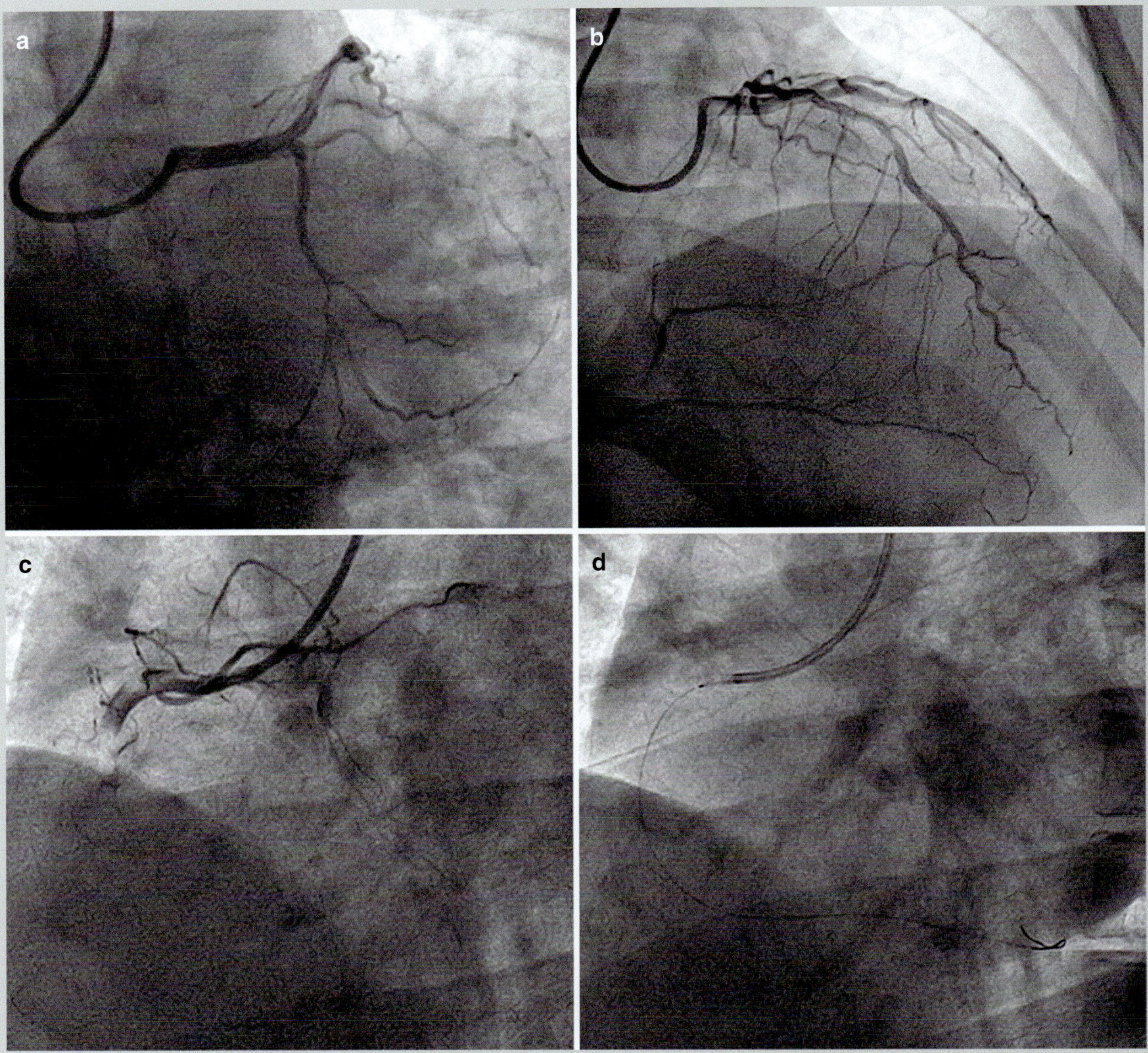

Fig. 14.13 Coronary angiogram showed moderate stenosis in distal-LCx (**a**) and mid-LAD with good collateral to visualize distal RCA (**b**), RCA was totally occluded in proximal segment with huge thrombus (**c**); thrombus aspiration was performed (**d**); and thrombi were retrieved (**e**); coronary angiography revealed thrombus present after aspiration (**f**); aspiration again and retrieval of larger thrombi (**g**); severe stentosis in mid-RCA (**h**); the lesion was predilated (**i**) and stented (**j**). *LCx* left circumflex, *LAD* left anterior ascending artey, *RCA* right coronary artery

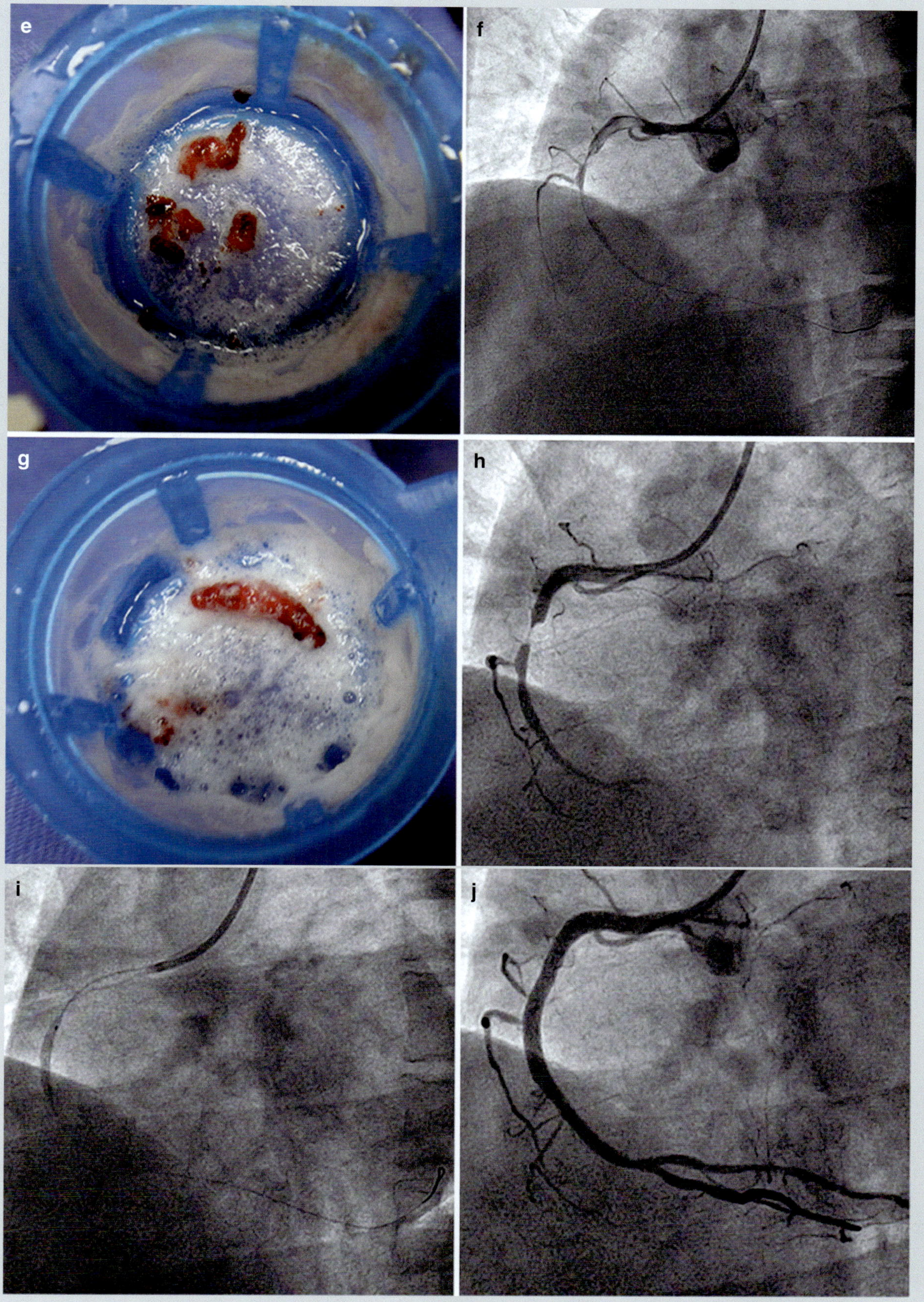

Fig. 14.13 (continued)

Case 4

A 46-year-old man experienced a constant, substernal, sharp, nonradiating chest pain of 2.5 h' duration, He denied previous chest discomfort. He was transferred to emergency department by ambulance. His heart rate was 64 beats per minute, with a blood pressure of 75/30 mmHg. Initial 12-lead ECG showed ST-segment elevation in leads aVL, aVR, V_{2-3} and ST segment depression in inferior leads (Fig. 14.14). Diagnosed with acute anterior myocardial infarction, he was treated with aspirin, clopidogrel and dopamine was intravenously given for hypotension. Coronary angiography was performed via right radial artery while IABP was inserted to support hemodynamic through right femoral artery access. RCA was engaged first using a single MAC3.5 guiding catheter and coronary angiography demonstrated that RCA was normal and dominant vessel, no collateral from RCA to LCA was found (Fig. 14.15a). The same guiding catheter was also engaged LCA and revealed that total occlusion of left main (Fig. 14.15b). After 0.014-in. wire passed the lesion and aspiration catheter aspirated, TIMI grade 3 flow was restored. After crossover stenting from left main to LAD (Fig. 14.15c, d), LCx ostium was jailed (Fig. 14.15e) which was predilated and stented (Fig. 14.15f). Post-dilation with kissing balloon technique was done in both left main-LAD and left main-LCx with good result (Fig.14.15g, h).

Comment: It is noteworthy that the use of the MAC guide catheter for both angiography and intervention in this acute left main occlusion case avoided time-consuming catheter exchanges.

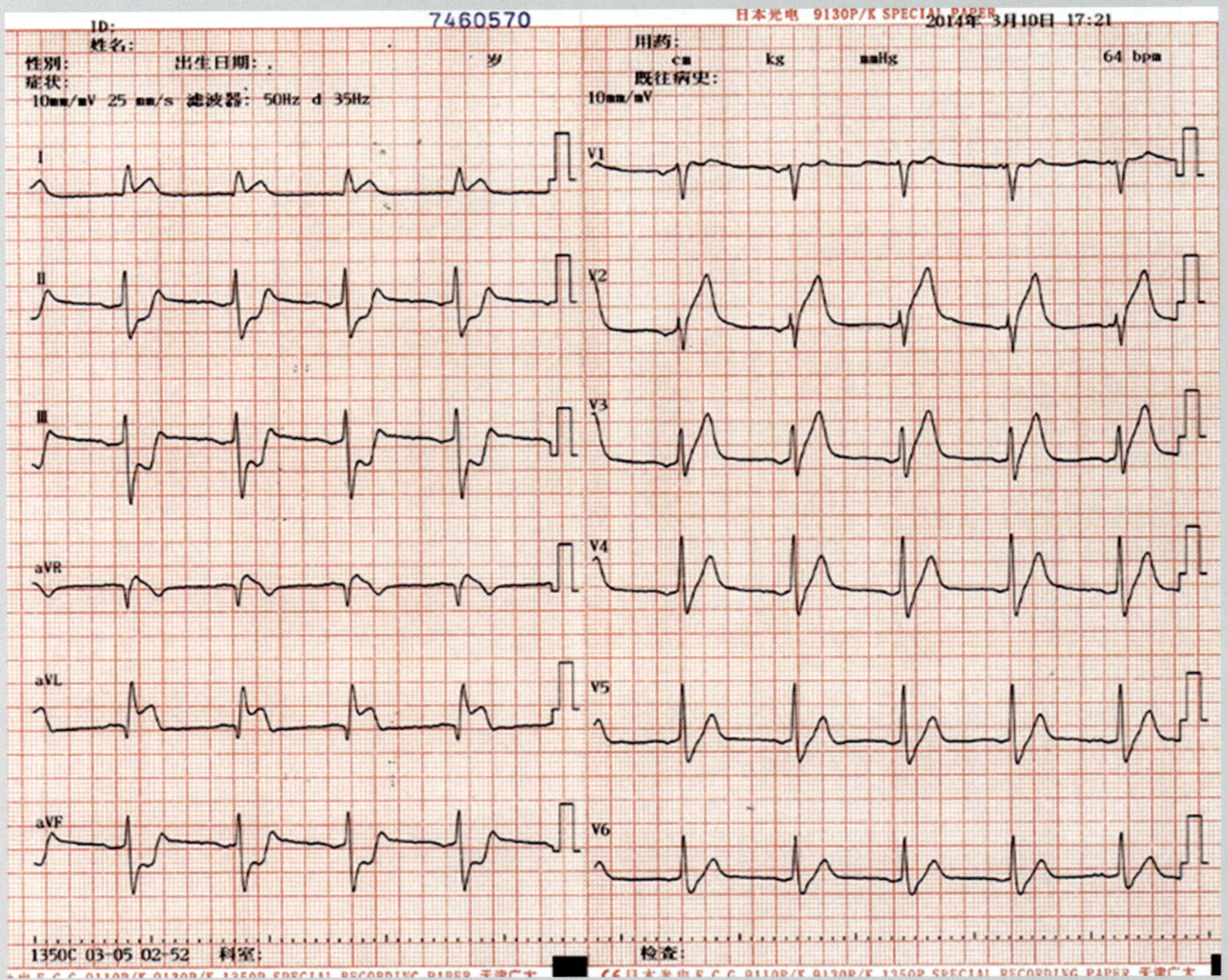

Fig. 14.14 Initial 12-lead ECG showed ST-segment elevation in leads aVL, aVR, V2-3 and ST segment depression in inferior leads (II, III, aVF)

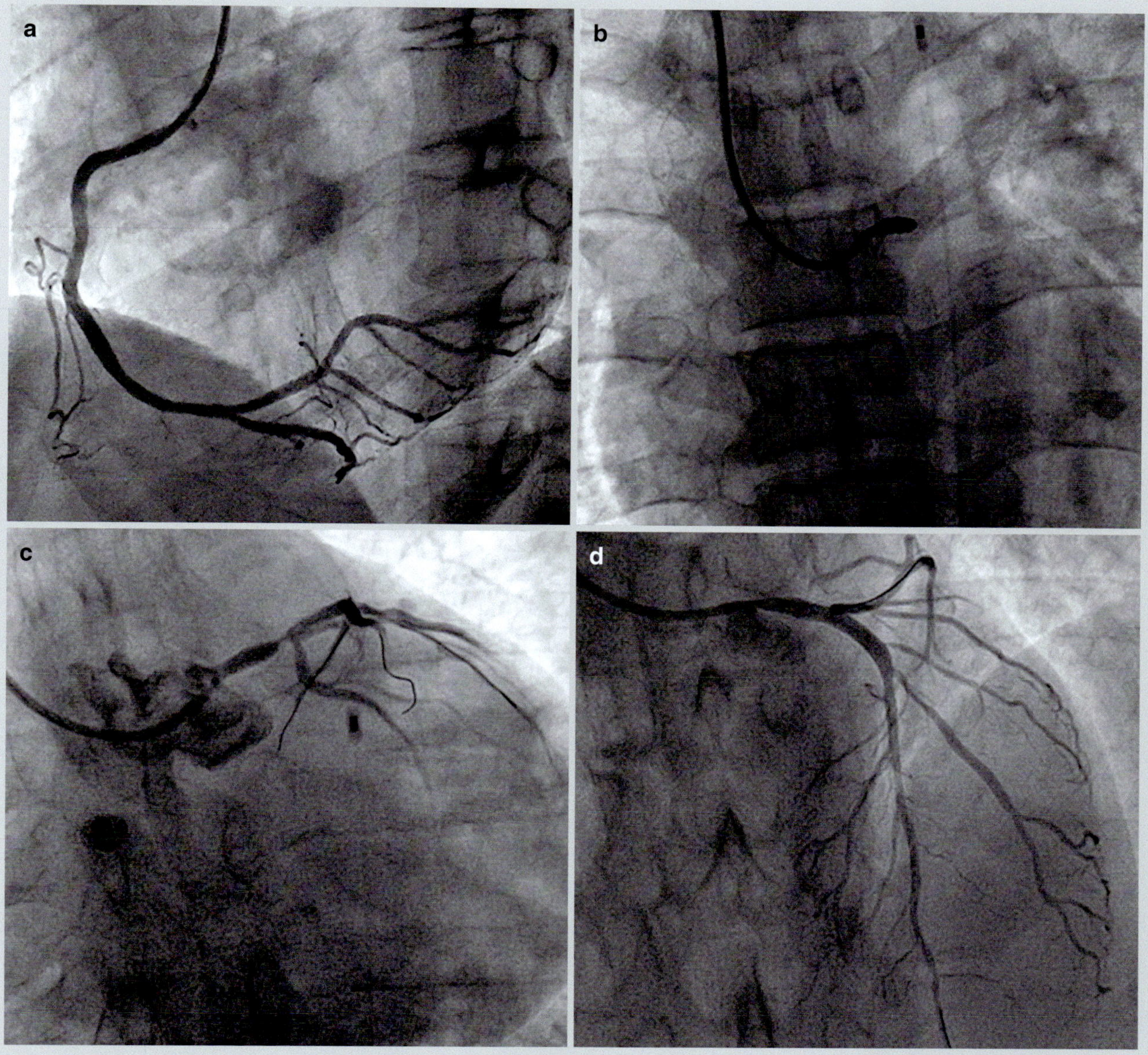

Fig. 14.15 The basal angiogram of RCA using MAC3.5 guiding catheter showed normal and dominant without collateral from right to left (**a**); the same guiding catheter for LCA showed total occlusion of the left main and IABP was inserted from right femoral artery (**b**); After thrombus aspiration, TIMI grade 3 flow was restored (**c**). crossover stenting from left main to LAD (**d**); LCx ostium was jailed (**e**); which was predilated and stented with final kissing balloon technique in both left main-LAD and left main-LCx with good result (**f–h**)

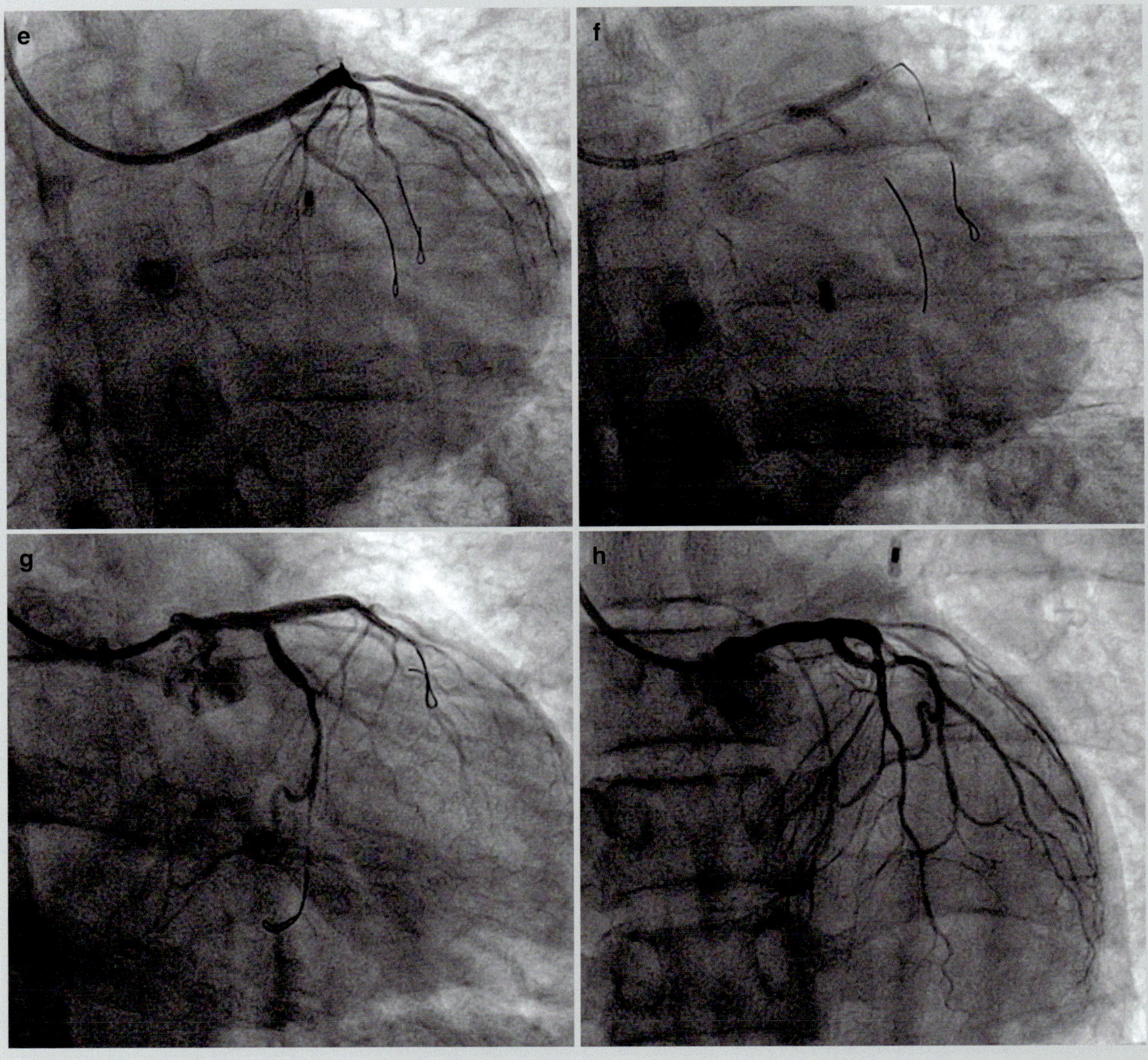

Fig. 14.15 (continued)

Case 5

A 48-year-old man with hypertension developed acute onset of substernal chest pain while he was watching television at 22:00, he presented to emergency department at 22:45, the initial ECG revealed inferior ST-segment elevation (Fig. 14.16). He was taken emergently to the cardiac catheterization laboratory for presumed occlusion of the RCA, where he was arrived at 23:00. A 6 Fr MAC3.5 guiding catheter was advanced over a 0.35_in guidewire into the ascending aorta. Angiography of the left coronary system revealed a severe stenosis in the mid-LAD (Fig. 14.17a) and normal LCx. The same catheter was redirected to the RCA which was severe stenosis in proximal segment and occluded in its distal portion with TIMI grade 0 flow (Fig. 14.17b). A 0.014-in. soft guidewire was easily passed through the occlusion into the distal vessel, after aspirate the thrombus and predilate with a 2.0 mm balloon TIMI grade 3 flow was restored (Fig. 14.17c), The culprit RCA was stented with a 2.75×33 mm drug-eluting stent (DES) in culprit lesion and 3.5×36 mm DES in proximal lesion with no residual narrowing and TIMI grade 3 flow (Fig. 14.17d, e). The patient remained hemodynamically stable, we decided to treat non-culprit vessel-LAD and a 3.0×18 mm DES was implanted into mid-LAD with good result (Fig. 14.17f).

Comment: It is very typical case of using a single MAC3.5 guiding catheter for both culprit RCA and non-culprit LAD PCI. Its advantage is to reduce catheter exchange and procedure time.

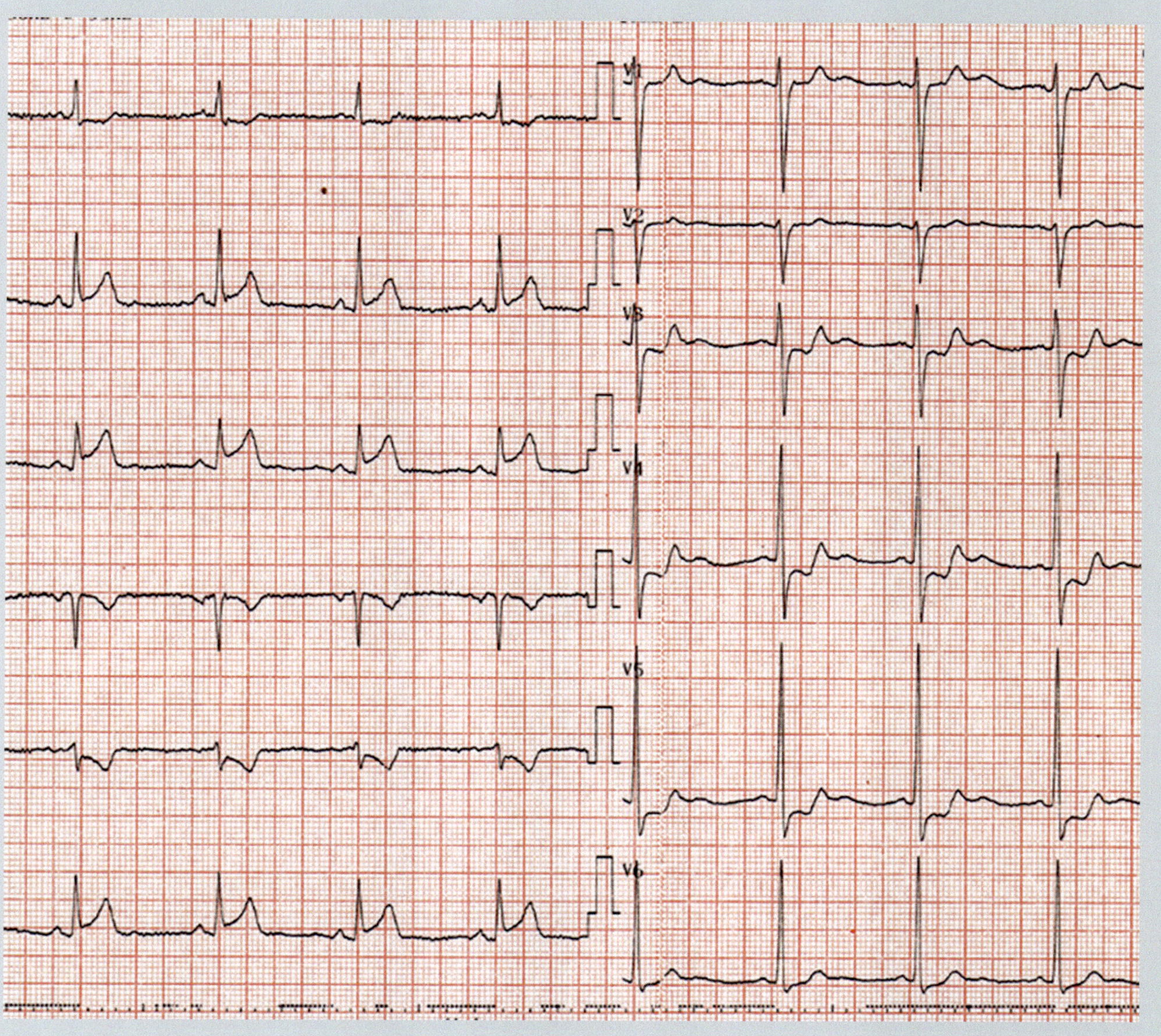

Fig. 14.16 A 12-lead ECG demonstrated ST segment elevation in leads II, III, aVF and depression in leads I, aVL, V_{3-5}

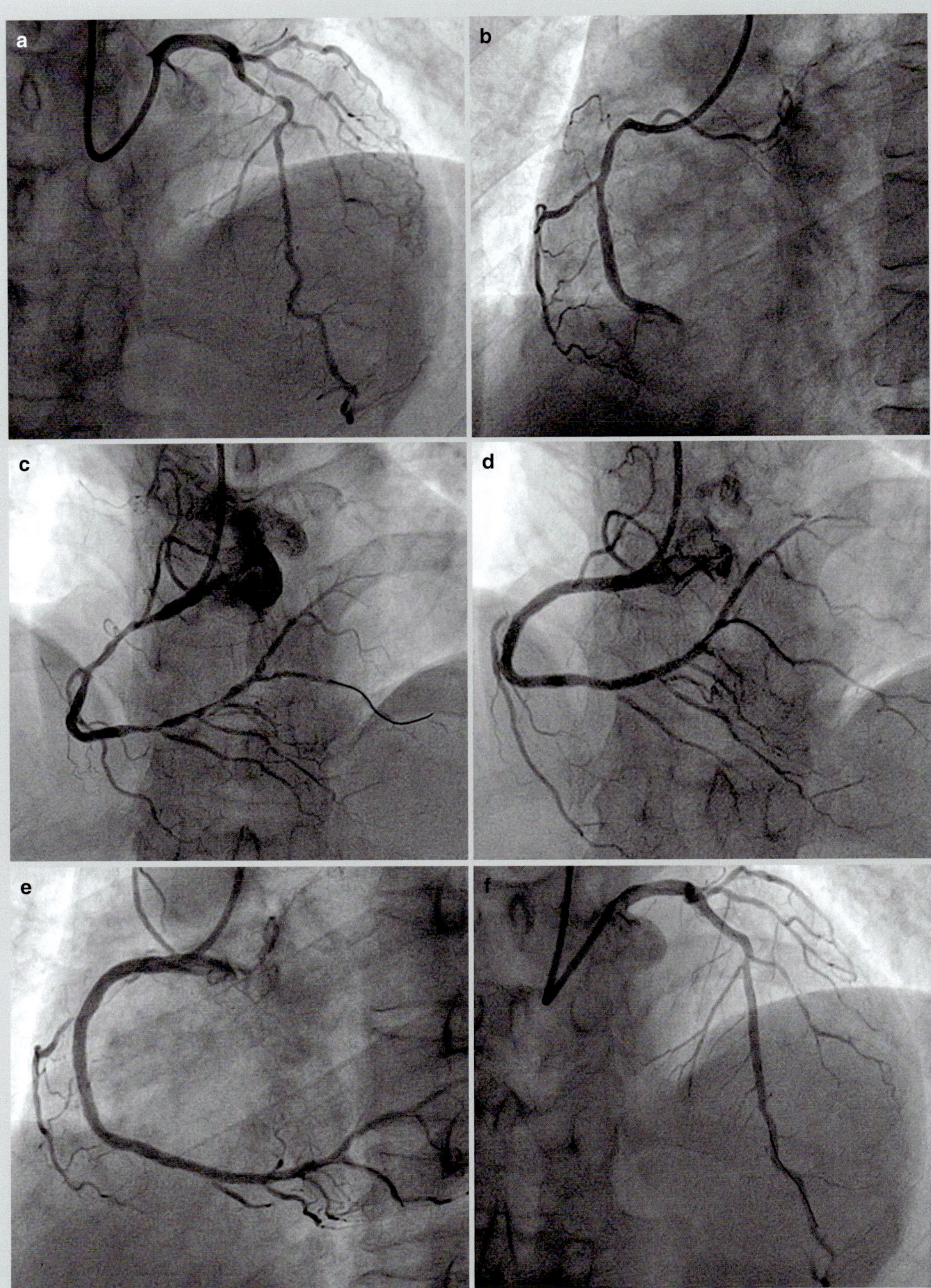

Fig. 14.17 Left coronary artery was first cannulated and revealed a severe stenosis in the mid-LAD (**a**) and normal LCX; distal RCA was totally occluded (**b**); long diffuse lesion in distal-RCA after thrombus aspiration and predilatation (**c**); proximal and distal lesion was stented (**d**, **e**); stenting the LAD lesion (**f**)

References

1. Kiemeneij F, Laarman GJ. Percutaneous transradial artery approach for coronary palmaz-schatz stent implantation. Am Heart J. 1994; 128:167–74.
2. Valgimigli M, Saia F, Guastaroba P, Menozzi A, Magnavacchi P, Santarelli A, Passerini F, Sangiorgio P, Manari A, Tarantino F, Margheri M, Benassi A, Sangiorgi MG, Tondi S, Marzocchi A. Transradial versus transfemoral intervention for acute myocardial infarction: a propensity score-adjusted and -matched analysis from the real (registro regionale angioplastiche dell'emilia-romagna) multicenter registry. JACC Cardiovasc Interv. 2012;5:23–35.
3. Mamas MA, Ratib K, Routledge H, Neyses L, Fraser DG, de Belder M, Ludman PF, Nolan J. Influence of arterial access site selection on outcomes in primary percutaneous coronary intervention: are the results of randomized trials achievable in clinical practice? JACC Cardiovasc Interv. 2013;6:698–706.
4. Windecker S, Kolh P, Alfonso F, Collet JP, Cremer J, Falk V, Filippatos G, Hamm C, Head SJ, Juni P, Kappetein AP, Kastrati A, Knuuti J, Landmesser U, Laufer G, Neumann FJ, Richter DJ, Schauerte P, Sousa Uva M, Stefanini GG, Taggart DP, Torracca L, Valgimigli M, Wijns W, Witkowski A. 2014 esc/eacts guidelines on myocardial revascularization: the task force on myocardial revascularization of the european society of cardiology (esc) and the european association for cardio-thoracic surgery (eacts)developed with the special contribution of the european association of percutaneous cardiovascular interventions (eapci). Eur Heart J. 2014;35:2541–619.
5. Bertrand OF, Belisle P, Joyal D, Costerousse O, Rao SV, Jolly SS, Meerkin D, Joseph L. Comparison of transradial and femoral approaches for percutaneous coronary interventions: a systematic review and hierarchical bayesian meta-analysis. Am Heart J. 2012;163:632–48.
6. Jolly SS, Yusuf S, Cairns J, Niemela K, Xavier D, Widimsky P, Budaj A, Niemela M, Valentin V, Lewis BS, Avezum A, Steg PG, Rao SV, Gao P, Afzal R, Joyner CD, Chrolavicius S, Mehta SR. Radial versus femoral access for coronary angiography and intervention in patients with acute coronary syndromes (rival): a randomised, parallel group, multicentre trial. Lancet. 2011;377:1409–20.
7. Baklanov DV, Kaltenbach LA, Marso SP, Subherwal SS, Feldman DN, Garratt KN, Curtis JP, Messenger JC, Rao SV. The prevalence and outcomes of transradial percutaneous coronary intervention for st-segment elevation myocardial infarction: analysis from the national cardiovascular data registry (2007 to 2011). J Am Coll Cardiol. 2013;61:420–6.
8. Bertrand OF, Rao SV, Pancholy S, Jolly SS, Rodes-Cabau J, Larose E, Costerousse O, Hamon M, Mann T. Transradial approach for coronary angiography and interventions: results of the first international transradial practice survey. JACC Cardiovasc Interv. 2010;3:1022–31.
9. Chiang A, Gada H, Kodali SK, Lee MS, Jeremias A, Pinto DS, Bangalore S, Yeh RW, Henry TD, Lopez-Cruz G, Mehran R, Kirtane AJ. Procedural variation in the performance of primary percutaneous coronary intervention for st-elevation myocardial infarction: a scai-based survey study of us interventional cardiologists. Catheter Cardiovasc Interv. 2014;83:721–6.
10. Plourde G, Abdelaal E, Bataille Y, MacHaalany J, Dery JP, Dery U, Larose E, De Larochelliere R, Gleeton O, Barbeau G, Roy L, Costerousse O, Bertrand OF. Effect on door-to-balloon time of immediate transradial percutaneous coronary intervention on culprit lesion in st-elevation myocardial infarction compared to diagnostic angiography followed by primary percutaneous coronary intervention. Am J Cardiol. 2013;111:836–40.
11. Jurado-Roman A, Garcia-Tejada J, Hernandez-Hernandez F, Granda-Nistal C, Rubio-Alonso B, Agudo-Quilez P, Velazquez-Martin M, Albarran-Gonzalez-Trevilla A, Tascon-Perez J. Does reducing ischemia time justify to catheterize firstly the culprit artery in every primary pci? Heart Vessels. 2016;31:1022–9.
12. Roberts EB, Wood A. Use of a single q guide catheter for complete assessment and treatment of both coronary arteries via radial access during acute st elevation myocardial infarction: a review of 40 consecutive cases. J Interv Cardiol. 2011;24:389–96.
13. Chow J, Tan CH, Tin AS, Ong SH, Tan VH, Goh YS, Gan HW, Tan KS, Lingamanaicker J. Feasibility of transradial coronary angiography and intervention using a single ikari left guiding catheter for st elevation myocardial infarction. J Interv Cardiol. 2012;25:235–44.
14. Malaiapan Y, Leung M, Ahmar W, Hutchison AW, Prasad S, Katticaran T, Cameron JD, Harper RW, Meredith IT. Guideline recommended door-to-balloon time can be achieved in transradial primary pci – the usefulness of a dedicated radial guide catheter. Cardiovasc Revasc Med. 2013;14:27–31.
15. Moon KW, Kim JH, Kim JY, Jung MH, Kim GH, Yoo KD, Kim CM. Reducing needle-to-balloon time by using a single guiding catheter during transradial primary coronary intervention. J Interv Cardiol. 2012;25:330–6.

15 Transradial Approach for Unprotected Left Main Lesions

Yujie Zhou and Wei Liu

Abstract

With the development of new technology and emergence of new generation drug eluting stent, unprotected left main coronary artery (ULMCA) is no longer a contraindication for percutaneous coronary intervention (PCI). Although most coronary lesions can now be successfully treated via the transradial approach (TRA), PCI for ULMCA disease is usually performed via transfemoral access (TFA) by using 7 or 8 French guiding catheter, because of the high rate of distal bifurcation lesion and the large diameter of the vessel.

In this chapter we will address the evidence of using TRA approach for ULM CA intervention procedures, as well as discuss the technical aspects in the subset of high risk and complex PCI.

15.1 Introduction

Coronary artery bypass grafting is currently the recommended choice for left main CAD [1]. However due to a high rate of atherosclerosis in vein grafts and a shortage in arterial grafts, more and more cardiologists are leaning towards percutaneous coronary intervention as an alternative method of revascularization for the left main coronary disease. Thanks to evolvement of technique and proficiency, the efficacy and safety of LM PCI has significantly improved. Introduction of drug eluted stents has dramatically decreased the rate of restenosis of LM, which used to be a major disadvantage of PCI. The syntax score is a grading system used to assess the complexity of coronary artery disease. It allows the interventionists to gage whether the PCI or CABG would be more beneficial for a patient with CAD. Left main patients with syntax score greater than 33 or with multi-vessel disease fared much better with CABG than PCI. On the other hand, patients with a lower syntax score did just as well with PCI plus had a lower stroke rate [2]. Outcomes of LM-PCI get better over time mainly due to the better concept and improved DES [3, 4].

The use of trans-radial approach (TRA) instead of trans-femoral approach (TFA) is becoming more and more popular amongst interventionists for left main coronary intervention. The introduction of larger lumen catheters that maintain a small overall diameter have also allowed for a higher procedural success rate in transradial PCI for LM [5].

15.2 Feasibility and Advantages of Transradial Over Transfemoral in LM Intervention

Many studies have systematically compared the feasibility of left main PCI based on vascular access with consistent results [6, 7].

A study was undertaken with 467 patients undergoing ULMS-bifurcation PCI, of which 221 underwent TFA and 224 underwent TRA. The TR procedure is used more significantly in both simple and complex procedures with fewer access site complications (2.0 % vs 6.3 % in TF, $p=0.02$), and has a reduction in NACE rate (16.9 % vs 15.7 %, $p=0.1$). TRA has similar prolonged ischemic complications as TFA, but with decreased access site complications, resulting in a significant reduction in NACE rate [8]. The current total outcome noted for patients with ULMS

Y. Zhou (✉) • W. Liu
Department of Cardiology, Beijing Anzhen Hospital, Capital Medical University, Beijing, China
e-mail: Azzyj12@163.com; Liuwei525@hotmail.com

Y. Zhou et al. (eds.), *Transradial Approach for Percutaneous Interventions*, DOI 10.1007/978-94-017-7350-8_15

bifurcation who have undergone PCI showed an increase in safety, feasibility and reasonable clinical efficacy for transradial procedures compared to transfemoral procedures. Transradial centers have notably started adopting large bulks of patients under the transradial approach for ULMS bifurcation PCI. Cardiogenic shock and unfavorable transradial anatomy are the only factors which at times give TF approach a slight advantage.

Another trial conducted involving 853 patients (out of which 212 were in the TR group and 641 were in the TF group) and compared TR and TF techniques using drug eluting stents for left main bifurcation disease. It showed no differences in prognosis (98.6 % vs 99.7 %; P=.07) and side branches (90.6 % vs 94.4 %; P=.05). They also demonstrated that use of thrombolysis for MI patients are less likely to have bleeding in TRA as compared to TFA (2.4 % vs 9.4 %; P=.01). The current trial shows TRA has less bleeding complication compared to TFA and also showed no difference in procedural success rate and good prognosis in LMCA bifurcation disease patient. So according to the results, we can choose TRA as the primary access site for LMCA bifurcation disease patients.

Further studies have been conducted in a higher volume transradial PCI center from China for patients with high risk left main coronary anatomy [9]. In a total of 821 patients with UPLM disease, revascularization was done by TRA in 353 patients and TFA in 486 patients. This study showed similar procedural time, which was 97 % in TFA and 96 % in TRA (p=0.57). It also showed that with TRA there was a reduction in the length of hospital stay, thrombosis in myocardial infarction and major or minor bleeding. They also compared the rate of cardiovascular death (TRA 1.2 % vs TFA 2.0 %, p=0.48), nonfatal myocardial infarction (TRA 4.7 % vs TFA 2.4 %, p=0.16), thrombosis due to stents (TRA 0.8 vs TFA 2.8 %, p=0.10) and revascularization of vessel (TRA 6.0 % vs TFA 6.7 %) showing similar statistical data with propensity score modelling.

These LM specific studies comparing transradial and transfermoral approaches are a definite eye opener in the field of interventional cardiology. These studies have shown that PCI via the TRA rather than the TFA results in a significant reduction in overall bleeding complications. With this advantage, interventionists may be more comfortable giving adequate anti-thrombotic therapy which is virtually important for LM-PCI. Accordingly, the lower risk of bleeding with TRA is linked to a reduction in the formation of thrombosis which could be fatal to the patient.

These studies also show that TRA is associated with a shortened hospital stay and similar procedural success rates compared to TFA. All in all, these studies show that TRA is a feasible and effective alternative for revascularization in LM ostial and body, along with LM bifurcation lesions.

15.3 How to Overcome the Disadvantages of Transradial Approach in LM Intervention

Transradial intervention to-date holds a steep learning curve. Limitations of the TRA for LM mainly involves the learning curve and the shortage in valid technology or services available, this being in comparison with the transfemoral approach. Primary factors which predict TRA failure involve gender, BMI, advanced age and lack of experience. Being able to negotiate and correctly manage the radial artery and aortic arch during the procedure for LM with guide wires and catheters, is technically more demanding than the femoral approach.

One of the major drawbacks faced by radial artery interventionists is the small diameter of the radial artery (range 1.8–3 mm), making it difficult to choose the befitting equipment to carry out the procedure, resulting in it becoming a different approach in comparison to transfemoral intervention (diameters 7.02 ± 0.85 mm). Due to an unappealing anatomic route and size of the radial artery, it is often incorrectly perceived that certain techniques are not feasible. Nevertheless, the most commonly used catheter sizes for TRA interventions performed today are done using 6 or 7-Fr guiding catheters. Using 6 Fr catheters, the interventionist can successfully perform even the most complex lesions, such as left main bifurcation or chronic total occlusion. Furthermore, rotational atherectomy or intravascular ultrasound can be performed flawlessly with these guides. Even so, there are some complexities that could arise by using smaller sized guides but they more often than not do not stand as a barrier against achieving successful left main coronary intervention.

The limitation of small sized radial lumen diameter can also be overcome with sheathless guiding catheter. Recent study showed that sheathless guide catheter by transradial approach is a feasible alternative for percutaneous treatment of LM coronary artery disease achieving 95 % of procedure success with no cross-over to transfemoral approach and no access complications [10].

15.4 The Technical Issues of Transradial Left Main Coronary Intervention

Left main disease is associated with higher mortality with PCI. 4–6 % patients undergoing coronary angiography fall into this subset of category. Left main lesions appear complex, because more than 50 % of the cases have calcification, more than 70 % have concomitant multi-vessel disease and more than 70 % have distal bifurcation LM lesion. The left main also appears in many size and shapes, supplies large area at risk, has risk of hemodynamic instability, allows short windows in case of complications thus making PCI more difficult to perform.

Anatomically the left main lesions can be divided into three parts, namely distal, mid-shaft and ostial lesions. According to the syntax studies, the incidence rate of ostial lesions is 22.1 %, the mid-shaft is 13.8 % and the distal bifurcation being 64.1 %. As stated by the delta registry, distal ULMCA PCI has a higher rate of MACE (HR 1.48 1.16–1.89 P<0.001) in comparison with ostial and mid-shaft LM lesions. On the other hand, ostial lesions treated with PCI have a comparably long term MACCE result when compared to CABG. However, CABG is more beneficial for the long term MACE when it comes to distal LM bifurcation lesions [11].

15.4.1 Ostial Left Main Lesions

Transradial PCI in ostial LMCA stenosis is technically challenging for several reasons:

1. Coronary angiogram in left main ostium has well-known limitations due to overlapping and foreshortening of vessel shadows, evidence of catheter artifact and reflux of contrast material in the sinus of the aorta during injection. This limitation could explain the difficulties of proper evaluation of ostium, as well as bifurcation, reference of diffuse disease.
2. Ostial left main lesion arises from 3 mm of origin of the aorta. Usually it is a part of aortic disease that is calcified and fibrotic, having resistant to dilatation and prevalence of recoil.
3. PCI of ostium LM is challenging because of difficulties in siting guiding catheter, obtaining adequate images, accurate positioning during stent placement, covering the lesion adequately and preventing stent migration. Different from the balloon dilatation in non-ostial LM which is more physiological resulting in well longitude stretching and expansion of vessel diameter, the strength of aortic tunica media contains collagen fibers, the dilation in the aortic-LM junction results in resistance and recoil thus need for careful lesion preparation; high pressure post dilation of stent is compulsory.

15.4.2 Guide Support

Engagement of guiding catheter to LM ostium could cause complete obstruction and result in global ischemia, hypotension and arrhythmia. The guiding catheter can also cause plaque shifting, spasm, dissection and obstruction. Special requirement of guiding catheter includes: Optimal positioning of catheter has to facilitate easy and gentle engagement and disengagement. The operator must use less aggressive, soft tip catheter and avoid deep intubation. The most frequently used guiding catheter in TRA -LM is JL 3.5 or 4 when strong backup is not needed. However, EBU is preferred if distal LM was involved. (EBU manipulation during ostium-LM PCI, please refer to Chapter). Strong large volume of contrast injection is not recommended. Close monitoring of blood pressure curve, numbers and ECG is obligatory. Sufficient support, better visualization, time limited engagement, avoiding risk of complications are key points for manipulating guiding catheter during transradial LM -intervention.

15.4.2.1 Guide Wire

Insertion of guidewire is not a problem for LM -ostium intervention, standard, workhorse wire is appropriate. Supportive wires are preferable if guiding catheter could not provide sufficient support. The common recommendation is to preload the wire in the guiding catheter in order to facilitate the rapid wiring and disengagement.

The guidewire provides additional function to facilitate engagement and disengagement of guiding catheter, and stability of the system.

15.4.2.2 Balloon

Lesion preparation is an obligatory part in PCI for LM -ostium intervention. Use of high pressure balloon, cutting and scoring balloon, and debunking is currently a common approach, the inflation time of pre-dilatation is usually short to limit the duration of myocardial ischemia but often requires multiple high pressure inflations. Advancement and retrieval of the balloon should be performed gently and with precautions, in case of thrombus and atherosclerotic plaque embolized proximally to cerebral artery causing stroke.

15.4.2.3 Stenting

Stent implantation is challenging because of difficulties in positioning the guide catheter, obtaining adequate images to enhance stent placement, ensuring proper stent position to cover the entire lesion adequately, and preventing stent migration. The main difficulty in deploying the stent is the determination of the exact stent positioning. Incorrect definition of LMCA ostium leads to incorrect stent position (uncovered ostium of LM or stent protrusion into aorta). Angulations, length and shape of LM segments influence the accuracy of stent to vessel apposition.

Evidence of partial protrusion of strut into the aorta is documented when the stent completely covered the ostium and angulation of the arising left main achieved 30° or more, this situation will subject to trauma by the guiding catheter, causing prolapse of stent and prevent further passage of balloon or other devices during the current procedure or in the future. The main difficulty in deploying the stent is exact stent positioning. Incorrect apposition or protruding of stent can lead to development of aortic disease, development of stent thrombosis or restentosis; Uncovering ostium will results in suboptimal angiographic outcome, need additional stenting of the balloon, lead to dissection which spreads to aorta and causes restenosis or thrombosis. 2D imaging of left main stenting is restrictive, with false shortening of shadow of coronary artery and overlapping of shadows of coronary artery over one another. To recognize the position of aorta-ostium junction, a non -foreshortend LAO projection with cranial inclination is preferred to obtain a better visualization; slowly removing the guide catheter during contrast injection to define the aorta-ostium junction; Free-floating wire technique with second wire inserted into the aortic cusp can function as origin of ostium and prevent the guide deep engagement to the vessel.

Another challenging part of accurate stent positioning is the swifting of stent during transradial aorta-ostium stenting, Stent inflation is non-predictable. SZABO technique could benefit in this situation. SZABO technique is a guide wire threaded through the most proximal stent cell, the stent moves ahead until it is stopped at the carina [12]. However, the latest bench top evaluation and clinical experiences at 6–8 month follow up showed that The SZABO technique is not a precise technique in which the proximal end of the stent undergoes significant and asymmetric deformation, protruding into the main branch. Additional concerns with this complex technique include the potential for stent damage or contamination before implantation and the risk of stent dislodgement. Thus, requires further attention when using this technique during left main ostial lesions intervention [13].

Lesion preparation, use of stents with a high radial support and high pressure balloon post dilatation are strongly recommended. IVUS is mandatory for evaluation of PCI results: ostium coverage, lesion coverage, stent to vessel apposition, stent deployment and position of its distal edge.

15.4.3 Left Main Body Lesions

Isolated left main bifurcation lesions is rare, and not a challenge for transradial PCI. However, the length of LM should be assessed, since the smallest stents commercially available is 8 mm in length. If the length of LM is less than 8 mm; either ostium or distal bifurcation will be covered. The diameters of LM and its branch should be evaluated to choose the strategy. Lesion should be prepared well before stent implantation; in case of implanting a short stent (8 mm) in large size vessel, Cautions should be taken for the possible migration and dislodgment of the stent. Stent dislodgement can be secondary to marked coronary angulation, coronary calcification, underestimation of stent size, inadequate coronary pre-dilation and direct stent. Thus a short tip, steady guide is preferred. The stent should be fully expanded and covering the lesion.

15.4.4 Left Main Bifurcation

Left main bifurcation is also different from other bifurcations lesions that poses specific challenges relevant to anatomy, plaque layout and composition, and the patient's clinical status. Transradial PCI of left main bifurcation lesions can be successfully accomplished in most cases, but this practice is still restricted in many centers worldwide due to the perceived technical challenges of guiding catheter support, limitations of catheter sizes, need for the simultaneous use of stents and balloons, and consequences of procedural failure. Bifurcations are not alike and may differ with regards to angle, burden of atherosclerotic lesion, relative involvement of LAD/LCX ostia, mismatch of LM and stemming arties diameters.

The Murray's law should be given adequate attention, due to its relatively large sized proximal main branch in comparison to the LCX or LAD, which makes it even more crucial to deliver the correct stent size. In most circumstances, the size of the crossover stent would be chosen according to the diameter of the distal reference; however it would push the carina away, which increases the risk of the side branch being occluded. Meanwhile the stent would be undersized proximally. Thus, the role of POT holds heavy importance. By using it, the correct size of the proximal part of the main branch will be achieved [14]. Some small study shows the clinical outcome to be quite different for when left main is treated with or without POT.

The T-shape angulation has a higher risk of events due to the difficult angulation. Secondly, because of the systolic and diastolic motion between the two stents, which creates an increased potential hazard of stent fracture? More so, accessing the side branch of the left main becomes difficult for which the systematic two wires technique should be applied. On the contrary, both the crush and Culotte techniques are not optimal due to the limitations that result in leaving of a gap.

The ostium being involved increases the rate for a potential risk of a geographical miss. Thus, the view of the left main ostium is an essential factor to assure that no area will be left neglected. In addition, there remains a risk of longitudinal compression that arises when pulling the balloon and the guiding catheter is retracted which could compress the stents. The same would apply when removing the jail wire.

The side branch of the LM is relatively large; therefore it must stay open at the end of the procedure. Consequently, it remains very critical to assess the patient's wellbeing before the decision of stenting of the side branch is made, especially in case of FFR.

During Left main intervention, a single stent provisional approach is the preferred strategy over 2 stents [15]. The

LCX is one of the key elements for indication of LMCA PCI, It depends on the size, area of jeopardized myocardium, ostial location of atheroma plaque, diffuse atheroma and bifurcation angle. However, a 2nd stent may be needed especially when: The LCX is large, the LCX is heavily diseased or the LMS angle is large. Choosing the 2-stent strategy depends on the angle and relies on good quality technique. If the SB angle is acute, modified T or TAP could be used, if not, other techniques, such as DK crush, mini crush, Culotte, will be useful. Single versus double stenting for unprotected left main coronary artery bifurcation lesions: a systematic review and meta-analysis. The 3-year follow-up results of the DKCRUSH-III study showed that Culotte stenting for LMDBLs was associated with significantly increased rates of MACE and ST. (Double Kissing [DK] Crush Versus Culotte Stenting for the Treatment of Unprotected Distal Left Main Bifurcation Lesions [16]. The use of IVUS and FFR-guidance is to be strongly encouraged [17], especially in two stents technique for LM bifurcation lesions.

15.5 Active Plaque Transfer Technique for Provisional Stenting of LM Bifurcation Lesions

A new method of side branch protection technique, which is known as active plaque transfer technique (ATP) described by us, currently is under investigation in PCI for LM bifurcation lesions. (clinicaltrials.gov NCT02127138) In the ATP treatment of true bifurcation lesions, by the balloon pre-dilation in the target side branch, the plaque will be actively transferred from side branch to main vessel. Subsequently, the plaque will be fixed by the expansive stent in main vessel. The technique was reported as Balloon-Stent Kissing Technique which applied to non – LM bifurcation lesions [18]. This could prevent side-branch occlusion, which is devastating in LM -bifurcation PCI. This can also prevent carina shifting caused by MV/MB stenting and facilitate rewiring of the SB as close as possible to the original carina position, thereby leading to better results.

The procedural steps are schematically illustrated as follows (Fig. 15.1):

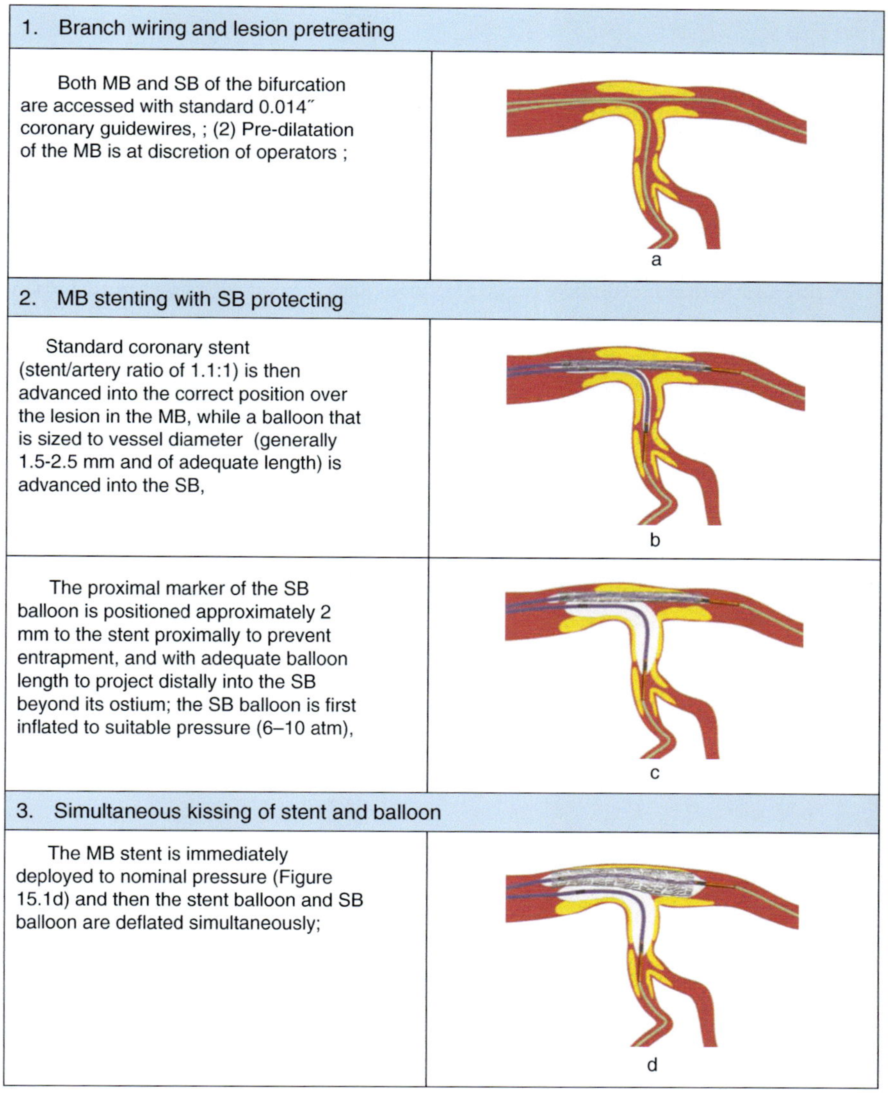

Fig. 15.1 Diagram of ATP procedural steps

Fig. 15.1 (continued)

<table>
<tr><td colspan="2">4. Reshaping of the main branch balloon</td></tr>
<tr><td>If the SB has not been compromised (i.e., TIMI-3 flow), then the trapped SB balloon and wire are removed. Thestent balloon is then fully expanded to moderate or high pressure as clinically indicated for the optimization of the MB stent apposition, and to correct any stent deformation as a result of the SB balloon inflation (e)</td><td>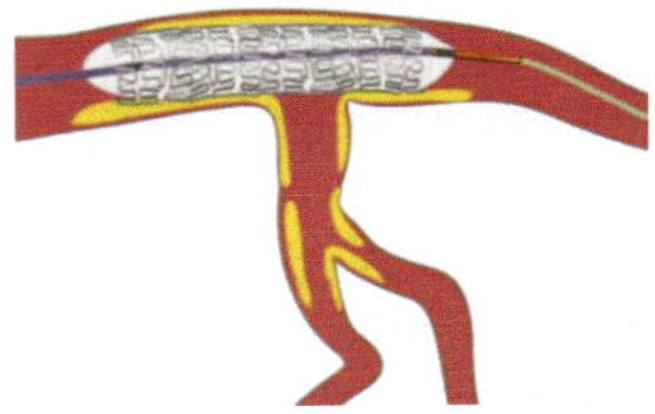
e</td></tr>
<tr><td colspan="2">5. Result of APT</td></tr>
<tr><td>Final angiography will then reveal whether or not re-crossing through the stent struts into the SB is necessary for provisional angioplasty and/or stenting</td><td>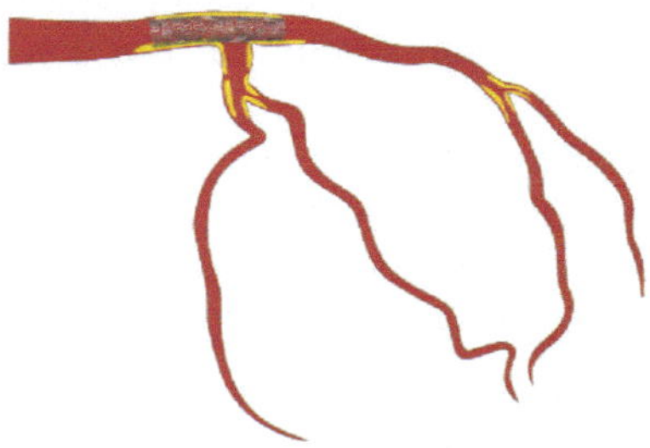
f</td></tr>
</table>

Case 15.1. Transradial LM Stenting in an Obese Patient with STEMI

This is a male patient, 31 years old, admitted due to anterior wall STEMI 1 week prior to admission. He had no hypertension, diabetes, but lead a sedentary life for 10 years, and had acute body weight gain over last 2 years with 167 kg, BMI 49.3. (A) He presented with cardiogenic shock with blood pressure of 70/50 mmHg, heart rate 140 bpm. Extensive ST elevation was noted through leads V1-5, Emergency PCI was performed under ECMO support.

Access: The right FA was occupied with ECMO units. The Left FA was too tortuous to push the catheter to descending aorta. The right radial artery was untouchable. Thus the only approach left was left radial artery.

Angiogram; CAG showed aneurysmal RCA and a LM occlusion at ostium with dissection and thrombus. Surgeon refused CABG (B).

PCI: (B) Through EBU 3.5 & JL4.0 Guiding catheter, it is difficult to advance Runthrough NS wire to cross the dissected LM due to enter into the false lumen. (C) A 6Fr JL 5 GC was exchanged, through which, two Runthrough NS wires were advanced into the distal D1 and LAD. Then D1 and LCX flow were recanalized. (D, E) The LM to LAD was pre-dilation with Ryujin 2.5 × 20 balloon at 16 atm, (F) Stenting to D1 was performed with 2.5 × 24 Partner stent at 14 atm. (G–I) LM-LAD stenting was performed with 3.5 × 29 Partner stent at 14 atm. After recanalization the heart rate was dropped to (120–100 bpm) immediately. Patient was recovered well.

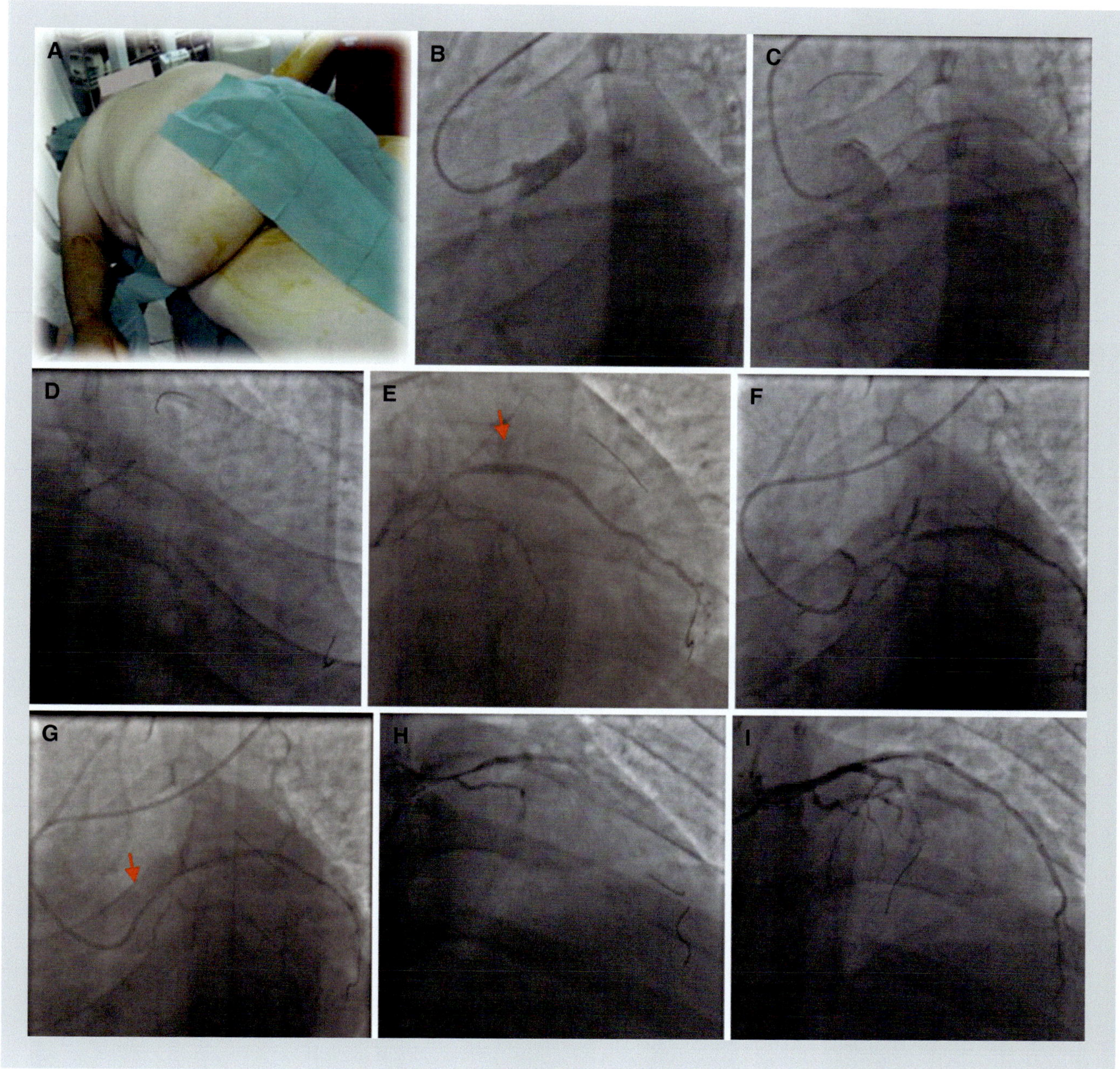
A
B
C
D
E
F
G
H
I

Case 15.2. LAD Bifurcation Lesion Treated with ATP Technique

This is a male patient, aged at 47 years with history of DM and hypertension, admitted due to exertional chest pain.

A: CAG showed a distal LM bifurcation lesion involving LAD and LCX (A, H). B: Lesion was pre-dilated with 2.0×20 mm balloon. C: A 3.5×24 mm Stent and 2.0×20 mm balloon were placed at LAD and LCX respectively. Initially, balloon in LCX was dilated. D: Then, the stent in LM-LAD and balloon in LM-LCX were dilated together at 10 atm E: LM-LCX balloon were pulled back. E: The stent was one more dilated with stent balloon at 14 atm. F: The proximal stent was further dialed with 4.0 mm NC Balloon at 14 atm. (POT) G, I: final result.

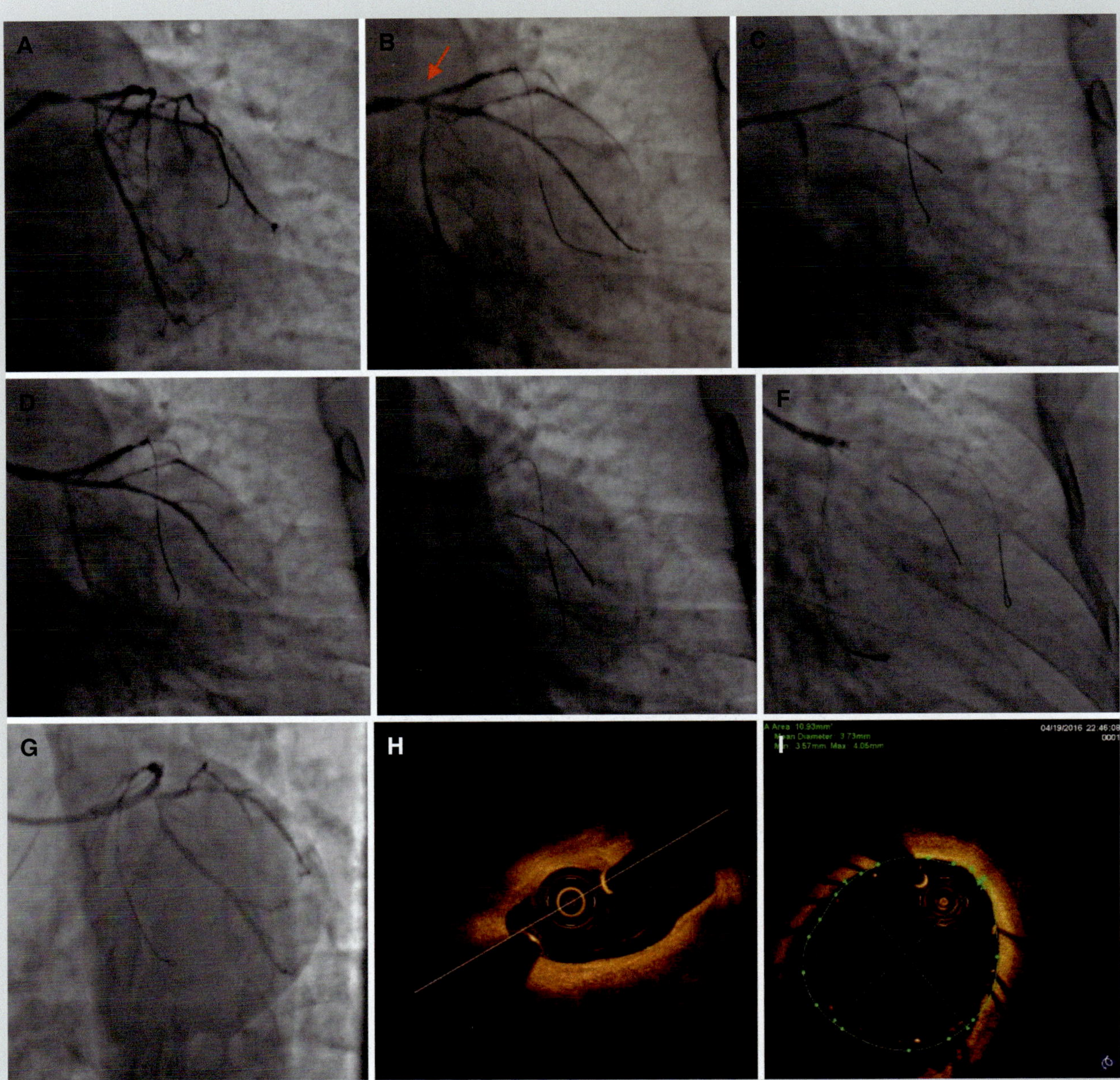

Case 15.3. LM Bifurcation Lesion Treated with Culotte Stenting, Restenosis at 9 Month Follow Up

This is a male patient, aged at 67 years, with history of hyperlipidemia and ex-smoker, admitted due to intermittent chest pain for two years. Angiogram on Sep 26 2013 showed DLM 50 %, o LAD 90 % o LCX 90 % (A). The LM lesion was treated by culottes double stenting technique with 3.5 × 18 mm XienceV at LM-LCX and 3.5 × 18 mm XienceV at LM-LAD (B–D); completed with double kissing (2 NC 3.5 × 12 mm balloon E, F). Angiogram at 14 month post-op showed restenosis at LM-Olad (G). Plaque transferred to LCX after balloon dilatation at LAD and reversely to LAD after balloon dilatation at LCX (H, I). The lesion was further treated with double kissing balloon (two NC balloon 3.5 × 12 mm) and cutting balloon (J, K), Completed by dilatation with 2 Drug eluting balloon (B Brwaun Melsungen Sequent Please 3 × 26 mm) at LAD and LCX respectively (L, M). Follow up at 1 years showing patent left main stent (N.O).

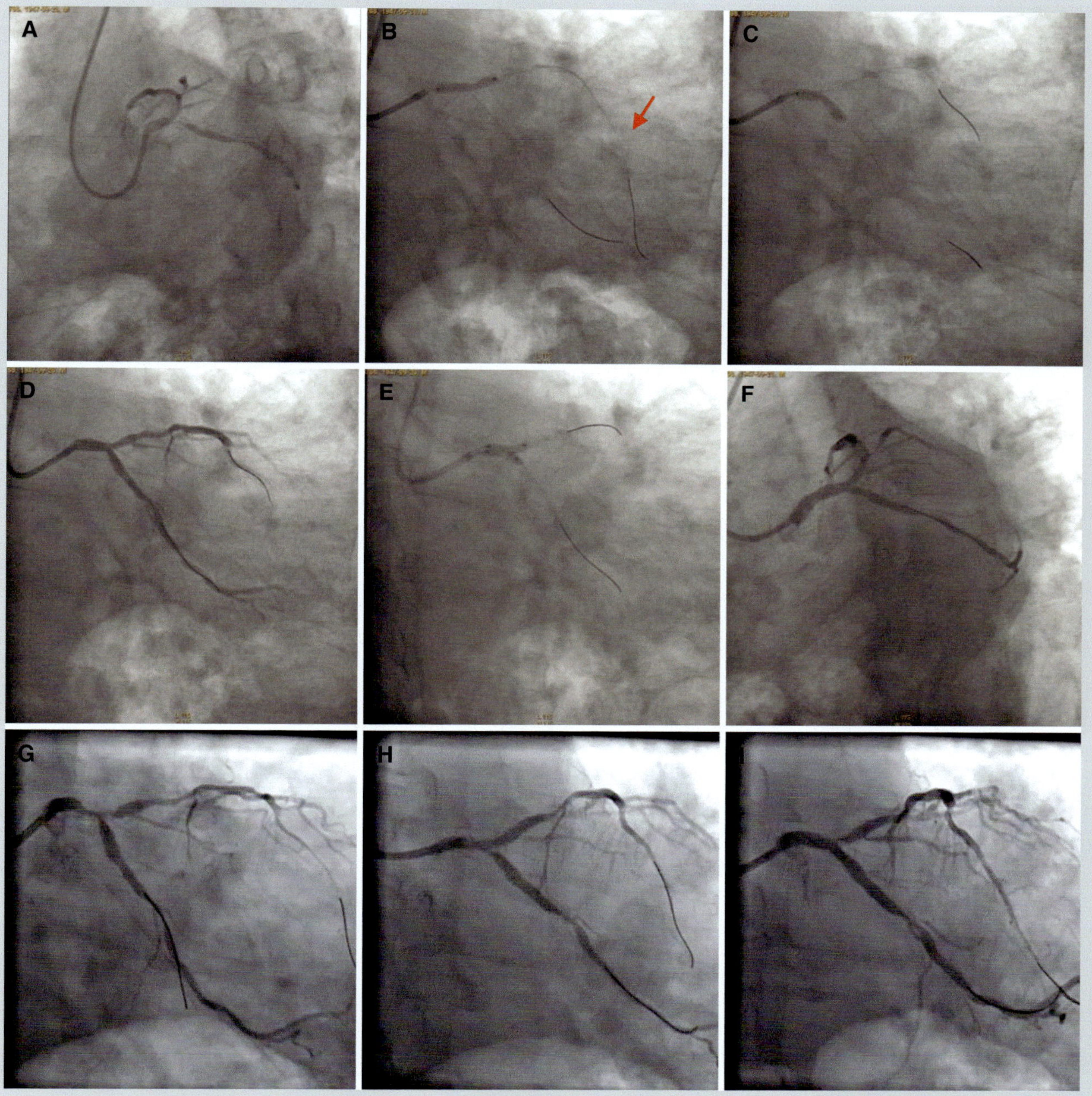

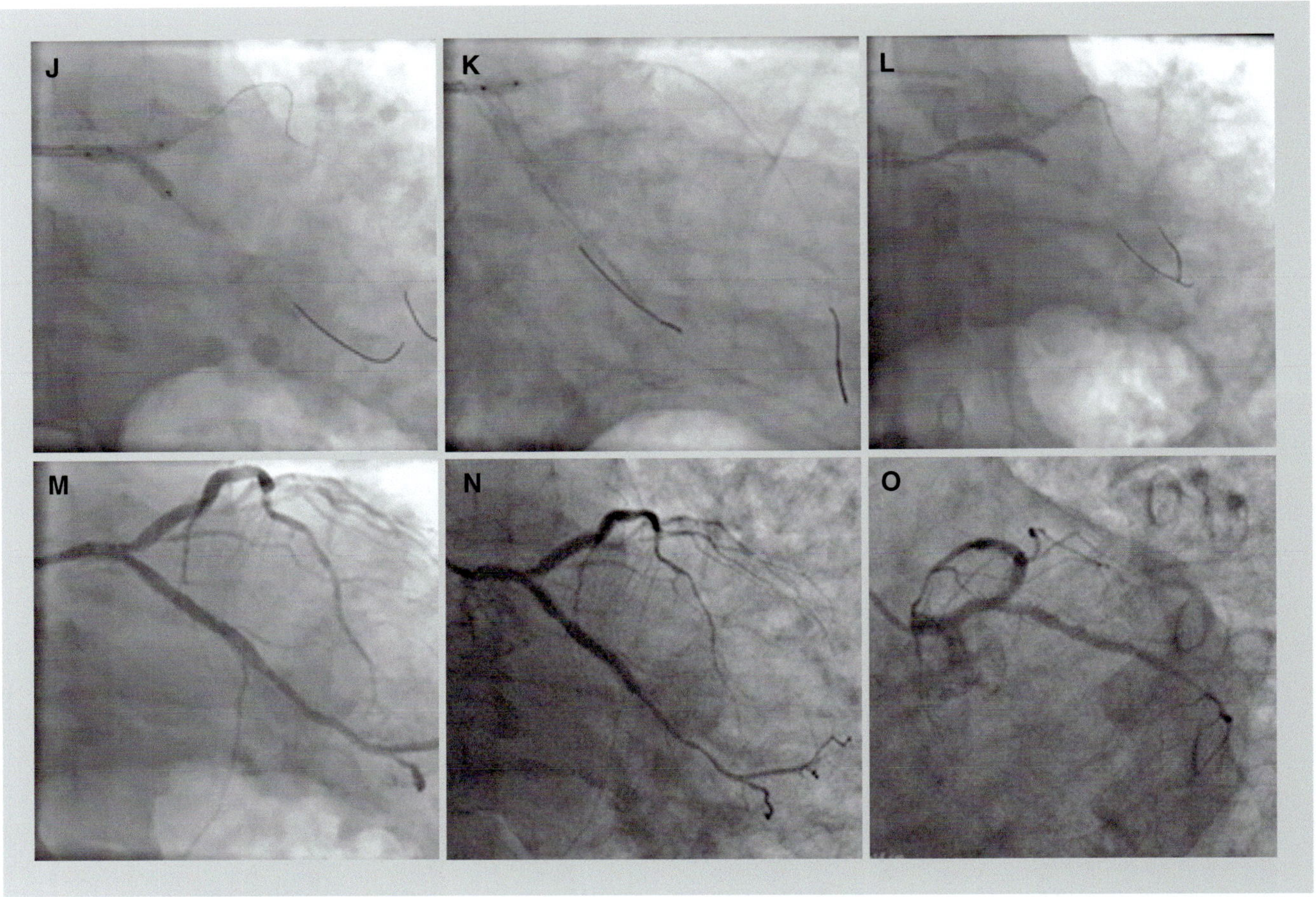
J
K
L
M
N
O

Case 15.4. LM Trifurcation Lesion Treated with 2 Step Mini Crush Stenting

This is 71 y.o. male presented with unstable angina complicated by cardiogenic shock. His euro score was 17 and SYNTAX Score was 34. A 6 Fr. VL 3.5 Guiding catheter (Mach 1, BSC) was used to engage the LM, Two BMW universal II (Abbott Vascular) guidewires were placed to LAD and IM respectively. A 3.0/13 mm Lacrosse NSE (Goodman) balloon was used to dilate LM to LAD lesion. 2.0/15 mm Tazuna (Terumo) was used to dilate at IM, (A–E). A XT-R (ASAHI INTECC) guidewire was used to cross the LCX, later was exchanged with BMW. The LCX was pre-dilated with a 2.0/15 mm TREK (Abbott Vascular) balloon; With a 2.5/15 mm Tazuna (Terumo) placed at IM, a 2.25/12 mm Promus Element (BSC) was deployed at LCX. The stent was later crushed by the 2.5 mm balloon dilatation (E–K). With a A 3.0/15 mm Hiryu (Terumo) (Terumo) placed at LAD, A 2.5/28 mm Promus Element (BSC) stent was deployed at IM, Then the stent was crushed by 3.0 mm balloon;(L–M), Stent: A 3.0/38 mm Promus Element (BSC) Balloon was deployed at LM-LAD (N, O): IM was recrossed with Runthrough wire and dilated 1.25/10 mm Sapphire (OrbusNeich) balloon. Kissing balloon was performed at LAD and LM by 3.0/15 mm Hiryu (Terumo) Balloon at LAD and 2.5/15 mm Emerge (BSC) at LM (P). Then Kissing balloon was performed at IM and LCX with 3.0/15 mm Hiryu (Terumo) at IM and a 1.25/10 mm Sapphire (OrbusNeich) balloon at LCX (Q). Final results presented well.

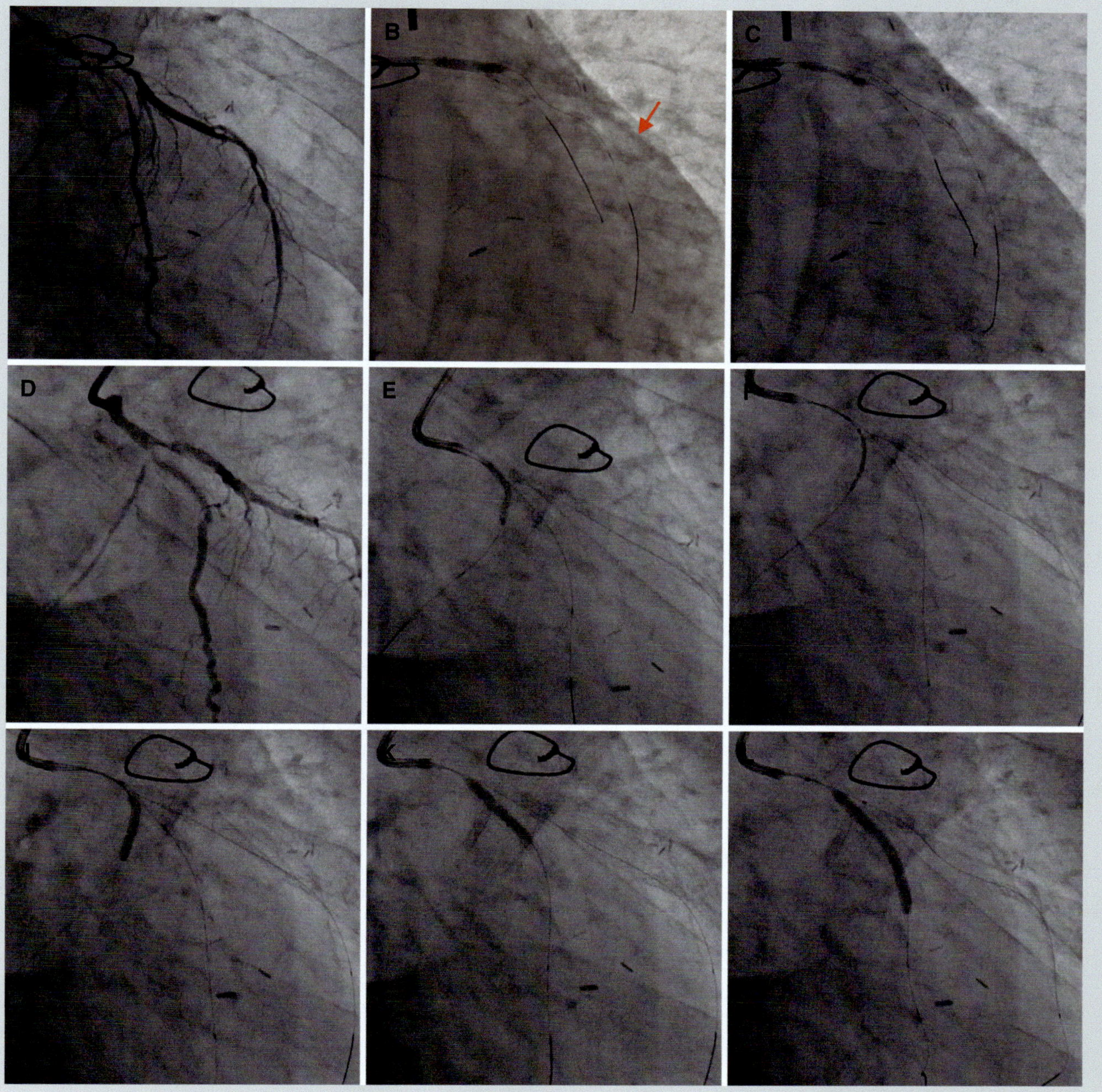

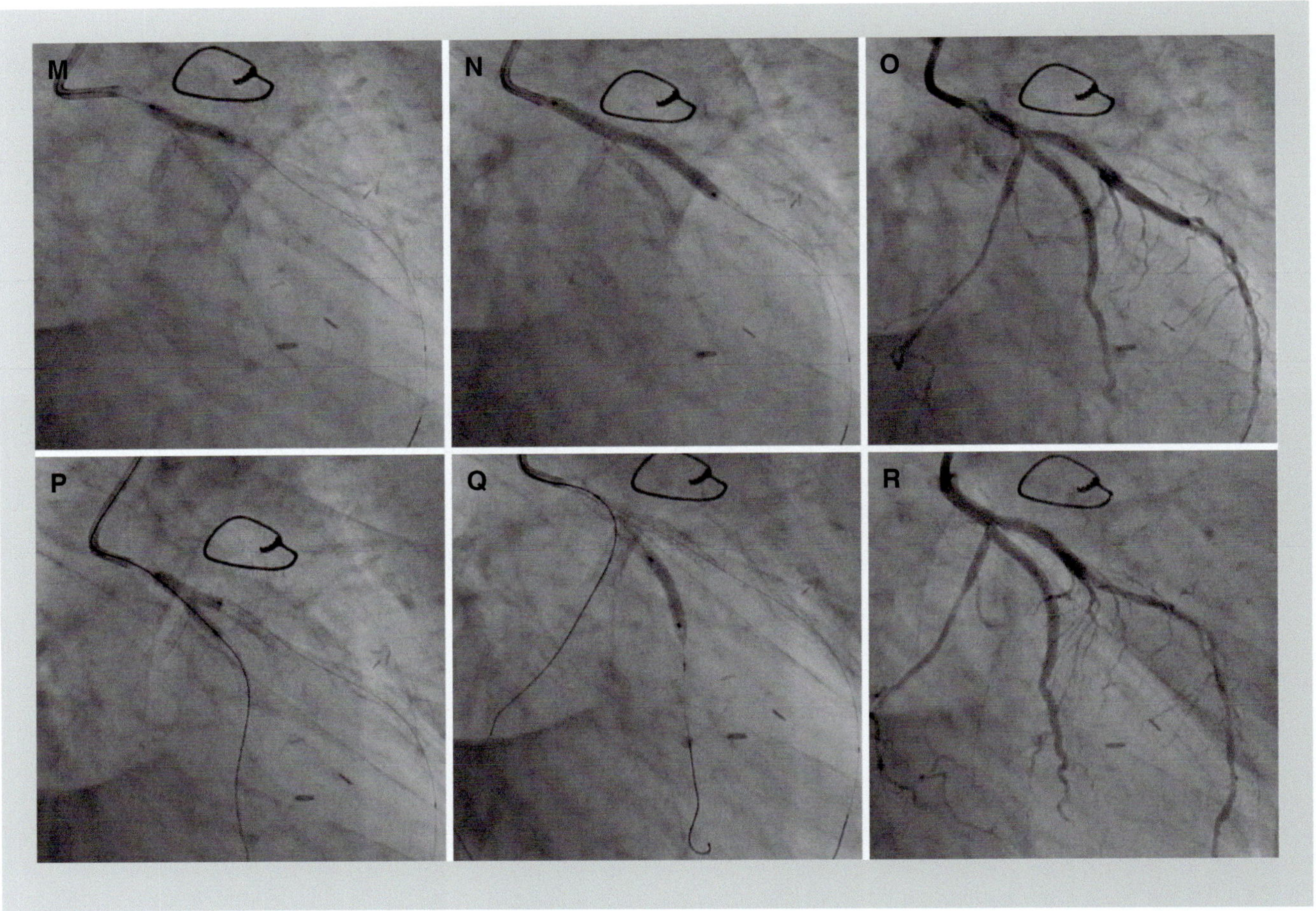

References

1. Serruys PW, Morice MC, Kappetein AP, Colombo A, Holmes DR, Mack MJ, et al. Percutaneous coronary intervention versus coronary-artery bypass grafting for severe coronary artery disease. N Engl J Med. 2009;360(10):961–72.
2. Morice MC, Serruys PW, Kappetein AP, Feldman TE, Stahle E, Colombo A, et al. Five-year outcomes in patients with left main disease treated with either percutaneous coronary intervention or coronary artery bypass grafting in the synergy between percutaneous coronary intervention with taxus and cardiac surgery trial. Circulation. 2014;129(23):2388–94.
3. Athappan G, Patvardhan E, Tuzcu ME, Ellis S, Whitlow P, Kapadia SR. Left main coronary artery stenosis: a meta-analysis of drug-eluting stents versus coronary artery bypass grafting. JACC Cardiovasc Interv. 2013;6(12):1219–30.
4. Park SJ, Ahn JM, Kim YH, Park DW, Yun SC, Yoon SH, et al. Temporal trends in revascularization strategy and outcomes in left main coronary artery stenosis: data from the ASAN Medical Center-Left MAIN Revascularization registry. Circ Cardiovasc Interv. 2015;8(3):e001846.
5. Chang K, Koh YS, Jeong SH, Lee JM, Her SH, Park HJ, et al. Long-term outcomes of percutaneous coronary intervention versus coronary artery bypass grafting for unprotected left main coronary bifurcation disease in the drug-eluting stent era. Heart. 2012; 98(10):799–805.
6. Cheng CI, Wu CJ, Fang CY, Youssef AA, Chen CJ, Chen SM, et al. Feasibility and safety of transradial stenting for unprotected left main coronary artery stenoses. Circ J Off J Jpn Circ Soc. 2007; 71(6):855–61.
7. Tomassini F, Gagnor A, Montali N, Gambino A, Bollati M, Infantino V, et al. Is percutaneous coronary intervention of unprotected left main coronary artery via transradial approach feasible for skilled transfemoral operators? Initial experience in an unselected population. Cardiovasc Revascu Med Mole Interv. 2013;14(4):193–6.
8. De Maria GL, Burzotta F, Trani C, Kassimis G, Pirozzolo G, Patel N, et al. Trends and outcomes of radial approach in left-main bifurcation percutaneous coronary intervention in the drug-eluting stent Era: a Two-Center Registry. J Invasive Cardiol. 2015;27(7):E125–36.
9. Yang YJ, Kandzari DE, Gao Z, Xu B, Chen JL, Qiao SB, et al. Transradial versus transfemoral method of percutaneous coronary revascularization for unprotected left main coronary artery disease: comparison of procedural and late-term outcomes. JACC Cardiovasc Interv. 2010;3(10):1035–42.
10. Garcia-Blas S, Nunez J, Carrillo P, Cordero A, Minana G, Frutos A, et al. Usefulness of sheathless guide catheter for the percutaneous coronary intervention of left main disease by radial approach. Int J Cardiol. 2016;211:49–52.
11. Naganuma T, Chieffo A, Meliga E, Capodanno D, Park SJ, Onuma Y, et al. Long-term clinical outcomes after percutaneous coronary intervention for ostial/mid-shaft lesions versus distal bifurcation lesions in unprotected left main coronary artery: the DELTA Registry (drug-eluting stent for left main coronary artery disease): a multicenter registry evaluating percutaneous coronary intervention versus coronary artery bypass grafting for left main treatment. JACC Cardiovasc Interv. 2013;6(12):1242–9.

12. Applegate RJ, Davis JM, Leonard JC. Treatment of ostial lesions using the Szabo technique: a case series. Catheter Cardiovasc Interv Off J Soc Cardiac Angiogr Interv. 2008;72(6):823–8.
13. Vaquerizo B, Serra A, Ormiston J, Miranda-Guardiola F, Webber B, Fantuzzi A, et al. Bench top evaluation and clinical experience with the Szabo technique: new questions for a complex lesion. Catheter Cardiovasc Interv Off J Soc Cardiac Angiogr Interv. 2012;79(3):378–89.
14. Lefevre T, Girasis C, Lassen JF. Differences between the left main and other bifurcations. EuroIntervention J EuroPCR Collab Working Group Interv Cardiol Eur Soc Cardiol. 2015;11 Suppl V:V106–10.
15. Karrowni W, Makki N, Dhaliwal AS, Vyas A, Blevins A, Dughman S, et al. Single versus double stenting for unprotected left main coronary artery bifurcation lesions: a systematic review and meta-analysis. J Invasive Cardiol. 2014;26(6):229–33.
16. Chen SL, Xu B, Han YL, Sheiban I, Zhang JJ, Ye F, et al. Clinical outcome after DK crush versus culotte stenting of distal left main bifurcation lesions: the 3-year follow-up results of the DKCRUSH-III study. JACC Cardiovasc Interv. 2015;8(10):1335–42.
17. de la Torre Hernandez JM, Baz Alonso JA, Gomez Hospital JA, Alfonso Manterola F, Garcia Camarero T, Gimeno de Carlos F. Clinical impact of intravascular ultrasound guidance in drug-eluting stent implantation for unprotected left main coronary disease: pooled analysis at the patient-level of 4 registries. JACC Cardiovasc Interv. 2014;7(3):244–54.
18. Jin Z, Li L, Wang M, Zhang S, Chen Z, Shen Z. Innovative provisional stenting approach to treat coronary bifurcation lesions: balloon-stent kissing technique. J Invasive Cardiol. 2013;25(11):600–4.

16 The Transradial Approach for Bifurcation Lesions

Yves Louvard and Thierry Lefevre

16.1 History of the Radial Approach and Review of its Benefits

The first non-selective coronary angiograms were carried out in Sweden at the end of WWII by S. Radner using a proximal radial cut-off and ligation technique [1].

The transradial route fell into disuse for the first time in 1953 with the advent of Seldinger's femoral technique [2]. Following the first transbrachial and transaxillary selective coronary angiograms performed by Sones in 1959 and Ricket and Abrams in 1963 [3, 4], respectively, Lucien Campeau re-introduced the transradial approach in 1964 using proximal cut-off and subsequent suturing [5]. The radial route was again discarded when the first sheaths became available in 1965 before being re-introduced for the second time by Campeau in 1986–1989 [6] for coronary angiography via the transradial distal approach using Potts-Cournand needles.

In 1992, Ferdinand Kiemeneij re-instated the distal transradial approach when 6 F angioplasty guiding-catheters were developed. Over the three following years, he carried out transradial balloon angioplasty [7], the first Palmaz-Schatz stent implantations [8, 9] and the first outpatient angioplasty procedures [10].

Around the same period, other individual operators started implementing this technique in Europe (France, Italy), North America (Canada) and Asia (Taiwan, Japan). As a result, a number of technical and anatomical issues in diagnostic angiography and PCI were identified and successfully addressed. These difficulties included spasm, antebrachial, brachial and subclavian loops, high take-off radial arteries, arteria lusoria [11] etc. Increasing operator experience also resulted in a marked improvement in the equipment used as well as the implementation of the transradial approach in the majority of clinical and angiographic settings [12–18] (AMI, patients under anticoagulation treatment, coronary bifurcation lesions, left main, etc..) using a variety of technical strategies such as rotablator [19] and thromboaspiration in most clinical settings.

The transradial route was subsequently shown to be associated with a reduction in vascular complications and procedural cost in addition to improved patient comfort compared with the transfemoral approach [20–25]. Longer procedural duration and increased X-ray exposure are directly related to insufficient operator experience [26–30].

The rapid progression of the radial approach recently observed in many countries has resulted in the publication of large-size trials which have pointed to a potential reduction in mortality rates compared to the femoral approach. The reported decrease in mortality is closely related to operator experience, especially in unstable clinical settings [31–33].

16.2 Limitations of the Transradial Approach in Coronary Angioplasty

Compared to the femoral artery, the radial artery is a small vessel which cannot always accommodate 6 F or even 5 F sheaths. Because of its small diameter, the radial artery can be difficult to puncture and its muscular nature and proneness to spasm can also hinder catheter advancement.

While certain acquired anatomical difficulties are predictable such as loops in patients with hypertension or calcifications in diabetics [34], congenital abnormalities cannot be easily identified before PCI and may considerably reduce procedural success [35, 36]. Acquired difficulties such as loops are less frequent in the left radial artery, but the left radial route is more uncomfortable for the operator.

The reduction in catheter diameter has two potential consequences: incompatibility with equipment and devices used for coronary angioplasty and a decrease in guiding-catheter support at the coronary ostium which is necessary in certain PCI settings such as chronic coronary occlusions.

Table 16.1 shows compatibility between guiding-catheter sizes and devices commonly used in PCI. When the

Y. Louvard (✉) • T. Lefevre
Institut Cardiovasculaire Paris Sud (ICPS), Hôpital Privé Jacques Cartier, Générale de Santé, Massy, France
e-mail: y.louvard@icps.com.fr

Y. Zhou et al. (eds.), *Transradial Approach for Percutaneous Interventions*, DOI 10.1007/978-94-017-7350-8_16

Table 16.1 Compatibility between the sheath size and the devices, techniques and radial arteries in a population of French patients (male and females)

Cath. size	Devices	Techniques	Radial compatibility[a] (%)
5F	Ballons ≤5 mm	No kissing balloon	100
	Microcatheter		
	Stents ≤4.5 mm		
	IVUS		
	Rota 1.25 mm		
6F	All coronary balloons	Kissing balloons (compliant or NC)	86.9
	All coronary stents	Two microcatheters	
	Cutting/scoring balloon	Microcatheter and monorail B.	
	Rota ≤1.75 mm	Anchoring balloon	
	Most protection devices		
	Tornus		
7F	Angioguard	Kissing stent	76.9
	Rota 2 mm	Microcatheter and IVUS	
8F	Rota >2 mm		64.7

[a]Y Louvard, Population of 150 french people with echographic diameter measurement of radial artery

radial artery cannot accommodate a 6 F sheath, certain PCI procedures can be performed with a 5 F guiding-catheter. In cases when procedures can only be carried out with 6 F guiding-catheters, the use of a sheathless guiding catheter [37] may be helpful as its inner lumen is larger than that of a conventional 6 F guiding catheter and its outer diameter is 1.5 F smaller compared to that of a 6 F introducer (equivalent to 8 F). The efficiency of these catheters is also enhanced by their trackability. The diameter of 7.5 Fr Sheathless guiding catheters is also slightly smaller than that of a 6 F introducer.

The support provided by a 6 or 5 F guiding-catheter at the level of the coronary ostium can be improved by active support maneuvers like deep intubation on a wire. A 5 F catheter with no specific shape, longer than the guiding-catheter can be inserted co-axially in the coronary artery (5 in 6, mother and child) [38]. Monorail catheter extensions can be used for the same purpose (Guideliner [39], Guidezilla Boston Sc). With their inner diameter equivalent to 5 F guiding-catheters, these catheters can facilitate stent delivery distally, but they cannot be used in the treatment of coronary bifurcations (no kissing balloon, but balloon or stent plus a wire is possible).

16.3 Angioplasty of Coronary Bifurcations

Coronary trees are pseudo-fractal objects with assymetric bifurcation self replication up to the level of myocardial penetration. Each bifurcation is an anatomo-functional entity whose 3 diameters are ruled by Murray's law [40, 41] modified by Huo-Kassab [42] and simplified by Finet [43].

In each of the three segments of a bifurcation there is a linear relation between the diameter, the length of the distal segment, flow, and the vascularized myocardial mass. Any anatomical variation may result in a functional change.

Coronary bifurcation sites are prone to the development of atheroma [44, 45]. Proximal to the bifurcation, blood flow is laminar with a transversal diastolic flow profile and maximal velocity in the mid-segment. Flow is less rapid along the vessel walls where a high level of friction exerts a protective effect against the atheroma. In coronary bifurcations, flow is rapid and wall shear stress is high at the level of the flow divider whereas flow is turbulent, recirculating with low wall shear stess on the walls of the main vesel (proximal and distal) and the side branch opposite the flow divider. This accounts for the fact that the flow divider is initially free of atheroma.

16.4 Definition, Classifications, Designation, Measurements and Imaging of Coronary Bifurcation Lesions

The European Bifurcation Club (EBC) adopted a simple and open definition: a coronary bifurcation lesion is a coronary artery narrowing occurring adjacent to and/or involving the origin of a significant side branch. A significant side branch is a branch that you do not want to lose in the context of a specific patient.

Medina's classification [46] (Fig. 16.1) proposed in 2006 and adopted by the EBC is simple and well suited to research purposes and provides a thorough description of lesion characteristics. In order to describe a bifurcation lesion accurately, it is necessary to designate the side branch (SB) from the two distal vessels. Coronary bifurcations can be described using Medina's classification (e.g., LM, Circ, LAD where LAD is considered as the SB) [47].

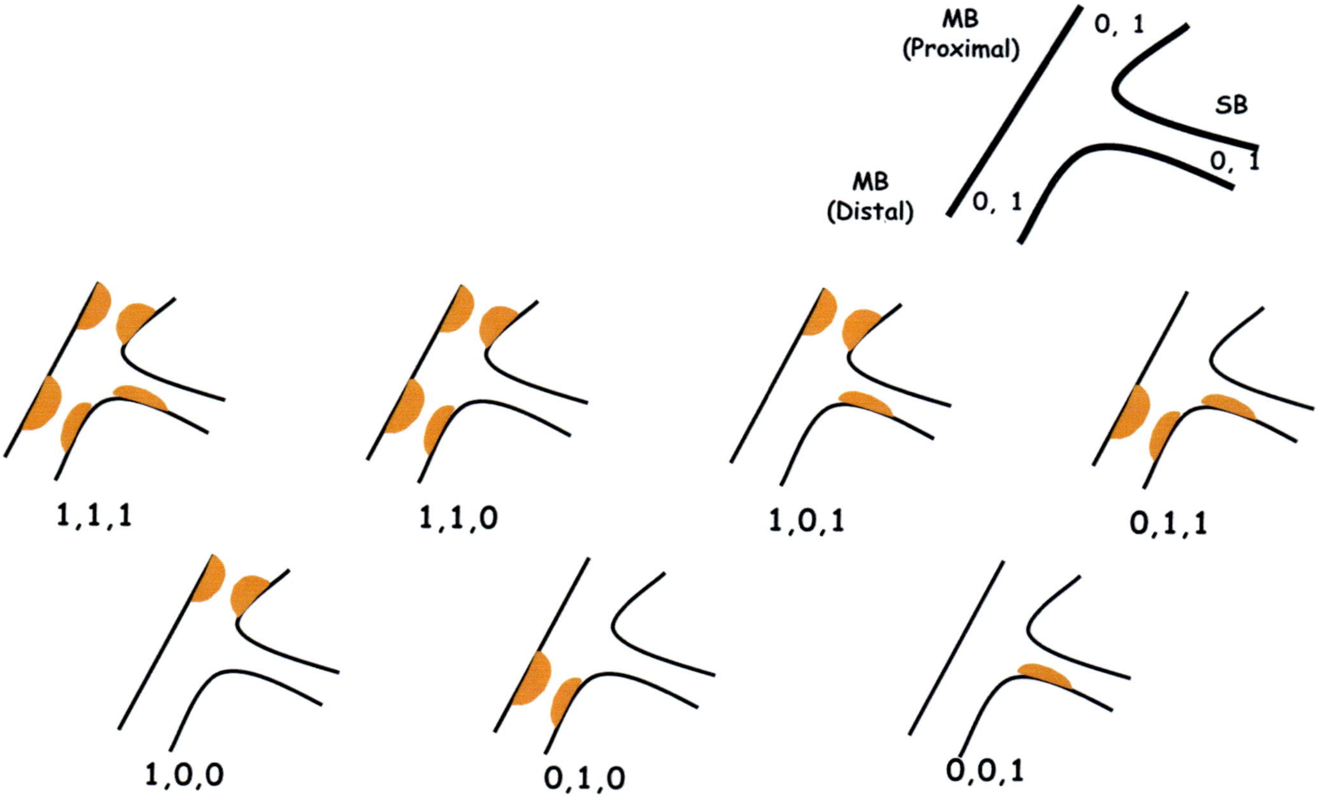

Fig. 16.1 Medina classification

A classification of the various bifurcation treatment strategies [48] (Fig. 16.2) was established by the EBC based on the positioning of the first stent (MADS). The techniques used are defined according to final stent positioning. This classification does not include balloon maneuvers such as kissing, or the Proximal Optimization Technique (POT) used to give a cross-over stent selected according to the distal diameter of the main vessel its proximal diameter corresponding to the proximal diameter of the vessel.

As described previously, coronary arteries do not have a linear reference diameter from the ostium to the distal segment but the diameter between two bifurcations is constant with a stepped reference function (Figs. 16.3 and 16.4). Conventional QCA software produce erroneous data on reference diameters (interpolated reference) especially in the vicinity of bifurcations and when the analysis is performed from the proximal segment of the vessel towards the SB [48]. There are currently at least two software programs dedicated to bifurcation lesion analysis [49, 50]. For some operators, angiographic data in bifurcations do not provide adequate information about the vessel wall and the extent of atheromatous plaque. However, although the benefit of endocoronary echography has been recently highlighted in a meta-analysis [51], potential improvements in the results of coronary bifurcation stenting under systematic IVUS guidance or CT scan have not yet been demonstrated in large randomized trials. Optical Coherence Tomography (OCT) could prove a useful tool for procedure guidance as this technique allows very rapid 3D reconstruction of the artery and the implanted stent [52].

16.5 One or two Stents in a Bifurcation?

This issue has generated a large number of publications involving bare metal stents and drug-eluting stents [53]. Of the seven randomized trials conducted with DES, six have shown that systematic double stenting does not provide any benefit [54–56].

A Chinese study (DK-Crush) on complex lesions (true bifurcation lesions with significant stenosis in both branches) showed a 1-year difference in terms of repeat revascularization in favor of the double stenting strategy following, however, systematic coronary angiography at 8 months (known to provoke a higher rate of reintervention) [57, 58].

Provisional SB stenting is currently the gold standard strategy for the treatment of bifurcation disease not involving the left main and when access to the SB is possible [59].

The results of several registries suggest that a similar approach to treatment of distal left main lesions could be considered [60, 61].

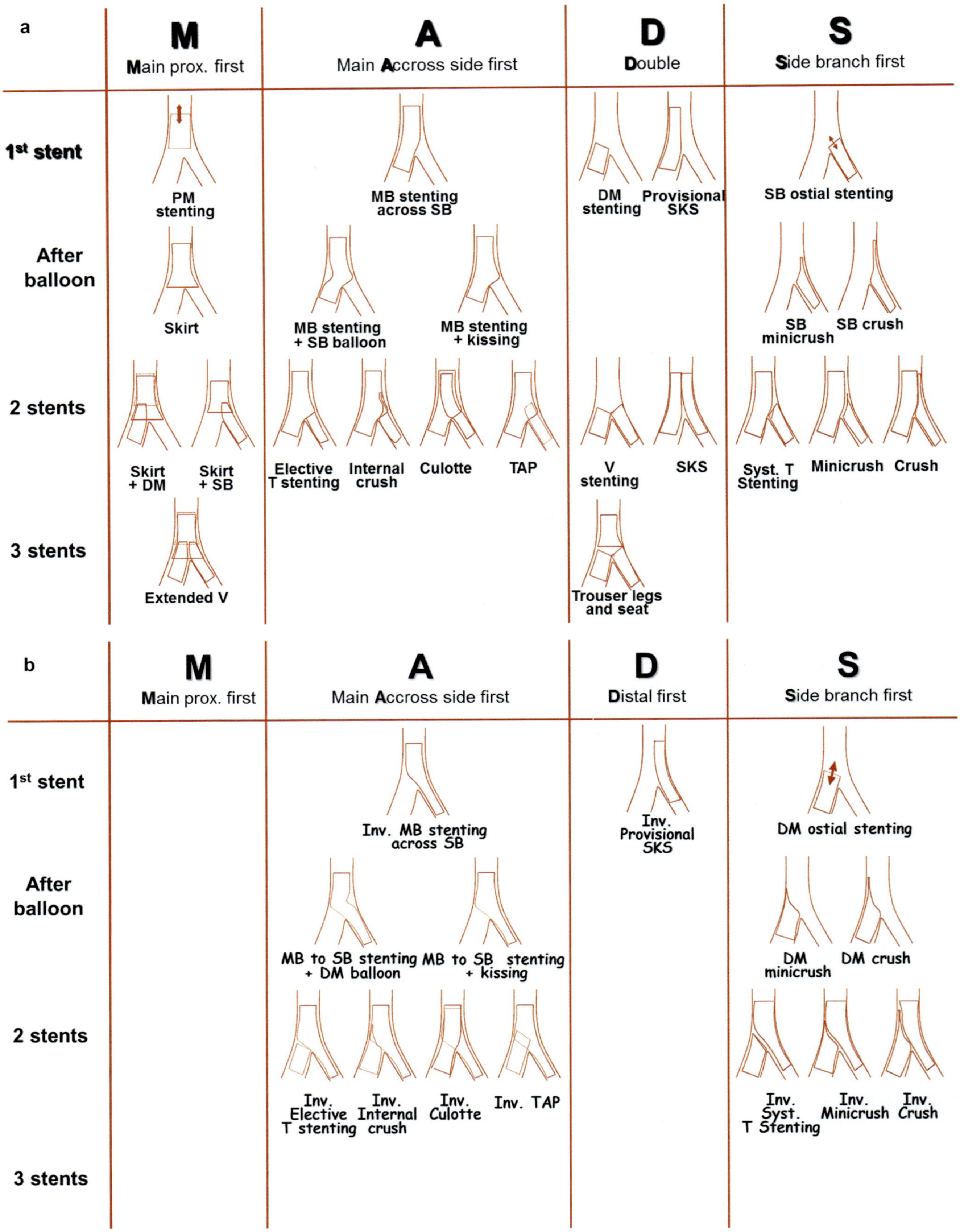

Figs. 16.2 (**a**) MADS classification based on the final position and the order of deploiement of stent(s) in a bifurcation. Bifurcation techniques are classified by stategy defined by the position of the first stent. All the techniques described have been published or reported. In the (**a**) figure are the "straight" techniques, in (**b**) are the "inverted" techniques, distal main vessel (normally the biggest, longest …) is exchanged with the side branch. Not all the wires and balloons maneuvers are described

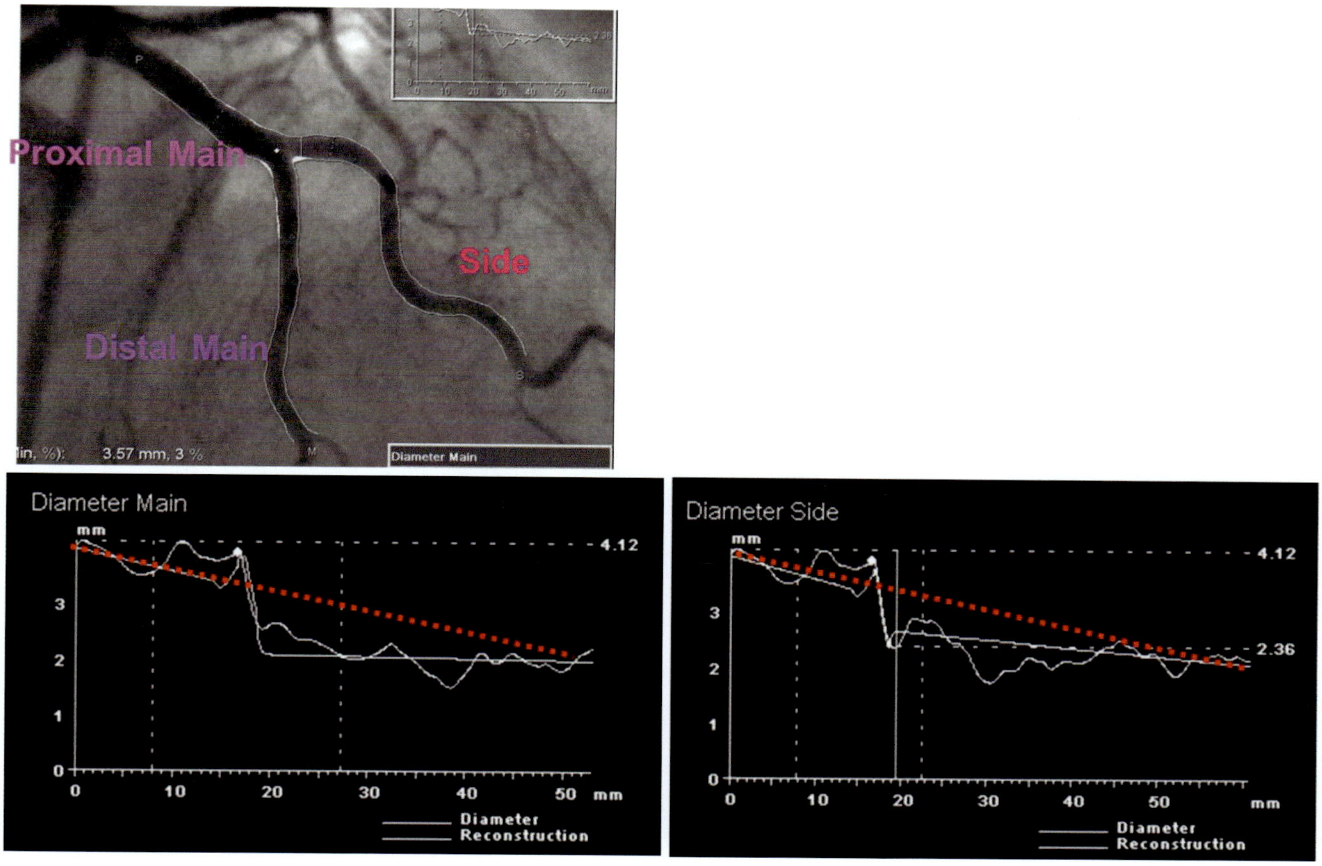

Fig. 16.3 Description of a dedicated bifurcation software. The reference diameter of the proximal main to distal main vessel (*left*) or proximal main vessel to side branch (*right*) is no more linearly decreasing like in former QCA software (*dotted red line*) but stepped at the level of the bifurcation (reconstruction). The diameter is deducted from the automatically detected vessel contour. The standard QCA software decreases the stenosis rate proximal to the bifurcation and strongly increases it distally specially when the design is done from proximal main vessel to side branch

16.6 How to Implement the Provisional Stenting Strategy

Figure 16.5 shows the different steps of this strategy. The first step consists in deploying a stent directly or following predilatation, in the main artery through the side branch into which a wire has been previously inserted. The stent size should be selected according to the distal diameter of the main branch in order to avoid carena shift towards the side branch and occlusion of the side branch. Predilatation of a diseased SB has long been the subject of debate, as it carries a risk of dissection potentially requiring a change of strategy. Following stent deployment, the proximal segment is inevitably malapposed in the proximal main vessel, which may require guide wire exchange outside the stent, and neutralize the biological effect of the DES whilst increasing the risk of thrombosis. In order to address this issue, it is necessary to implement the proximal optimization technique (POT) before any guide wire exchange. This technique consists in the complete deployment of the proximal stent segment using a balloon matching the proximal diameter of the vessel. The balloon must be short in order to prevent the occurrence of geographic miss. Any additional treatment of the SB depends on the results of subsequent angiographic examination, namely, the presence of symptoms, EKG changes, occurrence of dissection, or a suboptimal result in relation to the size of the vessel. Angiographic assessement of the result is always difficult due to the fact that the lumen of the SB ostium which is normally round, becomes oval or is reduced to a slit and is always visualized in the worst possible angiographic view. FFR [62, 63] measurement or OCT show that the SB lesion is not significant in most instances. In such cases, Kissing balloon inflation is carried out with balloon diameters matching the size of the two distal branches using a non-compliant balloon in the SB in order to avoid excessive dilatation [64]. The Kissing technique can be replaced by successive inflation of two balloons in order to avoid stent distortion due to inflation in the SB only.

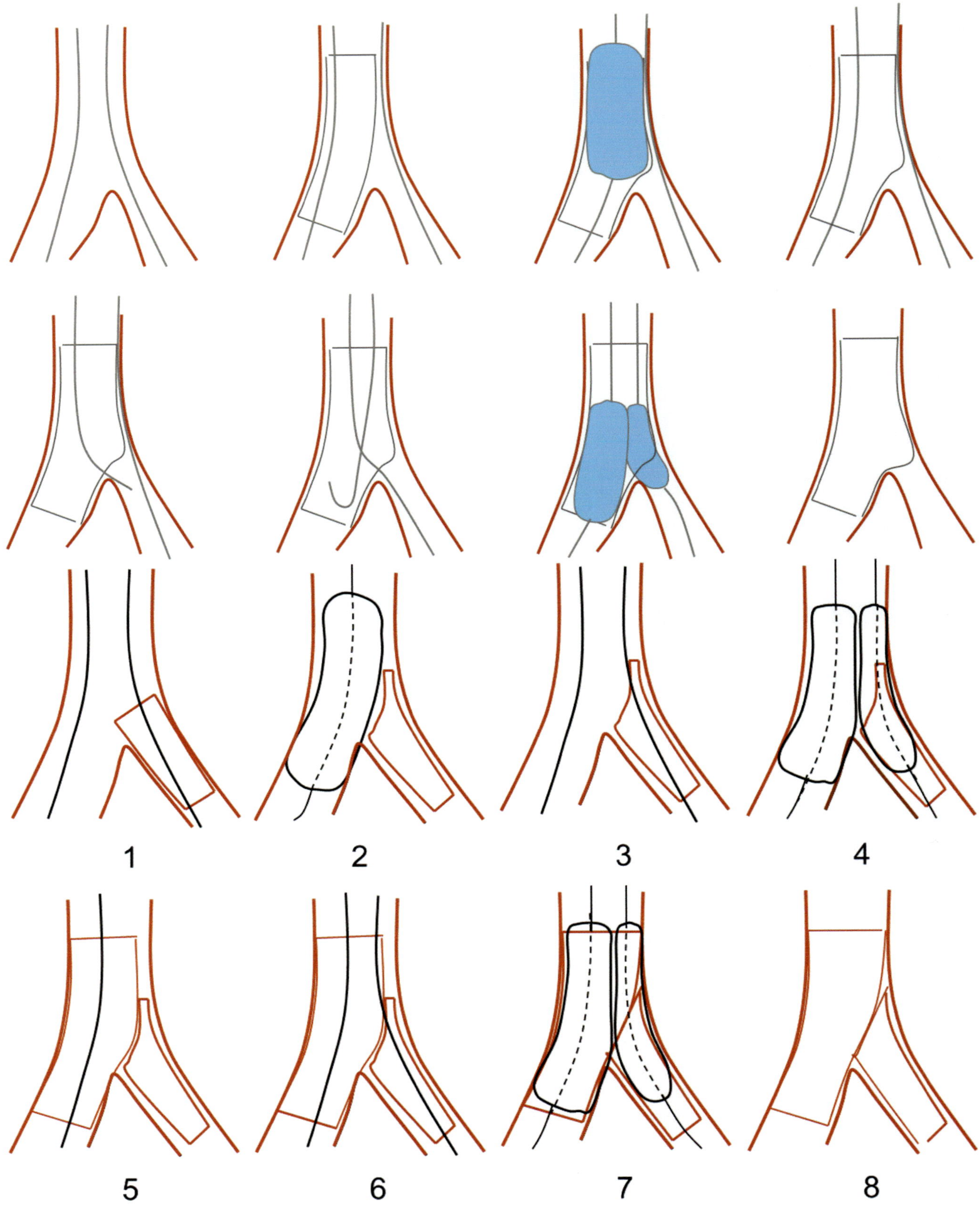

Fig. 16.4 Stepped of the provisional strategy. After wiring the two branches, a stent choosen from the diameter of the distal main vessel is implanted across the SB, then a big balloon according to the diameter of the proximal main vessel is deployed in the proximal part of the stent (distal marker in front of the carena), then the wires are safely exchanged, the main vessel wire prepared with a long shape is entering the side branch through the most distal stent cell and the SB wire is de-jailed and push in the main distal vessel (loop). Then a kissing balloon inflation can be performed with short and non-compliant balloons adapted to the two distal diameters. Finally a decision is taken about the need for stenting the side branch

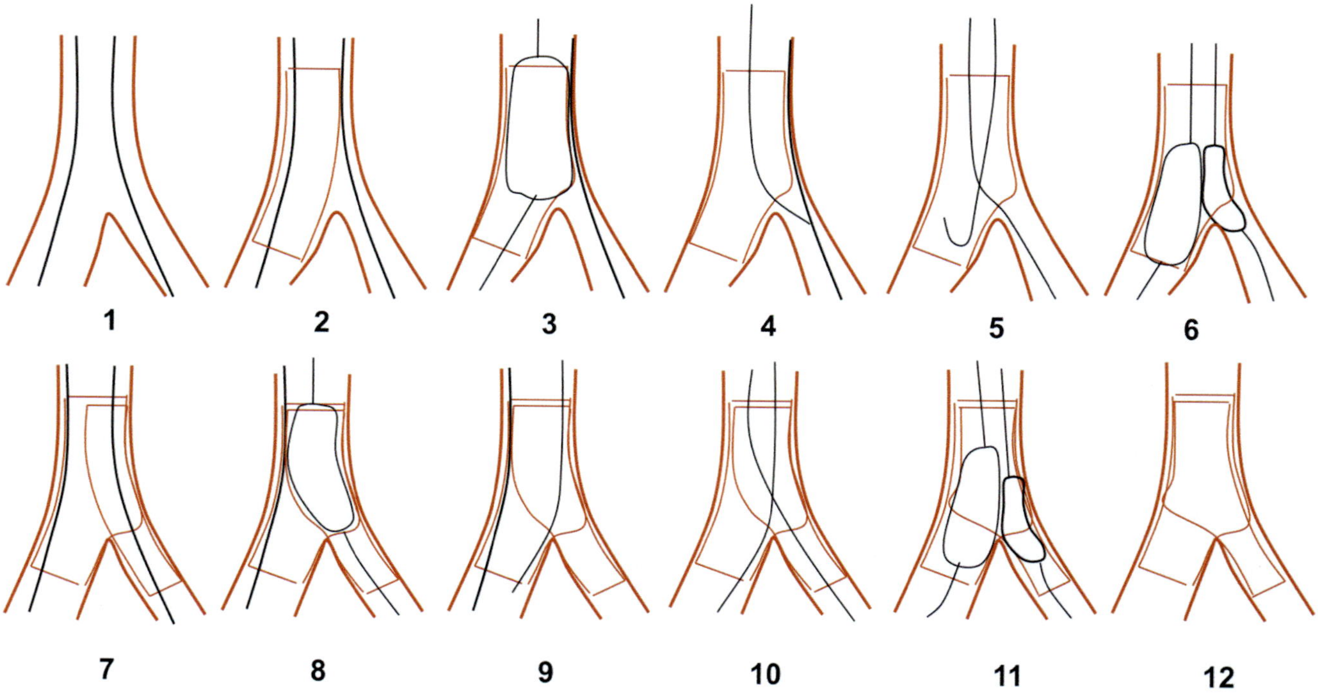

Fig. 16.4 (continued)

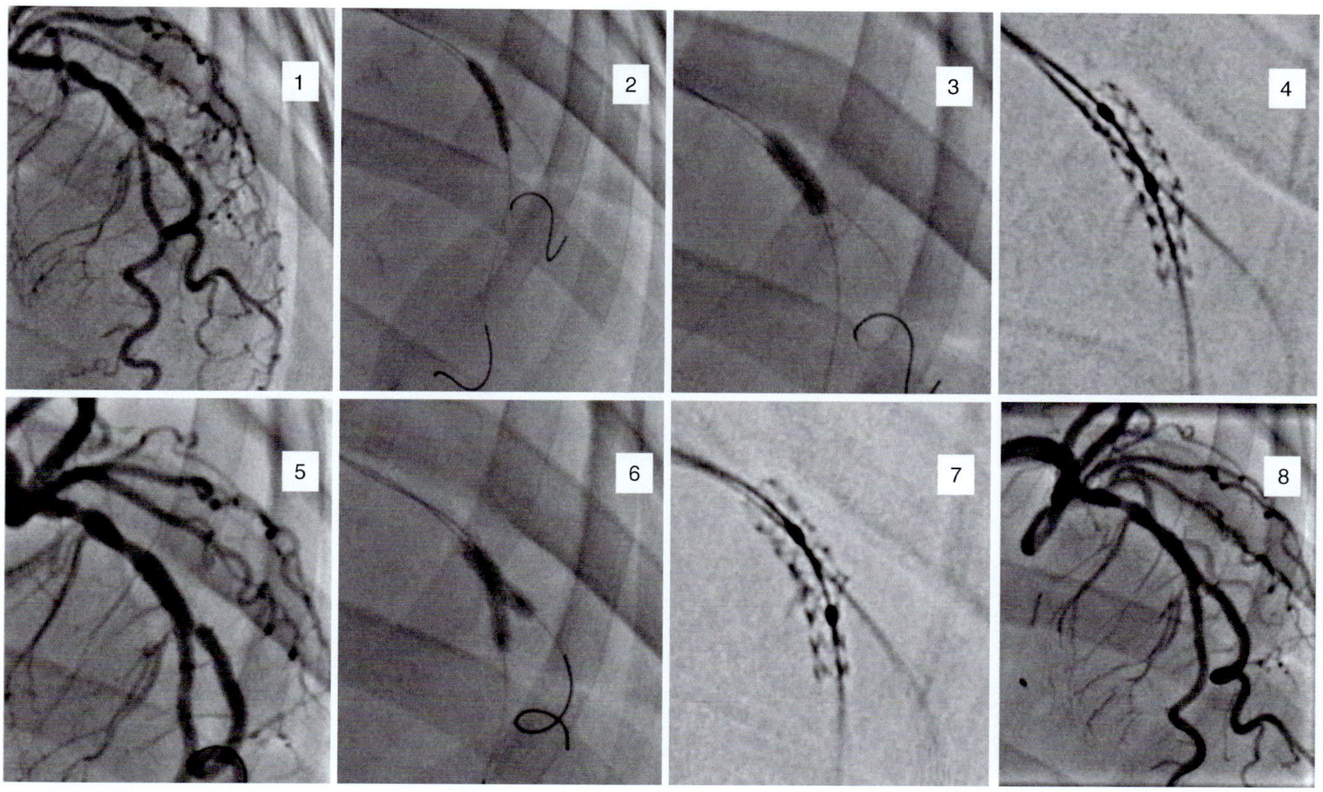

Fig. 16.5 Relative simplicity of the DK-Crush technique

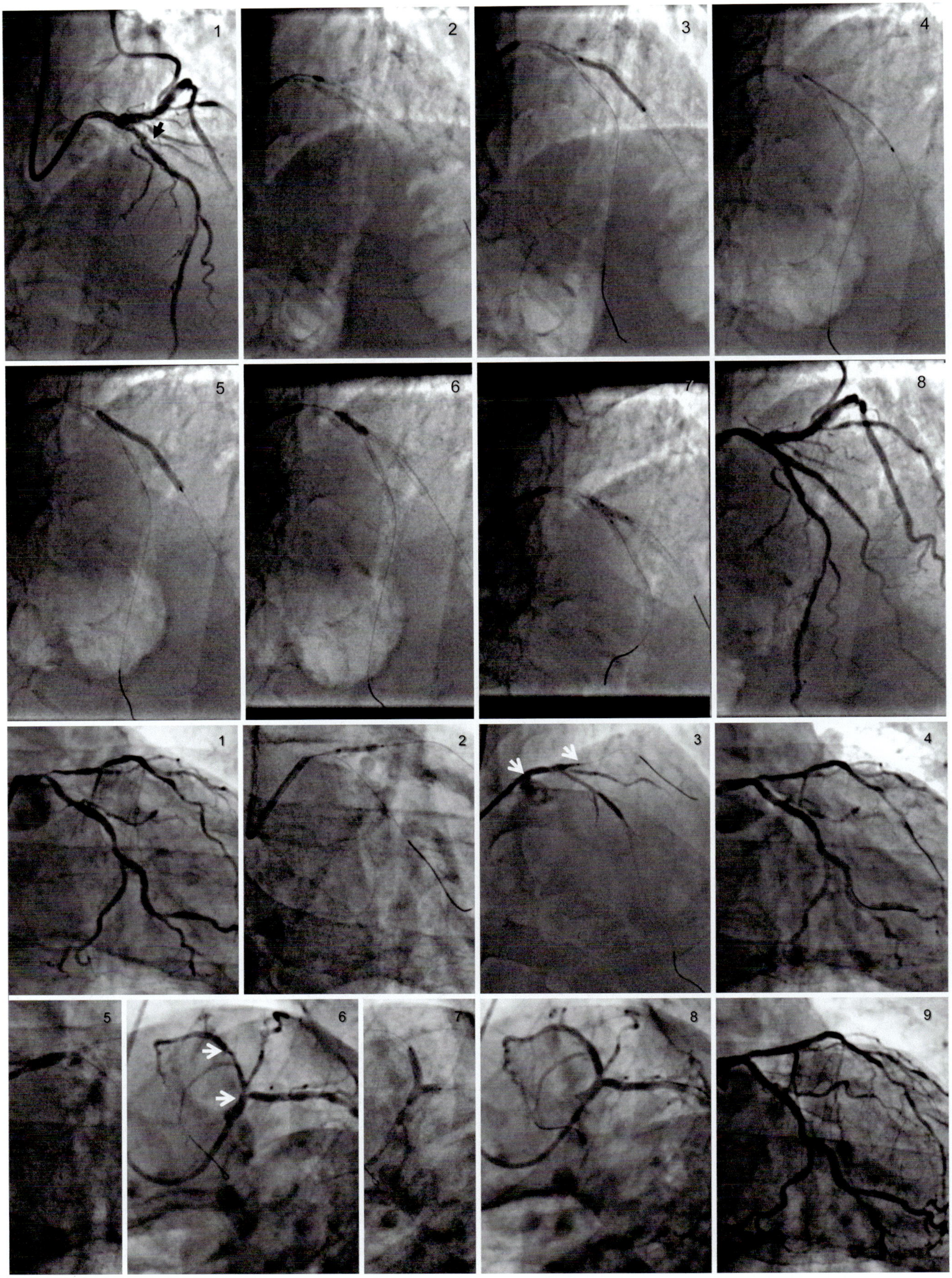

Fig. 16.5 (continued)

This strategy allows the deployment of a second stent in the SB when necessary, by using either the T stenting or the TAP technique (T and Protrusion) according to the partial protrusion of the main branch stent into the SB [65]. This can be clearly visualized using the stent enhancement technique [66].

16.7 Bifurcation Stenting Through Transradial Approach: Case Exemples

Most bifurcation techniques can be performed through transradial approach, including techniques beginning with side branch stenting. Some techniques are more comfortable with 7 F guiding catheters which can be used transradially (specially with a sheathless) like classical crush or TAP where a balloon is present in the main branch during stenting of the side branch. Classical crush is now clearly replaced by balloon crush technique or even better DK-crush technique. The only one technique that cannot be performed in 6 F is the SKS, simultaneous kissing stent, where two stents are delivered simultaneously with creation of a neo carena. This strategy has not been compared with other strategies in a randomized trial. We will illustrate the provisional stenting strategy in non-left main and left main bifurcation lesions with single or double stenting.

Case 1

(1) Right radial approach with 6 F sheth and EBU 3.5 guiding catheter. LAD2,LAD2,Diag2 0,1,0 bifurcation stenosis. 2. 2 wires, direct stenting with (2) 5 ×18 mm Xience. (3) Proximal optimization technique (POT) with a short 3.0 balloon (distal marker in front of the carena). (4) On the stent enhancement differences in cell opening distally and proximally are visible. (5) Angiographic result after POT, stenosis (moderate?) at the ostium of the diagonal. (6) After wire exchange kissing balloon with 2 × 2.5 short non compliant balloons. (7) Stent enhancement after kissing showing projection of struts inside the ostium of the SB (distal cell crossing). (8) Final result.

Case 2

(1) 6 F right radial approach. 0,0,1 proximal LAD bifurcation lesion. The ostial diagonal subocclusion (arrow) was created years earlier by a LAD BMS stenting without diagonal protection. The patient has effort angina with anterior ischemia on three segments during stress MRI. (2) After difficult wiring a rotablation is necessary to remove the blockage. (3) Predilatation of the diagoixnal branch with a long 2.5 balloon. (4) A long (2.5 ×38 Xience) stent is implanted as an inverted provisional strategy. (5) Stent deployment. (6) POT with a short 3.0 balloon. (7) Kissng balloon with 2 × 2.5 NC balloons. (8) Final result.

Case 3

(1) A 1,1,1 distal LM lesion in a male patient 69 yo. Right radial approach in 6 F, EBU 4 guiding catheter. (2) Predilation of the LAD. (3) Stenting from ostial LM to proximal Circonflex artery (Resolute 3.5 × 22) (arrows). In AP cranial incidence. (4) Result after LM to Circ. Stenting. (5) POT with a 4.5 short balloon. (6) After wire exchange and LAD ostium ballooning, implantation of a 2.75 × 26 mm Resolute stent in ostial LAD (elective T stenting). (7) Kissing balloon with 2 × 3.0 mm balloons. 8–9. Final result.

Case 4

(1) Distal LM bifurcation lesion 1,0,0 very calcified in a 86 yo lady with aortic stenosis. Right radial 6 F sheathless SPB 3.5 Asahi guiding catheter (severe friction with 5 F coronary angiograply). (2) Stent from LM ostium to Circonflex artery (Nobori 3.5 ×20). (3) Stent deploiementaccross LAD. 4. POT with a 4.0 mm short balloon at 20 athm. (5) Kissing balloon 3.0 mm (LAD)+3.5 mm (Circ.). 6–7. Final result. (8) Corevalve from femoral approach 1 week later.

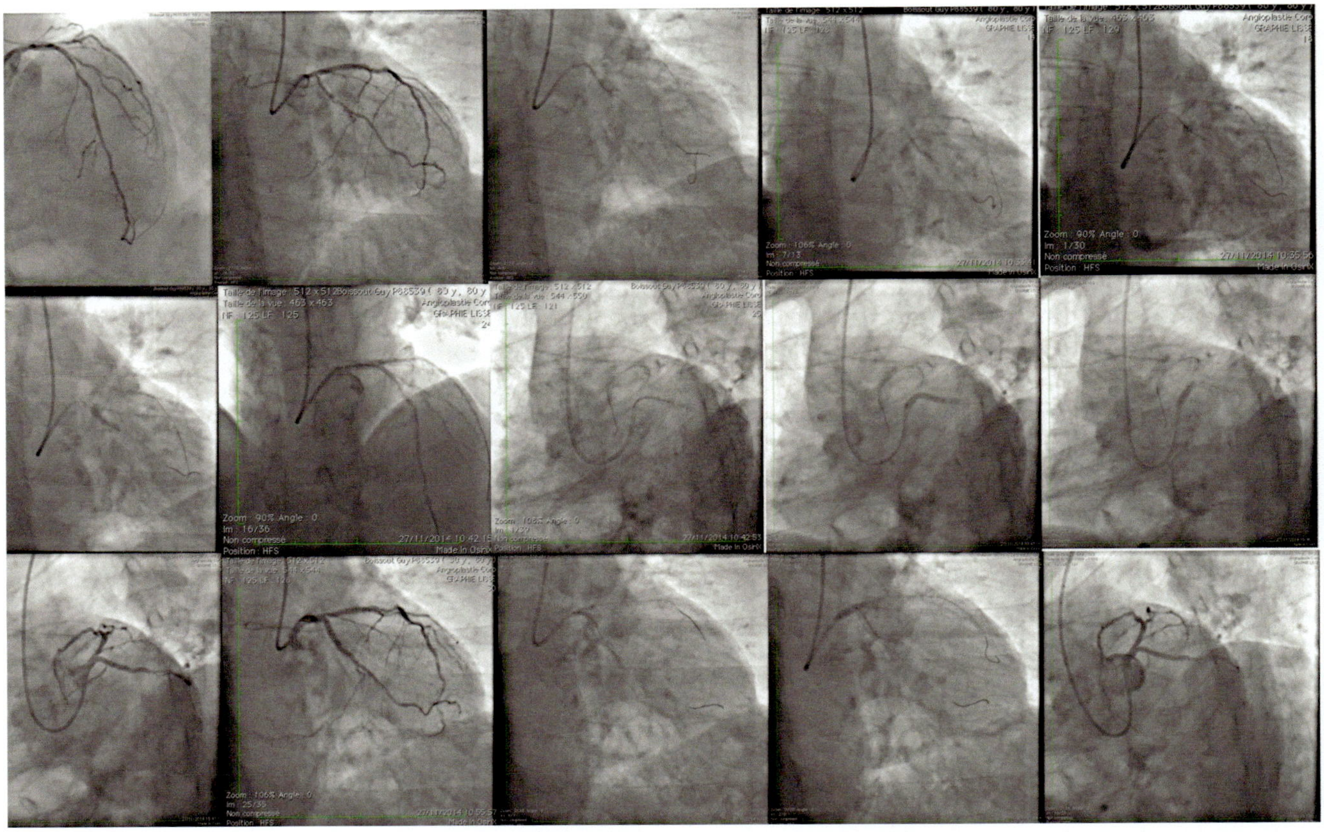

Fig. 16.6 Complexity of the Culotte technique (here the straight one, the inverted one being even more complex because of the diameter discrepancy between proximal and distal vessel)

Conclusion

Radial artery is now a widely accepted approach for coronary interventional cardiology. It is known to reduce the risk of vascular complications, increased patient comfort and the best support for outpatient diagnostic or interventions. This approach has been adapted since 20 years to most patients, clinical settings, lesions and techniques with a potential of life saving in ST elevated acute coronary syndroms.

Coronary bifurcation stenosis stenting has been during the last 15 years the field of intense clinical research and strong controversies. The actual consensus is to try to minimize the number of implanted stents. The best way to reach this goal is to use the provisional SB stenting strategy beginning by a crossover mainvessel stenting across the side branch. Most studies and meta-analysis show that systematic SB stenting first has no advantage over provisional strategy and may be responsible of a higher rate of stent thrombosis. In some situations (difficult SB access…) DK-crush technique or Culotte technique can provide effective and safe treatment (Fig. 16.6).

Radial approach in 6 F allow the use of most bifurcation techniques (excepted SKS). In case of small radial artery a sheathless guiding catheter can be used.

References

1. Radner S. Thoracal aortography by catheterization from the radial artery; preliminary report of a new technique. Acta Radiol. 1948;29(2):178–80.
2. Seldinger SI. Catheter replacement of the needle in percutaneous arteriography; a new technique. Acta Radiol. 1953;39(5):368–76.
3. Shirey EK, Sones FM. Retrograde transaortic and mitral valve catheterization. Physiologic and morphologic evaluation of aortic and mitral valve lesions. Am J Cardiol. 1966;18(5):745–53.
4. Ricketts HJ, Abrams HL. Percutaneous selective coronary cine arteriography. JAMA. 1962;181:620–4.
5. Campeau L. Entry sites for coronary angiography and therapeutic interventions: from the proximal to the distal radial artery. Can J Cardiol. 2001;17(3):319–25. Review.
6. Campeau L. Percutaneous radial artery approach for coronary angiography. Cathet Cardiovasc Diagn. 1989;16(1):3–7.
7. Kiemeneij F, Laarman GJ. Percutaneous transradial artery approach for coronary stent implantation. Cathet Cardiovasc Diagn. 1993;30(2):173–8. Erratum in: Cathet Cardiovasc Diagn 1993 Dec;30(4):358.
8. Kiemeneij F, Laarman GJ. Percutaneous transradial artery approach for coronary Palmaz-Schatz stent implantation. Am Heart J. 1994;128(1):167–74.
9. Kiemeneij F, Laarman GJ, de Melker E. Transradial artery coronary angioplasty. Am Heart J. 1995;129(1):1–7.
10. Kiemeneij F, Laarman GJ, Slagboom T, van der Wieken R. Outpatient coronary stent implantation. J Am Coll Cardiol. 1997;29(2):323–7.
11. Abhaichand RK, Louvard Y, Gobeil JF, Loubeyre C, Lefèvre T, Morice MC. The problem of arteria lusoria in right transradial

coronary angiography and angioplasty. Catheter Cardiovasc Interv. 2001;54(2):196–201.
12. Mann T, Cubeddu G, Bowen J, Schneider JE, Arrowood M, Newman WN, Zellinger MJ, Rose GC. Stenting in acute coronary syndromes: a comparison of radial versus femoral access sites. J Am Coll Cardiol. 1998;32(3):572–6.
13. Delarche N, Idir M, Estrade G, Leblay M. Direct Angioplasty for Acute Myocardial Infarction in Elderly Patients Using TransradialApproach. Am J Geriatr Cardiol. 1999;8(1):32–3.
14. Louvard Y, Ludwig J, Lefèvre T, Schmeisser A, Brück M, Scheinert D, Loubeyre C, Klinghammer L, Morice MC, Flachskampf FA, Daniel WG. Transradial approach for coronary angioplasty in the setting of acute myocardial infarction: a dual-center registry. Catheter Cardiovasc Interv. 2002;55(2):206–11.
15. Saito S, Tanaka S, Hiroe Y, Miyashita Y, Takahashi S, Tanaka K, Satake S. Comparative study on transradial approach vs. transfemoral approach in primary stent implantation for patients with acute myocardial infarction: results of the test for myocardial infarction by prospective unicenter randomization for access sites (TEMPURA) trial. Catheter Cardiovasc Interv. 2003;59(1):26–33.
16. Hildick-Smith DJ, Walsh JT, Lowe MD, Petch MC. Coronary angiography in the fully anticoagulated patient: the transradial route is successful and safe. Catheter Cardiovasc Interv. 2003;58(1):8–10.
17. Lim PO, Dzavík V. Balloon crush: treatment of bifurcation lesions using the crush stenting technique as adapted for transradial approach of percutaneous coronary intervention. Catheter Cardiovasc Interv. 2004;63(4):412–6.
18. Ziakas A, Klinke P, Mildenberger R, Fretz E, Williams MB, Della Siega A, Kinloch RD, Hilton JD. Comparison of the radial and femoral approaches in left main PCI: a retrospective study. J Invasive Cardiol. 2004;16(3):129–32.
19. Watt J, Oldroyd KG. Radial versus femoral approach for high-speed rotational atherectomy. Catheter Cardiovasc Interv. 2009;74(4):550–4.
20. Kiemeneij F, Laarman GJ, Odekerken D, Slagboom T, van der Wieken R. A randomized comparison of percutaneous transluminal coronary angioplasty by the radial, brachial and femoral approaches: the access study. J Am Coll Cardiol. 1997;29(6):1269–75.
21. Morice MC, Dumas P, Lefèvre T, Loubeyre C, Louvard Y, Piéchaud JF. Systematic use of transradial approach or suture of the femoral artery after angioplasty: attempt at achieving zero access site complications. Catheter Cardiovasc Interv. 2000;51(4):417–21.
22. Kiemeneij F, Hofland J, Laarman GJ, van der Elst DH, van der Lubbe H. Cost comparison between two modes of Palmaz Schatz coronary stent implantation:transradial bare stent technique vs. transfemoral sheath-protected stent technique. Cathet Cardiovasc Diagn. 1995;35(4):301–8.
23. Cooper CJ, El-Shiekh RA, Cohen DJ, Blaesing L, Burket MW, Basu A, Moore JA. Effect of transradial access on quality of life and cost of cardiac catheterization: A randomized comparison. Am Heart J. 1999;138(3 Pt 1):430–6.
24. Louvard Y, Lefèvre T, Allain A, Morice M. Coronary angiography through the radial or the femoral approach: The CARAFE study. Catheter Cardiovasc Interv. 2001;52(2):181–7.
25. Louvard Y, Benamer H, Garot P, Hildick-Smith D, Loubeyre C, Rigattieri S, Monchi M, Lefèvre T, Hamon M, OCTOPLUS Study Group. Comparison of transradial and transfemoral approaches for coronary angiography and angioplasty in octogenarians (the OCTOPLUS study). Am J Cardiol. 2004;94(9):1177–80.
26. Bertrand OF, Arsenault J, Mongrain R. Operator vs patient radiation exposure it transradial and transfemoral coronary interventions. Eur Heart J. 2008;29(20):2577–8.
27. Brueck M, Bandorski D, Kramer W, Wieczorek M, Höltgen R, Tillmanns H. A randomized comparison of transradial versus transfemoral approach for coronary angiography and angioplasty. JACC Cardiovasc Interv. 2009;2(11):1047–54.
28. Behan M, Haworth P, Colley P, Brittain M, Hince A, Clarke M, Ghuran A, Saha M, Hildick-Smith D. Decreasing operators' radiation exposure during coronary procedures: the transradial radiation protection board. Catheter Cardiovasc Interv. 2010;76(1):79–84.
29. Ratib K, Mamas MA, Fraser DG, Routledge H, Stables R, Nolan J. Operator experience and radiation exposure during transradial and transfemoral procedures. JACC Cardiovasc Interv. 2011;4(8):936–7.
30. Lo TS, Ratib K, Chong AY, Bhatia G, Gunning M, Nolan J. Impact of access site selection and operator expertise on radiation exposure; a controlled prospective study. Am Heart J. 2012;164(4):455–61.
31. Chase AJ, Fretz EB, Warburton WP, Klinke WP, Carere RG, Pi D, Berry B, Hilton JD. Association of the arterial access site at angioplasty with transfusion and mortality: the M.O.R.T.A.L. study (Mortality benefit Of Reduced Transfusion after percutaneous coronary intervention via the Arm or Leg). Heart. 2008;94(8):1019–25.
32. Jolly SS, Yusuf S, Cairns J, Niemelä K, Xavier D, Widimsky P, Budaj A, Niemelä M, Valentin V, Lewis BS, Avezum A, Steg PG, Rao SV, Gao P, Afzal R, Joyner CD, Chrolavicius S, Mehta SR, RIVAL trial group. Radial versus femoral access for coronary angiography and intervention in patients with acute coronary syndromes (RIVAL): a randomised, parallel group, multicentre trial. Lancet. 2011;377(9775):1409–20.
33. Romagnoli E, Biondi-Zoccai G, Sciahbasi A, et al. Radial versus femoral randomized investigation in ST-segment elevation acute coronary syndrome: the RIFLE-STEACS (Radial Versus Femoral Randomized Investigation in ST-Elevation Acute Coronary Syndrome) study. J Am Coll Cardiol. 2012;60:2481–9.
34. Nicolosi AC, Pohl LL, Parsons P, Cambria RA, Olinger GN. Increased incidence of radial artery calcification in patients with diabetes mellitus. J Surg Res. 2002;102(1):1–5.
35. Lo TS, Nolan J, Fountzopoulos E, Behan M, Butler R, Hetherington SL, Vijayalakshmi K, Rajagopal R, Fraser D, Zaman A, Hildick-Smith D. Radial artery anomaly and its influence on transradial coronary procedural outcome. Heart. 2009;95(5):410–5.
36. Burzotta F, Brancati MF, Trani C, Tommasino A, Porto I, Niccoli G, Leone AM, Coluccia V, Di Noi P, Crea F. Impact of radial-to-aorta vascular anatomical variants on risk of failure in transradialcoronary procedures. Catheter Cardiovasc Interv. 2012;80(2):298–303.
37. Cheaito R, Benamer H, Hovasse T, Tritar A, Hage F, Garot P, Lefèvre T, Unterseeh T, Chevalier B, Morice MC, Louvard Y. Feasibility and safety of transradial coronary interventions using a 6.5-F sheathless guiding catheter in patients with small radial arteries: a multicenter registry. Catheter Cardiovasc Interv. 2015;86(1):51–8. doi:10.1002/ccd.25508.
38. Takahashi S, Saito S, Tanaka S, Miyashita Y, Shiono T, Arai F, Domae H, Satake S, Itoh T. New method to increase a backup support of a 6 French guiding coronary catheter. Catheter Cardiovasc Interv. 2004;63(4):452–6.
39. Kumar S, Gorog DA, Secco GG, Di Mario C, Kukreja N. The GuideLiner "child" catheter for percutaneous coronary intervention–early clinical experience. J Invasive Cardiol. 2010;22(10):495–8.
40. Murray CD. The physiological principle of minimum work. I. The vascular system and the cost of blood volume. Proc Natl Acad Sci U S A. 1926;12:207–14.
41. Kassab GS. Scaling laws of vascular trees: of form and function. Am J Physiol Heart Circ Physiol. 2005;290:H894–903.
42. Huo Y, Kassab G. A scaling Law of vascular volume. Biophysical J. 2009;96:347–53.
43. Finet G, Gilard M, Perrenot B, Rioufol G, Motreff P, Gavit L, Prost R. Fractal geometry of arterial coronary bifurcations: a quantitative coronary angiography and intravascular ultrasound analysis. EuroIntervention. 2008;3(4):490–8.

44. Chatzizisis YS, Coskun AU, Jonas M, Edelman ER, Feldman CL, Stone PH. Role of endothelial shear stress in the natural history of coronary atherosclerosis and vascular remodeling: molecular, cellular, and vascular behavior. J Am Coll Cardiol. 2007;49(25):2379–93. Epub 2007 Jun 8. Review.
45. Nakazawa G, Yazdani SK, Finn AV, Vorpahl M, Kolodgie FD, Virmani R. Pathological findings at bifurcation lesions: the impact of flow distribution on atherosclerosis and arterial healing after stent implantation. J Am Coll Cardiol. 2010;55(16):1679–87.
46. Medina A, Suárez de Lezo J, Pan M. A new classification of coronary bifurcation lesions. Rev Esp Cardiol. 2006;59(2):183.
47. Louvard Y, Thomas M, Dzavik V, Hildick-Smith D, Galassi AR, Pan M, Burzotta F, Zelizko M, Dudek D, Ludman P, Sheiban I, Lassen JF, Darremont O, Kastrati A, Ludwig J, Iakovou I, Brunel P, Lansky A, Meerkin D, Legrand V, Medina A, Lefèvre T. Classification of coronary artery bifurcation lesions and treatments: time for a consensus! Catheter Cardiovasc Interv. 2008;71(2):175–83.
48. Lansky A, Tuinenburg J, Costa M, Maeng M, Koning G, Popma J, Cristea E, Gavit L, Costa R, Rares A, Van Es GA, Lefevre T, Reiber H, Louvard Y, Morice MC. Quantitative angiographic methods for bifurcation lesions: a consensus statement from the European Bifurcation Group. European Bifurcation Angiographic Sub-Committee. Catheter Cardiovasc Interv. 2009;73(2):258–66.
49. Goktekin O, Kaplan S, Dimopoulos K, Barlis P, Tanigawa J, Vatankulu MA, Koning G, Tuinenburg JC, Mario CD. A new quantitative analysis system for the evaluation of coronary bifurcation lesions: comparison with current conventional methods. Catheter Cardiovasc Interv. 2007;69(2):172–80.
50. Ramcharitar S, Onuma Y, Aben JP, Consten C, Weijers B, Morel MA, Serruys PW. A novel dedicated quantitative coronary analysis methodology for bifurcation lesions. EuroIntervention. 2008;3(5):553–7.
51. Ahn JM, Kang SJ, Yoon SH, Park HW, Kang SM, Lee JY, Lee SW, Kim YH, Lee CW, Park SW, Mintz GS, Park SJ. Meta-analysis of outcomes after intravascular ultrasound-guided versus angiography-guided drug-eluting stent implantation in 26,503 patients enrolled in three randomized trials and 14 observational studies. Am J Cardiol. 2014;113(8):1338–47.
52. Di Mario C, Lakovou I, Van der Giessen WJ, Foin N, Adrianssens T, Tyczynski P, Ghilencea L, Viceconte N, Lindsay AC. Optical coherence tomography for guidance in bifurcation lesion treatment. EuroIntervention. 2010;6(Suppl J):J99–106.
53. Zamani P, Kinlay S. Long-term risk of clinical events from stenting side branches of coronary bifurcation lesions with drug-eluting and bare-metal stents: an observational meta-analysis. Catheter Cardiovasc Interv. 2011;77(2):202–12.
54. Katritsis DG, Siontis GC, Ioannidis JP. Double versus single stenting for coronary bifurcation lesions: a meta-analysis. Circ Cardiovasc Interv. 2009;2(5):409–15.
55. Behan MW, Holm NR, Curzen NP, Erglis A, Stables RH, de Belder AJ, Niemelä M, Cooter N, Chew DP, Steigen TK, Oldroyd KG, Jensen JS, Lassen JF, Thuesen L, Hildick-Smith D. Simple or complex stenting for bifurcation coronary lesions: a patient-level pooled-analysis of the Nordic Bifurcation Study and the British Bifurcation Coronary Study. Circ Cardiovasc Interv. 2011;4(1):57–64.
56. Zimarino M, Corazzini A, Ricci F, Di Nicola M, De Caterina R. Late thrombosis after double versus single drug-eluting stent in the treatment of coronary bifurcations: a meta-analysis of randomized and observational Studies. JACC Cardiovasc Interv. 2013;6(7):687–95.
57. Chen SL, Santoso T, Zhang JJ, Ye F, Xu YW, Fu Q, Kan J, Paiboon C, Zhou Y, Ding SQ, Kwan TW. A randomized clinical study comparing double kissing crush with provisional stenting for treatment of coronary bifurcation lesions: results from the DKCRUSH-II (Double Kissing Crush versus Provisional Stenting Technique for Treatment of Coronary Bifurcation Lesions) trial. J Am Coll Cardiol. 2011;57(8):914–20.
58. Gao XF, Zhang YJ, Tian NL, Wu W, Li MH, Bourantas CV, Jiang XM, Wang ZM, Li B, Mao WX, Zhang JJ, Chen SL. Stenting strategy for coronary artery bifurcation with drug eluting stents: a meta-analysis of nine randomised trials and systematic review. EuroIntervention. 2014;10(5):561–9.
59. Lassen JF, Holm NR, Stankovic G, Lefèvre T, Chieffo A, Hildick-Smith D, Pan M, Darremont O, Albiero R, Ferenc M, Louvard Y. Percutaneous coronary intervention for coronary bifurcation disease: consensus from the first 10 years of the European Bifurcation Club meetings. EuroIntervention. 2014;10(5):545–60.
60. Toyofuku M, Kimura T, Morimoto T, Hayashi Y, Shiode N, Okimoto T, Otsuka M, Tamekiyo H, Tamura T, Kadota K, Inoue K, Mitsudo K, j-Cypher Registry investigators. Comparison of target-lesion revascularisation between left main coronary artery bifurcations andleft anterior descending coronary artery bifurcations using the one and two stent approach with sirolimus-eluting stents. EuroIntervention. 2011;7(7):796–804.
61. Palmerini T, Marzocchi A, Tamburino C, Sheiban I, Margheri M, Vecchi G, Sangiorgi G, Santarelli A, Bartorelli A, Briguori C, Vignali L, Di Pede F, Ramondo A, Inglese L, De Carlo M, Falsini G, Benassi A, Palmieri C, Filippone V, Sangiorgi D, Barlocco F, De Servi S. Impact of bifurcation technique on 2-year clinical outcomes in 773 patients with distal unprotected left main coronary artery stenosis treated with drug-eluting stents. Circ Cardiovasc Interv. 2008;1(3):185–92.
62. Koo BK, Kang HJ, Youn TJ, Chae IH, Choi DJ, Kim HS, Sohn DW, Oh BH, Lee MM, Park YB, Choi YS, Tahk SJ. Physiologic assessment of jailed side branch lesions using fractional flow reserve. J Am Coll Cardiol. 2005;46(4):633–7.
63. Nam CW, Hur SH, Koo BK, Doh JH, Cho YK, Park HS, Yoon HJ, Kim H, Chung IS, Kim YN, Fearon WF, Tahk SJ, Kim KB. Fractional flow reserve versus angiography in left circumflex ostial intervention after left main crossover stenting. Korean Circ J. 2011;41(6):304–7.
64. Mylotte D, Hovasse T, Ziani A, Lefèvre T, Dumonteil N, Louvard Y, Carrie D. Non-compliant balloons for final kissing inflation in coronary bifurcation lesions treated with provisional side branch stenting: a pilot study. EuroIntervention. 2012;7(10):1162–9.
65. Burzotta F, Gwon HC, Hahn JY, Romagnoli E, Choi JH, Trani C, Colombo A. Modified T-stenting with intentional protrusion of the side-branch stent within the main vessel stent to ensure ostial coverage and facilitate final kissing balloon: the T-stenting and small protrusion technique (TAP-stenting). Report of bench testing and first clinical Italian-Korean two-centre experience. Catheter Cardiovasc Interv. 2007;70(1):75–82.
66. Silva JD, Carrillo X, Salvatella N, Fernandez-Nofrerias E, Rodriguez-Leor O, Mauri J, Bayes-Genis A. The utility of stent enhancement to guide percutaneous coronary intervention for bifurcation lesions. EuroIntervention. 2013;9(8):968–74.

Transradial Approach for Bifurcation Lesions: Chinese Experiences

17

Shao-Liang Chen, Jun-Jie Zhang, and Liang Long Chen

Abstract

Percutaneous coronary intervention (PCI) in coronary bifurcation lesions is relatively common in daily practice which accounts for approximately 1/5 of all the PCI procedures. Transradial PCI of left main or non–left main bifurcation lesions can be successfully accomplished in most cases, but this practice is still restricted in many centers worldwide due to the perceived technical challenges of guiding catheter support, limitations of catheter sizes, need for the simultaneous use of stents and balloons, and consequences of procedural failure. In the past few years, Chinese interventionists have developed a few techniques, such as double kissing crushing technique, double kissing mini culotte stenting technique to increase the procedural success rate and improve the long-term prognosis of complex bifurcation intervention. In this chapter, we will give a detailed description of those bifurcation intervention techniques via transradial approach.

17.1 Part 1: Double Kissing Crush – Its Advantage and Long Term Results in Transradial Intervention

Shao-Liang Chen and Jun-Jie Zhang

Percutaneous treatment of coronary bifurcations is a challenge for interventional cardiology. Drug-eluting stents (DES) reduce restenosis in coronary bifurcation lesions compared with historical bare metal stent (BMS) controls. For the majority of bifurcation lesions, provisional side branch (SB) stenting is considerate to be the default strategy [1, 2]. However, if the SB is large and has long segment disease extending beyond the vessel ostium, the 2-stent technique is usually reasonable [3]. Crush stenting, a modified T stenting technique, was introduced by Colombo and his colleagues in 2004 [4], with aim of fully covering the ostial SB. Originally, crush stenting technique consisted of stenting SB, stenting main vessel (MV) and final kissing balloon inflation (FKBI). One of the beauty of crush stenting is that SB is never lost, which is a main concern during stenting complex bifurcation lesions. However, several limitations of this technique were recognized in clinical practice: (1) a 7 F guiding catheter was required for two stents simultaneously positioned in both MV and SB, (2) impossible cross-over from provisional stenting to crush stenting. As a result, there are some alternatives of crush stenting techniques, including balloon crush, inner crush. Balloon crush needs simultaneously to advance one balloon in MV and one stent in SB, thus, a 6 F guiding catheter is sufficient to accommodate these two devices. Moreover, first crush is performed immediately after stenting SB. Inner crush is, in fact, a rescue crush similar to rescue (or provisional) T stenting. Once there are anatomical requirements after stenting MV, including severely pinched SB, dissection or even acute closure of SB, rescue stenting (provisional T or inner crush) for SB is recommended. Inner crush has relative long protrusion of SB stent into MV compared to rescue T. In order to minimize the negative impact of long protrusion into MV, balloon crush in MV is necessary, followed by a FKBI. Of note, the protruded

S.-L. Chen, MD (✉) • J.-J. Zhang, PhD
Department of Cardiology, Nanjing First Hospital, Nanjing Medical University, Nanjing, China
e-mail: chmengx@126.com

L.L. Chen
Union Hospital, Fujian Medical University, Fu Jian, China

Y. Zhou et al. (eds.), *Transradial Approach for Percutaneous Interventions*, DOI 10.1007/978-94-017-7350-8_17

SB stent struts are easily malapposed [5], even after FKBI. Indeed, all those crush stenting techniques are renamed as classic crush stenting.A body of studies have reported that classic crush stenting, in particular if FKBI was not successfully performed, was associated with a high rate of stent thrombosis (ST) and in-stent restenosis (ISR) which was most commonly seen at ostial SB [6]. Although the rate of FKBI failure was around 20~25% after classic crush stenting [7], the underlying reasons still remained unclear. Bench test showed that stent platform, irregular and small stent cell, severe distortion of MV stent, and presence of three layers of stent struts irregularly overlapping are potential factors affecting the successful rate of FKBI [8]. To overcome these disadvantages of classic crush, double kissing and double kissing (DK) crush stenting technique (Fig. 17.1) was introduced by our group in 2005 [9]. DK crush introduces two times kissing and includes the following steps: stenting SB (with 2–3 mm protrusion), balloon crush, first kissing, stenting MV, and FKBI. The main difference between classic and DK crush is the use of first kissing. After balloon crush of the implanted SB stent, there are two layers of stent struts from ostial SB to MV. Thus, first kissing can not only optimize the distorted SB stent and leave only one layer of metal struts at ostial SB, but also minimize repeated distortion of ostial SB stent when MV stent deployment, which probably facilitate the second kissing after stenting MV. In other words, first kissing re-builds the shape of bifurcation anatomy. Another advantage of DK crush over classic crush is 6Fr guiding catheter compatible, which can facilitate radial approach.

However, things are not easier than you think. As we found from the bench test for classic crush that rewiring SB is necessary to repair distorted SB stent [8]. Operators always need to pay more attention to rewire SB from proximal MV stent cell. As rewiring SB from distal MV stent cell could increase the possibility of wire going between stent and vessel wall, which will leave a gap at the ostium after balloon crushing (Fig. 17.2) [8]. The methods to confirm the exact position of SB wire are as following: visual assessment from fluoroscopy (Orthogonal projections to confirm SB rewiring from the proximal MV stent cell, online video), guidance with intravascular ultrasound (IVUS) or optical coherence tomography (OCT) from MV. Sometimes, it is difficult to advance balloon to SB after wire position in the true lumen of SB stent. One alternative is to inflate a balloon in distal MV to provide extra support (namely, balloon anchoring technique). Otherwise, minimal size balloon (such as, 1.5 mm) can be tried, followed by relative large one. Alternative inflation using non-compliant balloon (with the balloon/stent ratio of 1:1) at ≥16 atm starting from SB is recommended before first kissing and FKBI. Two non-compliant balloons are usually inflated at ≥12 atm during FKBI [10]. Proximal optimization technique (POT) is mandated to achieve well apposition of proximal MV stent unless IVUS or OCT confirms no presence of stent strut malapposition at proximal MB. Flow-limiting dissection at proximal, distal edge of MV, or distal edge of SB entails bail-out stent.

Clinical data, comparing DK crush versus either classic crush or other stenting techniques mainly come from the serial randomized DKCRUSH trials. Initially, we reported that FKBI was successfully performed in 100% by DK crush [5], compared to 80% in classic crush. In DKCRUSH-I study, we demonstrated that DK crush was associated with a significant reduction of ST, ISR and major adverse cardiac events (MACE) in treating patients with true bifurcation lesion compared to classic crush [11]. Interestingly, DKCRUSH-II trial [10] for the first time showed a significant low rate of target lesion revascularization (TLR) after DK crush for complex bifurcation lesions at 1-year follow-up, compared to provisional T stenting technique. Recently, the DKCRUSH-III study including patients with distal left main bifurcation lesions showed that 3-year clinical outcomes and 13-month angiographic results were in favor of DK crush when compared with culotte stenting technique [12, 13] in term of TVR, MI, ST and MACE. Furthermore, IVUS analysis confirmed better strut apposition in DK crush stenting group [14]. In addition, clinical results from the studies also supported the priority of DK crush to other stenting techniques for left main bifurcation lesions at long-term follow-up [11, 15]. Taking insight analysis from those DKCRUSH trials, it is too early to admire that DK crush is the best mousetrap for stenting bifurcation lesions. Actually, whether DK crush can achieve favorable outcomes in patients with more frequent morbidities (myocardial infarction, left ventricular dysfunction), longer SB lesion length and more complex lesions (chronic total occlusion, calcified and thrombus containing lesions) has not yet defined. Furthermore, no two bifurcation lesions are identical. It sounds superficial if we consider that all true bifurcation lesions belong to complex lesions. By our DEFINITION study [16] relying on anatomical variables from 3660 patients with Medina 1,1,1 and 0,1,1 bifurcations and SB diameter minimal 2.5-mm, complex bifurcation lesions only account for 30% among all true bifurcation lesions, with 70% classified in simple bifurcation lesions. All two-stent techniques did not show any benefits over one-stent approach for the simple bifurcation lesions. In contrast, two-stent techniques for complex bifurcation lesions were associated with less in-hospital mortality and 1-year MACE than one-stent technique. Apparently, before making final decision of the stenting technique selection, lesions stratification with this novel method is recommended. Of course, the superiority of DK crush over provisional stenting or other complex stenting techniques for the new defined complex lesion needs to be tested in the following randomized studies.

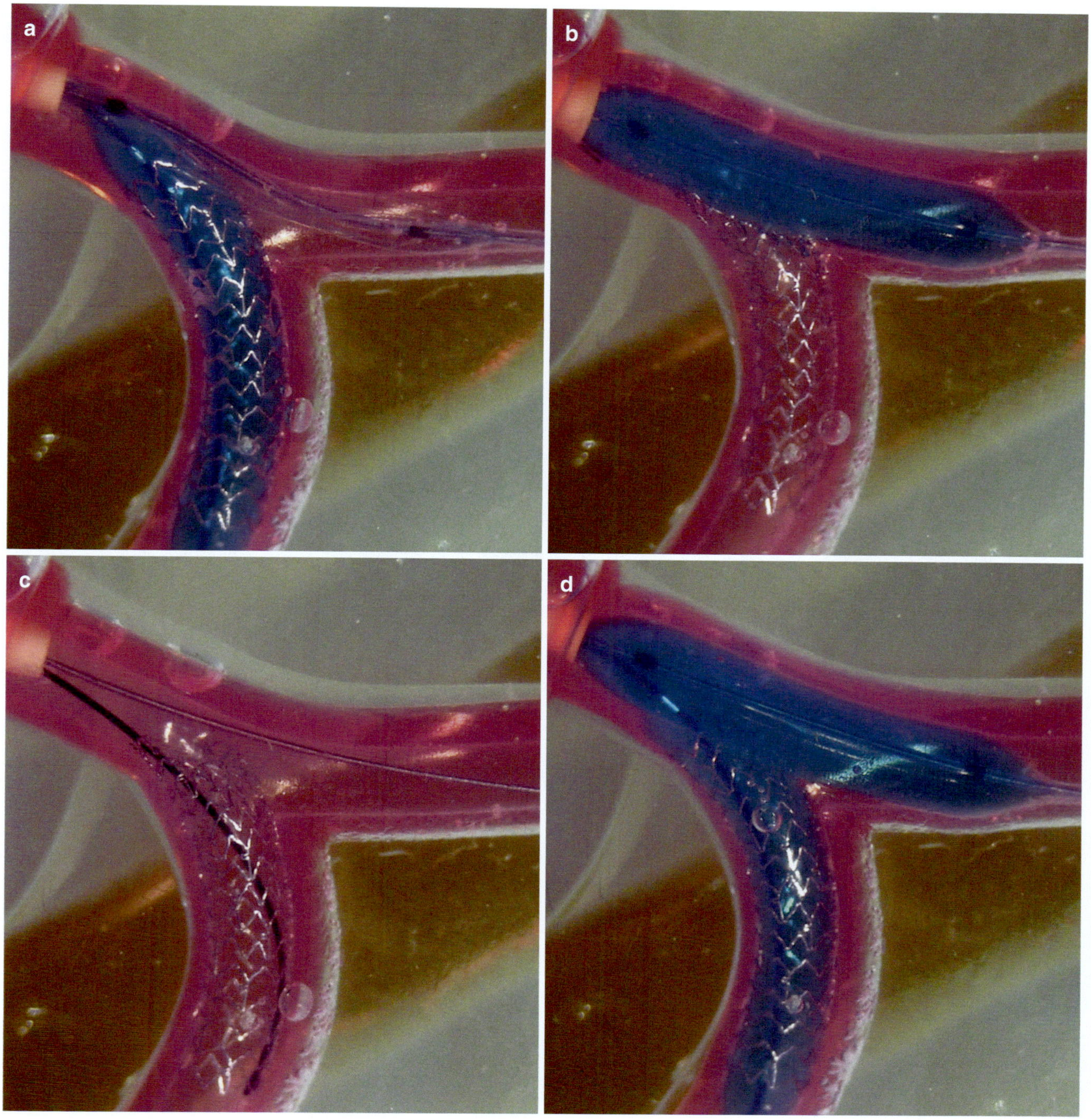

Fig. 17.1 Double kissing (*DK*) crush stenting (proximal SB re-crossing) for distal LM bifurcation (distal bifurcation angle of 90°). (**a**) SB stent deployment. (**b**) The balloon in the MV was inflated to crush the SB stent. (**c**) Proximal SB re-crossing. (**d**) First kissing balloon inflation. (**e**) MV stent deployment. (**f**) Proximal-middle SB re-crossing. (**g**) SB balloon dilation. (**h**) MV balloon dilation. (**i**) FKBI. (**j**) Proximal optimization technique (*POT*). (**k**, **l**) The stent strut of SB ostium was well appositioned without gap formation. (**m–o**) The electronically cut stents show a clear viewing of the SB ostium. *MV* main vessel, *SB* side branch, *FKBI* Final kissing balloon inflation (Acknowledgement: Reprinted from Jun Jie Zhang [17])

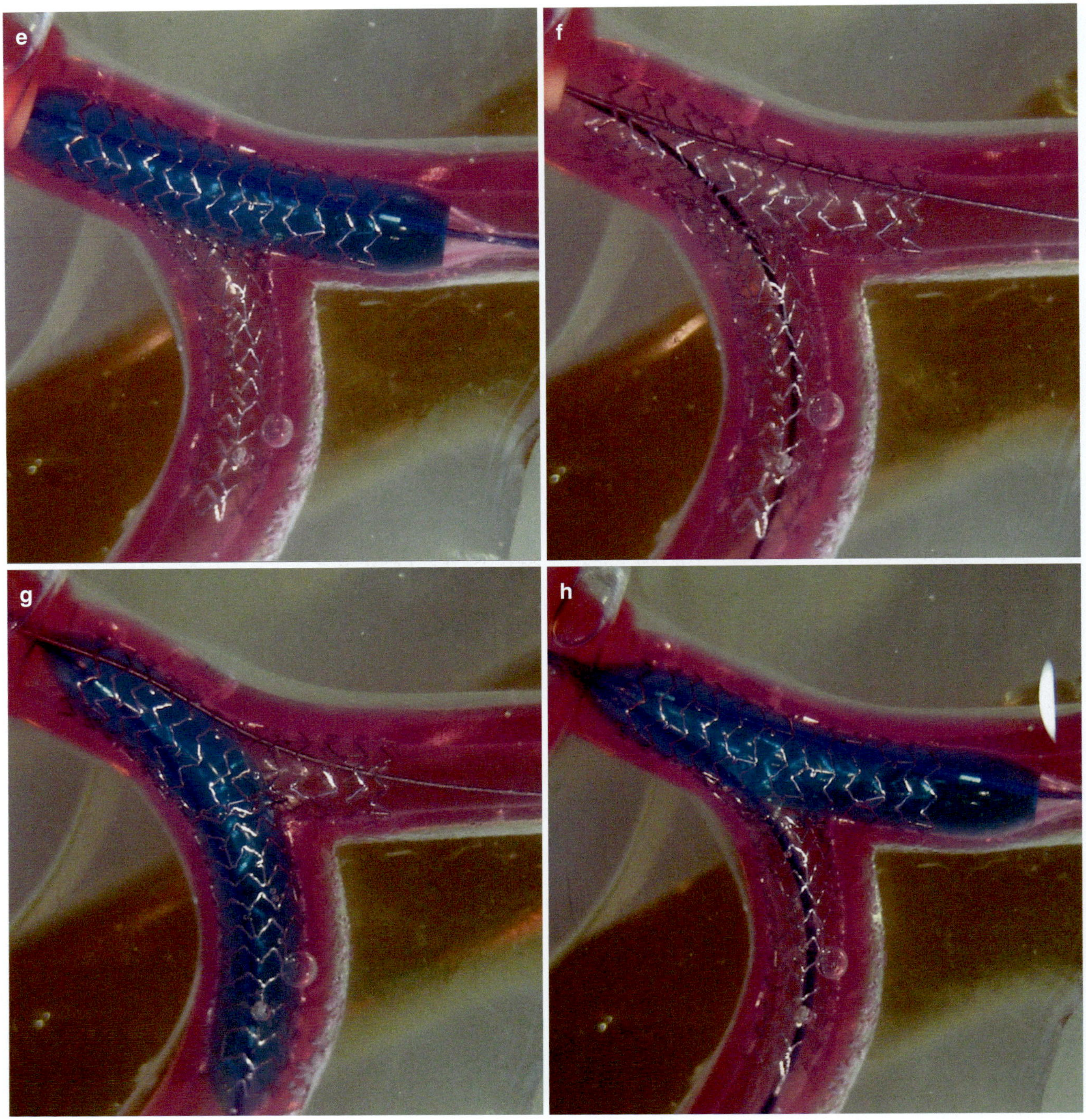

Fig. 17.1 (continued)

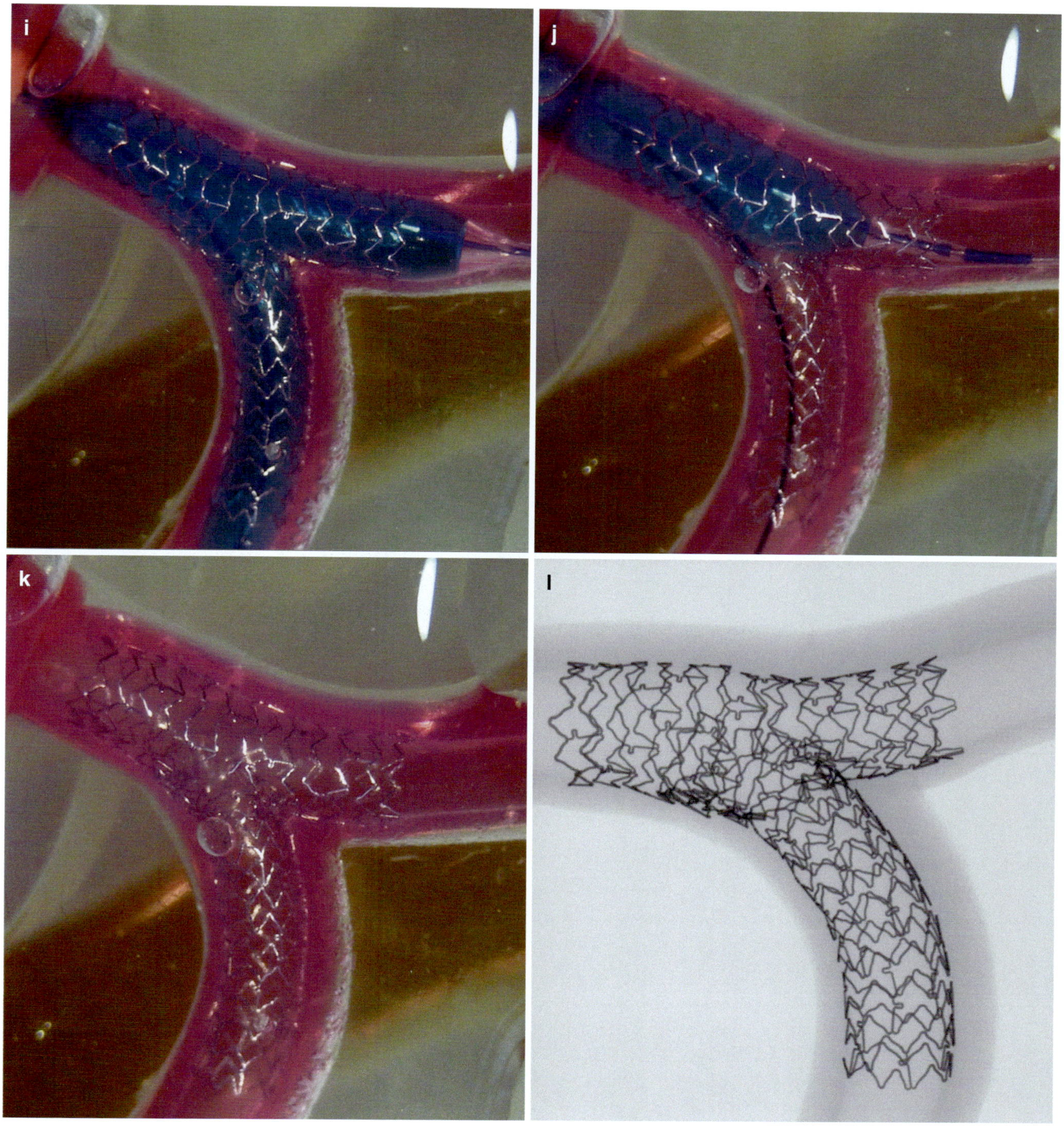

Fig. 17.1 (continued)

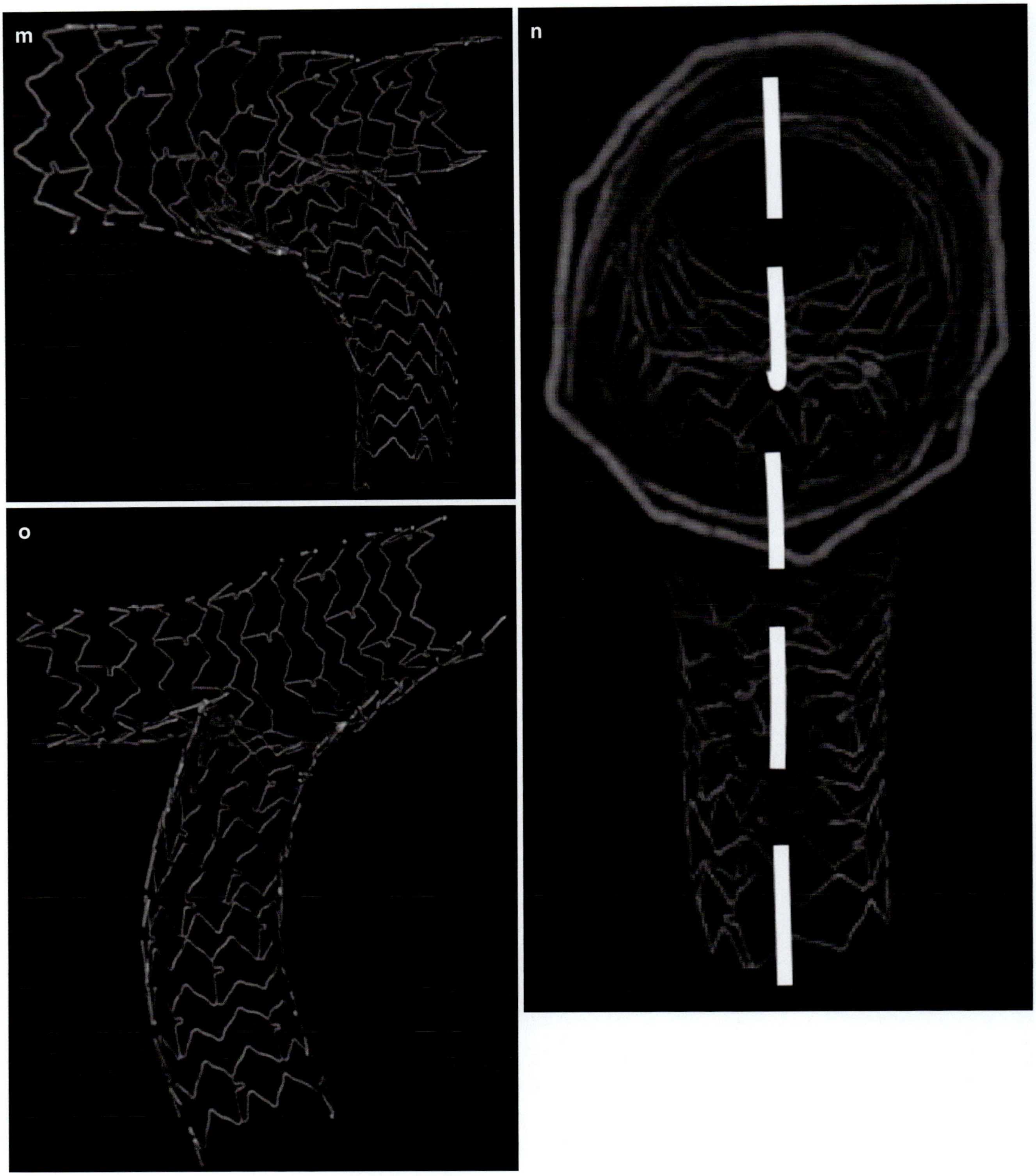

Fig. 17.1 (continued)

In summary, available clinical data supported the advantages of DK crush over other stenting techniques for more complex coronary bifurcation lesions. This technique consists of stenting SB, balloon crush, first kissing, stenting MV, and FKBI. Carefully rewiring from proximal cell of MV stent and maintaining the wire in the true lumen of SB stent is critical for optimal angiographic results at follow-up. Balloon anchoring from MV, alternative inflation and each kissing inflation using large enough non-compliant balloons at high pressure, and POT technique are mandatory to improve both angiographic and clinical outcomes. Imagining modalities are useful to guide SB rewiring and assessment of procedure quality. Stratification of a given bifurcation lesions is recommended before decision-making.

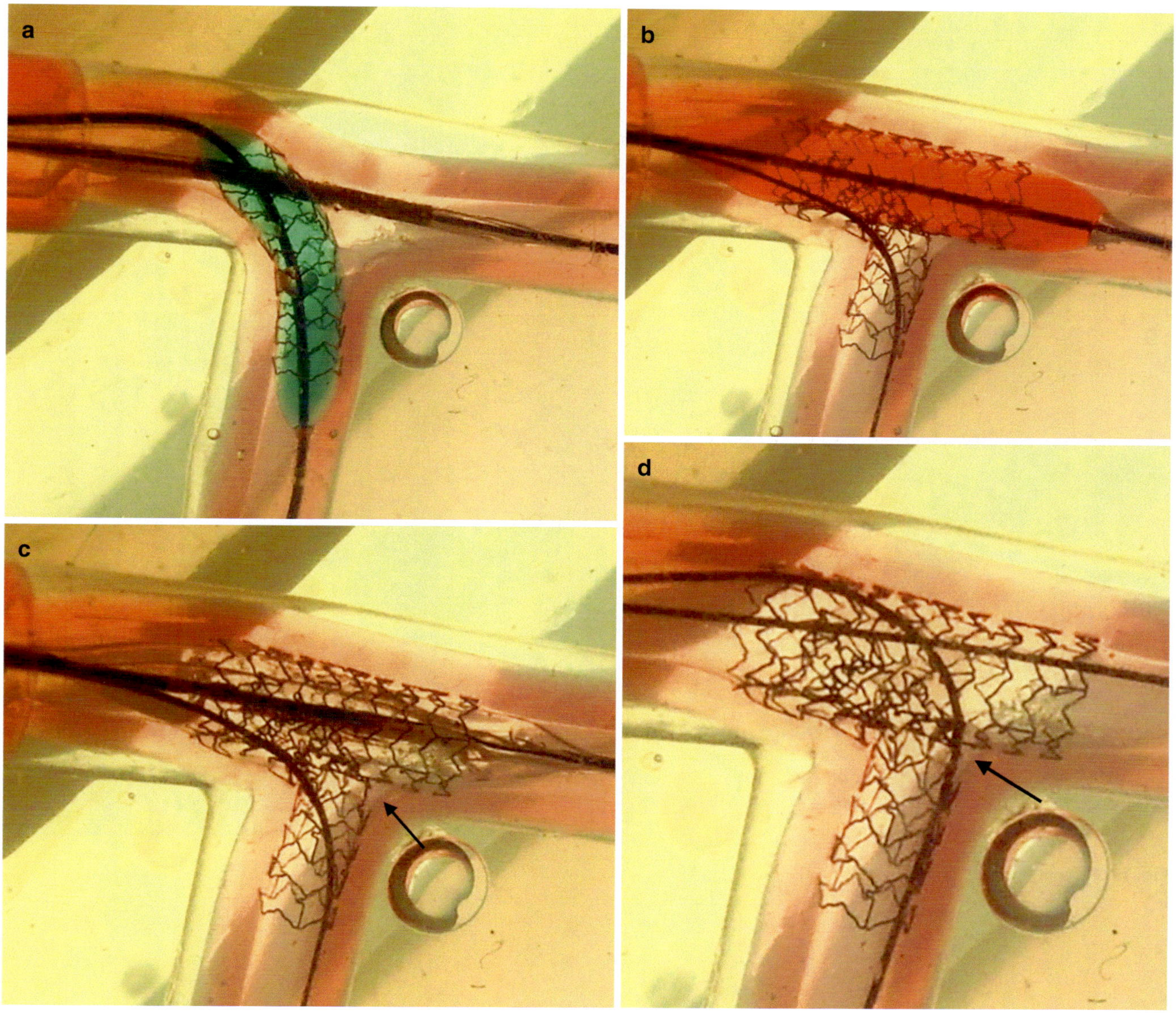

Fig. 17.2 Classic crush stenting (distal re-crossing SB) for distal LM bifurcation (distal bifurcation angle of 90°). (**a**) SB stent deployment. (**b**) MV stent deployment to crush the SB stent. (**c**) Gap formation near the carina (*arrow*). (**d**) Distal SB re-crossing, wire going between the SB stent and vessel wall. (**e**) SB balloon dilation. (**f**) Final kissing balloon inflation. (**g**, **h**) Leaving a significant gap near carina (*arrow*). *MV* main vessel, *SB* side branch, *FKBI* Final kissing balloon inflation (Acknowledgement: Reprinted from Jun Jie Zhang [18], with permission from Europa Digital & Publishing)

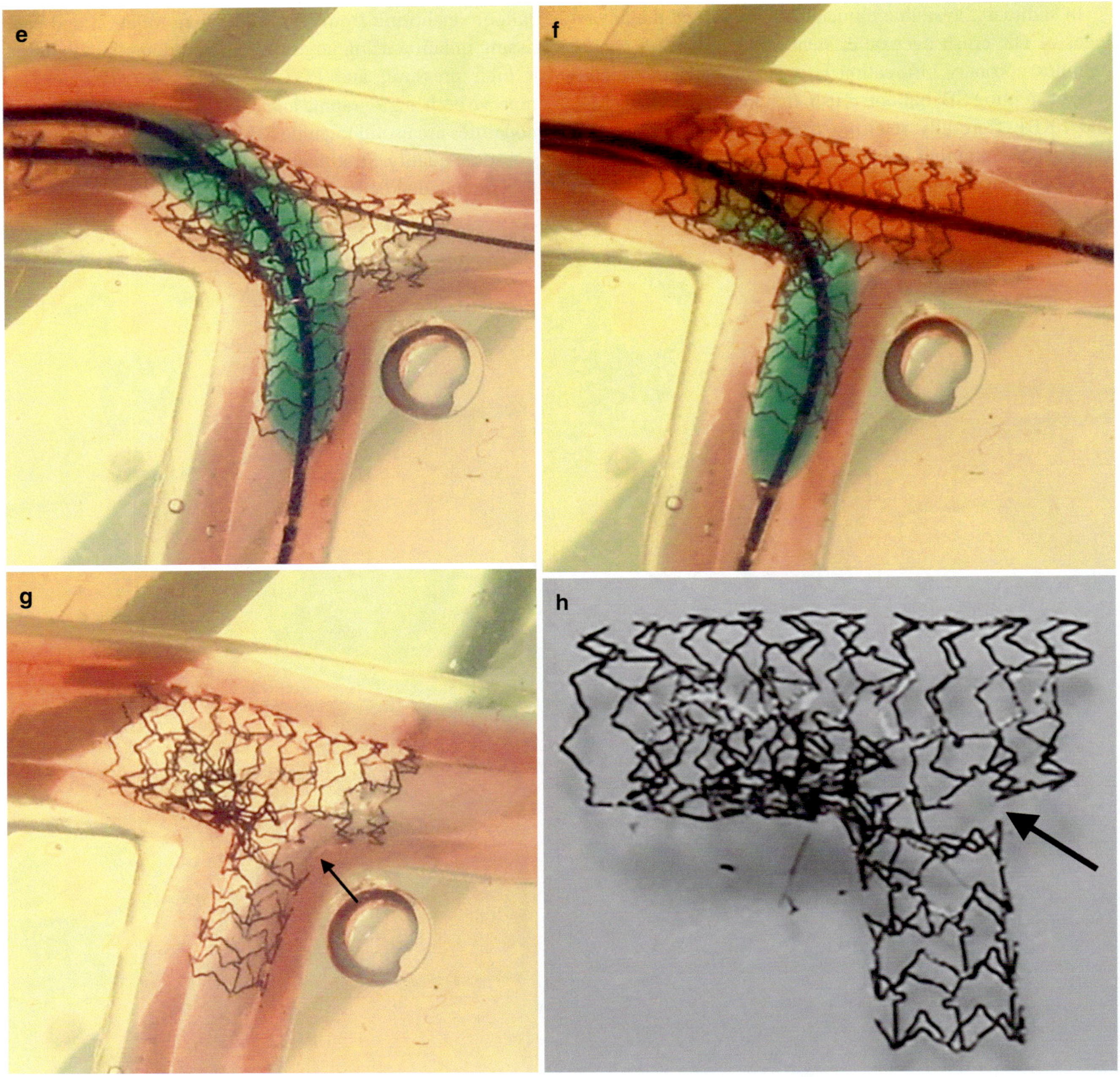

Fig. 17.2 (continued)

Fig. 17.3 DK crush stenting through radial approach for distal LM bifurcation lesion case: (**a**) A 1,1,1 distal LM lesion. 6 Fr GC through left radial approach. (**b**) SB stent deployment. (**c**) 3.5 mm balloon in MV inflation to crush SB stent. (**d**) Rewiring SB from proximal cell. (**e**) First kissing balloon inflation. (**f**) MV stent deployment. (**g**) Non-compliant balloon in SB inflation at 20 atm. (**h**) Non-compliant balloon in MV inflation at 20 atm. (**i**) Final kissing balloon inflation. (**j**) Final result. (**k**) Thirteen-month angiographic FU

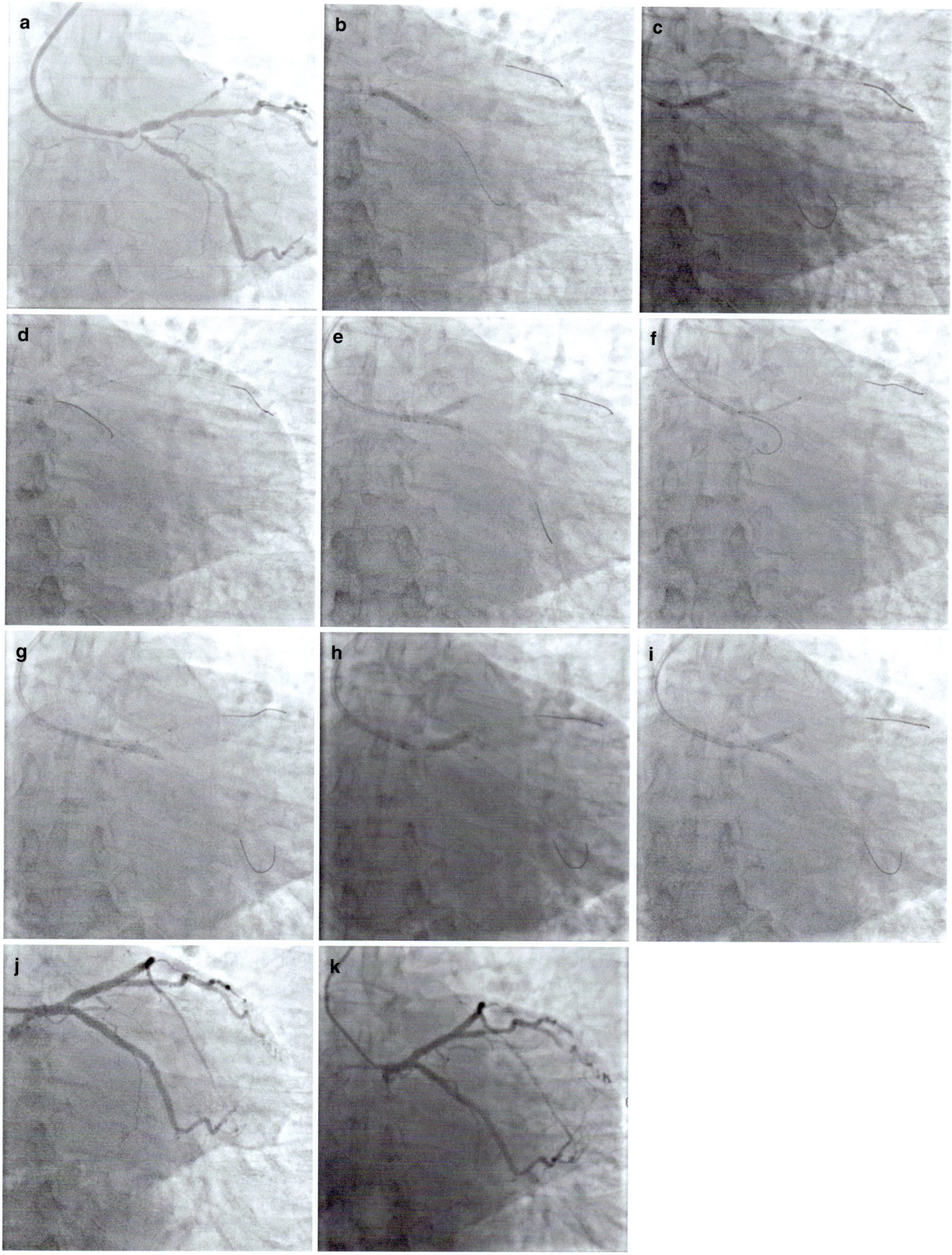
a
b
c
d
e
f
g
h
i
j
k

17.2 Part 2: Optimized Provisional Stenting for Treatment of Coronary Bifurcation Lesions

Liang Long Chen

17.2.1 The Procedural Essence

The optimized provisional T-stenting (OPT) distinguished itself from the classic provisional T-stenting (CPT) mainly in adoption of the ostial optimization technique (OOT), which can efficiently solve the dilemma in stent positioning and coverage of the SB ostium as rescue SB stenting is indicated, resulting in seamless connection between the two bifurcated stents.

17.2.2 The Procedural Indications

All CBLs can be treated with OPT on the premise of a reliable SB protection. OOT is able to turn the redundant MB struts over the SB ostium onto its upper ostial rim (struts ectropion), facilitating subsequent stent positioning and implanting if necessary for rescue SB stenting, or achieving "2-stent effect with 1-stent implantation" if not necessary for rescue SB stenting.

17.2.3 The Procedural Steps

OPT can be performed either via radial or femoral approach. 6–7 Fr. Guiding catheters with bigger lumen, open-cell stents with larger cell, and guiding wires with better shaping and recovering memory are preferred for the procedure. The procedural steps are schematically illustrated as follows (Fig. 17.4):

17.2.4 The Key Steps: Tricks and Points

1. Pre-imbedded balloon for prevention of SB occlusion or carina shifting

   Pre-imbedded balloon in the SB prior to the MB stenting is most effective for preventing its intra-procedural occlusion irrespective of occupying some catheter lumen. If used, the balloon should be stayed aside the MB stent, and then inflated simultaneously with the MB stenting and deflated after deflation of MB balloon, such a maneuver can prevent SB occlusion and/or carina shifting caused by MV/MB stenting, ensure rewiring the SB as closer as possible to the original carina position, thereby leading to a better result of OOT.
2. SiKBD for optimization of ostial SB

   As the most crucial step, SiKBD can be achieved by firstly inflating of the SB balloon followed by inflating of the MB balloon such that a better resultant direction of expanding-force can be generated to turn the abundant MB struts over the SB ostium onto its upper ostial margin, resulting in better effect of strut ectropion or better result of OOT.

17.2.5 The Typical Cases of OPT

The following case examples (Figs. 17.5, 17.6, and 17.7) demonstrate that OPT has broad indications for treating various CBLs including different anatomy (Y-/T-angulation and/or great BDD) and lesion locations [left main coronary artery (LM) or non-LM CBL] and also illuminate how to properly complete OPT by addressing the frequent problems and their solutions.

Figure 17.5 illustrates all procedural steps of OPT particularly the key steps (e.g., balloon branch protection, U-bend wiring technique and siKBD) in treatment of a LM-CBL patient with great DBA. Figures 17.6 and 17.7 exhibits OOT is able to achieve "2-stent effect with 1-stent implantation", thus avoiding rescue SB stenting (OOT only).

17.2.6 Provisional Stenting Family and Clinical Relevance of OPT

The provisional T-stenting offers an option between 1- and 2-stent techniques. If used properly, CPT is an efficacious treatment with reasonable cost [19–25]. However, there are two unresolved issues associated with CPT [24, 25]: (1) the potential risk of SB occlusion, (2) difficulty in stent positioning and coverage of the ostial SB as requiring the rescue T-stenting. The former has been solved by pre-imbedded protecting balloon technique [26, 27], whereas the later has not regardless of lots attempting. As well known, when the rescue T-stent is required for the SB with using CPT, it is difficult to accurately position the stent at ostial SB, particularly in Y-type lesion. If the proximal stent edge is aligned with inferior margin of the SB ostium, then there are no struts covering the superior margin of the SB ostium, thus being prone to develop in-stent restenosis. On the contrary, if the proximal stent edge is aligned with superior margin of the SB ostium, then the SB stent has to protrude into the MV, thereby resulting in suspension of partial stent inside the MV, thereby increasing the potential risk of in-stent thrombosis. Accordingly, several techniques, such as the T and small protrusion stenting (TAP), inner crush stenting, conventional culotte stenting and so on, have been used as alternatives for the rescue SB stenting with expectation of more complete coverage of the bifurcated area and less difficulty in ostial stent positioning. TAP, as used for the rescue SB stent, has been demonstrated to be easier in positioning of the SB stent and more complete in stent covering of the bifurcated lesion with favorable long-term clinical outcomes [28–30]. However, theoretically, all these techniques will introduce new problems due to increasing the metallic or drug burden at the bifurcated area or altering the bifurcated vessel/stent configuration or local hemodynamics, likewise leading to increasing the risks of in-stent restenosis and thrombosis.

The proximal optimization technique (POT) was introduced mainly for improving proximal stent lumen with somehow optimizing the SB ostium [31]. Despite that POT favored rewiring the SB and rewiring it closer to the carina so that the resultant stenting quality may be improved, the optimization afforded by POT alone is imperfect: (1) it is difficult to achieved "2-stent effect with 1-stent implanting" owing to the limited strut ectropion from the MB stent into the ostial SB, thus remaining at risk of acute branch occlusion, residual stenosis and in-stent restenosis, (2) it is still difficult to accurately position ostial SB stent as requiring a rescue T-stent.

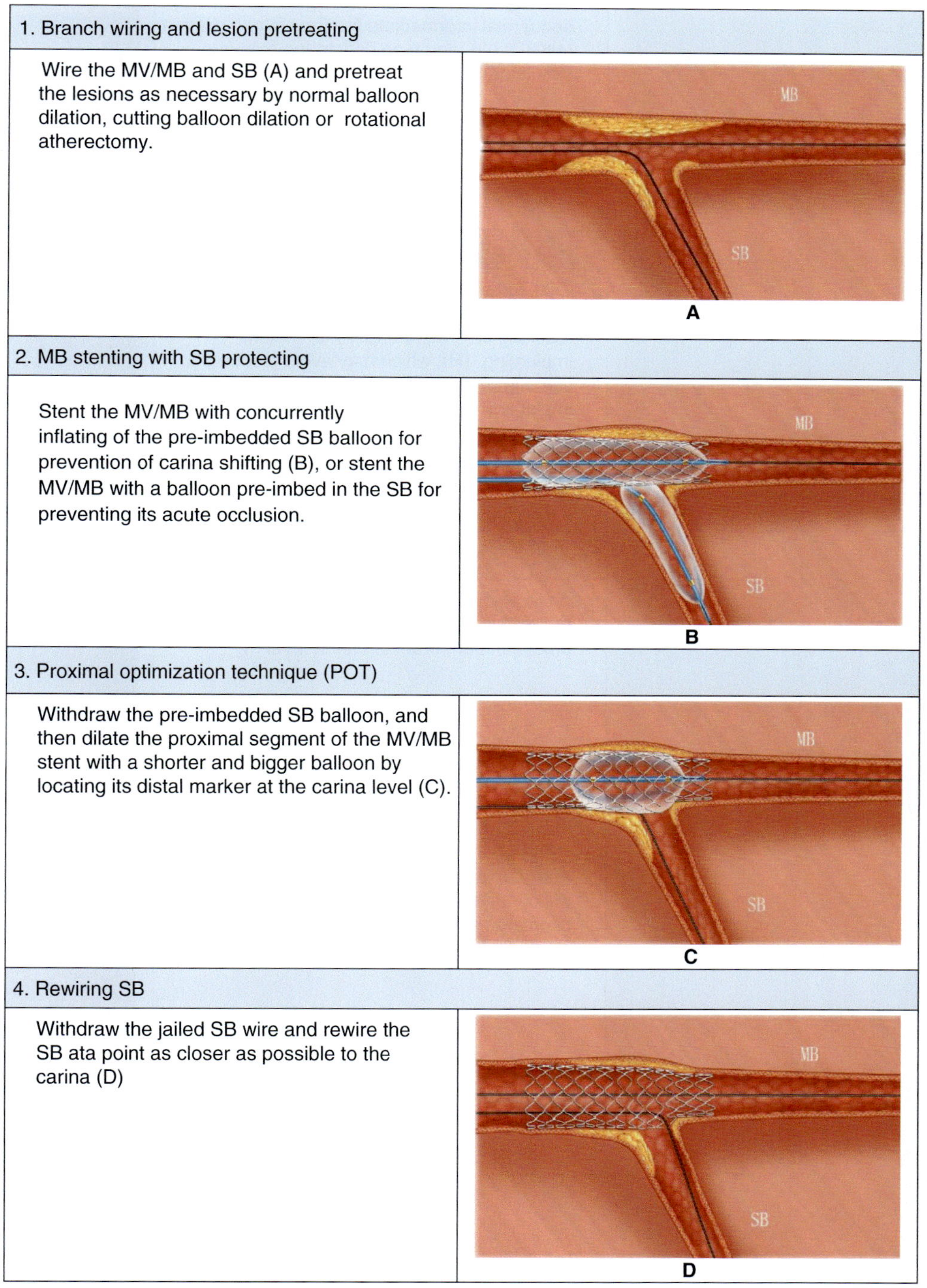

Fig. 17.4 Diagram of OPT procedural steps (Image provided courtesy of Medtronic Inc. © Medtronic Inc. All rights reserved)

Fig. 17.4 (continued)

5. Ostial optimization technique (OOT)	
Advance two balloons respectively over the MB and SB wires and align their proximal markers at the level of the polygon of confluence (POC) (E).	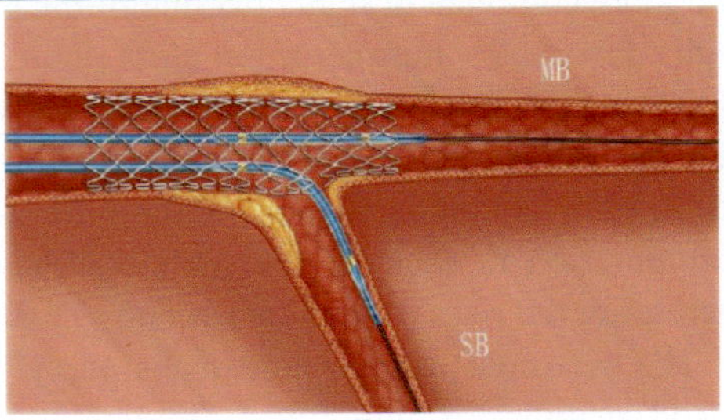 E
Inflate the SB balloon first (F), followed by inflating of the MB balloon to perform a sequential intermediate kissing balloon dilation (siKBD) (G), and then deflate the balloons simultaneously.	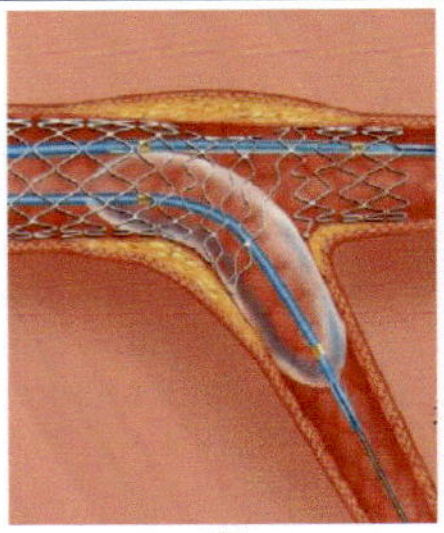 F 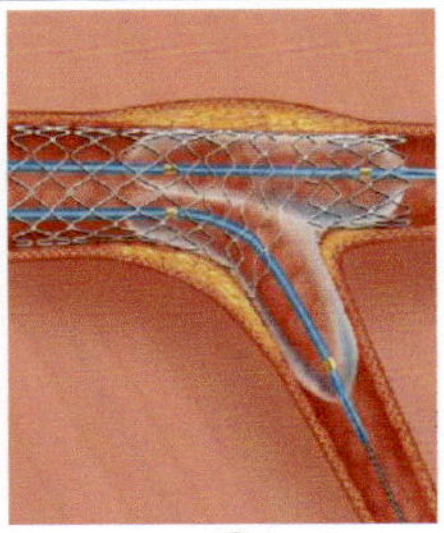 G
6. Result of OOT	
OOT turns the redundant MB struts over the SB ostium onto its upper rim (ectropion), resulting in “2-stent effect with 1-stent implanting” (H), which may avoid rescue SB stenting or facilitate stent positioning and implanting if necessary for rescue SB stenting.	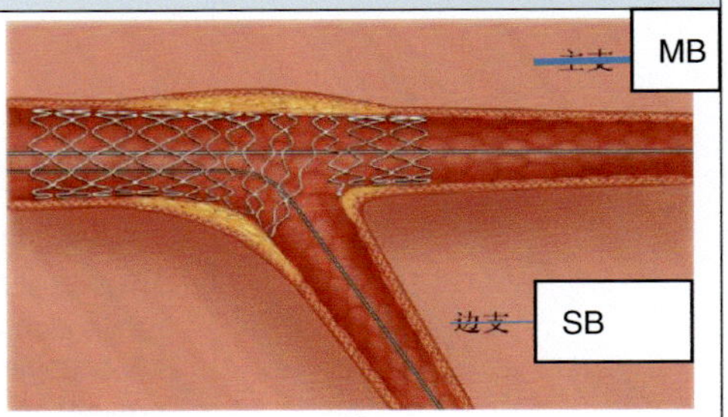 H
7. Rescue SB stenting	
As indicated for rescue SB stenting, it’s easy to position SB stent just by localizing its proximal marker at the carina level (I).	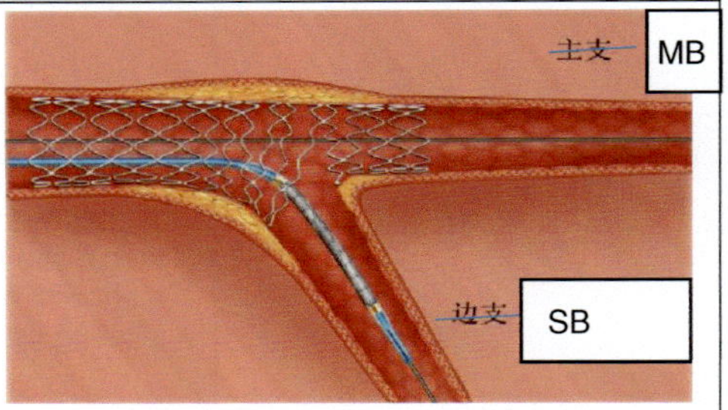 I
After deploying the SB stent, the two stents will connect seamlessly and cover the whole bifurcated area without protrusion of the SB stent into the MV (J).	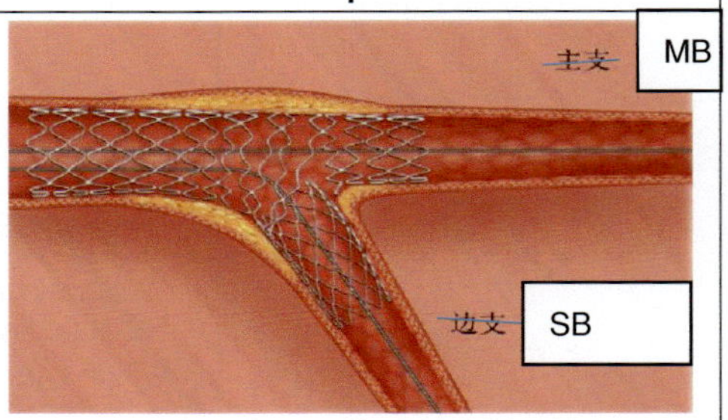 J

Fig. 17.4 (continued)

8. Final kissing balloon dilation (fKBD)	
Advance 2 non-compliance balloons (used for siKBD) respectively over the MB and SB wires and align their proximal markers at thelevel of POC and then perform fKBD to end the procedure (K)	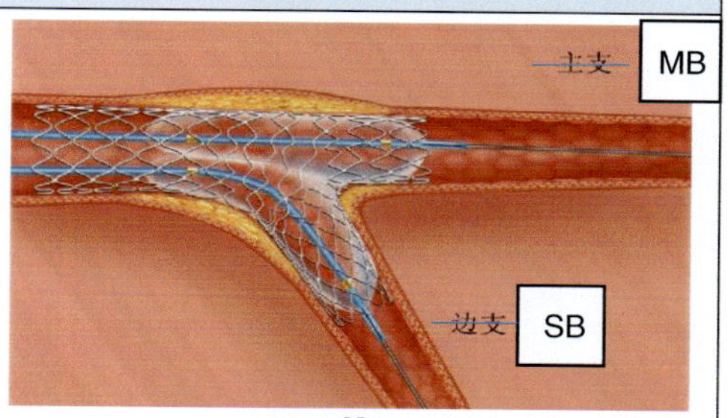 K
9. Final results	
OPT can result in excellent bifurcated stent morphology in terms of full lesion coverage and seamless connection between the two bifurcated stents without protrusion of the SB stent into the MB (L).	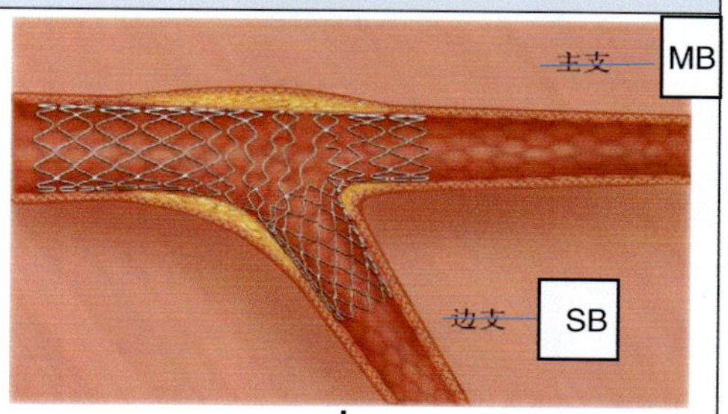 L

Besides POT, we first proposed OOT to optimize the ostial SB after MB stenting. OOT is characterized by siKBD or snuggling balloon dilation. Briefly, for 1-stent or CPT without requirement of a rescue SB stent, a smaller SB balloon (balloon/SB diameter of 0.75 or less), and for CPT with requirement of a rescue SB stent, a bigger SB balloon (balloon/SB diameter of 1.0 or bigger) should be chose to perform siKBD with the MB balloon. After OOT, the redundant MB stent struts over the SB ostium can be overturned into (strut ectropion) and cover the upper margin of the SB ostium, resulting in somehow "2-stent effect with 1-stent implanting" if not necessary for a rescue SB stent, or facilitating subsequent stent positioning and implanting if necessary for a rescue SB stent. Our in vitro study demonstrated that OOT are associated with more benefits as compared to TAP or CPT, for examples, technically easier to perform, more accurately to position the SB stent, better stent coverage of the ostial SB, less metal and/or drug burden in the bifurcated arena, better bifurcated vascular or stent configuration and local hemodynamics, which may be expected to reduce in-stent restenosis and thrombosis. In fact, our initial clinical application also shown that after OOT it was so easy to position a rescue SB stent just by positioning the stent proximal marker at the carina level such that accurate connection between the SB and MB stents could be readily achieved, thereby effectively avoiding stent over-protrusion or incomplete coverage.

Moreover, when using 1-stent technique or CPT as the initial interventional strategy, it is uncertain whether fKBD is necessary [32–35]. Currently available data showed that there was no significant difference of MCAE between fKBD and non-fKBD [33, 34]. Moreover, there were some drawbacks with conventional fKBD as using 1-stent technique or CPT: (1) causing local deformation or abnormal hemodynamics of MB stent, (2) leading to injury of the SB osium, (3) probably increasing in-stent restenosis and thrombosis. Conventional fKBD aimed to enlarge the SB ostium with using bigger compliance balloon for dilation, seldom considering optimized dilation, which may explain its poor results. Conversely, OOT aimed to overturn the abundant struts over the SB ostium to cover the ostial SB with using smaller non-compliance balloon for the SB dilation and unique siKBD. Therefore, OOT is expected to improve long-term outcomes in addition to reducing residual stenosis.

In conclusion, OPT distinguished itself from CPT by adding OOT, which is able to optimize the ostial SB, resulting in "2-stent effect with 1-stent implanting" if not necessary for rescue SB stenting, or facilitating stent positioning and implanting if necessary for rescue SB stenting. OPT should become the mainstream therapy and be served as the defaulted strategy for all CBLs on the premise of a reliable SB protection.

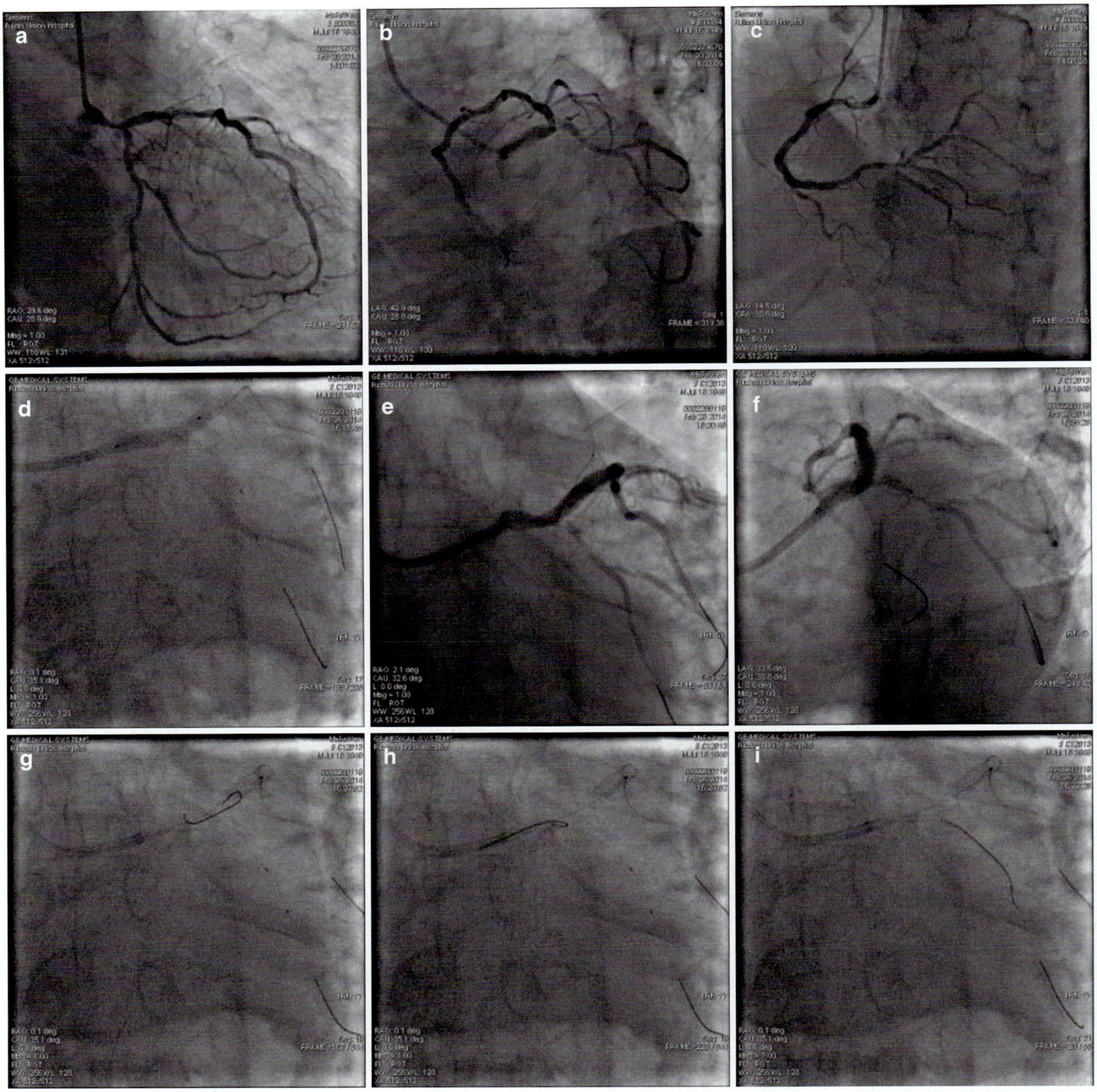

Fig. 17.5 LM bifurcation lesion treated with OPT. This was a male patient, aged at 65 years, admitted due to NSTEMI. Extensive ST depression was noted in leads V_{1-9}, I and aVL with ST elevation in lead aVR. Echocardiography detected left ventricular ejection fraction of 45 % with extensive left ventricular hypokensia. (**a–c**) CAG shows a true LM CBL with severe stenosis in distal LM, ostial LCX and moderate stenosis at ostial and proximal LAD, and a roughly normal RCA. (**d**) After pre-dilating LAD and LCX, stent LAD-LM first with a balloon deeply imbedded in LCX for branch protection. (**e, f**) Stenting LAD leads to severe pinching of ostial LCX but normal TIMI flow. (**g–i**) U-bend wiring technique for rewiring LCX: Slightly rotate and advance the U-bend wire into LAD deeply or at least over the carina level (**g**); pull the wire back to the carina level and then steer the wire to LCX direction (**h**); and finally, rewire LCX at a point as closer as possible to the carina (**i**). (**j**) OOT technique: align the proximal markers of the two balloons at POC level and perform siKBD to optimize ostial LCX. (**k**) Residual stenosis still exists at ostial LCX. (**l**) Position LCX stent by aligning its proximal marker at the carina level. (**m, n**) After LCX stenting, there is residual stenosis at ostial LCX due to hard plaque. (**o**) Perform fKBD with two non-compliance balloons to end the procedure. (**p–r**) There is no more residual stenosis at ostial LCX and seamless connection between the two stents can be reached without protrusion of the LCX stent into LM. *CAG* coronary angiography, *LM* left main coronary artery, *LAD* left anterior descending artery, *LCX* left circumflex artery, *OOT* ostial optimization technique, *POC* polygon of confluence, *siKBD* sequential intermediate balloon dilation, *fKBD* final kissing balloon dilation. Abbreviations are similar in the following cases unless noted otherwise

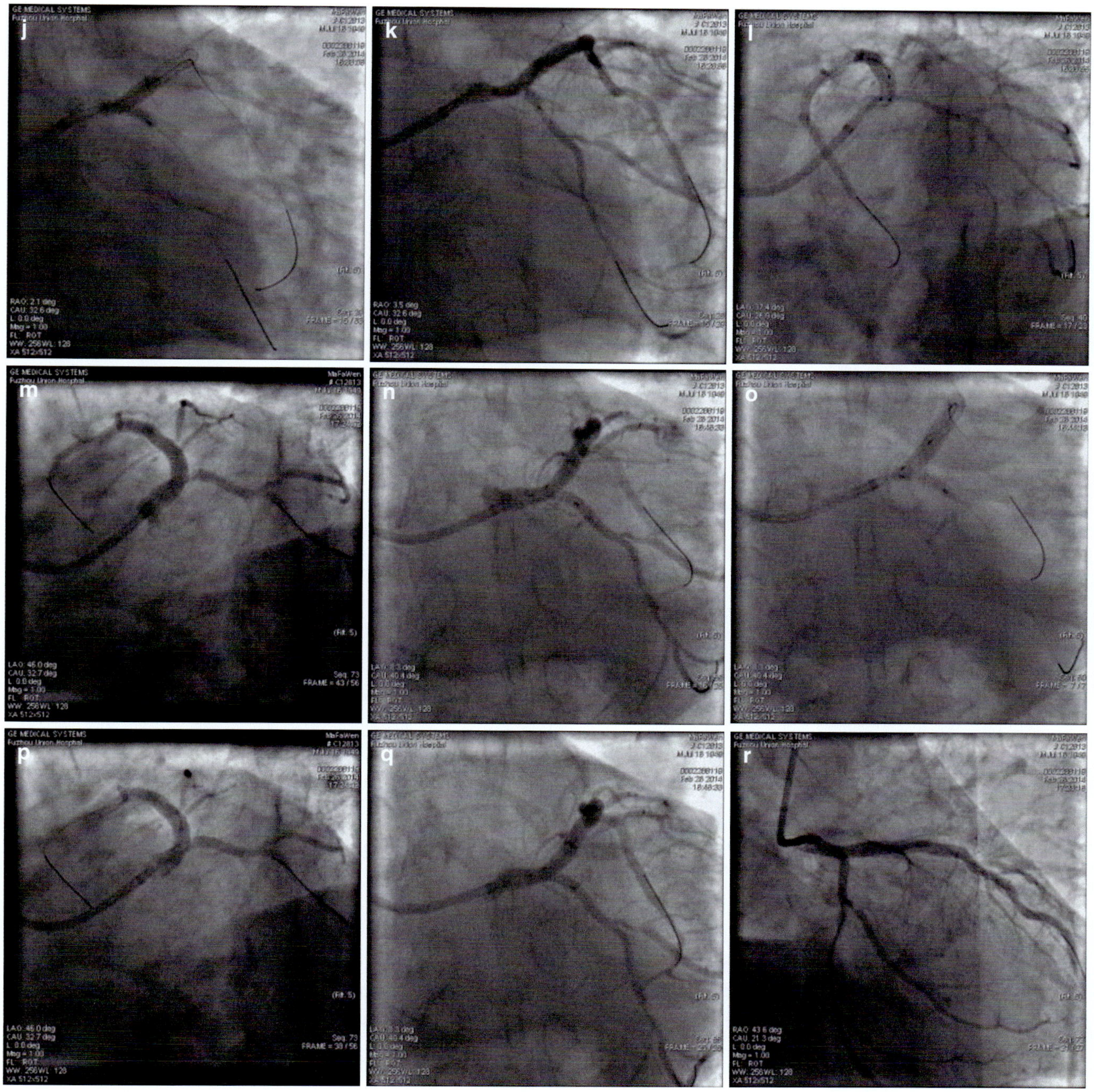

Fig. 17.5 (continued)

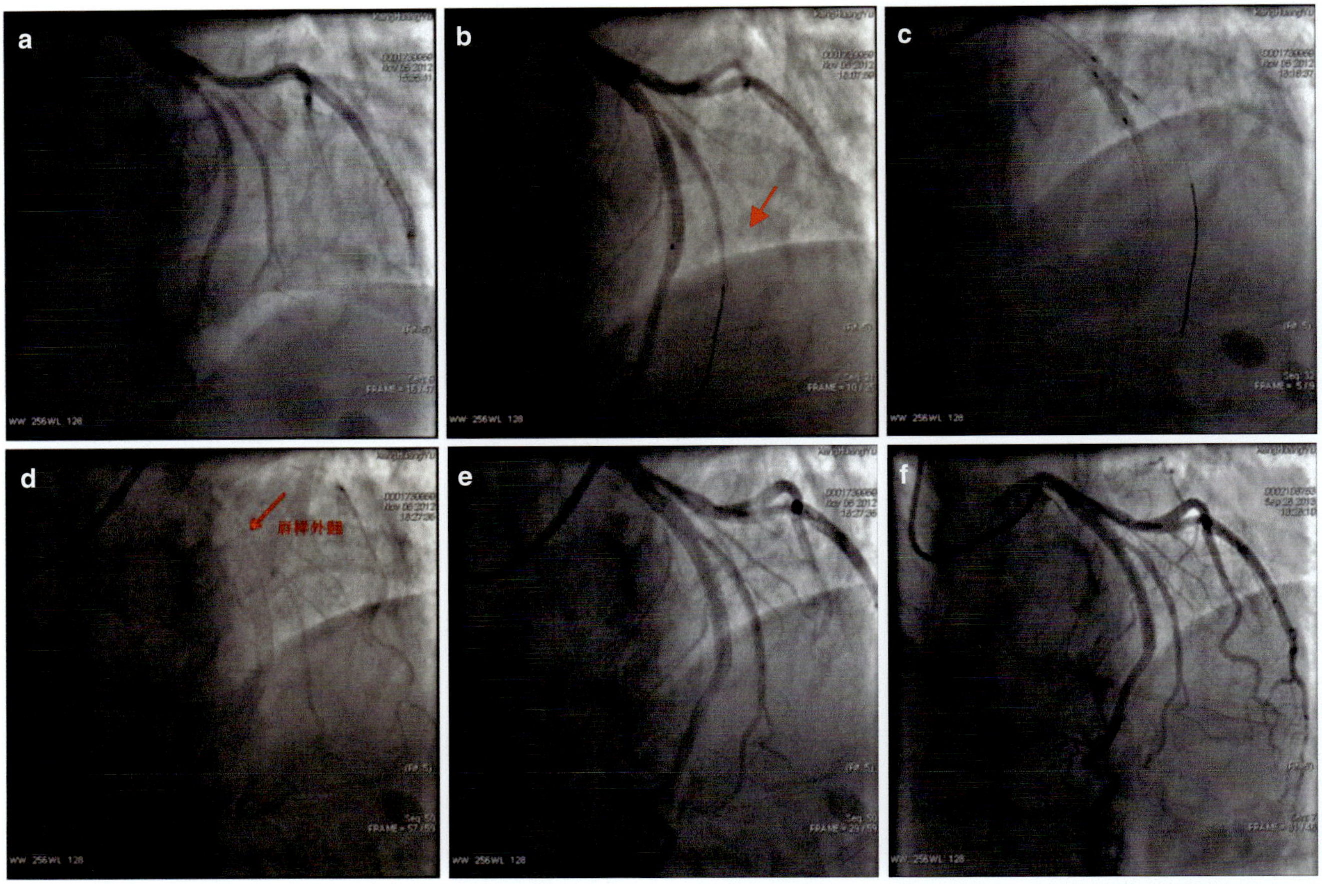

Fig. 17.6 LAD bifurcation lesion treated with OOT. This was a female patient, aged at 53 years, admitted due to exertional chest pain. ST depression was noted in leads V_{2-6} and left ventricular ejection fraction was 63 % assessed echocardiographically. (**a**) CAG shows a true CBL involving LAD and the first diagonal branch (D1). (**b**) Pre-imbed a balloon in D1 (*arrow*), and then stent LAD, which severely pinches D1 with TIMI flow <3. (**c**) Rewire D1 at a point close to the carina, and then perform siKBD. (**d**) The redundant LAD struts over the D1 ostium are turned onto the upper rim of D1 ostium (*arrow*). (**e**) Ostial pinching is lessened with only focally mild residual stenosis. (**f**) The result is well maintained as shown in angiographic follow up at 12 month

17.3 Part 3: Double Kissing Mini Culotte Stenting for Treatment of Complex Coronary Bifurcation Lesions

17.3.1 The Procedural Essence

The double kissing mini culotte stenting (DK-MCS) is characterized by three key points: (1) mini-protruding the side branch (SB) stent into the main vessel/main branch (MV/MB), (2) adding sequential intermediate kissing balloon dilation (siKBD) prior to MB stenting, and (3) pre-imbedding a balloon for MB protection.

17.3.2 The Procedural Indications

DK-MCS is suitable for true coronary bifurcation lesions (CBLs) particularly in setting of greater branch diameter difference (BDD). Compared to conventional mini culotte, DK-MCS has no strict requirement of similar branch size, thus broadening indications of the culotte-based stenting techniques (CBSTs) for treatment of CBLs.

17.3.3 The Procedural Steps

DK-MCS can be performed either by radial or femoral approach. 6–7 Fr. Guiding catheters with bigger lumen, open-cell stents with larger cell, and guiding wires with better shaping and recovering memory are preferred for the procedure. The procedural steps are schematically illustrated in Fig. 17.8.

17.3.4 The Key Steps: Tricks and Points

1. Pre-imbedded balloon and MB protection

   Pre-imbedded balloon is most effective technique for the MB protection regardless of occupying some catheter

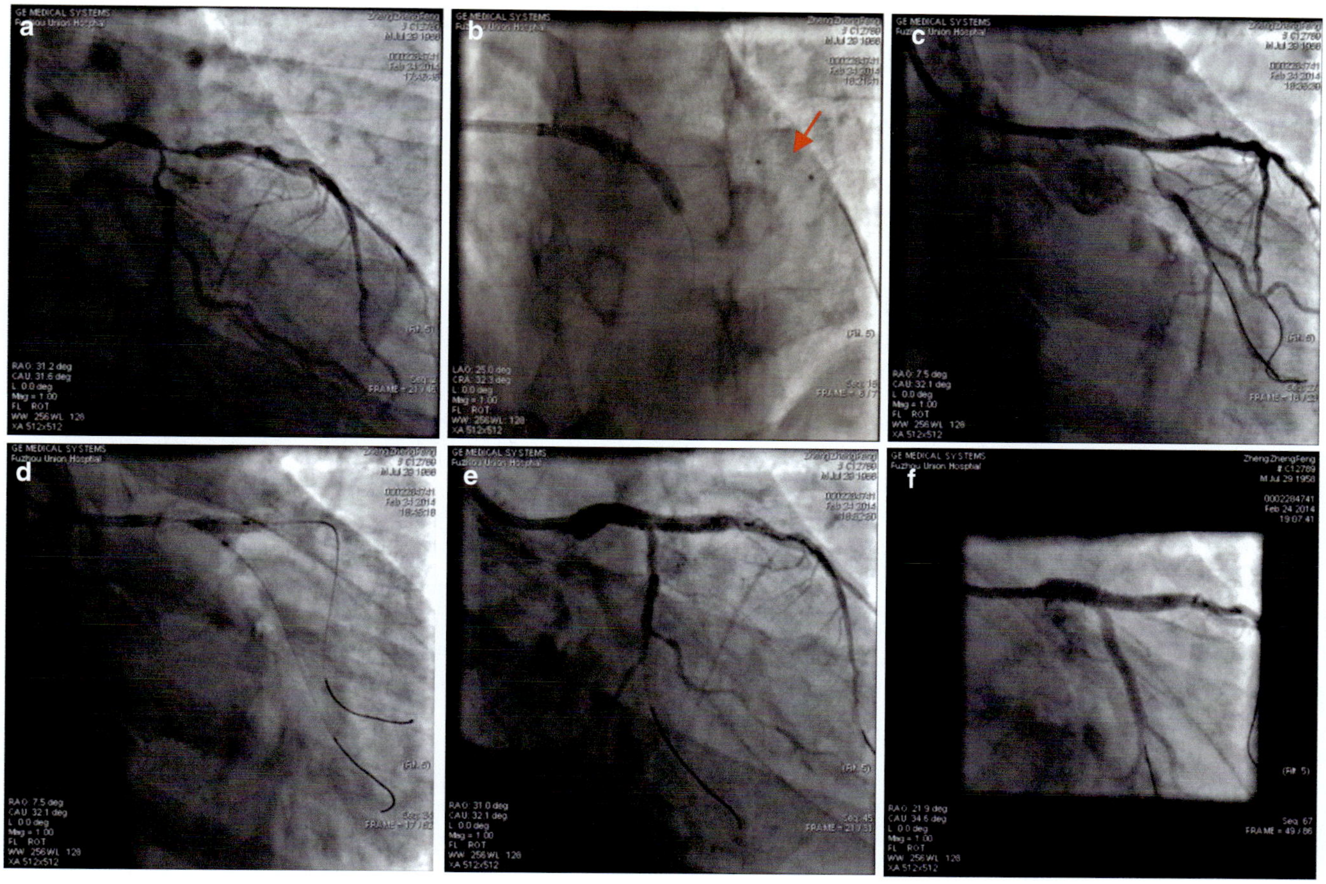

Fig. 17.7 LM bifurcation lesion treated with OOT. This was a male patient, aged at 56 years, admitted due to unstable angina. Extensive ST depression was noted in leads V_{1-9}, I and aVL and left ventricular ejection fraction was 51 % echocardiographically. (**a**) CAG shows a true LM CBL with severe stenosis involving ostial and proximal LAD and LCX. (**b**) Stent LAD after predilating LAD and LCX, which jails the balloon still stayed in LCX as shown in left anterior oblique projection (*arrow*). (**c**) Rewire LCX at a point as closer as possible to the carina and then withdraw the jailed balloon and wire. (**d**) OOT technique: advance 2 balloons respectively over LAD and LCX wires with aligning their proximal markers at the POC level, and then perform siKBD. (**e**, **f**) Rescue T-stenting is not indicated due to no residual stenosis at ostial LCX

lumen and should be reasonable particularly in case of high risk of intra-procedural MB occlusion or unexperienced operators. If used, the balloon should be stayed deeply in the MB rather than just aside the SB stent so that the harder segment of the balloon stem instead of the softer segment of the balloon itself will be jailed after the SB stenting.

2. Mini-protrusion

   Mine-protrusion technique shortens the stent overlapping zone, thus minimizing the width and severity of stent under-expansion band (SUEB), a unique phenomenon associated with culotte stenting. Despite that there are no criteria for mini-protrusion, 1–2 mm is reasonable for clinical practice since too short protrusion may cause rewiring difficulty.

3. The U-bend wiring technique

   During MB rewiring, due to possible suspension of the protruded SB stent inside the MV, the routine wiring technique may go a wrong way, resulting in unexpected or evenly disaster results, while the U-bend wiring technique can completely avoid such trouble. The technique seems to be difficult but easy. To handling the U-bend wiring technique, select a wire with good shaping and recovering memory, pre-shape it to form a small U-bend corresponding to the SB stent size, insert the pre-shaped wire unto the ostial SB stent, slightly rotate and advance the wire deeply into the SB or at least over the carina level, and then pulled it back to the carina level and rewire the MB at a point close to the carina.

4. SiKBD

   As the most crucial step, SiKBD can be achieved by firstly inflating of the SB balloon with higher pressure to fix the ostial SB stent, followed by inflating of the MB balloon with lower pressure. SiKBD can fully open the side-hole of the SB stent, well expanded mini-protruding part of the stent, and effectively prevent the ostial SB stent from distortion so that SUEB in the stent overlapping segment around the bifurcated area can be eliminated and incomplete bifurcated stent coverage near the ostial SB and carina be efficiently avoided evenly in case of greater BDD.

17.3.5 The Typical Cases of DK-MCS

The following case examples (Figs. 17.9, 17.10, 17.11, 17.12, and 17.13) demonstrate that DK-MCS has broad indications for treating various CBLs including different anatomy (Y-/T-angulation and/or great BDD) and lesion locations

1. Lesion pretreating:	
Wire the MV/MB and SB (A); pretreat the lesions by using normal balloon dilation, cutting balloon dilation or rotational atherectomy as necessary.	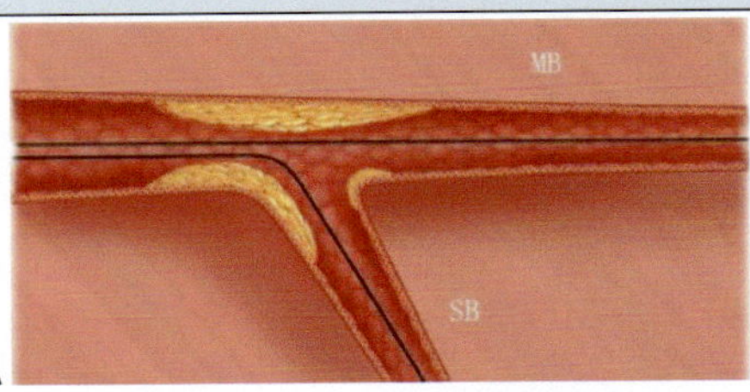 A
2. MB protection and SB stent mini-protrusion:	
Preimbed a balloon in the MB for preventing its acute occlusion in case of high risk of CBLs, and position the SB stent with mini-protrusion (1-2 mm) into the MV (B).	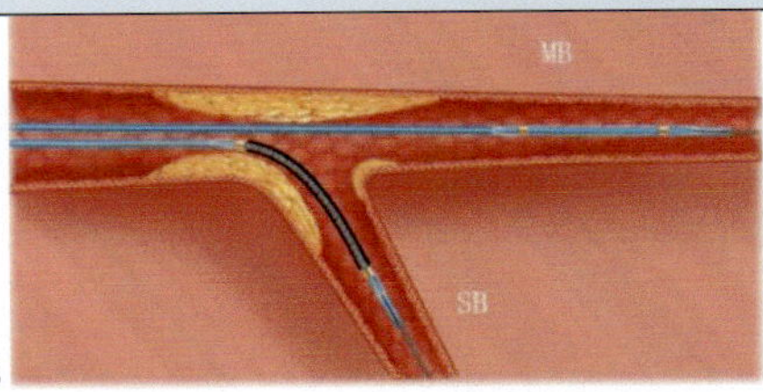 B
3. SB stenting techniques:	
1) Firstly stent the SB (reverse culotte) with nominated pressure, which will jail the MB protecting balloon when used (C).	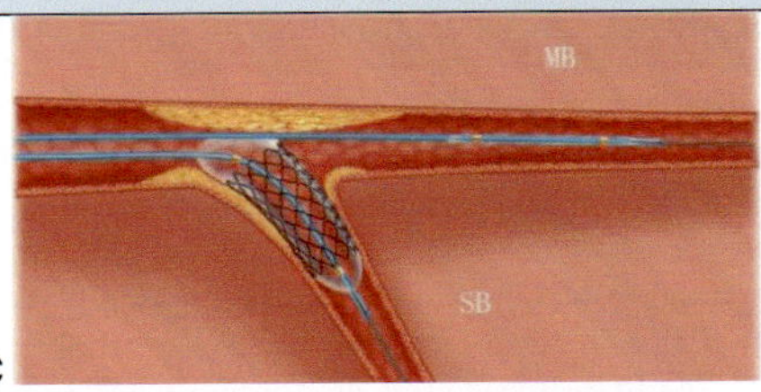 C
2) Slightly pull back the stent balloon and then inflate it with high pressure to fully expand the proximal SB stent or the protruded segment and to facilitate the subsequent MB rewiring (D).	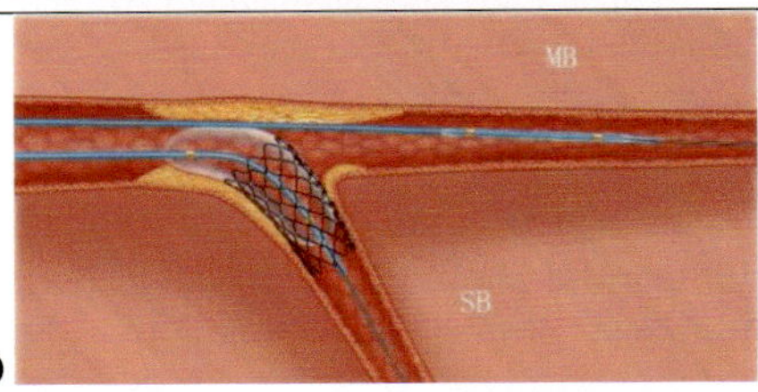 D
4. MB rewiring techniques:	
1) Advance the stent balloon distally to the SB stent, and then insert a new wire with a pre-shaped U-bend unto the ostial SB stent (E)	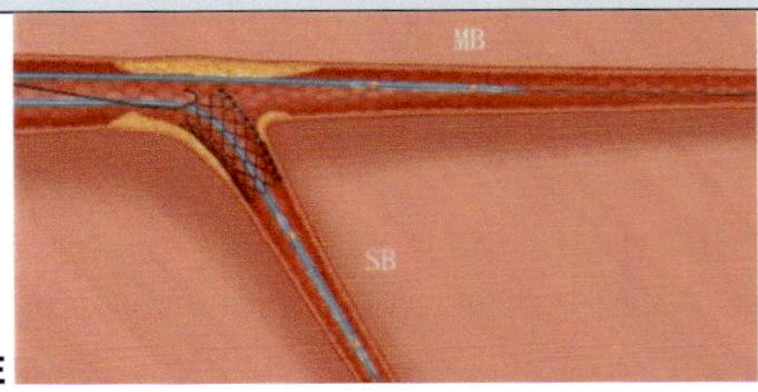 E

Fig. 17.8 Diagram of DK-MCS procedural steps (Image provided courtesy of Medtronic Inc. © Medtronic Inc. All rights reserved)

Fig. 17.8 (continued)

2) Slightly rotate and advance the U-bend wire into the SB deeply or at least over the carina level (F).	F 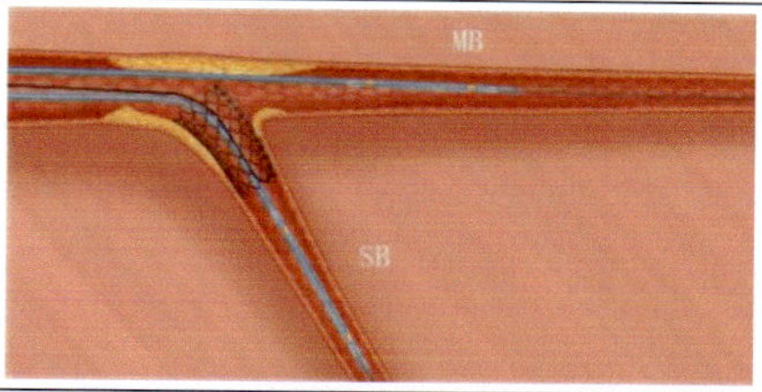
3) Pull the wire back to the carina level and then steer the wire to MB direction (G).	G 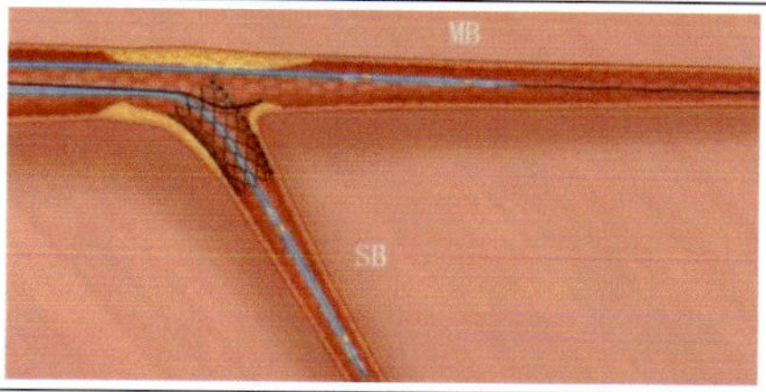
4) Finally, rewire the MB at a point as closer as possible to the carina (H).	H 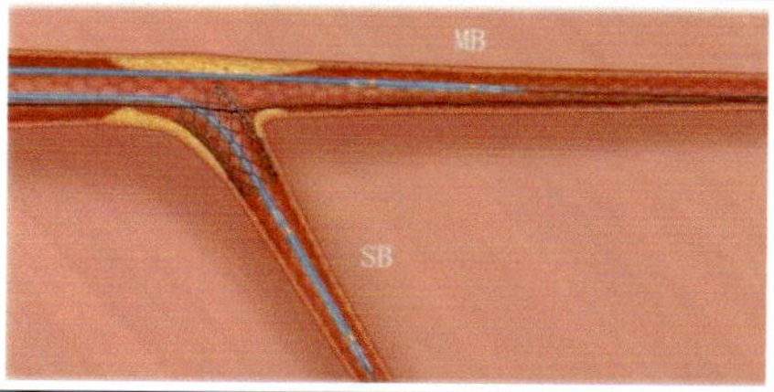
5. Sequential intermediate kissing balloon dilation (siKBD):	
1) Remove out the MB protecting balloon if used, and useit to pre-dilate side-hole of the SB stent with lower pressure if necessary (I).	I 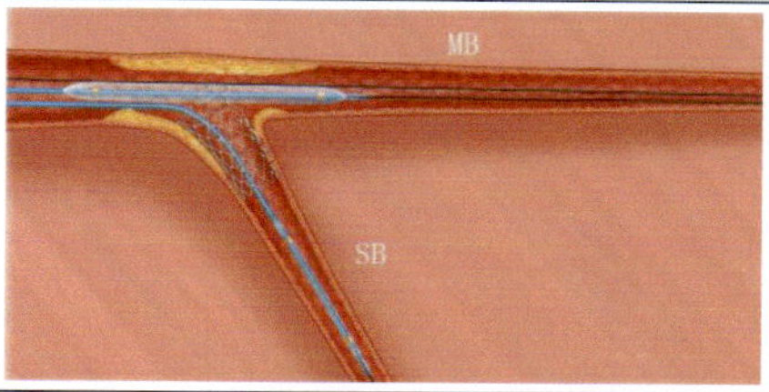
2) Pull back the SB stent balloon and insert a non-compliance balloon over the MB wire and aligned their proximal markers at the level of the polygon of confluence (POC)(J).	J 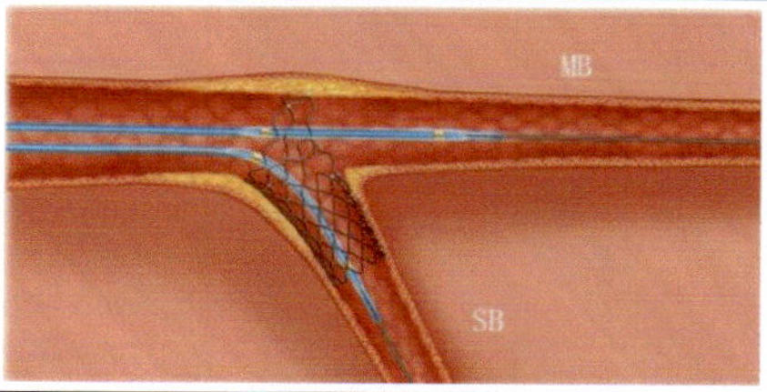
3) Firstly inflate the SB balloon with higher pressure to fix the ostial SB stent in order to prevent ostial SB stent deformation in the following kissing balloon dilation (K);	K 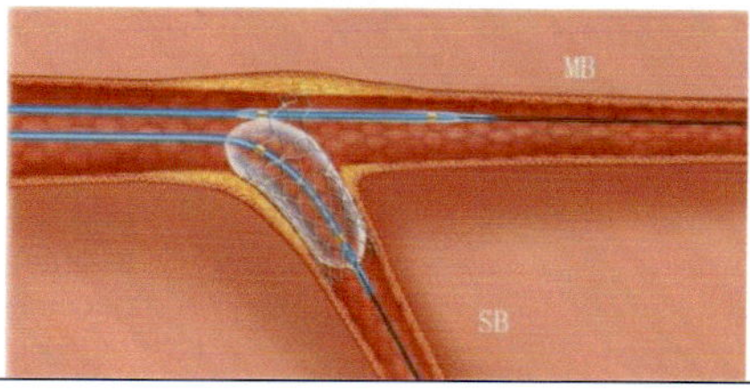

Fig. 17.8 (continued)

4) and then inflate the MB balloon with lower pressure to perform sequential intermediate kissing balloon dilation (siKBD) (L).	L 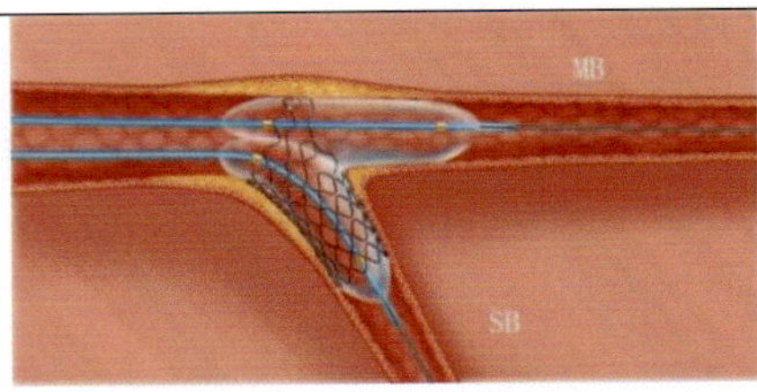
6. MB stenting:	
1) Withdraw the two balloons and SB wire, and then insert the MB stent (M).	M 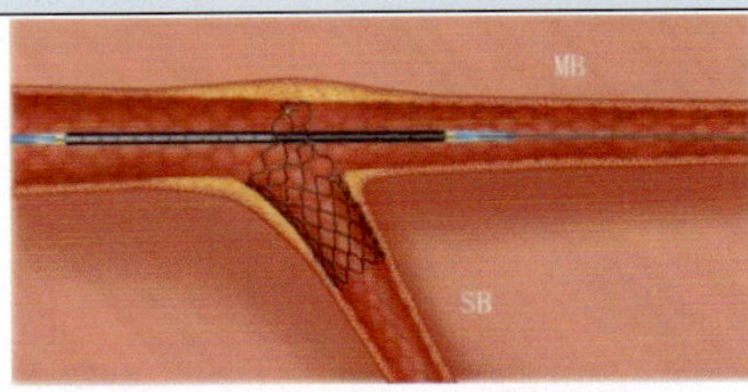
2) Deploy the MB stent and then withdraw the stent balloon (N).	N 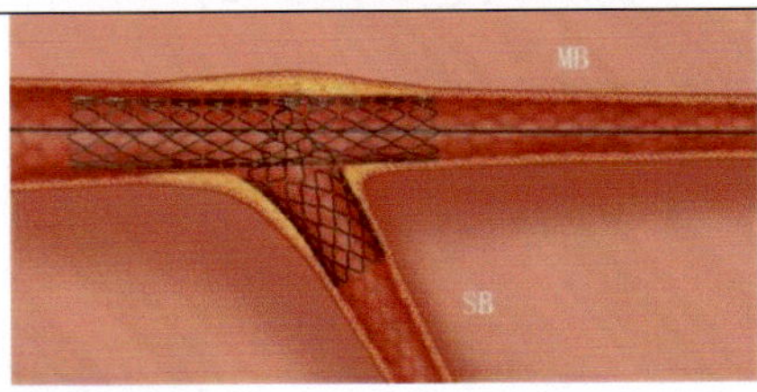
7. Rewiring SB:	
Rewire SB at a point close to carina by using U-bend wiring technique similar to MB rewiring (O).	O 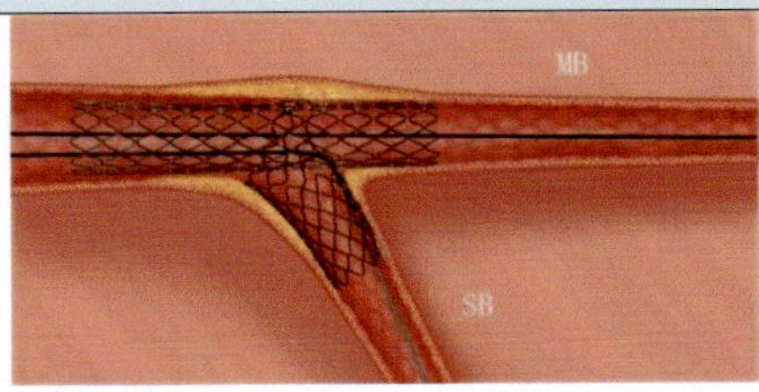
8. Final kissing balloon dilation (fKBD):	
Pre-dilate the side-hole of the MB stent with a smaller balloon as necessary and then perform the final kissing balloon dilation (fKBD) with two non-compliance balloons with their proximal markers at the POC level (P).	P 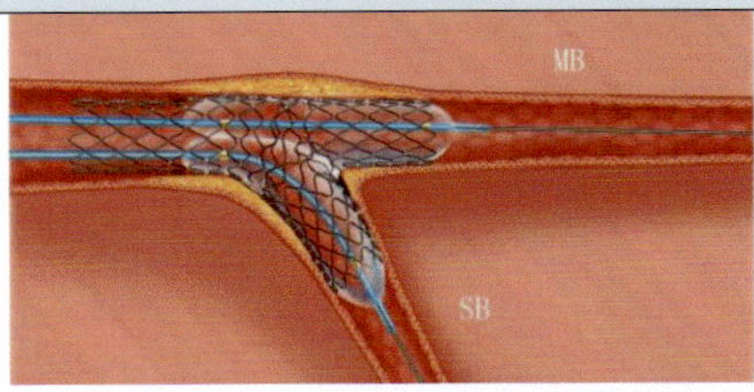
9. Proximal stent optimization:	
Use a short and big non-compliance balloon to optimize the proximal MB stent as necessary to end the procedure (Q).	Q 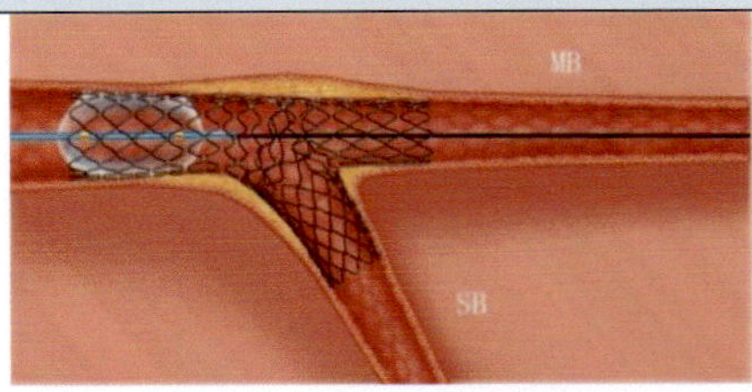
10. Final results:	
Usually, DK-MCS can result in excellent bifurcated stent morphology in terms of stent expansion and coverage (R).	R 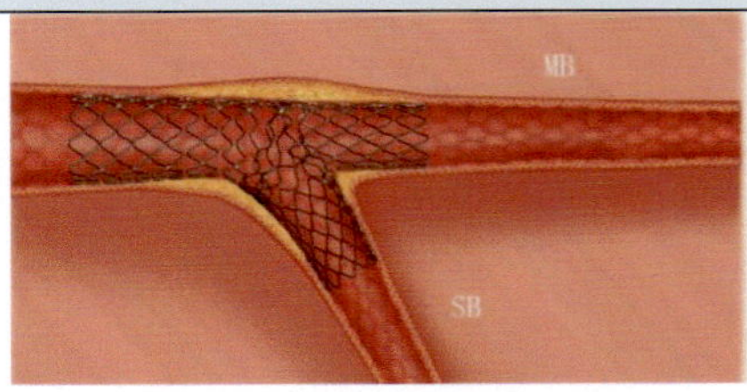

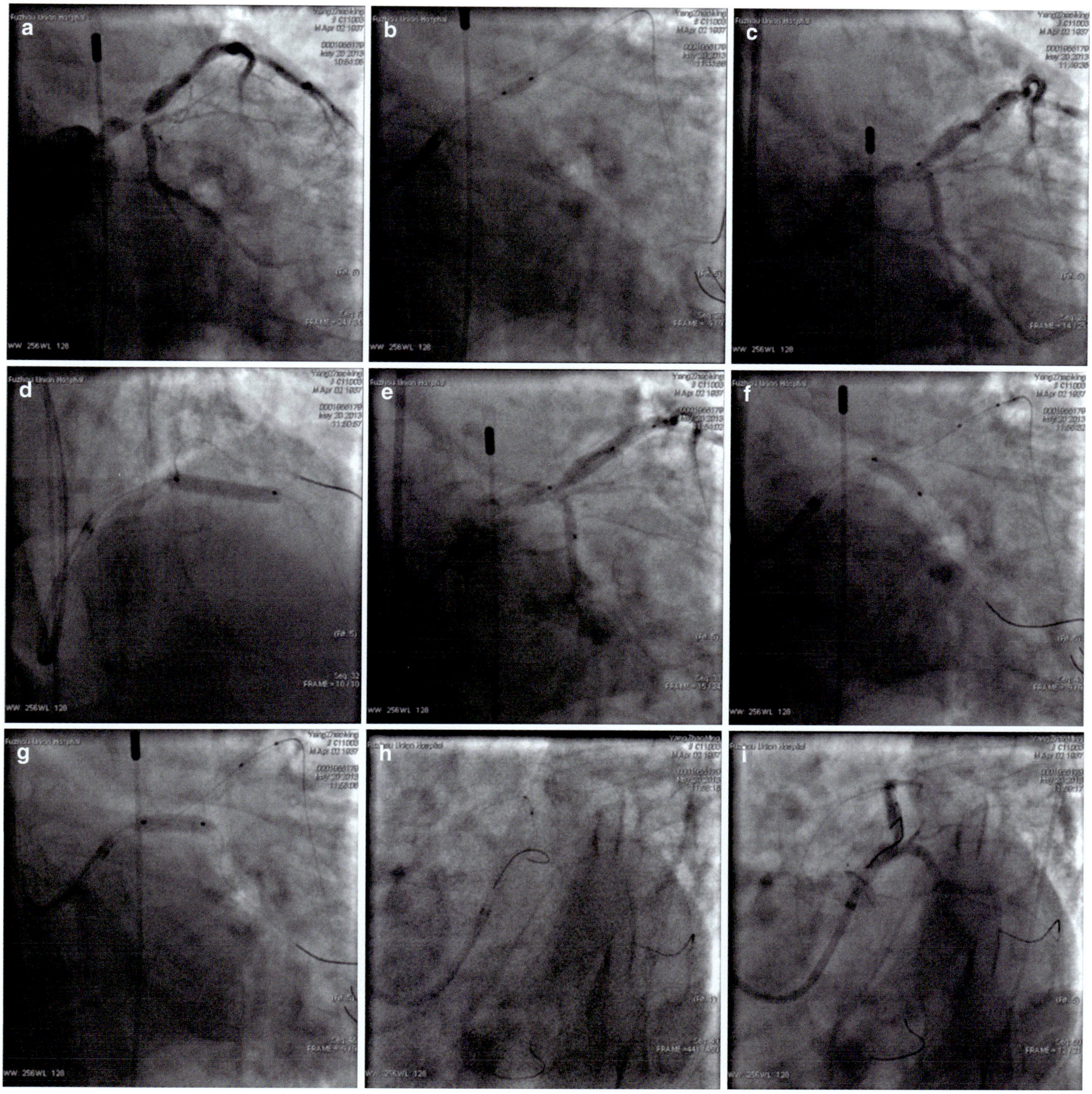

Fig. 17.9 LM bifurcation lesions treated with DK-MCS. This was a male patient, aged at 76 years, admitted due to NSTEMI complicating by cardiogenic shock. Because of hemodynamics instability and low oxygen saturation, IABP and mechanical ventilator were installed prior to coronary intervention. Extensive ST depression was noted in leads V_{1-9}, I and aVL and left ventricular ejection fraction was 40% with extensive left ventricular hypokinesia echocardiographically. (**a**) CAG shows a true distal LM CBL with severely calcified and tightly bifurcated stenosis, and also with huge BDD of 2.75 mm and DBA of 115° between LAD and LCX. (**b**) Pre-treat the lesions with a 3.5 mm cutting balloon due to severely calcified lesions. (**c**) Severe dissection is noted in the pretreated segments after cutting balloon dilation. (**d**) Implant a stent for treatment of the mid-proximal LAD lesion. (**e**) Position the LCX stent with the stent mini-protrusion into LM. (**f**) Pre-imbed a balloon in LAD and deploy LCX stent first with lower pressure. (**g**) Slightly withdraw the stent balloon and re-inflate with high pressure to fully expand the protruded stent segment. (**h, i**) U-bend wiring technique: advance a pre-shaped U-bending wire deeply into LCX (H); pull back the U-bend wire up to the carina level and rewire LAD at a point close to the carina (**i**). (**j**) After successfully rewiring of LAD, withdraw the protecting balloon and then perform siKBD. (**k**) The stent side-hole and protruded part are fully expanded by SiKBD without proximal LCX stent distortion. (**l**) Implant a stent to cover the proximal LAD and the whole LM. (**m**) Rewire LCX at a point close to the carina. (**n**) Perform fKBD with two non-compliance balloons to end the procedure. (**o**) No SUEB and residual stenosis are found angiographically in the bifurcated area. P-S: Cross-sectional stent area measured by IVUS is 12.9 mm² at ostial LAD (**p**), 10.8 mm² at ostial LCX (**q**), 19.6 mm² at POC level (**r**) and 21.2 mm² at mid-LM level (**s**). *Abbreviations*: *CAG* coronary angiography, *LM* left main coronary artery, *LAD* left anterior descending artery, *LCX* left circumflex artery, *BDD* branch diameter difference, *DBA* distal bifurcation angle, *POC* polygon of confluence, *siKBD* sequential intermediate kissing balloon dilation, *fKBD* final kissing balloon dilation. Abbreviations are the same as in the next case examples unless otherwise indicated

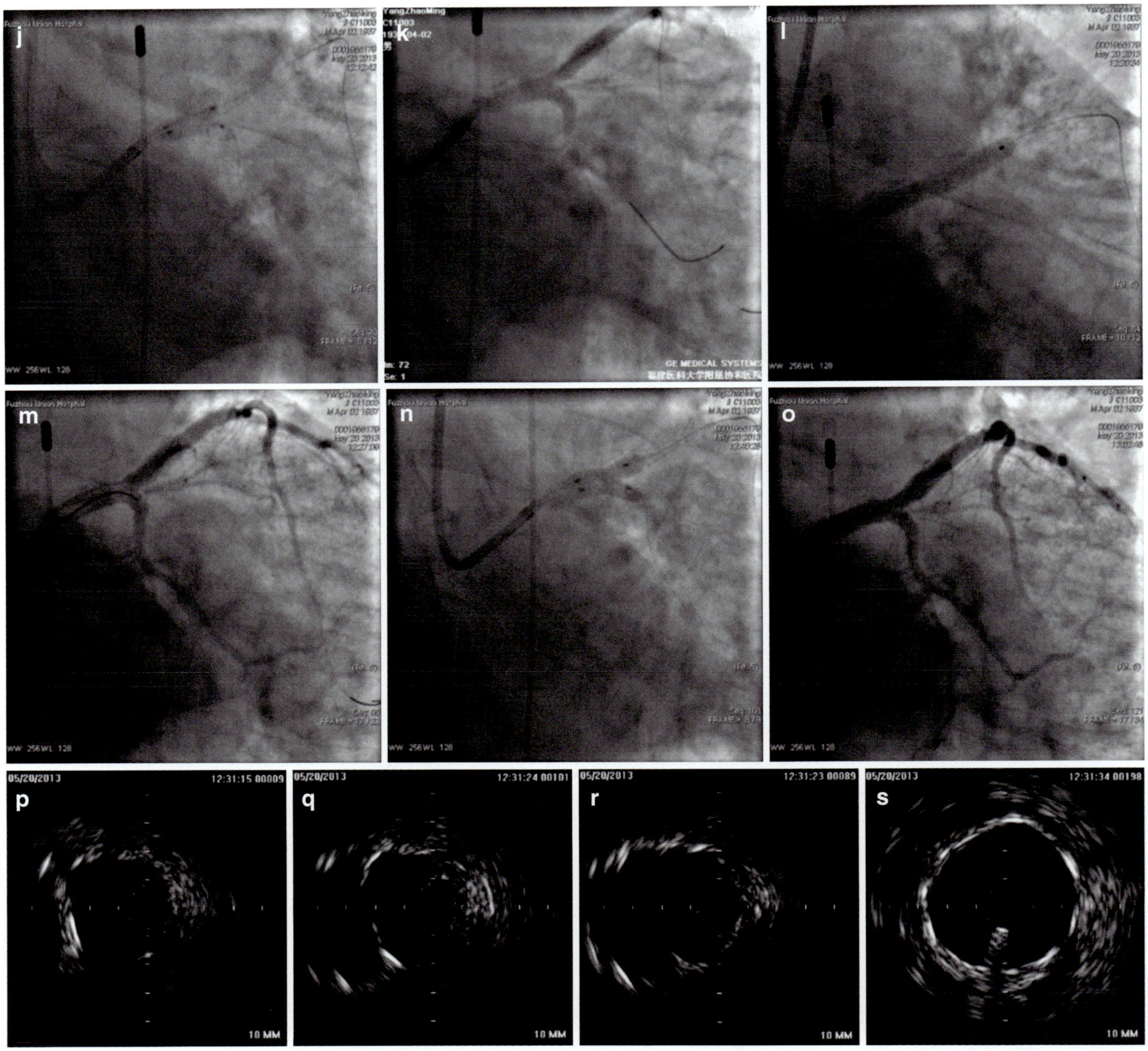

Fig. 17.9 (continued)

[left main coronary artery (LM) or non-LM CBL] and also illuminate how to properly accomplish DK-MCS by addressing the frequent problems and their solutions. Figure 17.9 illustrates all procedural steps of DK-MCS particularly the key steps (e.g., balloon branch protection, mini-protrusion technique, U-bend wiring technique, and siKBD) in treatment of a LM-CBL patient with vast BDD and DBA. Figures 17.10, 17.11, 17.12, and 17.13 show that DK-MCS can be used to treat non-LM-CBL patients with Y-/T-type lesion and/or great BDD, and also show how to rescue a branch from impending occlusion (Fig. 17.10) or how to prevent a branch from acute occlusion (Figs. 17.9, 17.10, 17.11, 17.12, and 17.13) intra-procedurally by using pre-imbedded balloon protection technique.

17.3.6 Culotte Stenting Family and Clinical Relevance of DK-MCS

Firstly introduced by Chevalier et al. [36] for treatment of CBLs, conventional culotte stenting has undergone numerous minor and major modifications in an attempt to improve safety and efficacy [37–43]. Up to date, CBSTs have become a big family with technical similarity but procedural heterogeneities.

The first major modification shifted from culotte to reverse culotte or from inner to outer culotte. The inner culotte was to stent the MB/MV first, and then the SB, whereas the outer culotte to stent SB first and then MB/MV. Whatever inner or outer culotte being used, SUEB in the stent overlapping segment around the bifurcated area

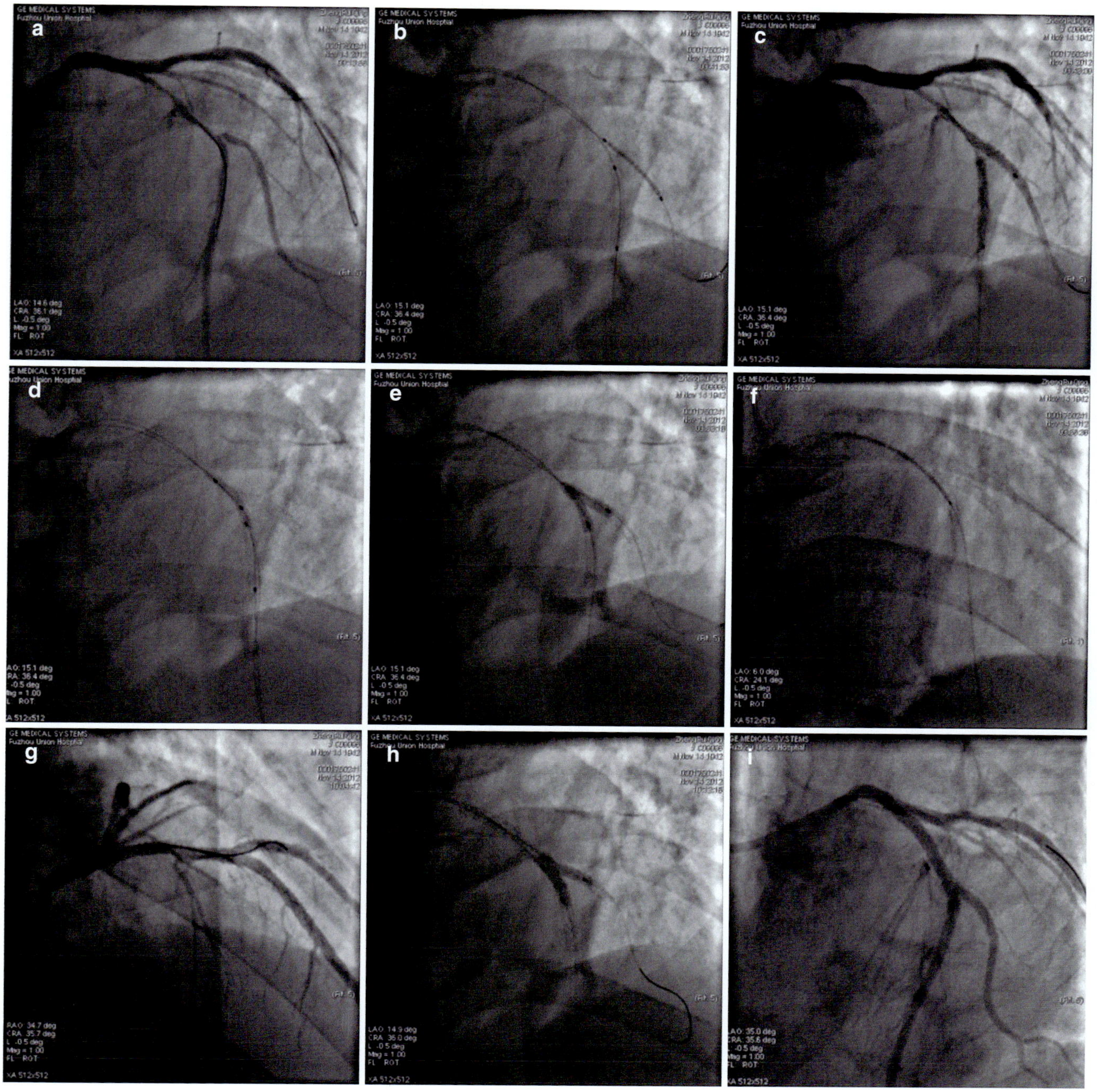

Fig. 17.10 LAD-D1 bifurcation lesions treated with DK-MCS. This was a male patient, aged at 70 years, admitted due to NSTEMI. Significant ST depression was noted in leads V_{1-6} and left ventricular ejection fraction was 53 % measured echocardiographically. (**a**) CAG shows a true Y-type CBL involving LAD and the first diagonal branch (D1) with defuse LAD disease and focally ostial D1 stenosis. (**b**) Stent the mid-LAD and keep the sent balloon in LAD for its protection and then position D1 stent (2.75 × 18 mm) with mini-protrusion into LAD. (**c**) Deploy the SB stent, and then slightly pull back the stent balloon and re-inflate with higher pressure, which compromise LAD and cause severe angina and low blood pressure. (**d**) Move the stent balloon stayed in LAD backward and forward to quickly restore the LAD flow; after successfully rewiring of LAD, insert a balloon to dilate LAD. (**e**) Withdraw the stent balloon still stayed inside LAD, and then perform siKBD. (**f**) Stent proximal LAD (3.5 × 36 mm stent) to cover the whole lesion. (**g**) Rewire D1 at a point close to the carina. (**h**) Perform fKBD by using two non-compliance balloons to end the procedure. (**i**) Excellent bifurcated stent configuration is noted angiographically without SUEB and residual ostial stenosis both in LAD and D1

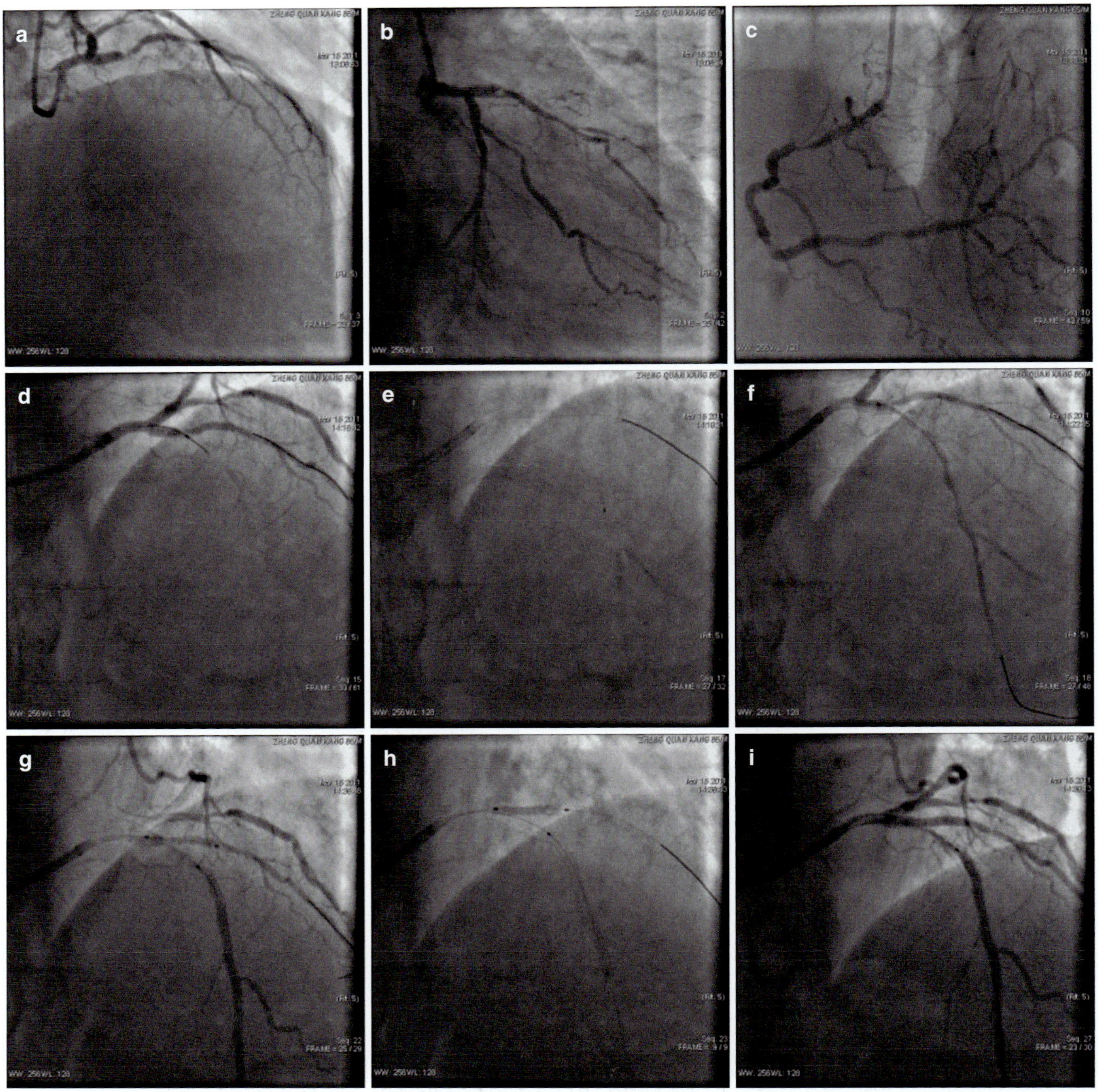

Fig. 17.11 LAD-D1 bifurcation lesions treated with DK-MCS. This was a male patient, aged at 55 years, admitted due to exertional chest pain. He had prior myocardial infarction. Smaller r-waves with ST depression were noted in leads V_{1-4} and left ventricular ejection fraction was 50 % with anterior, antero-septal and apical hypokinesis detected by echocardiography. (**a–c**) CAG shows a true T-type CBL located at LAD and D1 with totally occluded LAD and severe ostial D1 stenosis, and with greater BDD of 1.25 mm and DBA of 70° between LAD and D1; additionally, CAG also detects multiple focal tight stenosis along RCA and well-developed collateral circulation to the occluded LAD dominated by RCA. (**d–f**) Re-cannulate the occluded LAD under the assistance of a micro-catheter. (**g**) Stent the mid-LAD and keep the stent balloon inside LAD, and then position D1 stent (2.5 × 18 mm) with mini-protrusion (1.0 mm) into LAD. (**h**) Deploy the SB stent with lower pressure, and then slightly pull back the stent balloon and re-inflate with higher pressure. (**i**) Full expansion of the proximal D1 stent is noted with the LAD stent balloon still jailed in LAD. (**j**) After successfully rewiring of LAD, insert a balloon over the wire and then withdraw the stent balloon jailed in LAD. (**k**): Perform siKBD. (**l**) Expand the stent side-hole and protruded part by siKBD without proximal D1 stent distortion. (**m, n**) Implant the proximal LAD stent (3.5 × 24 mm). (**o**) Rewire the SB close to the carina level. (**p**) Perform fKBD to end the procedure. (**q, r**) Satisfactory stenting result was noted angiographically in antero-posterior and left anterior oblique projections

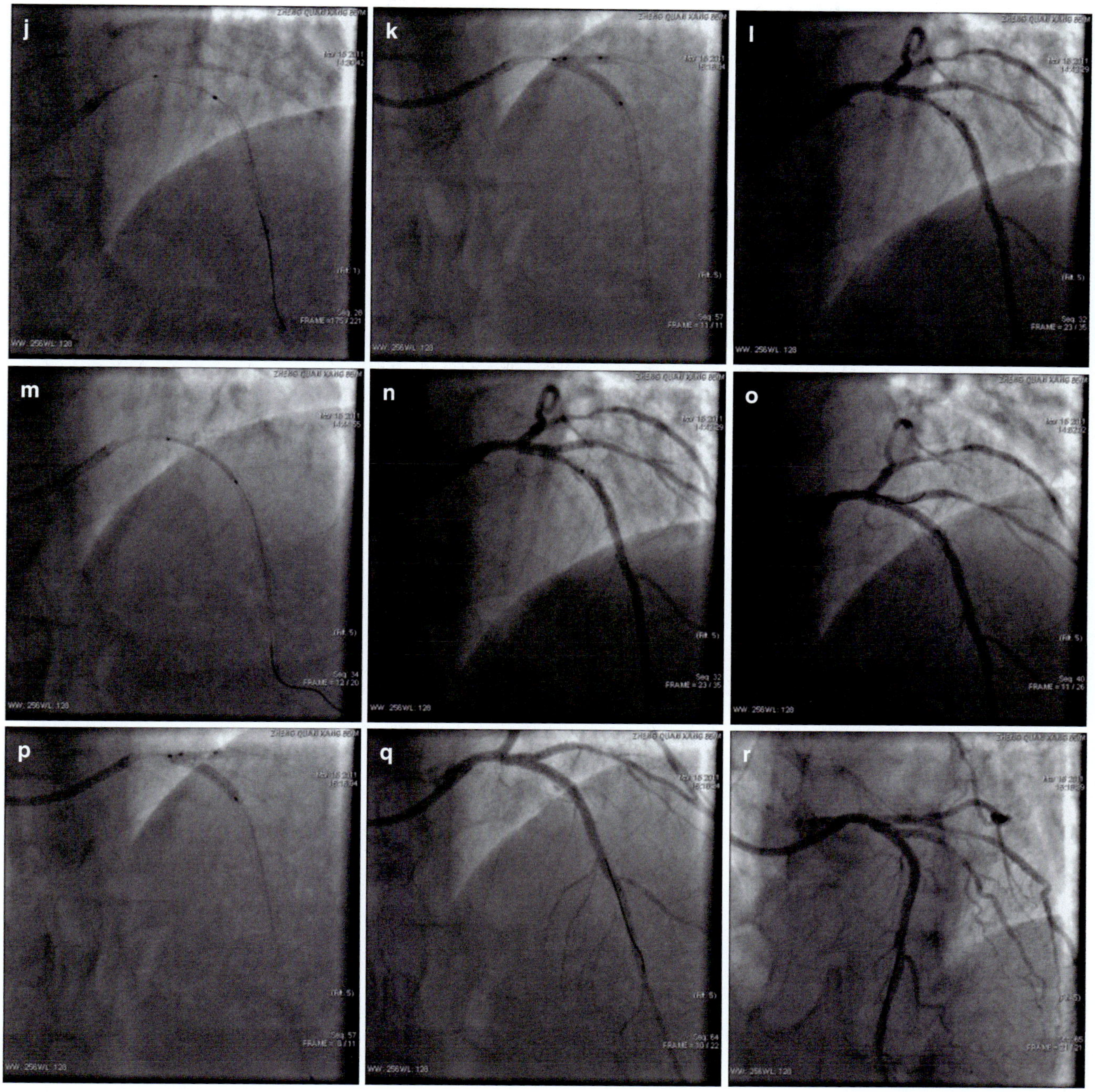

Fig. 17.11 (continued)

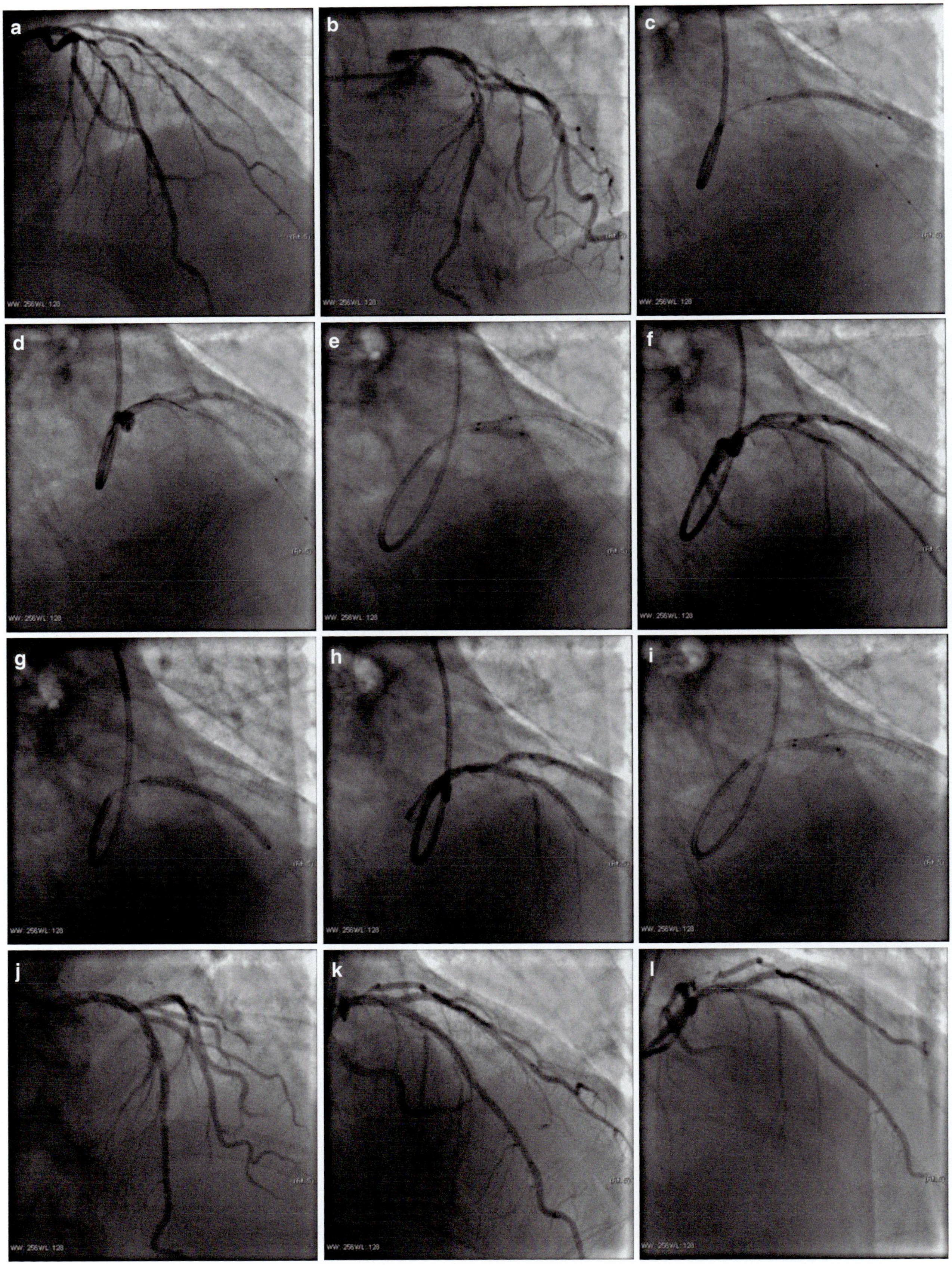
a
b
c
d
e
f
g
h
i
j
k
l

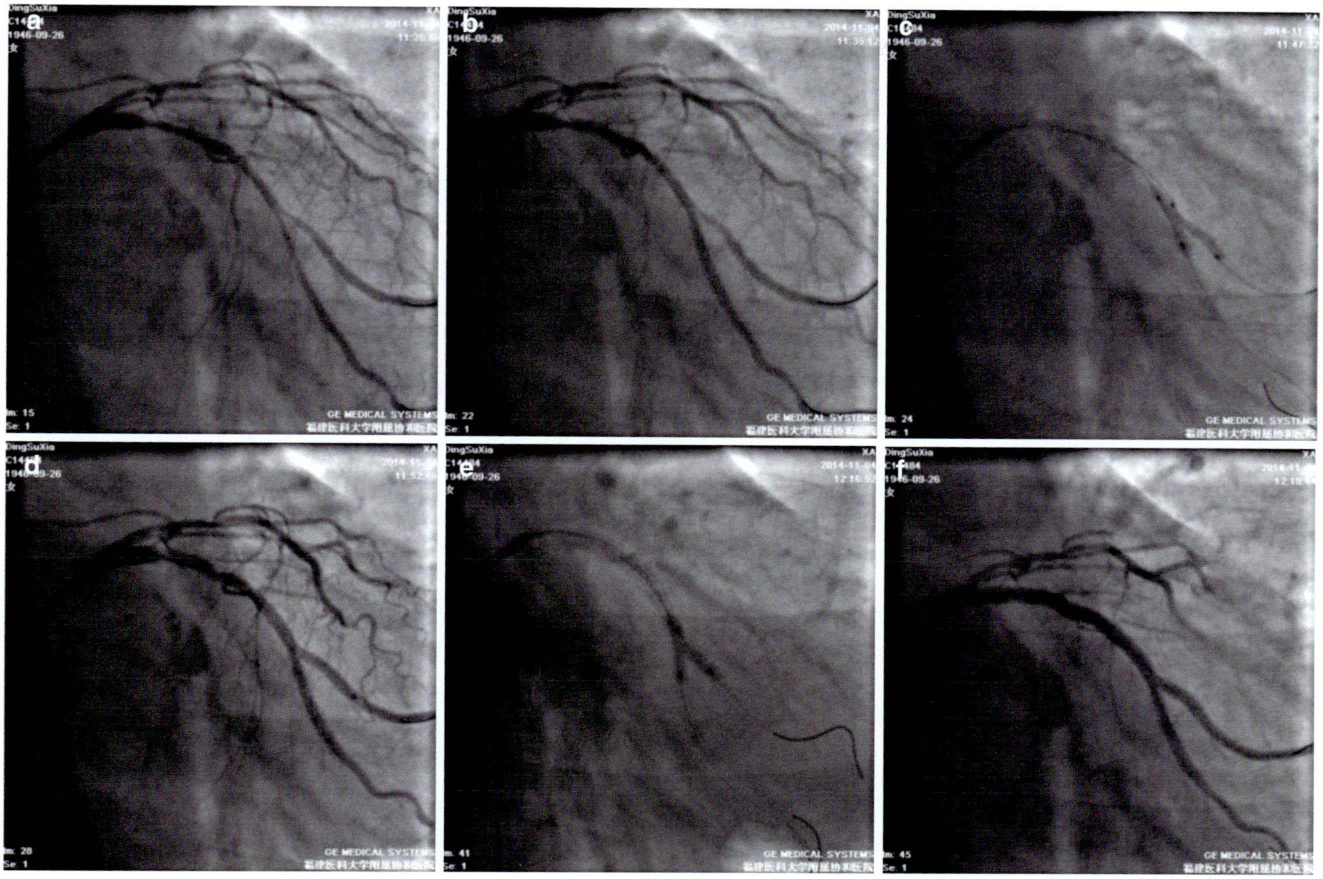

Fig. 17.13 PDA-OM bifurcation lesions treated with DK-MCS. This was a male patient, aged at 68 years, admitted due to unstable angina. ST depression was noted in leads $V_{7–9}$ and left ventricular ejection fraction was 68 % measured echocardiographically. (**a**) CAG shows a true LCX CBL with small DBA of 30° between posterior descending artery (*PDA*) and obtuse marginal branch (*OM*). (**b**) Stent PDA first. (**c**) Rewire OM at a point close to the carina and then perform siKBD. (**d**) Implant a long stent to cover all OM-LCX lesions. (**e**) Rewire D1 at a point close to the carina and then perform fKBD with two non-compliance balloons to end the procedure. (**f**) No SUEB and residual stenosis are detected in the bifurcated area in the final angiography

Fig. 17.12 LAD-D1 bifurcation lesions treated with DK-MCS. This was a male patient, aged at 67 years, admitted due to unstable angina. He had risk factors of hypertension, hyperlipidemia and EX-smoking. ST depression was noted in leads $V_{1–6}$ and left ventricular ejection fraction was 63 % echocardiographically. (**a**, **b**) CAG showed a true LAD-D1 CBL with greater BDD of 1.0 mm and DBA of 85° between LAD and D1. (**c**) Stent the SB first. (**d**) Rewire LAD at a point close to the carina. (**e**) Perform siKBD. (**f**) Expand the stent side-hole and protruded part by siKBD without proximal D1 stent distortion. (**g**, **h**) Implant a long stent to cover all LAD lesions. M: Rewire D1 at a point close to the carina. (**i**) Perform fKBD with two non-compliance balloons to end the procedure. (**j**, **k**) No SUEB and residual stenosis are observed in the bifurcated area in two angiographic projections. (**l**) Stent restenosis are not found in bifurcated area but in mid-LAD stent at 12 month angiographic follow-up may be produced particularly in case of greater BDD. SUEB will cause stent-stent (inner culotte) or stent-vessel (outer culotte) malopposition, leading to residual ostial stenosis, in-stent thrombosis or in-stent restenosis. Therefore, conventional culotte stenting had very limited anatomic indications with strict requirement of similar branch size.

The second major modification aimed to lessen SUEB in order to broaden the clinical utility in the stetting of greater BDD. By shortening of the SB stent protrusion into the MV, the mini-culotte stenting [31] or single string culotte technique [36, 37] was able to diminish but not eliminate SUEB even after successful fKBD, while by performing intermediate kissing balloon dilation (iKBD) before MB stenting, DK-MCS could efficiently lessen SUEB, but might induce ostial SB stent distortion. Hence, SUEB and its associated drawbacks remain the unsolved issues especially in the setting of greater BDD evenly using mini-culotte stenting for treatment of CBLs.

The third major modification addressed the stent coverage in addition to stent expansion. Irrespective of reducing SUEB, iKBD in DK-MCS might induce ostial SB stent distortion, which was not allowable for culotte stenting since its basic concept was to complete cover the SB ostium and carina. By performing sequential rather than simultaneous iKBD, DK-MCS could avoid ostial SB stent deformation. Our previous study demonstrated that DK-MCS was more efficient in improvement of bifurcated stent configurations in the bench testing and in reduction of SB restenosis and TVR/TLR in clinical application [32].

Therefore, DK-MCS is associated with not only better stent expansion but also better stent coverage especially in the treatment of CBLs with great BDD, thus broadening the anatomic indications of CBSTs.

Conflict of Interest Statement The authors have no conflicts of interest to declare.

References

Part 1: Double Kissing Crush – Its Advantage and Long Term Results in Transradial Intervention

1. Steigen TK, Maeng M, Wiseth R, et al. On behalf of the Nordic PCI Study Group, Randomized study of simple versus complex stenting of coronary artery bifurcation lesions: the Nordic bifurcation study. Circulation. 2006;114:1955–61.
2. Behan MW, Holm NR, Curzen NP, et al. Simple or complex stenting for bifurcation coronary lesions: a patient-level pooled-analysis of the Nordic Bifurcation Study and the British Bifurcation Coronary Study. Circ Cardiovasc Interv. 2011;4:57–64.
3. Erglis A, Kumsars I, Niemela M, et al. Randomized comparison of coronary bifurcation stenting with the crush versus the culotte technique using sirolimus-eluting stents: the Nordic stent technique study. Circ Cardiovasc Interv. 2009;2:27–34.
4. Colombo A, Moses JW, Morice MC, et al. Randomized study to evaluate sirolimus-eluting stents implanted at coronary bifurcation lesions. Circulation. 2004;109:1244–9.
5. Costa RA, Mintz GS, Carlier SG, et al. Bifurcation coronary lesions treated with the "crush" technique: an intravascular ultrasound analysis. J Am Coll Cardiol. 2005;46:599–605.
6. Ge L, Airoldi F, Iakovou I, et al. Clinical and angiographic outcome after implantation of drug-eluting stents in bifurcation lesions with the crush stent technique: importance of final kissing balloon post-dilation. J Am Coll Cardiol. 2005;46:613–20.
7. Hildick-Smith D, de Belder AJ, Cooter N, et al. Randomized trial of simple versus complex drug-eluting stenting for bifurcation lesions: the British Bifurcation Coronary Study: old, new, and evolving strategies. Circulation. 2010;121:1235–43.
8. Ormiston JA, Webster MW, Webber B, et al. The "crush" technique for coronary artery bifurcation stenting: insights from micro-computed tomographic imaging of bench deployments. JACC Cardiovasc Interv. 2008;1:351–7.
9. Chen SL, Ye F, Zhang JJ, et al. DK crush technique: modified treatment of bifurcation lesions in coronary artery. Chin Med J (Engl). 2005;118:1746–50.
10. Chen SL, Santoso T, Zhang JJ, et al. A randomized clinical study comparing double kissing crush with provisional stenting for treatment of coronary bifurcation lesions: results from the DKCRUSH-II (Double Kissing Crush versus Provisional Stenting Technique for Treatment of Coronary Bifurcation Lesions) trial. J Am Coll Cardiol. 2011;57:914–20.
11. Chen SL, Zhang JJ, Ye F, et al. Study comparing the double kissing (DK) crush with classical crush for the treatment of coronary bifurcation lesions: the DKCRUSH-1 Bifurcation Study with drug-eluting stents. Eur J Clin Invest. 2008;38:361–71.
12. Chen SL, Xu B, Han YL, et al. Comparison of double kissing crush versus Culotte stenting for unprotected distal left main bifurcation lesions: results from a multicenter, randomized, prospective DKCRUSH-III study. J Am Coll Cardiol. 2013;61:1482–8.
13. Chen SL, Xu B, Han YL, et al. Clinical outcome after DK crush versus culotte stenting of distal left main bifurcation lesions: the 3-year follow-up results of the DKCRUSH-III study. JACC Cardiovasc Interv. 2015;8:1335–42.
14. Chen SL, Mintz G, Kan J, et al. Serial intravascular ultrasound analysis comparing double kissing and classical crush stenting for coronary bifurcation lesions. Catheter Cardiovasc Interv. 2011;78:729–36.
15. Chen SL, Zhang Y, Xu B, et al. Five-year clinical follow-up of unprotected left main bifurcation lesion stenting: one-stent versus two-stent techniques versus double-kissing crush technique. EuroIntervention. 2012;8:803–14.
16. Chen SL, Sheiban I, Xu B, et al. Impact of the complexity of bifurcation lesions treated with drug-eluting stents: the DEFINITION study (Definitions and impact of complEx biFurcation lesIons on clinical outcomes after percutaNeous coronary InterventTIOn using drug-eluting steNts). JACC Cardiovasc Interv. 2014;7:1266–76.
17. Jun Jie Z. Two-stent techniques for coronary artery bifurcation stenting: insights from imaging of bench deployments. JCIC. 2016;1:12–9.
18. Jun Jie Z. Classic crush and DK crush stenting techniques. EuroIntervention. 2015;11:V102–5. V104.

Part 2: Optimized Provisional Stenting for Treatment of Coronary Bifurcation Lesions

19. Hildick-Smith D, de Belder AJ, Cooter N, et al. Randomized trial of simple versus complex drug-eluting stenting for bifurcation lesions: the British Bifurcation Coronary Study: old, new, and evolving strategies. Circulation. 2010;121(10):1235–43.
20. Stankovic G, Lefèvre T, Chieffo A, European Bifurcation Club, et al. Consensus from the 7th European Bifurcation Club meeting. EuroIntervention. 2013;9(1):36–45.
21. Levine GN, Bates ER, Blankenship JC, et al. 2011 ACCF/AHA/SCAI Guideline for Percutaneous Coronary Intervention. A report of the American College of Cardiology Foundation/American Heart Association Task Force on Practice Guidelines and the Society for Cardiovascular Angiography and Interventions. J Am Coll Cardiol. 2011;58(24):e44–122.
22. Behan MW, Holm NR, Curzen NP, et al. Simple or complex stenting for bifurcation coronary lesions: a patient-level pooled-analysis of the Nordic Bifurcation Study and the British Bifurcation Coronary Study. Circ Cardiovasc Interv. 2011;4(1):57–64.
23. Grundeken MJ, Stella PR, Wykrzykowska JJ. Why the provisional single-stent approach is not always the right strategy; arguments for the development of dedicated bifurcation devices. EuroInterv. 2012;7(11):1249–53.
24. Moussa ID. Coronary artery bifurcation interventions: the disconnect between randomized clinical trials and patient centered decision-making. Catheter Cardiovasc Interv. 2011;77(4):537–45.
25. Páez L, Moreno R, Alcocer A, et al. Side branch occlusion during direct stent implantation. Incidence and related factors. Arch Cardiol Mex. 2005;75(3):252–9.
26. Chen LL, Fan L, Chen ZY, et al. Modified culotte stenting for treatment of complex coronary bifurcation lesions: immediate and 9-month outcomes in a pilot study. Chin Med J (Engl). 2011;124(13):1943–50.
27. Fan L, Chen L, Luo Y, et al. DK mini-culotte stenting in the treatment of true coronary bifurcation lesions: a propensity score matching comparison with T-provisional stenting. Heart Vessels. 2016;31:308–21.
28. Burzotta F, Gwon HC, Hahn JY, et al. Modified T-stenting with intentional protrusion of the side-branch stent within the main vessel stent to ensure ostial coverage and facilitate final kissing balloon: the T-stenting and small protrusion technique (TAP-stenting). Report of bench testing and first clinical Italian-Korean two-centre experience. Catheter Cardiovasc Interv. 2007;70(1):75–82.
29. Naganuma T, Latib A, Basavarajaiah S, et al. The long-term clinical outcome of T-stenting and small protrusion technique for coronary bifurcation lesions. JACC Cardiovasc Interv. 2013;6(6):554–61.
30. Lee MS, Finch W. Stenting techniques for patients with bifurcation coronary artery disease. Rev Cardiovasc Med. 2011;12(4):231–9.
31. Mylotte D, Routledge H, Harb T, et al. Provisional side branch-stenting for coronary bifurcation lesions: evidence of improving procedural and clinical outcomes with contemporary techniques. Catheter Cardiovasc Interv. 2013;82(4):E437–45.
32. Hariki H, Shinke T, Otake H, et al. Potential benefit of final kissing balloon inflation after single stenting for the treatment of bifurcation lesions--insights from optical coherence tomography observations. Circ J. 2013;77(5):1193–201.
33. Niemela M, Kervinen K, Erglis A, et al. Randomized comparison of final kissing balloon dilatation versus no final kissing balloon dilatation in patients with coronary bifurcation lesions treated with main vessel stenting: the Nordic-Baltic Bifurcation Study III. Circulation. 2011;123(1):79–86.
34. Biondi-Zoccai G, Sheiban I, De Servi S, et al. To kiss or not to kiss? Impact of final balloon kissing inflation on early and long-term results of PCI for bifurcation lesions. Heart Vessels. 2014;29(6):732–42.
35. Yamawaki M, Muramatsu T, Kozuma K, et al. Long-term clinical outcome of a single stent approach with and without a final kissing balloon technique for coronary bifurcation. Circ J. 2014;78(1):110–21.

Part 3: Double Kissing Mini Culotte Stenting for Treatment of Complex Coronary Bifurcation Lesions

36. Chevalier B, Glatt B, Royer T, et al. Placement of coronary stents in bifurcation lesions by the "culotte" technique. Am J Cardiol. 1998;82:943–9.
37. Chen LL, Fan L, Chen ZY, et al. Modified culotte stenting for treatment of complex coronary bifurcation lesions: immediate and 9-month outcomes in a pilot study. Chin Med J (Engl). 2011;124:1943–50.
38. Fan L, Chen LL, Luo YK, et al. DK mini-culotte stenting in the treatment of true coronary bifurcation lesions: a propensity score matching comparison with T-provisional stenting. Heart Vessels. 2014;17 [Epub ahead of print].
39. Kaplan S, Barlis P, Dimopoulos K, et al. Culotte versus T-stenting in bifurcation lesions: immediate clinical and angiographic results and midterm clinical follow-up. Am Heart J. 2007;154(2):336–43.
40. Tiroch K, Mehilli J, Byrne RA, ISAR-LEFT MAIN Study Investigators, et al. Impact of coronary anatomy and stenting technique on long-term outcome after drug-eluting stent implantation for unprotected left main coronary artery disease. JACC Cardiovasc Interv. 2014;7(1):29–36.
41. Erglis A, Kumsars I, Niemela M, et al. Randomized comparison of coronary bifurcation stenting with the crush versus the culotte technique using sirolimus eluting stents. (Nordic bifurcation II study). Circ Cardiovasc Interv. 2009;2:27–34.
42. Kawasaki T, Koga H, Serikawa T. Modified culotte stenting technique for bifurcation lesions: the cross-stenting technique. J Invasive Cardiol. 2010;22(5):243–6.
43. G Toth G, Pyxaras S, Mortier P, et al. Single string technique for coronary bifurcation stenting: detailed technical evaluation and feasibility analysis. JACC Cardiovasc Interv. 2015;8(7):949–59.

Transradial Approach for Chronic Total Occlusion of Coronary Arteries: Its Advantages and Disadvantages

18

Shigeru Saito

Abstract

Since the introduction of transradial coronary intervention (TRI) by Kiemeneij, its advantages over transfemoral coronary intervention (TFI) have been shown in many clinical situations. TRI can reduce the incidence and severity in the bleeding complications through arterial access site [1], which result in the reduction in mortality, length of hospital stay and cost after percutaneous coronary intervention (PCI). Since TRI is more patients' friendly, most of the patients, who have received both TRI and TFI, prefer to the former from next session.

The major disadvantage of TRI is its limitation in the size of guiding catheter due to the smaller diameter of radial compared to femoral arteries. The distribution of radial artery diameter in Japanese patient population has been reported [2]. This limitation first results in the reduced backup support achieved by the guiding catheters. Secondly, it limits the use of several devices or the simultaneous use of several devices. This, in turn, limits the use of several techniques, which have been developed in angioplasty for chronic total occlusion (CTO) lesions.

In this chapter, various techniques for CTO angioplasty will be first described. Then, the feasibilities in their application in TRI will be discussed.

18.1 Basic Knowledge Before Stating Angioplasty for CTO Lesions

18.1.1 Simultaneous Bilateral Angiography

If coronary anatomy distal to the CTO lesion is not clearly visualized by ipsilateral coronary angiography, contralateral dye injection is essential. Even if the anatomy distal to the lesion can be identified through the ipsilateral collateral feeding bridging the lesion, it is better to prepare for contralateral coronary angiography. During the antegrade manipulation of guidewires, ipsilateral bridging collateral may be damaged, which may result in unclear imaging for distal anatomy.

S. Saito, MD, FACC, FSCAI, FJCC
Division of Cardiology and Catheterization Laboratories, Shonan Kamakura General Hospital, Kamakura, Japan
e-mail: cto.expert@gmail.com

18.1.2 Biplane Fluoroscopy

Biplane fluoroscopy is useful to save the procedure time. If angiography is done by biplane machine, the amount of contrast dye can also be saved.

However, the use of biplane fluoroscopy tends to increase the radiation dose. Immediately after successful crossing the lesion with a guidewire, it is necessary to switch the machine from biplane to monoplane mode.

18.1.3 Selection of Guiding Catheters

In order to achieve strong backup support, EBU (Medtronic), XB (Cordis), VL (Boston) or BL (TERUMO) with side holes is recommended for left coronary artery. JR or Amplatz Left with side holes is recommended for right coronary artery. Regular Amplatz Left has too long distal tip for Asian patients. Thus, SAL1.0 or AL0.75 (Medtronic) is

Y. Zhou et al. (eds.), *Transradial Approach for Percutaneous Interventions*, DOI 10.1007/978-94-017-7350-8_18

recommended to avoid the intimal dissection caused by the tip of the guiding.

18.1.4 Consideration for the Radial Access Side

The subclavian artery may show excessive tortuosity especially in the elder patients. This situation can be negotiated by using a stiff guidewire such as 0.063-in. J guidewire or by the use of double wire technique using two 0.032 or 0.035-in. guidewires through a 6 French guiding catheter. By using these maneuvers, guiding catheters can be successfully engaged into the target coronary artery. If you are targeting the lesions other than CTO, you will be successful in doing angioplasty. However, in case of targeting CTO lesion, the situation is totally different. The tortuosity of the subclavian artery will reduce the torque transmission ability of PCI guidewires, especially in using stiff guidewires for CTO lesions. Thus, encountering very tortuous subclavian artery, switching to the opposite side of radial artery may be considered (Fig. 18.1).

18.1.5 Use of Microcatheter

In angioplasty for CTO lesions, guidewire should be used not with "bare-wire technique" but always with microcatheter. This is recommended because;

1. Guidewires can be changed quickly and easily.
2. Reshaping of the tip of guidewires is easy.
3. By adjusting the length of guidewire protruding out of microcatheter, tip stiffness of guidewires can be controlled.
4. Better torque transmission to the distal tip of guidewire can be achieved especially through tortuous coronary arteries.

Between the over-the-wire balloon catheter and microcatheter, the use of latter one is my recommended, because its tip is softer and guidewire manipulation is easier than the first in general.

18.1.6 Guidewire Selection

Guidewires specifically designed for CTO lesions can be classified into 3 major groups;

1. Category I: Plastic-jacket hydrophilic tapered-tip guidewires: Fielder-XT, -XTR, -XTA (ASAHI Intecc), Wizard-78, -1, 3 (Japan Lifeline), etc.
2. Category II: Non-plastic jacket blunt end guidewires: Miracle-3, -6, -12, -Ultimate (ASAHI Intecc)
3. Category III: Non-plastic jacket tapered-tip guidewires: Gaia-First, -Second, -Third, Conquest-Pro 9, 12, 8–20 (ASAHI Intecc)

Based on the pathological findings in CTO lesions (described bellow), it is rational to start from plastic-jacket hydrophilic tapered-tip soft-end guidewires, which include Fielder-XT, -XTR or –XTA in Category I [3]. If these wires cannot pass the lesion, the wires should be quickly changed to Category II or III wires according to the lesion characteristics felt by the tip of Category I guidewires. If the lesion contains much calcification, Category II guidewires are preferred. Instead, if the lesion does not contain much calcification or target distal artery is clear, Category III guidewires are chosen.

18.2 Various Techniques in Angioplasty for CTO Lesions

18.2.1 Double Guidewire (Parallel Guidewire) Technique

Pathological examination of CTO lesions indicate the presence of small vascular channels partly or completely connecting from the proximal to the distal ends of the CTO lesions [4]. Their diameters are ranging between 160 and 230 μm. The channels are frequently ends at the sidewall of the coronary artery or connecting to the side branches far proximal to the distal end of the CTO lesion. The channels themselves cannot bee seen on fluoroscopy because of tiny diameters. Computed tomography of coronary arteries may be helpful especially to identify the presence of calcification within the lesion [5] (Fig. 18.2). A PCI guidewire can easily advance into these micro channels, which are ending at the sidewall of the coronary artery and results in forming intimal dissection.

Double guidewire technique is the best way to overcome this situation. If the guidewire goes into the false lumen or side branches, do not pull out but leave it there. While leaving the 1st guidewire there, you have to take the 2nd guidewire. You have to train yourself hard, so that you can trace the exactly same pathway by the 2nd guidewire as the 1st guidewire. After the tip of the 2nd guidewire reaches the point, where the 1st guidewire seems diverting from the true lumen, you intentionally direct the tip of the 2nd guidewire into the true lumen. This is the concept of "Double Guidewire Technique" (Fig. 18.3).

Three rationales can be listed for the mechanism of double guidewire technique. First, the 1st guidewire occludes the entry into the false lumen, and the 2nd guidewire can

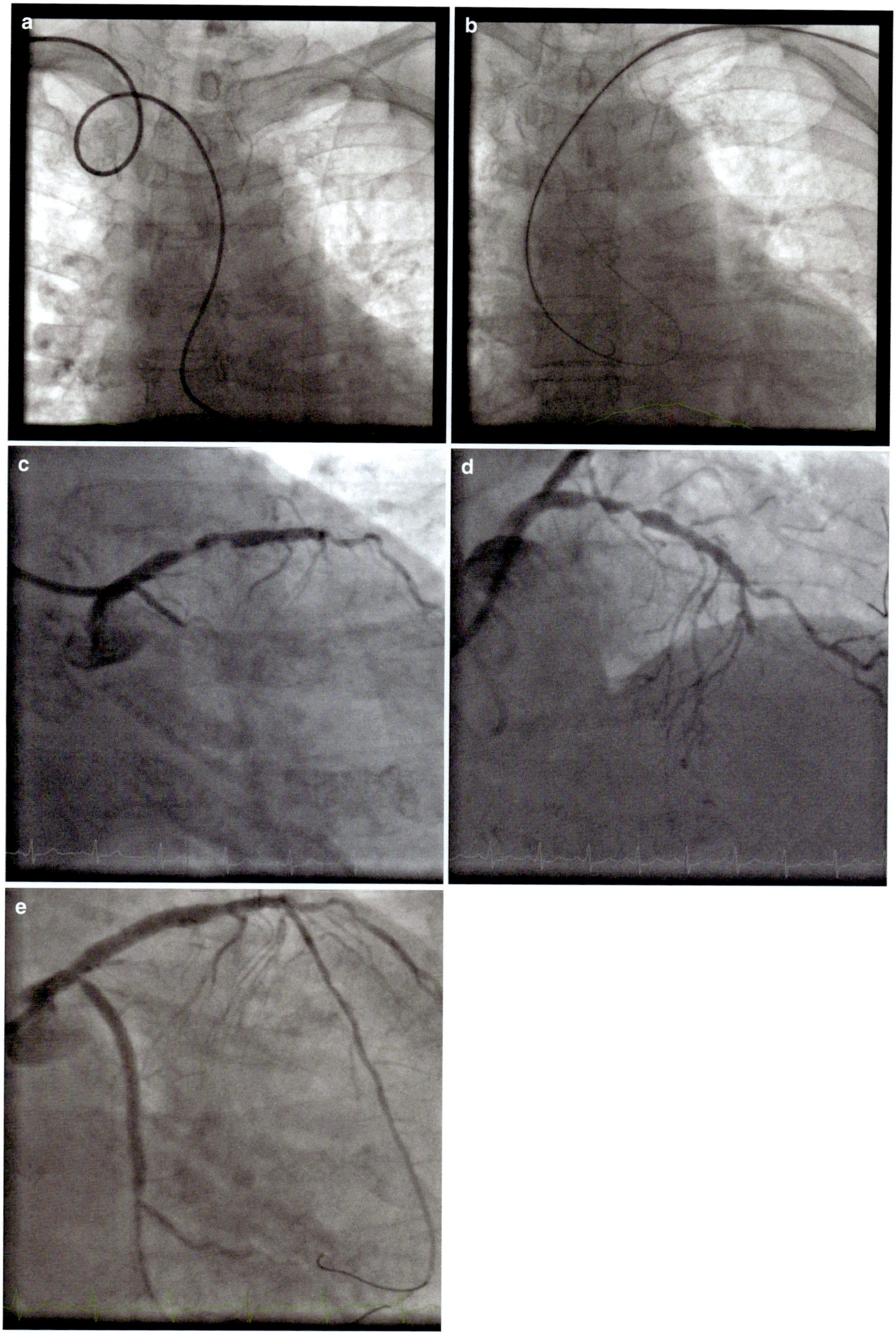

Fig. 18.1 (**a**) 73-year old female patient. Right subclavian artery showed marked tortuosity and loop. (**b**) However, the left subclavian artery was relatively straight. (**c**) The LCA was cannulated by a 6 French EBU 3.5 guiding catheter (Launcher) through the left radial artery. Two CTO lesions were in the proximal LCX and distal LAD. (**d**) LAD also showed 2 critical narrowings in the proximal and 1 CTO lesion in the distal parts. (**e**) Final angiogram after stenting for both arteries

Fig. 18.2 Tapered-tip guidewire in PCI for CTO Lesions

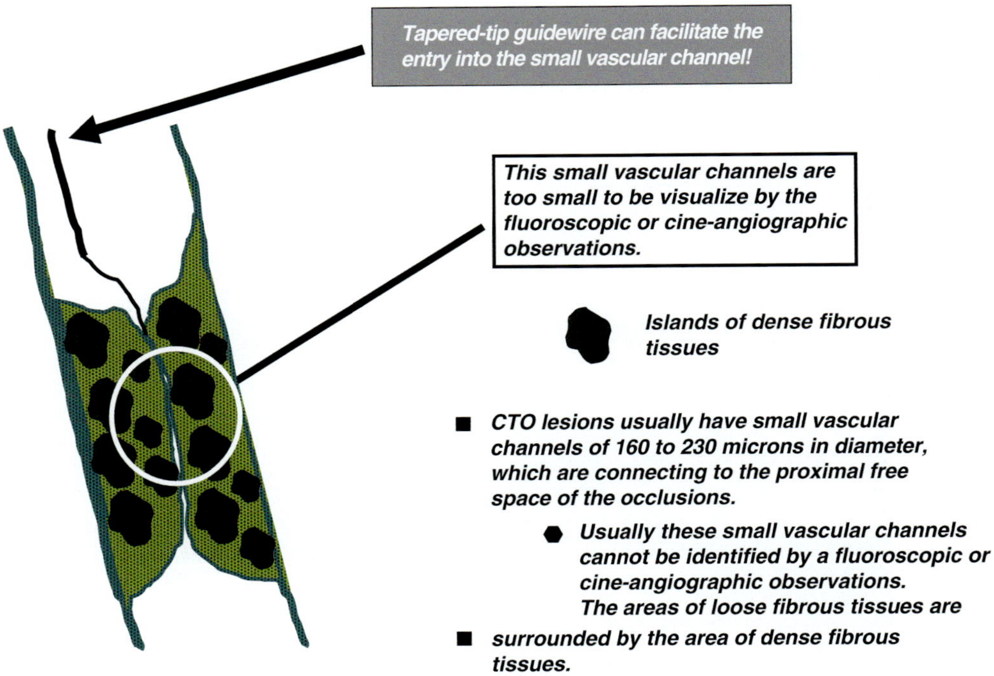

advance along the true lumen. Second, the 1st guidewire works as a landmark for the manipulation of the 2nd guidewire. Last, the 1st guidewire can straighten the tortuous coronary artery or change its geometry, which makes the guidewire manipulation easier.

Considering these three rationales, the proper strategies in double guidewire technique can be reached as follows:

1. Do not manipulate the 1st guidewire too much within the false lumen. This maneuver will expand the subintimal space, and the subsequent attempts by using the 2nd guidewire to find the true lumen become more difficult.
2. Take the penetrating technique for the 2nd guidewire to find the true lumen even after the drilling technique for the 1st guidewire.
3. Take the 2nd guidewire stiffer than the 1st one in order to achieve the better torque transmission and penetration abilities.
4. Always take a microcatheter with the 2nd guidewire. The use of the microcatheter prevents the twisting of the two guidewires and enables the fine torque control for the 2nd guidewire.

18.2.2 Triple Guidewire Technique (Fig. 18.4)

If the double guidewire technique fails, the 3rd guidewire can be applied while leaving the previous two guidewires in the false lumen. The handling of the 3rd guidewire is more difficult compared to double guidewire technique, since the guidewires easily tend to be twisted each other. To prevent this twisting, the simultaneous use of two or three microcatheters is necessary, which requires at least six French (for two microcatheters) or seven French (for tree microcatheters) guiding catheters.

18.2.3 Side Branch Technique (Fig. 18.5)

If a guidewire successfully penetrates the proximal cap of the CTO lesion and entered into the side branch but not crossed the lesion completely, it is recommended to take a 1.5-mm balloon and dilate the lesion to the side branch. After this balloon dilatation, you can ensure the route at lest to the side branch, and the re-wiring to the distal true lumen becomes easier. Important tips for the side branch technique include:

1. Before you get convinced that the guidewire is really in the lumen of a side branch, do not attempt this technique.
2. Always take a 1.5-mm balloon but not 1.25- or 2.0-mm balloons. A 1.25-mm balloon is too small for the next rewiring, and a 2.0-mm balloon is so big that it may destroy the route to the distal true lumen.
3. Always take the double guidewire technique while leaving a guidewire in the side branch.

18.2.4 Anchoring Balloon Technique

18.2.4.1 Co-axial Anchoring Technique

If the lesion is too stiff to be penetrated by any stiff guidewire, we can take an over-the-wire (OTW) balloon catheter over the guidewire. The inflation of the balloon proximal to the CTO lesion, very strong penetration power can be generated at the tip of the guidewire [6]. Instead of OTW balloon, we can use an adequate size of monorail balloon to utilize this technique. Parallel to the combination of a microcatheter and CTO guidewire, we can place a monorail balloon with or without a guidewire inside. Inflating this balloon, we can utilize the similar effect with OTW balloon anchoring technique (Fig. 18.6).

18.2.4.2 Side-Branch Anchoring Technique

If there is a side branch proximal to the CTO lesion, we can place a guidewire and an adequate size of balloon in it.

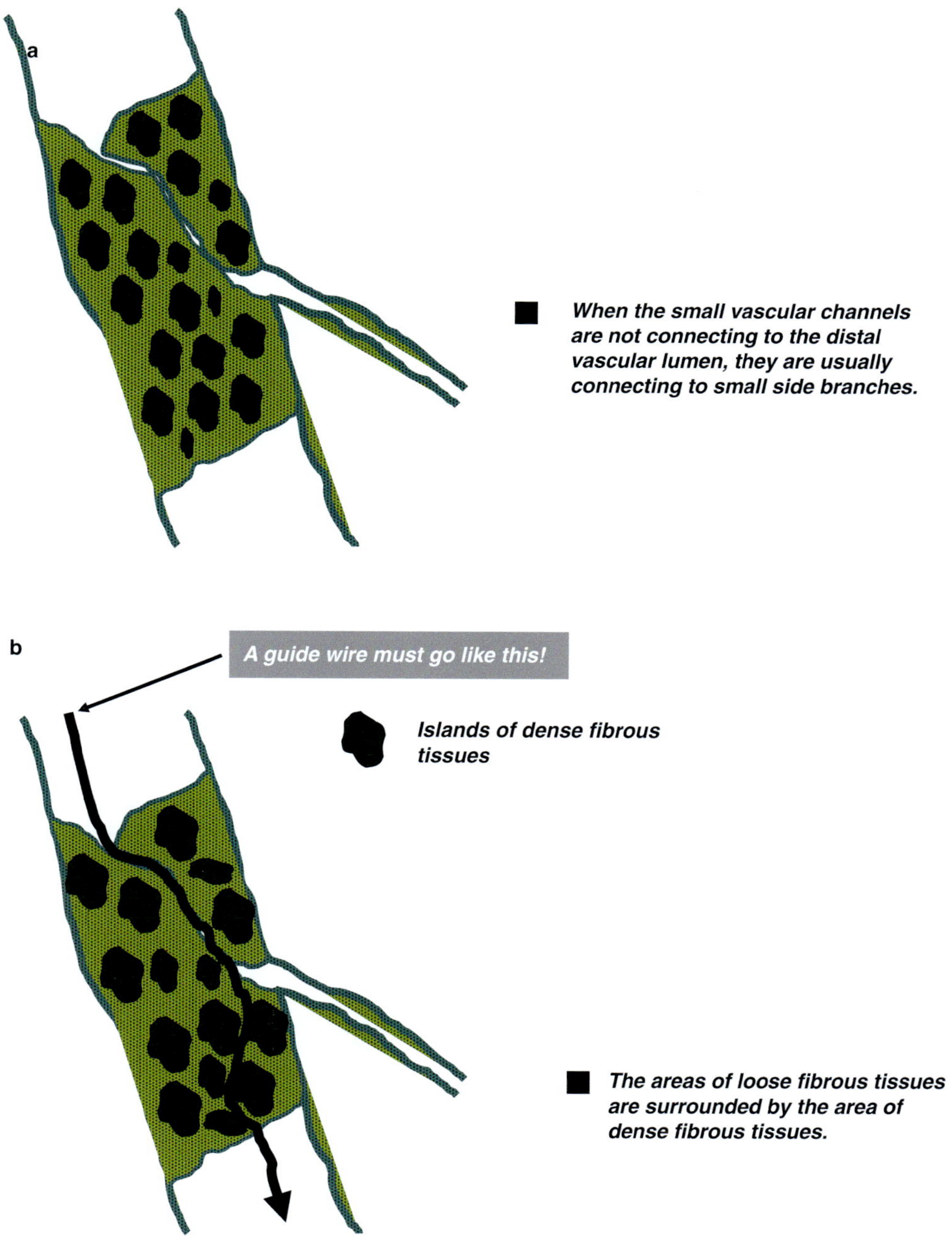

Fig. 18.3 Double Guidewire Technique in CTO Lesions

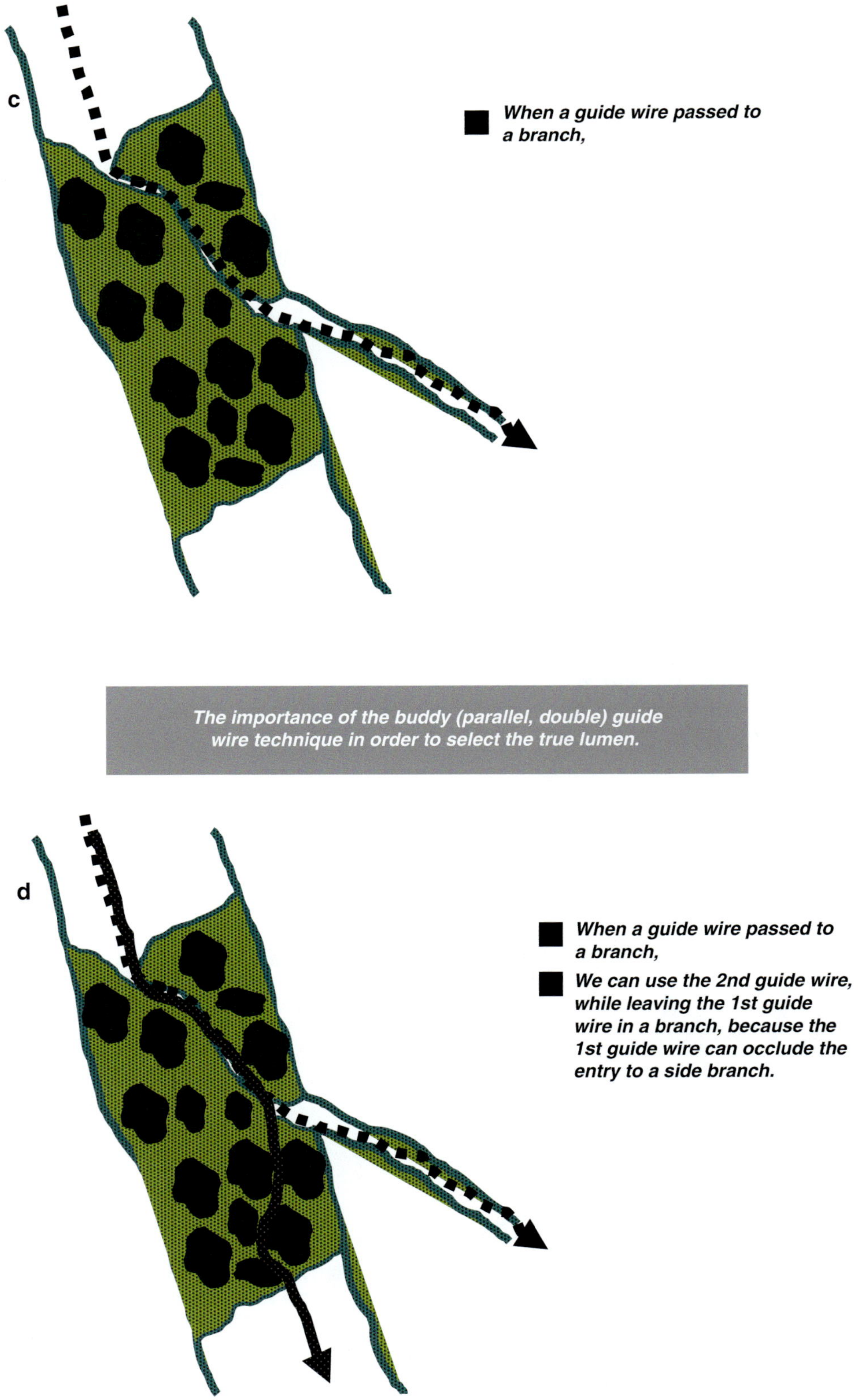

Fig. 18.3 (continued)

e

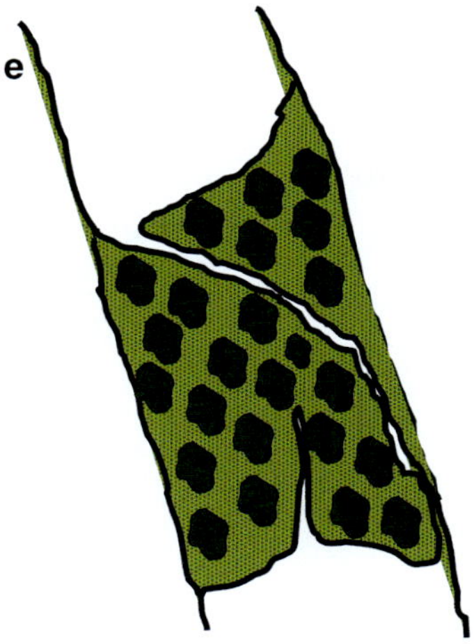

f

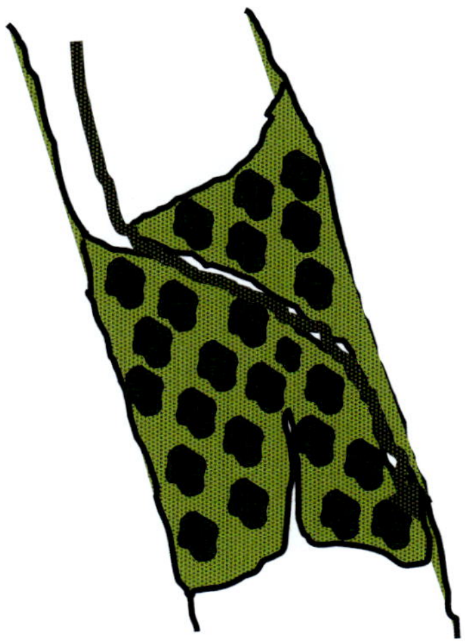

g

The importance of the buddy (parallel, double) guide wire technique in order to select the true lumen.

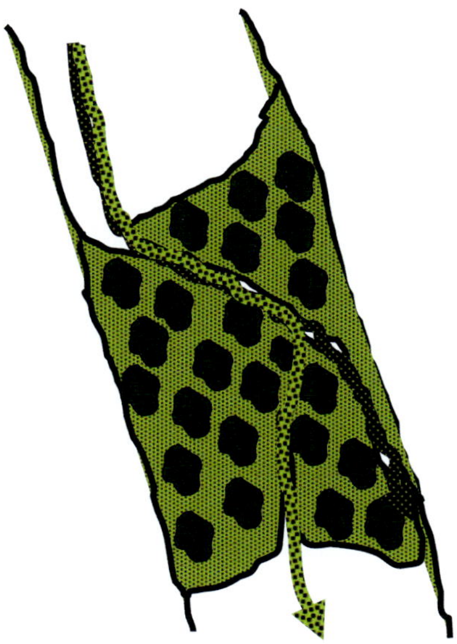

Fig. 18.3 (continued)

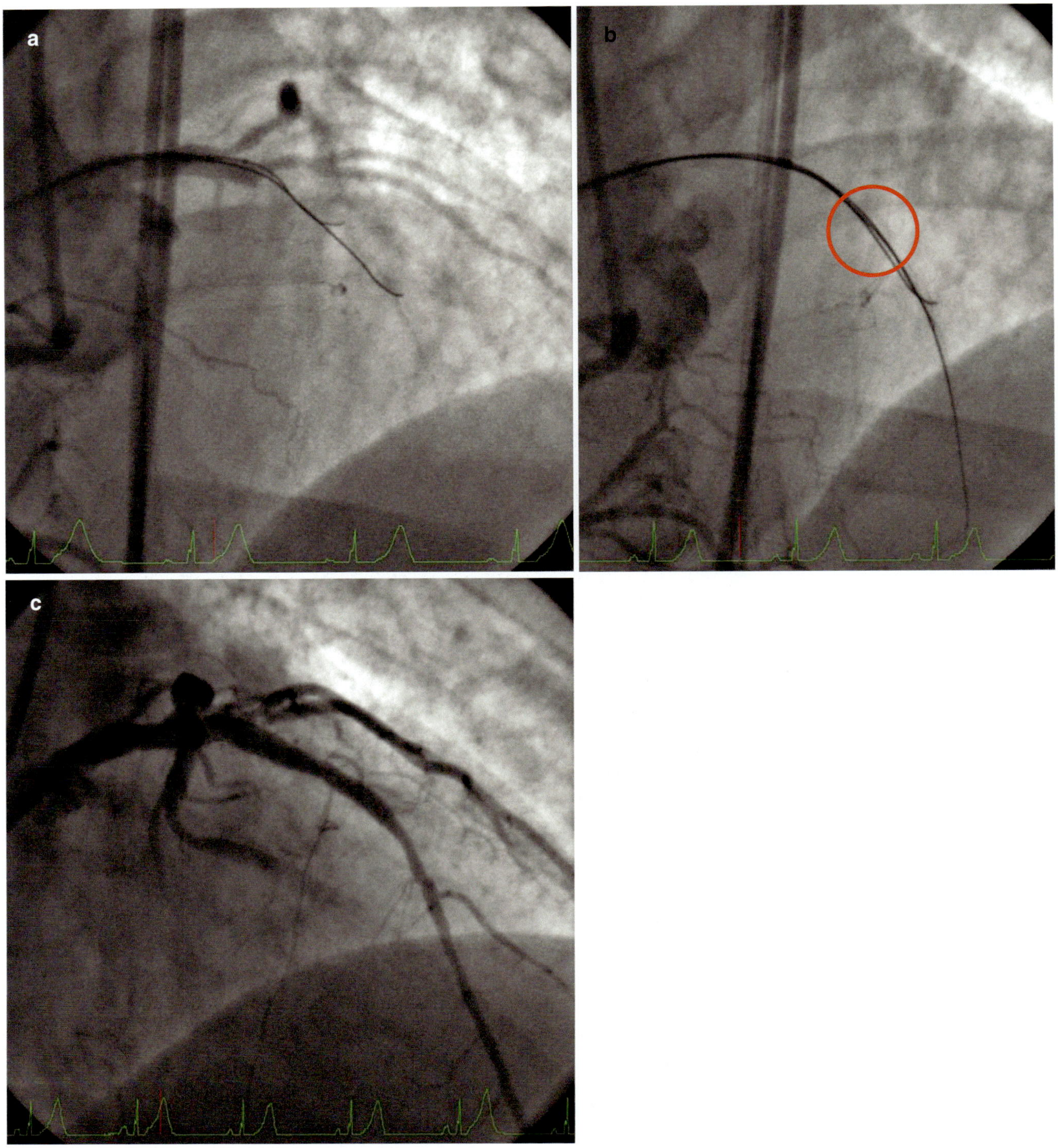

Fig. 18.4 Triple Guidewire Technique (**a**) Both two wires are in the false lumen. (**b**) Three wires are overlayed within the circle. (**c**) After successful stenting

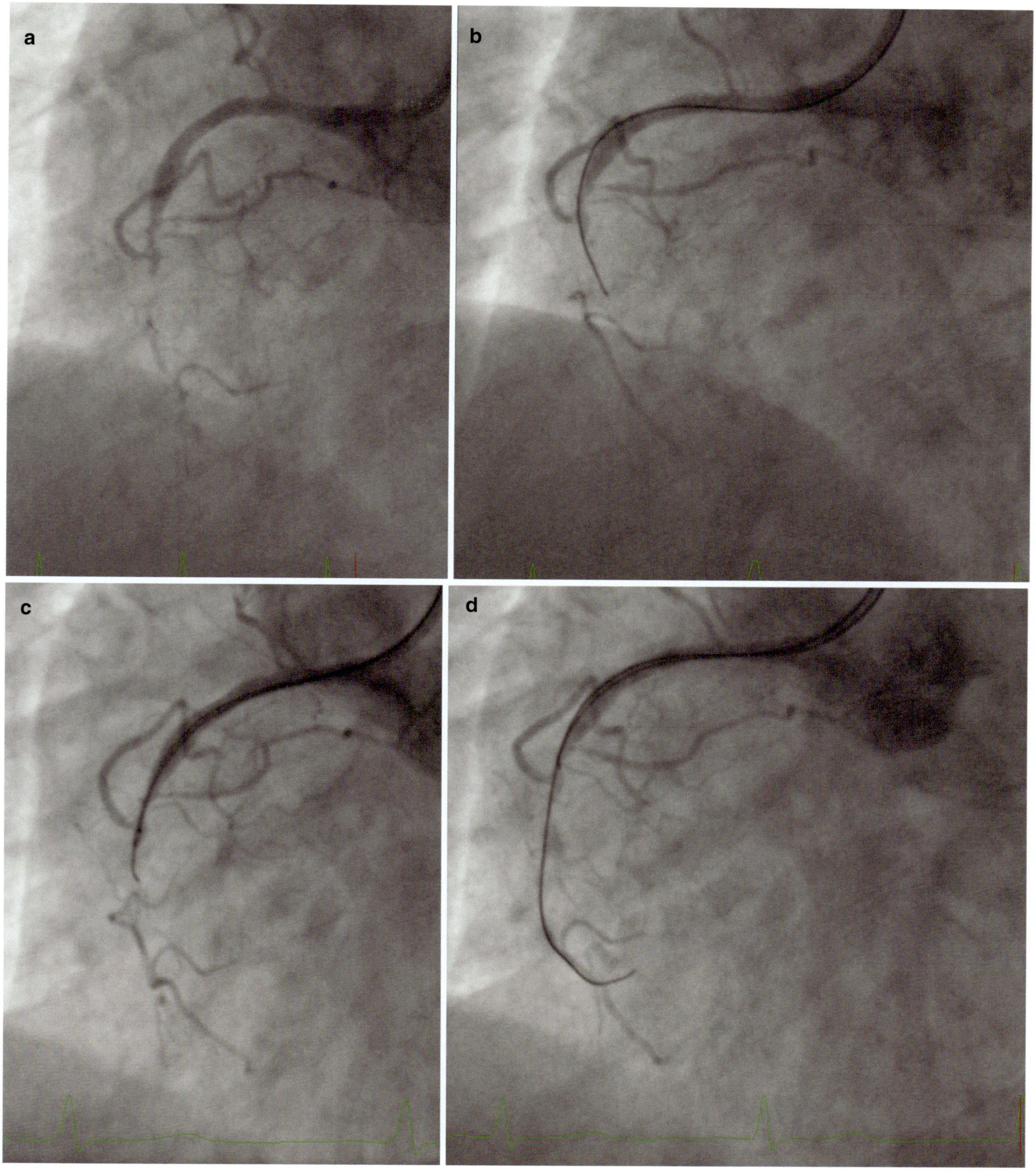

Fig. 18.5 Side-Branch Technique (**a**) CTO lesion in mid right coronary artery. (**b**) Antegrade approach with a stiff guidewire. (**c**) Starting double wire technique. (**d**) One of the double wires passed into a side branch distal to the CTO lesion. (**e**) The wire was clearly in the right ventricular branch. Dissection is clearly identified. (**f**) A 1.5-mm balloon dilated to the branch. (**g**) After the balloon dilatation with a 1.5-mm balloon to the side branch. Faint antegrade filling through the CTO lesion can be seen. (**h**) Final angiogram

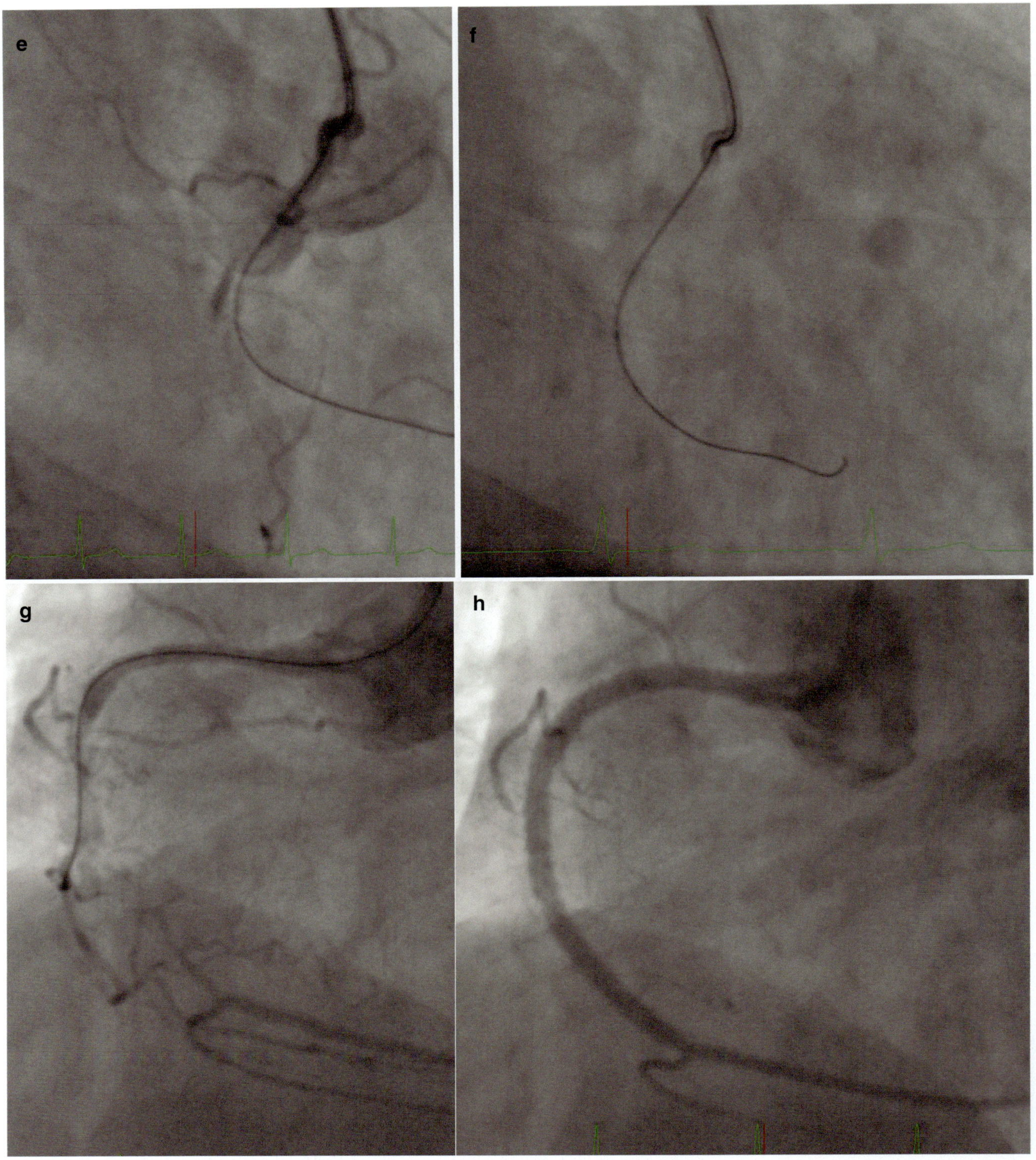

Fig. 18.5 (continued)

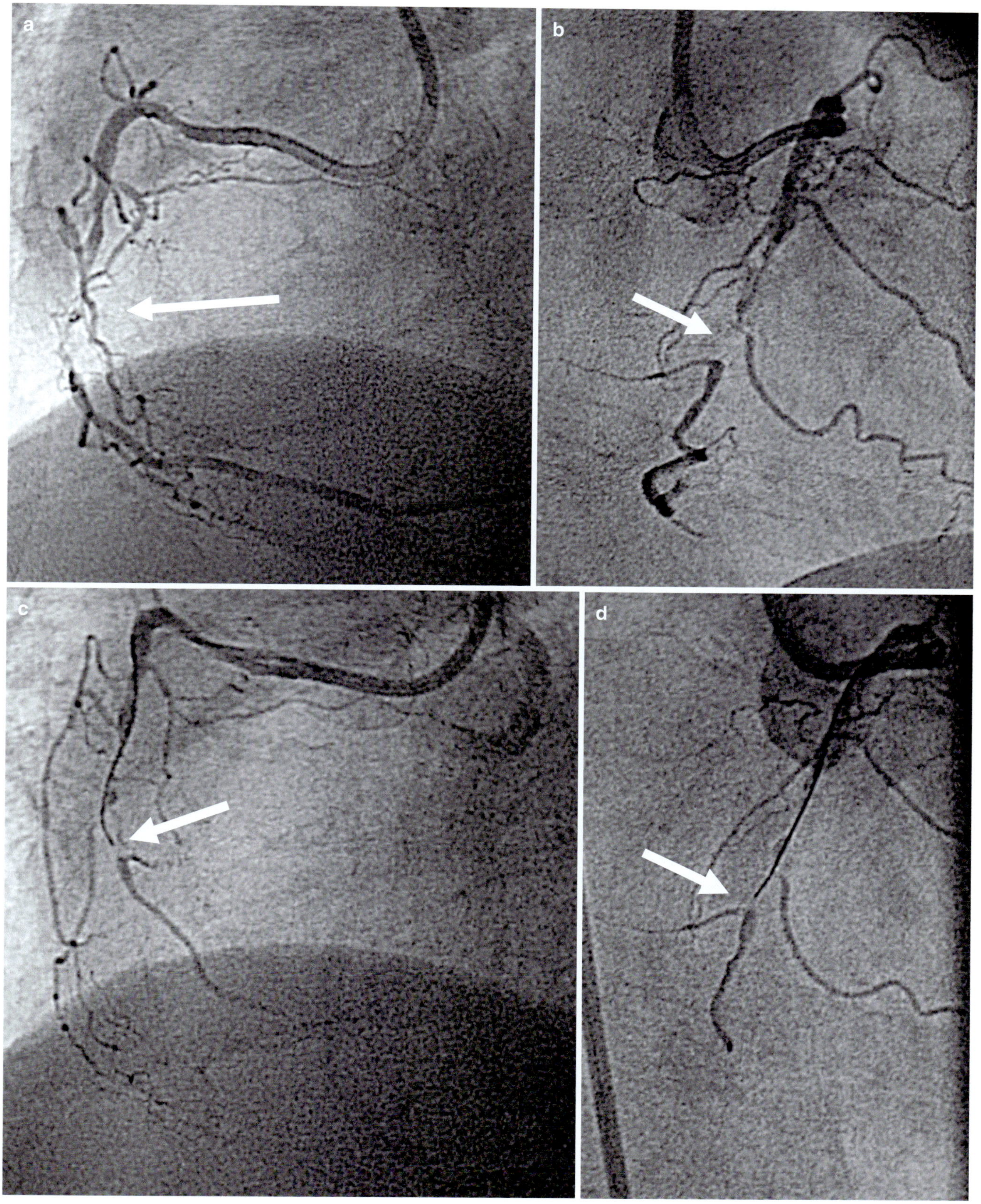

Fig. 18.6 Co-axial Anchoring Balloon Technique. (**a**, **b**) *Arrow* indicates a short chronic total occlusion in the mid right coronary artery. (**c**, **d**) A tapered-tip stiff guidewire (Conquest) could not pass through the lesion even under the strong back-up support by seven French left Amplatz guiding catheter. (**e**, **f**) By inflating a 2.5 mm balloon proximal to the CTO lesion, the tapered-tip stiff guidewire (Conquest) could be successfully passed through the lesion. (**g**, **h**) By inflating a 2.5 mm balloon proximal to the CTO lesion, the tapered-tip stiff guidewire (Conquest) could be successfully passed through the lesion. (**i**) The lesion was successfully opened and stented

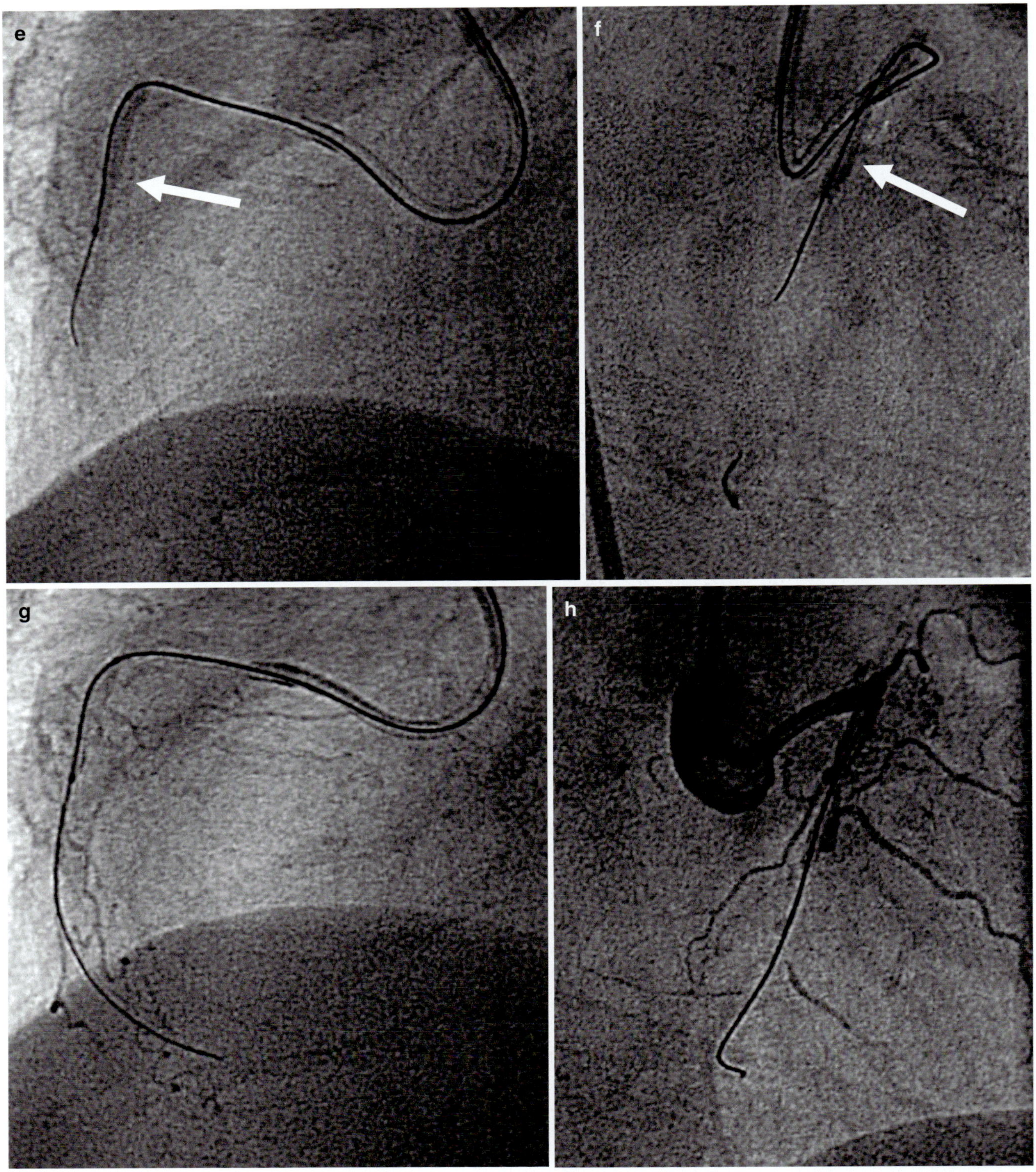

Fig. 18.6 (continued)

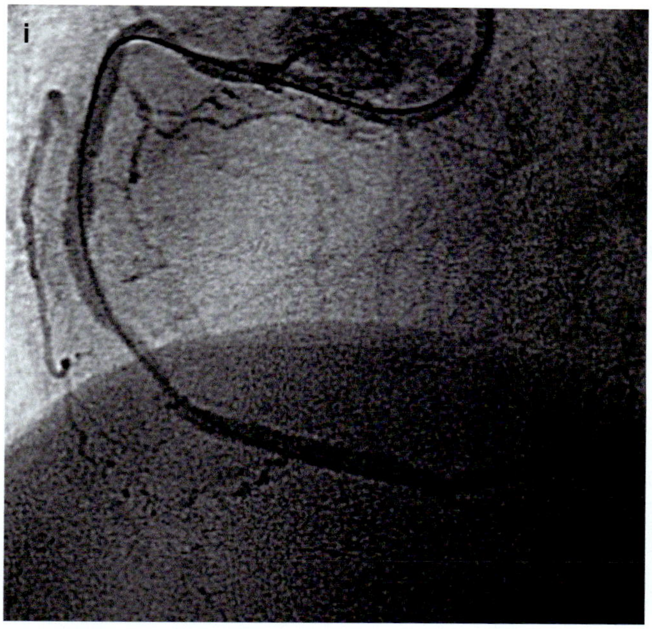

Fig. 18.6 (continued)

The balloon inflation at 4–6 ATM in the side branch can fix a guiding catheter into the coronary ostium. In this situation, the combination of a microcatheter and a stiff guidewire can generate very strong penetration power against the CTO lesion [7] (Fig. 18.7).

18.2.5 Mother-and-Child Technique [8–10]

It is sometimes encountered that even the smallest size of balloon cannot pass the lesion after the successful penetration of a guidewire through it, when TRI is applied with a six French guiding catheter for CTO angioplasty. In this situation we can take Mother-and-Child technique besides anchoring technique. Original one of these techniques is using a straight five French guiding catheter (ST01, TERUMO), which has the total length 10 CM longer than conventional six French guiding catheters. By putting this longer child catheter into the mother six French catheters, the distal end of the first one can protrude out of the distal end of the latter one, and engage deeply in the coronary artery. This protrusion and engagement can provide strong backup support.

From in-vitro experiments, this system can provide the back-up force even stronger than a seven French guiding catheter alone, when the tip of the child-catheter is protruding from the mother six French mother guiding catheters into the coronary artery by 5 mm or more.

In order to secure enough length of the child-guiding catheter, which can be protruded into the coronary artery, we have to exchange the regular Y-adapter, which was connected with the six French outer guiding catheters, with a short stopcock. In order to minimize the bleeding from the catheter while changing the system, the child catheter is being put though the short stop cock so that 1 or 2 CM of the tip of inner catheter should penetrating the stopcock. Next, the regular Y-adapter, which has been already attached to the mother-guiding catheter, is detached quickly while the PCI guidewire kept in position. Then, the child-guiding catheter is put over the distal end of the PCI guidewire, and inserted deeply within the mother-guiding catheter. Finally, the regular Y-adapter is attached to the end of the child-guiding catheter. By following these procedures, the regular guiding catheter system can be quickly changed to the mother-and-child one with minimal bleeding.

18.2.6 Open Sesame Technique [11]

When a side branch is bifurcating at the proximal end of the CTO lesion, this technique [Article] can be applied. Briefly mentioned, when the tip of any stiff guidewires cannot enter into the lesion, by putting stiff wires with or without small sized balloon into the side branch, the entry of the tip of guidewire can be easier. This is possible, because putting stiff wires or balloons into the side branch changes the geometry between the proximal hard plaque and the true lumen within the CTO lesion (Fig. 18.8).

18.2.7 Retrograde or Bi-directional Approach [12–15]

Retrograde approach is getting more popular for CTO lesions, especially after failed attempt of antegrade approach. Almost in every case, retrograde approach needs bi-

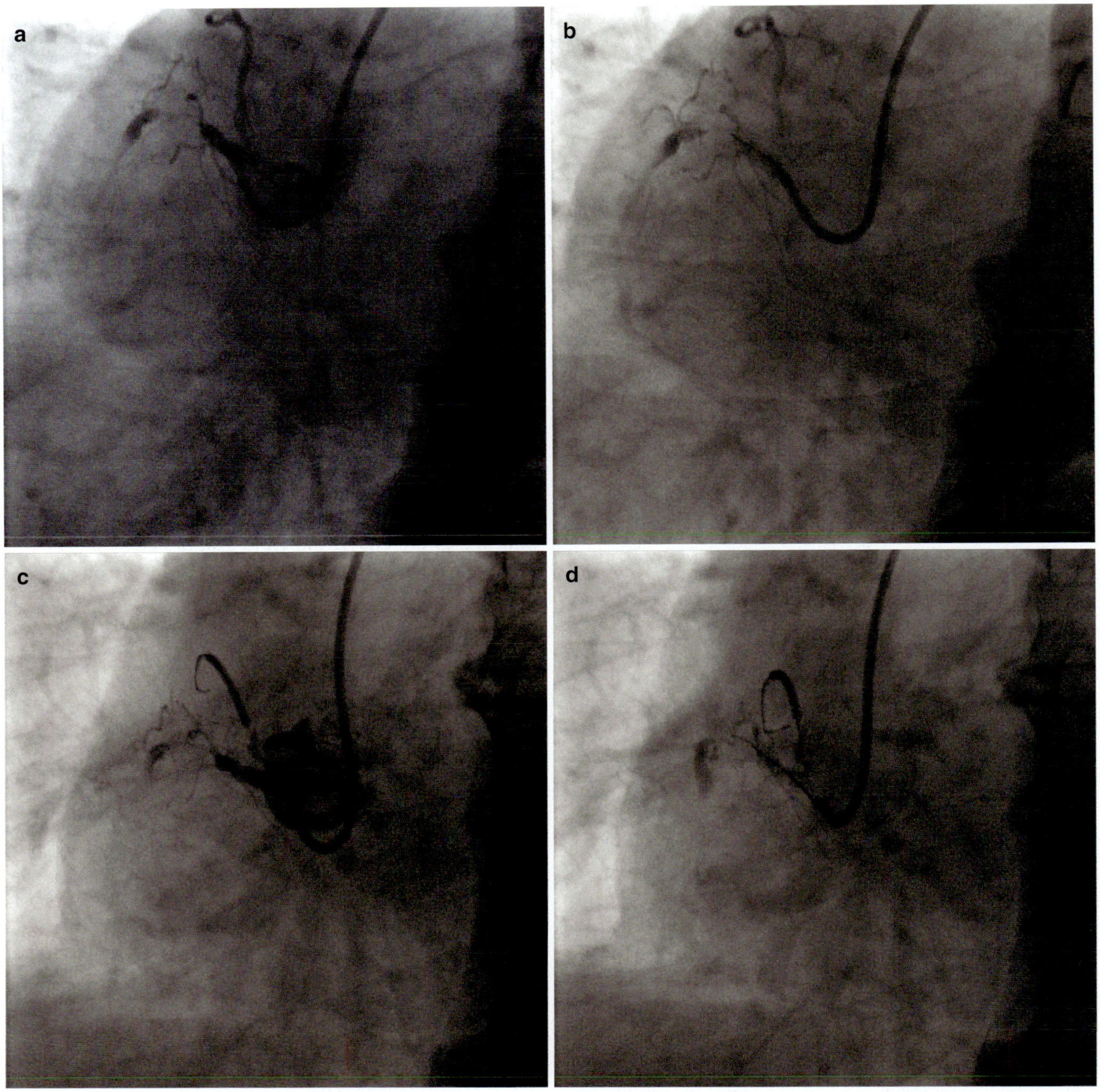

Fig. 18.7 Anchoring Balloon Technique (**a**) Proximal RCA shows CTO. I used a 6 French SAL 1.0 guiding catheter (Launcher, Medtronic) through the right radial approach. (**b**) When I push a stiff guidewire (Magic-18), the guiding catheter is pushed back away from the coronary ostium. (**c**) I put a 2.0-mm balloon in the conus branch and inflated it by 4 atm. (**d**) The balloon anchoring in the conus branch kept the tip of guiding catheter against the RCA, and the stiff guidewire could gradually advance through the CTO lesion. (**e**) Finally, the guidewire passed through the lesion. (**f**) Final result after stenting. This case might be unsuccessful without Side-branch Anchoring Technique in the conus branch through the radial approach

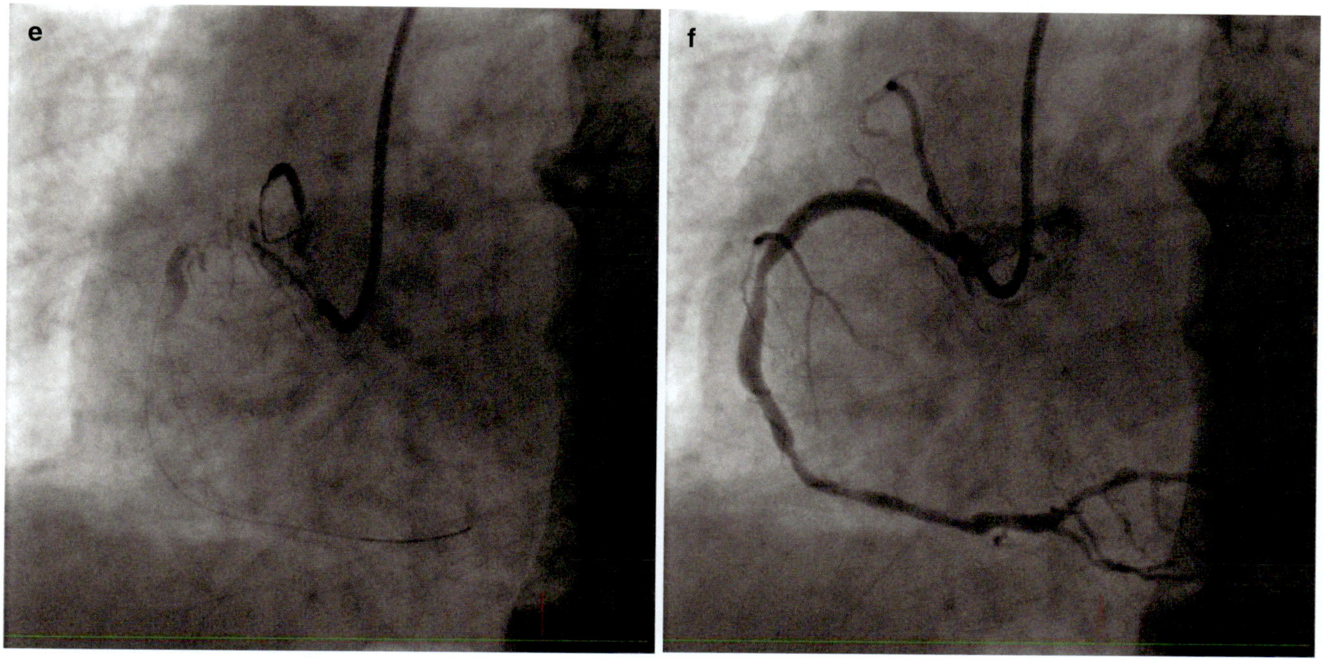

Fig. 18.7 (continued)

directional approach. This means correct terminology shall be "Bi-directional approach". By using bi-radial approach, we can use this technique in TRI.

18.2.8 IVUS-guided PCI for CTO Lesions

Intravascular ultrasound examination (IVUS) is helpful to identify the entry point of the lumen to the CTO lesion, when it can be inserted into the side branch proximal to the lesion. It is also helpful to identify which direction the true lumen is present, when it can be inserted into the false lumen, which was aerated by previous antegrade wire manipulation [16].

18.3 Feasibility of Various Techniques for CTO Angioplasty in TRI

Most of the above-mentioned techniques can be applied through six French guiding catheters and TRI. Triple guidewire technique using three microcatheters together needs at least seven French guiding catheters. IVUS-guided technique, which was not described above, needs at least seven French and hopefully eight French guiding catheters. When you plan the PCI strategy for the specific lesion before starting the case, if your plan includes IVU-guided technique, you should switch to transfemoral approach using eight French guiding catheters.

Conclusion

PCI for CTO lesions through transradial approach needs enough experiences of both transradial approach itself and PCI for CTO lesions through transfemoral approach. However, its success rate has been definitely being improved due to the continuous advent in various techniques and accumulation of skillful operators' experiences [17] [18]. It also needs the most sophisticated techniques developed for PCI for CTO lesions as well. I can tell that PCI for CTO lesions through transfemoral approach can be performed by any operator. However, PCI for CTO lesions through transradial approach can be performed only by limited operators. I wish you would be one of them.

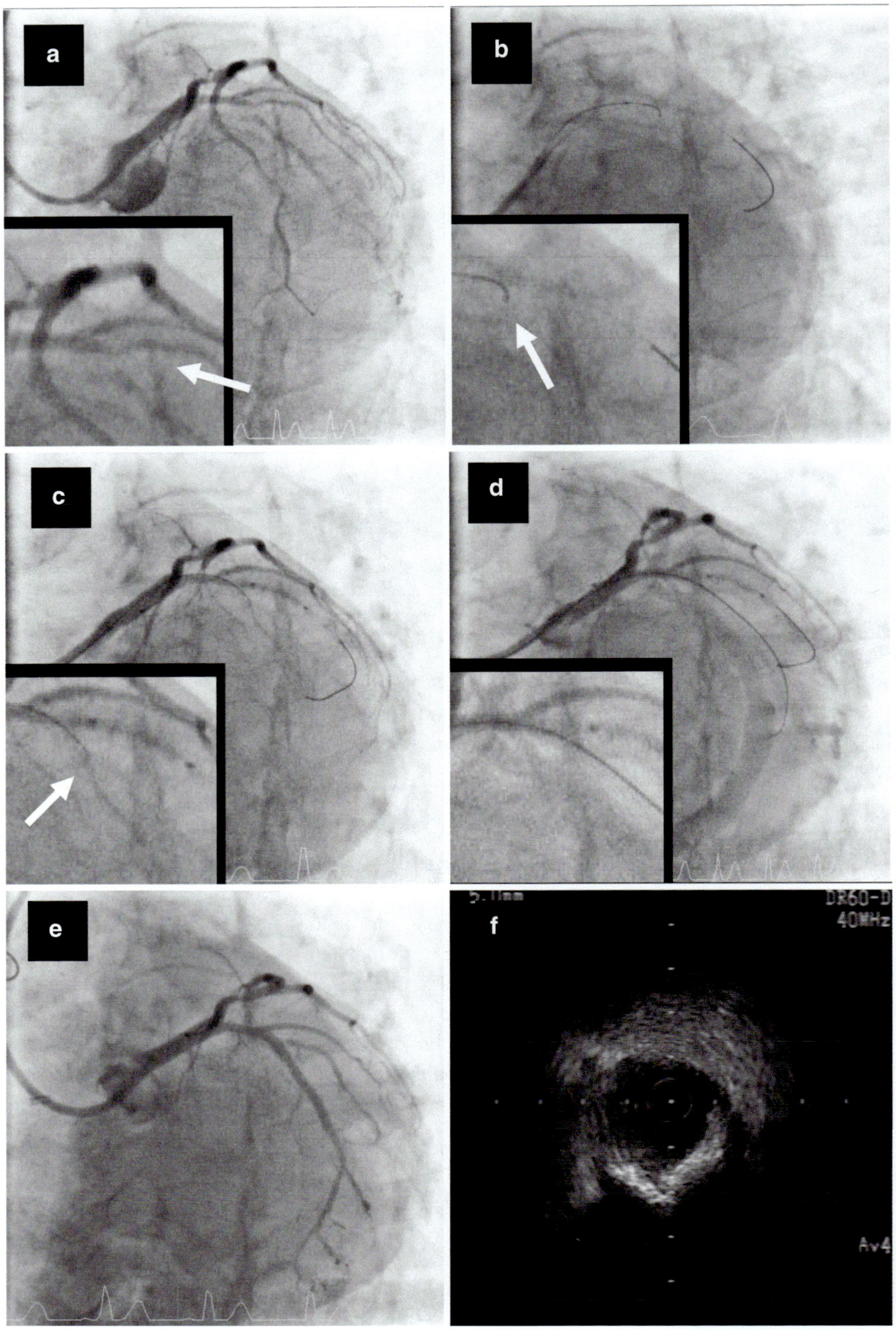

Fig. 18.8 (**a**) *Arrow* indicates a short CTO lesion in the proximal circumflex artery. (**b**) an Antegrade attempt with a stiff guidewire failed due to inability of wire crossing. (**c**) A 2.0-mm balloon catheter was inflated in the side branch proximal to the CTO lesion. Then, the same stiff guidewire easily entered into the lesion (*Arrow*). (**d**) The wire completely crossed the lesion. (**e**) The final result after stenting. (**f**) IVUS examination after ballooning revealed a dense calcification at the ostium of the lesion

References

1. Saito S, Miyake S, Hosokawa G, Tanaka S, Kawamitsu K, Kaneda H, Ikei H, Shiono T. Transradial coronary intervention in Japanese patients. Catheter Cardiovasc Interv. 1999;46:37–41.
2. Saito S, Ikei H, Hosokawa G, Tanaka S. Influence of the ratio between radial artery inner diameter and sheath outer diameter on radial artery flow after transradial coronary intervention. Catheter Cardiovasc Interv. 1999;46:173–8.
3. Saito S, Tanaka S, Hiroe Y, Miyashita Y, Takahashi S, Satake S, Tanaka K. Angioplasty for chronic total occlusion by using tapered-tip guidewires. Catheter Cardiovasc Interv. 2003;59:305–11.
4. Katsuragawa M, Fujiwara H, Miyamae M, Sasayama S. Histologic studies in percutaneous transluminal coronary angioplasty for chronic total occlusion: comparison of tapering and abrupt types of occlusion and short and long occluded segments. J Am Coll Cardiol. 1993;21:604–11.
5. Kaneda H, Saito S, Shiono T, Miyashita Y, Takahashi S, Domae H. Sixty-four-slice computed tomography-facilitated percutaneous coronary intervention for chronic total occlusion. Int J Cardiol. 2007;115:130–2.
6. Hirokami M, Saito S, Muto H. Anchoring technique to improve guiding catheter support in coronary angioplasty of chronic total occlusions. Catheter Cardiovasc Interv. 2006;67:366–71.
7. Fujita S, Tamai H, Kyo E, Kosuga K, Hata T, Okada M, Nakamura T, Tsuji T, Takeda S, Bin Hu F, Masunaga N, Motohara S, Uehata H. New technique for superior guiding catheter support during advancement of a balloon in coronary angioplasty: the anchor technique. Catheter Cardiovasc Interv. 2003;59:482–8.
8. Takahashi S, Saito S, et al. New method to increase a backup support of a 6 French guiding coronary catheter. Catheter Cardiovasc Interv. 2004;63:452–6.
9. Takeshita S, Shishido K, Sugitatsu K, Okamura N, Mizuno S, Yaginuma K, Suenaga H, Tanaka Y, Matsumi J, Takahashi S, Saito S. In vitro and human studies of a 4F double-coaxial technique ("mother-child" configuration) to facilitate stent implantation in resistant coronary vessels. Circ Cardiovasc Interv. 2011;4:155–61.
10. Shishido K, Takeshita S, Tanaka Y, Saito S. The 4 Fr mother-child technique with side-branch protection for treatment of complex bifurcation lesions. EuroIntervention. 2012;8:634–7.
11. Saito S. Open Sesame Technique for chronic total occlusion. Catheter Cardiovasc Interv. 2010;75:690–4.
12. Saito S. Different strategies of retrograde approach in coronary angioplasty for chronic total occlusion. Catheter Cardiovasc Interv. 2008;71:8–19.
13. Kaneda H, Takahashi S, Saito S. Successful coronary intervention for chronic total occlusion in an anomalous right coronary artery using the retrograde approach via a collateral vessel. J Invasive Cardiol. 2007;19:E1–4.
14. Taketani Y, Kaneda H, Saito S. Successful coronary intervention for chronic total occlusion using a retrograde approach with biradial arteries. J Invasive Cardiol. 2007;19:E281–4.
15. Matsumi J, Adachi K, Saito S. A unique complication of the retrograde approach in angioplasty for chronic total occlusion of the coronary artery. Catheter Cardiovasc Interv. 2008;72:371–8.
16. Matsubara T, Murata A, et al. IVUS-guided wiring technique: promising approach for the chronic total occlusion. Catheter Cardiovasc Interv. 2004;61(3):81–6.
17. Matsumi J, Saito S. Progress in the retrograde approach for chronic total coronary artery occlusion: a case with successful angioplasty using CART and reverse-anchoring techniques 3 years after failed PCI via a retrograde approach. Catheter Cardiovasc Interv. 2008;71:810–4.
18. Tanaka Y, Takeshita S, Takahashi S, Matsumi J, Mizuno S, Yamanaka F, Sugitatsu K, Nomura Y, Imori Y, Shishido K, Tobita K, Saito S. Comparison of short- and long-term outcomes of percutaneous coronary intervention for chronic total occlusions between patients aged ≥75 years and those aged <75 years. Am J Cardiol. 2013;112:761–6.

Special Technique and Case Illustrations of CTO Intervention via Transradial Approach

19

Ramesh Daggubati, Dan Le, and Pierfrancesco Agostoni

Abstract

Part 1: Bilateral Transradial Approach for Chronic Total Occlusion Percutaneous Coronary Interventions

Chronic total occlusion is a well-known challenge for interventional cardiologists and it occurs in approximately 30–50 % of all patients with significant coronary stenosis (Christofferson, et al. Am J Cardiol 95:1088–91, 2005). Transradial coronary intervention (TRI) is growing in the United States and has become a worldwide popular approach. The reasons for this increased use of the TRI have been broadly published and include lower risk of access site complications, early mobilization, increased patient comfort, lower costs, and hence shortening of hospital stay compared to the traditional transfemoral intervention (TFI) (Lotan, et al. Transradial approach for coronary angiography and angioplasty. Am J Cardiol 76:164–7, 1995).

The purpose of this chapter is to discover the opportunity that the bilateral transradial approach (TRA) can offer in the CTO interventions.

Part 2: Single Transradial Guiding Catheter for Retrograde Recanalization of Left Coronary Artery Chronic Total Occlusions with Ipsilateral Collaterals

Coronary chronic total occlusions (CTO) are challenging in interventional cardiology. The most common cause of procedural failure in percutaneous coronary intervention (PCI) for CTO is the inability to cross the CTO lesion with the wire. The developments in technology and material and new techniques developed to perform PCI via retrograde collaterals have definitely improved the success rate of CTO PCI. In order to pass the retrograde channels, multiple arterial puncture sites are frequently needed. The routine is to perform these procedures using large guiding catheters (7–8 French [F]) via a bilateral femoral approach. Moreover, the bifemoral approach is commonly used also due to the perception of reduced guiding catheter support from the radial approach. Radial approach and downsizing in retrograde CTO PCI appears challenging. However, a number of publications has demonstrated the feasibility of radial approach for CTO PCI even with retrograde approach using a biradial access). Besides, some CTO present **ipsilateral collaterals**. In these **selected anatomies**, the procedure may be simplified using a single catheter for both antegrade and retrograde approach. In these **selected anatomies**, one single six French transradial guiding catheter can be used to perform retrograde recanalization of left sided CTO via ipsilateral epicardial or septal collateral channels. The following case series confirms this.

R. Daggubati, MD, FACC, FSCAI (✉) • D. Le, MD
Brody School of Medicine East Carolina University, Greenville, NC, USA
e-mail: daggubatir@ecu.edu

P. Agostoni, MD, PhD (✉)
Department of Cardiology, St. Antonius Hospital, Nieuwegein, The Netherlands
e-mail: agostonipf@gmail.com

Y. Zhou et al. (eds.), *Transradial Approach for Percutaneous Interventions*, DOI 10.1007/978-94-017-7350-8_19

19.1 Part 1: Bilateral Transradial Approach for Chronic Total Occlusion Percutaneous Coronary Interventions

19.1.1 Definition

Coronary chronic total occlusion (CTO) was defined as a lesion with total occlusion exhibiting a Thrombolysis in Myocardial Infarction (TIMI) flow grade 0 in a native vessel for more than 3 months. Estimation of the occlusion duration was based on first onset of anginal symptoms, prior history of myocardial infarction in the target vessel territory, or comparison with a prior angiogram. The lesion length was measured from the total occlusion site to the collateral flow, or the length of significant stenosis after predilatation. Procedure success was defined as wiring across the CTO lesion with a resultant residual diameter stenosis <30 % and TIMI 3 flow following angioplasty or stenting without any major cardiovascular complications. Clinical success was defined as successful percutaneous coronary intervention (PCI) with the patient discharged alive.

19.1.2 Advantages of TRA for CTO Interventions

As radial artery is in superficial location, easy access, compressibility, easy control of bleeding, somewhat isolation from adjacent veins, and dual palmar blood supply; hence, the most vascular complications seen with the TFA, such as access-site bleeding, pseudoaneurysms, arteriovenous fistulas, and limb ischemia are markedly decreased with the TRA [3].

In the patient with common femoral artery disease, TRA avoids excessive manipulation of catheters in atherosclerotic aortas through a diseased femoral artery, and the potential complications at the TFA site.

Finally, using TRA patient comfort is superior by the ability to sit up and ambulate early after the procedure that also reduces potential complications and expenses.

Therefore, patients undergoing CTO interventions would benefit from TRA. However, it has not yet been established with large randomized trials.

19.1.3 Disadvantages of TRA for CTO Interventions

Small radial artery size, arterial spasm, anatomic variants, and severe tortuosity may make procedural challenges for advancement of guide catheter. As the radial artery has high spasm tendency, patient must receive spasmolytic cocktails and well sedation during procedures. TRA for CTO PCI was associated with similar success and complication rates as transfemoral but with longer procedural and fluoroscopy times [4].

Guiding catheter (GC) size is one of the major limitations of TRI. In general population, the average diameter of the upper end of the RA at styloid process is 2.7 mm [5], so a 6-Fr (outer diameter 2.6 mm) sheath is predominantly used for TRI. However, complex lesions like CTO may require the use of a larger GC (7 or 8 Fr). Of note, several benefits of using large GCs in CTO PCI such as accommodation of two guide-wires or two microcatheters, application of balloon anchoring technique, and better back-up support have been known [6].

TRA for CTO intervention requires different strategies such as a retrograde approach, crossing collateral channels, kissing guiding wires, controlled antegrade and retrograde subintimal tracking (CART) or reverse CART, and techniques like the use of an anchoring balloon and a reverse anchoring balloon [7]. All these techniques may increase the final success rate to 84 % [8]. The use of equipment such as IVUS and rotablator also contributes to the success of CTO interventions [8]. These techniques and devices usually require a larger diameter GC (7 Fr), but a TRA with a routine sheath system may limit the GC size, especially in females and Asians.

19.1.4 Transradial Approach for Chronic Total Occlusion Percutaneous Coronary Interventions: Technical Aspects

19.1.4.1 General Considerations

The forearm and hand of the selected side were shaved and stabilized and the skin area around the selected puncture site was sterilized and anesthetized. A 6 Fr radial artery sheath was inserted into the radial artery using the Seldinger technique. Patient must receive spasmolytic cocktails and well sedation during procedures to prevent arterial spasm. On insertion of the sheath, 5000 units of heparin were routinely administered. After the diagnostic procedure, an additional bolus of 5000 units of heparin was administered just before starting PCI.

Engagement of the left coronary artery (LCA) or right coronary artery (RCA) for diagnostic angiography was generally attempted using a Kimny mini guiding catheter (Boston Scientific, Natick, MA, U.S.A.), because a single Kimny catheter can be used to engage either the LCA or RCA orifice and can also serve as a guiding catheter for PCI. If further support was required during PCI, the Kimny guiding catheter was replaced with another guiding catheter.

There are numerous techniques for CTO PCI including simultaneous contralateral coronary angiography, double guidewire technique and five in six guiding catheter technique. Thus, different guiding catheters, guidewires (soft, stiff, hydrophilic, Miracle series, and tapering tip guidewires), supporting catheters and over-the-wire (OTW) balloons were used. However, decisions on how to cross the CTO lesion and selection of the equipment were at the discretion of the individual operator.

TRA for CTO intervention is represented by the need of GC back up to push wires, microcatheters and balloons across the occlusive lesion. The "passive" back up is the support offered by the GC itself and is increased with increasing GC size. Of difference compared to femoral operators, TRA interventional cardiologists use to gain the maximal "active" backup from the usually smaller GC.

The procedure should be stopped in the following circumstances such as use of excessive contrast medium; prolonged procedure time; patient intolerance; failure of a guidewire, balloon, or stent to cross the lesion despite optimal support; or complications (e.g., false lumen wiring, perforation, extravasation, tamponade or unstable hemodynamics).

19.1.4.2 Technical Aspects

The radial approach is associated with some specific technical characteristics that make the PCI procedure quite different from the femoral approach for CTO intervention. The main differences are related to the knowledge of materials and the familiarity with the technique of "active" guiding catheter support, owing to the need to use smaller guiding catheters than for the transfemoral approach.

19.1.5 Gaining Active Backup By the Guiding Catheter Using Transradial Approach

Placing large GCs in the radial artery may be feasible, but large sheaths may not be and may increase the risk of radial artery damage and postcatheterization occlusion [9]. As a consequence, the interventional cardiologist adopting TRA for CTO usually tries to gain the maximal 'active' backup from small GCs and reserves the usage of large GCs only for the specific techniques that require bulky materials.

To achieve the best active support, it is important to select the best radial artery entry site (the left radial artery is better for right coronary artery CTO and the right radial artery is better for left coronary artery CTO) for extra backup GC shapes, a strong support.

Furthermore, when selecting the GC shape, it should be recognized that, even if "passive" backup is always higher by TFA, some GC shapes (e.g., Ikari and Amplatz Left) have been demonstrated to have a smaller difference in provided support by radial or femoral approaches compared with other curves (e.g., Judkins family) [10].

During the GC selection for TRA CTO PCI, an important point is to look for the possibility of having shapes suitable for the deep intubation technique [11]. Actually, deep intubation may allow very strong support in specific phases of the CTO PCI (e.g., balloon crossing of the lesion) and may be facilitated by the selection of smaller GCs with smoother curves (e.g., JR 4 for deep intubation on the right coronary artery).

It should be highlighted that specific devices have been designed to improve the support of small sized GC. Among these, the "five in six technique" (or "mother and child technique") has been reported to be effective in the setting of CTO interventions [12]. This technique is facilitated by the availability of specifically designed 5 Fr GC compatible with 6 Fr GC (Heartrail Terumo). Of note, the use of such devices may be facilitated by less complex guiding catheter curves (e.g., JR 4 instead of Amplatz for RCA CTO).

Finally, when deep intubation is not feasible (e.g., in CTOs close to the coronary ostia or CTOs located downstream of severe, diffuse disease of the proximal coronary segment), the GC may be stabilized using the anchoring balloon technique [13].

The retrograde approach for PCI of CTO has helped to improve the success rate. It is usually performed through collateral connections that originate from the contralateral coronary artery to the occluded one and by using two arterial accesses and two guiding catheters.

Over the past few years, both the miniaturization of CTO-dedicated devices and the tremendous improvement of techniques for complex PCI have largely improved the success rate of CTO intervention by using bilateral transradial approach [14].

19.1.6 Bilateral Transradial Approach for Retrograde Techniques

The feasibility of the bilateral radial approach for CTO PCI with a retrograde technique using a 6 Fr (or 7 Fr) GC for antegrade artery and a 6 Fr (or 7 Fr) GC for retrograde artery with a success rate of approximately 80.6 % without any in-hospital major adverse cardiac events [15].

The retrograde approach requires a special step in which a wire is passed retrogradely through the collateral channels with the support of a small size balloon or a microcatheter until it reaches the distal end of the CTO (Figs. 19.1–19.4). The presence of suitable collateral is the key to the success of this approach.

19.1.7 Conclusion

Use of bilateral transradial approach for CTO PCI is safe and feasible and there are several advantages, beyond the well-established lower risk of post-procedural bleeding, but requires a specific learning phase and careful case selection. Compared with the transfemoral approach, the transradial approach for CTO PCI has an equally high success rate; thus, bilateral transradial approach for CTO PCI should be

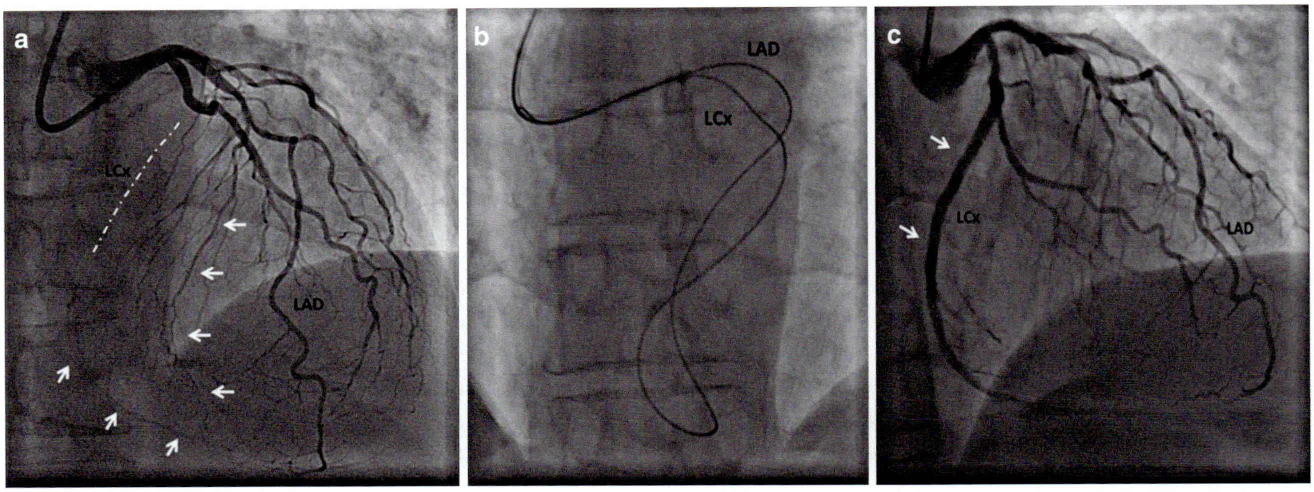

Fig. 19.1 (**a**) Chronic total occlusion (*CTO*) of a dominant left Circumflex (*LCx*) artery (*dotted line*) with retrograde septal collaterals from the left anterior descending (*LAD*) artery (*white arrow*). (**b**) Externalization of the 330 mm RG3 wire. The Corsair microcatheter makes a loop back to the guiding catheter through the septal collaterals. (**c**) Final result after successful recanalization of the CTO (*white arrow*)

considered first. If this approach fails due to poor back up support from the guiding catheter, the transfemoral approach can be attempted with a larger guiding catheter.

19.1.8 Future Perspective

The upcoming improvements of miniaturized angioplasty equipment for TRA CTO PCI will allow an extension of the number of techniques that can be performed through small sheaths. Both GCs and wire–balloon systems are undergoing a miniaturization process.

19.2 Part 2: Single Transradial Guiding Catheter for Retrograde Recanalization of Left Coronary Artery Chronic Total Occlusions with Ipsilateral Collaterals

Case 1

A woman with a non-ST elevation myocardial infarction after orthopedic surgery underwent a coronary angiogram showing a CTO of the dominant Left Circumflex (LCx) artery in its distal segment, just after a large marginal branch, and a severe lesion of the mid Left anterior descending (LAD) artery. The proximal cap of the CTO was ambiguous (blunt stump), meanwhile significant retrograde septal collaterals to the distal LCx were noticed from the LAD (Fig. 19.1a). The heart-team decided to aim at complete revascularization, in first instance via a percutaneous approach. A direct retrograde approach to tackle the LCx CTO was attempted. A Sion Blue wire supported by a 150 cm Corsair microcatheter was passed through the septal channels into the distal LCx. The occlusion was then passed with a Pilot 200 wire. The Corsair microcatheter was then advanced up to the guiding catheter, making a loop out of it (Fig. 19.1b). Then a 330 cm RG3 wire was externalized. The Corsair microcatheter was then removed and the procedure was successfully completed via the antegrade route on the RG3 wire, with implantation of two overlapping drug eluting stents (Fig. 19.1c). The patient was subsequently treated also in the LAD with success.

Case 2

A man with history of previous anterior myocardial infarction presented with angina pectoris and anteroseptal inducible ischemia around the old infarcted area. The coronary angiogram showed single vessel disease with CTO in the mid-LAD and retrograde epicardial collaterals from a large obtuse marginal (OM) artery. There was a clear proximal stump at the level of the CTO (Fig. 19.2a). Antegrade approach was attempted with a Sion Blue wire and microcatheter support. However, the wire went into a diagonal artery and the distal part of the CTO was not crossed. A retrograde approach was directly attempted. A Pilot 200 wire successfully passed via the OM and the epicardial collaterals to the apical LAD and a 150 cm Corsair microcatheter was advanced through this way. The LAD CTO was successfully passed using a Miracle 12 wire. Then the Corsair microcatheter was advanced up to the left main. It was then possible to externalize a 330 cm RG3 wire (Fig. 19.2b). In order to exchange the RG3 wire for a normal antegrade wire, two FineCross microcatheters inserted from both ends of the RG3 wire were used, and the microcatheter tips "kissed" at the distal part of the target vessel. It was possible to remove the RG3 wire via the retrograde collaterals, protected by the retrograde FineCross microcatheter, and the antegrade channel was preserved by the antegrade FineCross microcatheter. An Extra-support wire was inserted via the antegrade microcatheter and the LAD was successfully treated with four overlapping drug eluting stents (Fig. 19.2c).

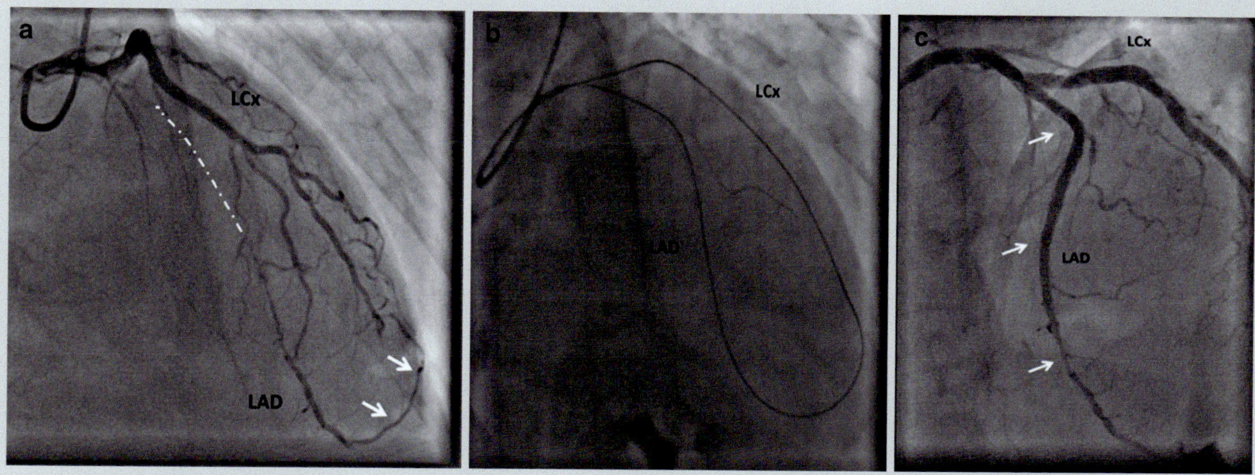

Fig. 19.2 (**a**) Chronic total occlusion (*CTO*) of the proximal left anterior descending (*LAD*) artery (*dotted line*) with retrograde epicardial collaterals from the left circumflex (*LCx*) artery through a large obtuse marginal branch (*white arrow*). (**b**) Externalization of the 330 mm RG3 wire. The Corsair microcatheter makes a loop almost back to the guiding catheter through the epicardial collaterals. (**c**) Final result after successful recanalization of the CTO (*white arrow*)

Case 3

A man with history of previous myocardial infarction and previous PCI of the left main-Ramus intermedius (RI) branch, known CTO of the mid-LAD and reduced left ventricular function, presented with out-of-hospital cardiac arrest. An implantable cardioverter-defibrillator (ICD) was implanted for secondary prevention. A magnetic resonance imaging, performed before ICD implantation, showed a large area of viability in the anterior wall. The coronary angiogram showed a patent stent in the left main-RI and the known mid-LAD CTO with retrograde epicardial collaterals from the RI. The proximal entry stump of the LAD CTO was ambiguous due to a septal branch at this level (Fig. 19.3a). Direct retrograde approach was chosen. A Sion Blue wire was brought to the distal LAD via the retrograde collaterals followed by a 150 cm Corsair microcatheter. A Miracle six wire successfully passed the CTO lesion. The Corsair was then advanced from the distal LAD up to the guiding catheter (Fig. 19.3b), then a 330 cm RG3 wire was externalized. The procedure was successfully concluded with implantation of two drug eluting stents from the ostium of the LAD (T-stenting technique with the old left main-RI stent) up to the mid-segment. Final kissing balloon was performed in the left main-LAD-RI with two balloons over the antegrade and retrograde part of the same RG3 wire. The final angiogram showed a good result and no damage of the collaterals (Fig. 19.3c).

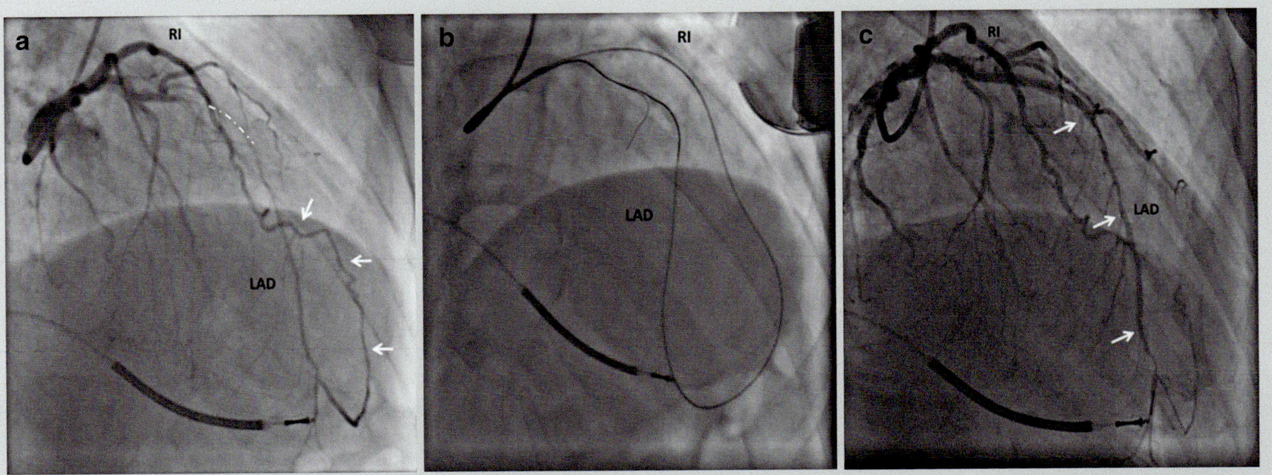

Fig. 19.3 (**a**) Chronic total occlusion (*CTO*) of the mid-left anterior descending (*LAD*) artery (*dotted line*) with retrograde epicardial collaterals from the ramus intermedius (*RI*) branch (*white arrow*). (**b**) Externalization of the 330 mm RG3 wire. The Corsair microcatheter makes a loop back to the guiding catheter through the epicardial collaterals. (**c**) Final result after successful recanalization of the CTO (*white arrow*)

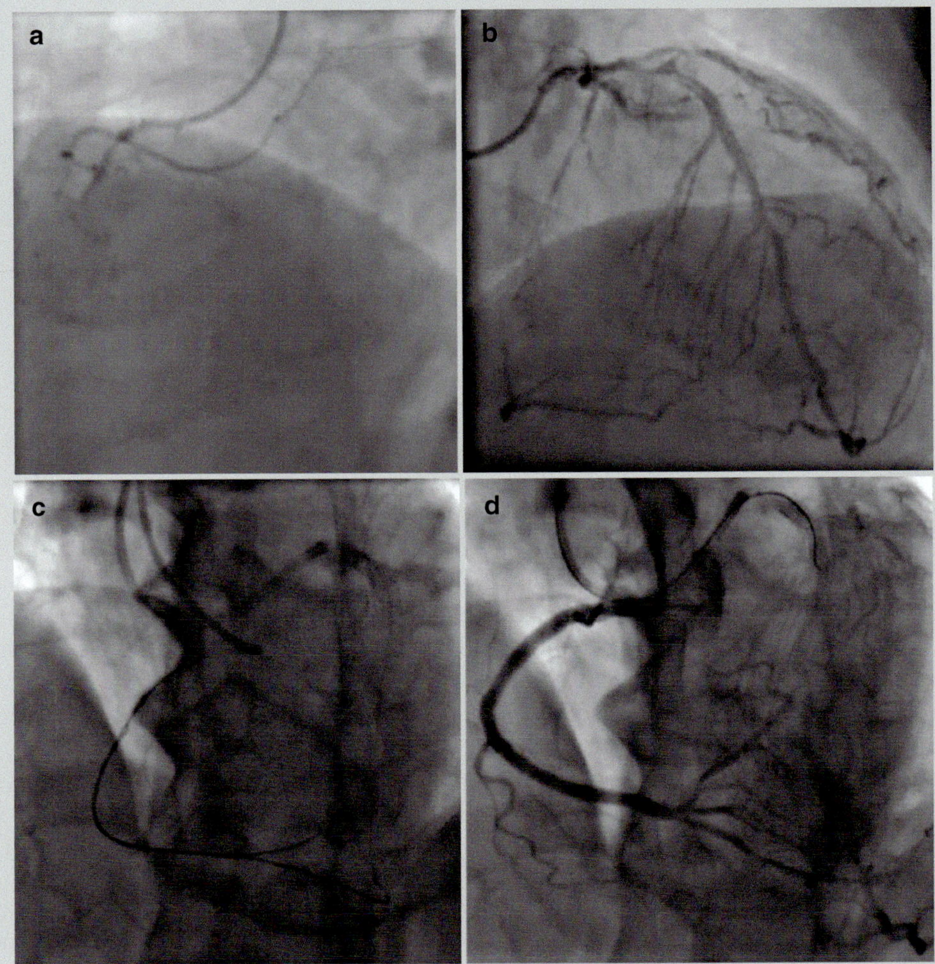

Fig. 19.4 Bilateral TRA for RCA CTO PCI. (**a**) Proximal RCA CTO. (**b**) Collaterals from LCA. (**c**) A miracle 6 guidewire passed antegrade into PDA using OTW anchoring balloon at proximal RCA and guided by the retrograde wire. (**d**) Final angiography after stenting showed good result

19.2.1 In Summary

Our case series support the concept of using a single guiding catheter for radial approach for **selected** left coronary artery CTO lesions with **ipsilateral collaterals**. It should be kept in mind that the 6 F guiding catheter, due to its small caliber, cannot accommodate all the needed tools after placement of the Corsair microcatheter. The Corsair microcatheter needs to be removed to give space to other devices needed to complete the procedure successfully. One solution is to complete the procedure with a single RG3 wire with both ends being externalized from the same guiding, and this gives also good support. A microcatheter should be reinserted via the retrograde channel after completion of the procedure for protection of the retrograde vessel during removal of RG3 wire. Otherwise, exchange of the externalized wire with an antegrade wire to complete the procedure is also an option. In conclusion, in **selected** CTO anatomies with **ipsilateral collaterals**, a retrograde recanalization procedure can be performed with a single 6 F guiding catheter through the radial approach.

References

1. Christofferson RD, Lehmann KG, Martin GV, Every N, JH C- w, Kapadia SR. Effect of chronic total coronary occlu- sion on treatment strategy. Am J Cardiol. 2005;95:1088–91.
2. Lotan C, Hasin Y, Mosseri M, et al. Transradial approach for coronary angiography and angioplasty. Am J Cardiol. 1995;76:164–7.
3. Jolly SS, Yusuf S, Cairns J, et al. Radial versus femoral access for coronary angiography and intervention in patients with acute coronary syndromes (RIVAL): a randomized, parallel group, multicenter trial. Lancet. 2011;377:1409–20.
4. Alaswad K, Menon RV, Christopoulos G, et al. Transradial approach for coronary chronic total occlusion interventions: insights from a contemporary multicenter registry. Catheter Cardiovasc Interv. 2015;85(7):1123–9.
5. Chang TS, Zhu SX, Wang ZC. Forearm flap transplant. In: Chang TS, editor. Principles, techniques and applications in microsurgery. Sigapore: World Scientific; 1986.
6. Ungvari T, Hoye A. Percutaneous Treatment of Chronic Total Occlusion. Catheter-Based Cardiovascular Interventions Springer Berlin Heidelberg; 2013:593–609.
7. Saito S. Different strategies of retrograde approach in coronary angioplasty for chronic total occlusion. Catheter Cardiovasc Interv. 2008;71:8–19.4.
8. Wu CJ, Fang HY, Cheng CI, Hussein H, Abdou SM, Youssef AA, Bhasin A, Yang CH, Chen CJ, Hsieh YK, Yip HK, Fang CY. The safety and feasibility of bilateral radial approach in chronic total occlusion percutaneous coronary intervention. Int Heart J. 2011;52:131–8.
9. Saito S, Ikei H, Hosokawa G, Tanaka S. In uence of the ratio between radial artery inner diameter and sheath outer diameter on radial artery ow after transradial coronary intervention. Catheter Cardiovasc Interv. 1999;46(2):173–8.
10. Ikari Y, Masuda N, Matsukage T, et al. Backup force of guiding catheters for the right coronary artery in transfemoral and transradial interventions. J Invasive Cardiol. 2009;21(11):570–4.
11. Saito S, Tanaka S, Hiroe Y, et al. Angioplasty for chronic total occlusion $_{25}$ by using tapered-tip guidewires. Catheter Cardiovasc Interv. 2003;59(3):305–11.
12. Takahashi S, Saito S, Tanaka S, et al. New method to increase a backup support of a 6 French guiding coronary catheter. Catheter Cardiovasc Interv. 2004;63(4):452–6.
13. Hirokami M, Saito S, Muto H. Anchoring technique to improve guiding catheter support in coronary angioplasty of chronic total occlusions. Catheter Cardiovasc Interv. 2006;67(3):366–71.
14. Galassi AR, Tomasello SD, Reifart N, et al. In-hospital outcomes of percutaneous coronary intervention in patients with chronic total occlusion: insights from the ERCTO (European Registry of Chronic Total Occlusion) registry. EuroIntervention. 2011;7(4):472–9.
15. Wu CJ. Feasibility of bilateral radial access antegrade and retrograde approach for CTO lesions: single center experience. Presented at: Transcatheter Cardiovascular Therapeutics 2008. Washington, DC, USA, 12 Oct 2008.

Transradial Approach for Calcified and Tortuous Lesions

20

Kenji Wagatsuma

Abstract

The size of the guiding catheter (GC) commonly used in transradial coronary intervention (TRI) is 6 Fr or smaller. Since this size inevitably provides less backup support than a 7Fr or 8 Fr GC, even in institutions that have taken up TRI, operators may often select transfemoral coronary intervention (TFI) over TRI for procedures requiring sufficient backup support because it facilitates the use of large diameter GCs.

Calcified and tortuous lesions—the topic of this manuscript—are representative of lesions that often require strong GC backup support. In order to treat such lesions through TRI, operators would need to master several techniques that are key to achieving backup support of 6Fr.GCs equal to or better than that of 7 Fr GCs.

In the following sections, proper understanding of GC selection and, moreover, the techniques that could be powerful tools in achieving GC backup support in the treatment of severely calcified lesions and tortuous lesions by TRI, will be briefly explained while citing cases. Unless otherwise noted, all of the case studies presented here are TRI cases that were conducted with a 6 Fr GC.

20.1 Basic GC Selection

Regarding the size and shape of the GC, although this is not without exception as it also depends on the policy of the operator, 6 Fr GCs are generally the global standard for TRI, with 6 Fr believed to be the most widely used GC size in TRI. In recent years, centering in Japan, GCs with outer diameters of 5 Fr or smaller have been clinically introduced, but there are still technical limitations in the use of GCs of 5 Fr or smaller, and, moreover, the backup support provided by these GCs themselves are, in general, considerably inferior to that of 6 Fr GCs. But, on the other hand, from the fact that small diameter GCs provide ease in performing the deep engagement technique (to be explained later), it is believed that with the appropriate selection of cases, these small diameter GCs could be used to treat calcified lesions and tortuous lesions as well. However, in general terms, it is felt that a 6 Fr GC should be used in the treatment of such lesions.

With regard to the shape of the GC, more backup support than that of the common Judkins type GC can be achieved if an extra back-up type, namely a long-tip GC or Amplatz type, is used to engage the LCA, and if the Amplatz type is used for the RCA. However, when the deep engagement technique, as explained in the next section, is necessary, the Amplatz type GC would not only be difficult to use but its shape could also easily damage the ostium of the coronary artery. Therefore, we primarily use an extra back-up type GC for the LCA, and in over 90 % of RCA cases, regardless of calcification or tortuosity of the lesion, we use Wave 3S (Terumo, Heartrail II), a long-tip GC with a special 3-dimensional shape that we developed (Fig. 20.1). A long-tip GC can easily be used for the deep engagement technique when necessary, and on the other hand, it also provides a certain extent of back-up support in conventional engagement.

In PCI, it is important to achieve coaxiality of the GC and coronary artery in order to gain backup support. But there was no optimal GC to use in cases presenting difficulty in

K. Wagatsuma, MD, PhD, FACC, FSCAI, FESC,FAPSC
Tsukuba Heart Center, Tsukuba Memorial Hospital, Tsukuba, Ibaraki, Japan
e-mail: thc-wagatsuma@tsukuba-kinen.or.jp

Y. Zhou et al. (eds.), *Transradial Approach for Percutaneous Interventions*, DOI 10.1007/978-94-017-7350-8_20

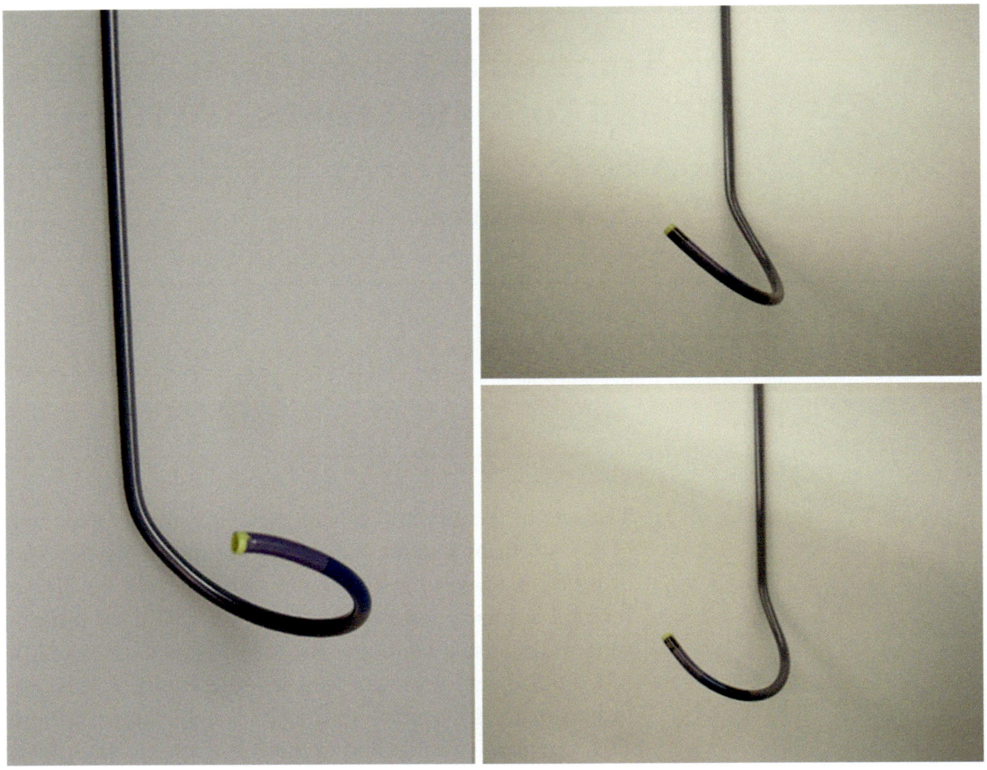

Fig. 20.1 Configuration of the Wave 3S (Terumo, Heartrail II)

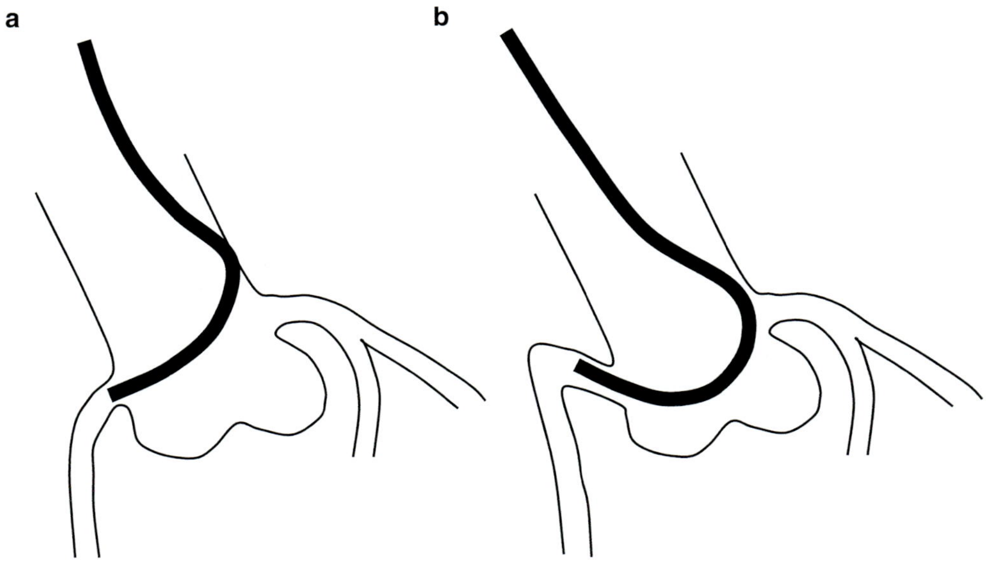

Fig. 20.2 Wave 3S coaxiality by difference in RCA origin as viewed from the left anterior oblique view. (**a**) Low takeoff. (**b**) High takeoff

engagement because of, in particular, the many varieties in origin and course of the RCA compared to the LCA, and moreover, in the case of TRI, reasons such as tortuosity of the subclavian artery. This was the situation behind the development of the Wave 3S GC. As can be seen in Fig. 20.2, this GC can be used for various takeoffs and courses of the RCA.

Because there are times when it is difficult to achieve sufficient backup support when the RCA is treated by right TRI, some operators favor treating the RCA by left TRI, and the LCA by right TRI. However, as the radial artery pulsation becomes weakened by multiple punctures, and because there are more than a few cases where it is not possible to puncture both the right and left radial arteries, it is believed that operators need to be trained to achieve backup support regardless of whether the approach is from the right or left radial artery.

In order to achieve sufficient GC backup support, a GC with a large-sized curve should generally be selected. For instance, in treatment that conventionally uses a JL4.0, if engagement using a GC with a one-size larger curve, such as a JL4.5, is possible, the second curve can touch the opposite side of the aortic wall to increase support.

20.2 Deep Engagement Technique

No matter what shape or size of GC is used, we sometimes experience cases in treatment of calcified lesions and highly tortuous lesions where stent delivery, and at times, even balloon delivery, is difficult due to insufficient backup support. As mentioned above, although TRI basically uses a 6 Fr GC, by acquiring proficiency in the deep engagement technique it would become possible to achieve stronger backup support than conventional use of a 7 Fr GC.

The deep engagement technique is often used in a tortuous RCA. In recent years, the delivery performance of balloons and stents have improved, and also small diameter inner catheters are able to reach deeper into the coronary artery using the mother-child catheter technique, which will be explained later. Due to these reasons, the employment of extreme deep engagement (Fig. 20.3) is decreasing. In general, in the deep engagement technique, after crossing a guidewire, the GC is advanced into the coronary artery while a balloon is inflated to provide anchoring. Because this poses the risk of dissection at the coronary ostium, it would be important to identify the coronary artery's characteristics, course and morphology. When there is a stenosis at the coronary ostium, the operator may start by implanting a stent, which could make it easier to deeply engage the catheter, but on the other hand, the proximal stent could hamper distal stent delivery.

20.3 Parallel Wire Technique

The parallel wire technique is a conventional technique that is used when difficulty is encountered in device delivery during the treatment of tortuous lesions and calcified lesions. With only the additional insertion of a wire, the procedure itself is not a difficult one, making it an easy-to-select option when stent delivery is difficult in TRI as well. However, it must be understood that its effects are limited. It is also often effective in the tortuous lesions of flexible coronary arteries that can be straightened to some extent when a wire is inserted. On the other hand, in severely calcified lesions, this technique is often not successful even when there is no tortuosity present (Fig. 20.4).

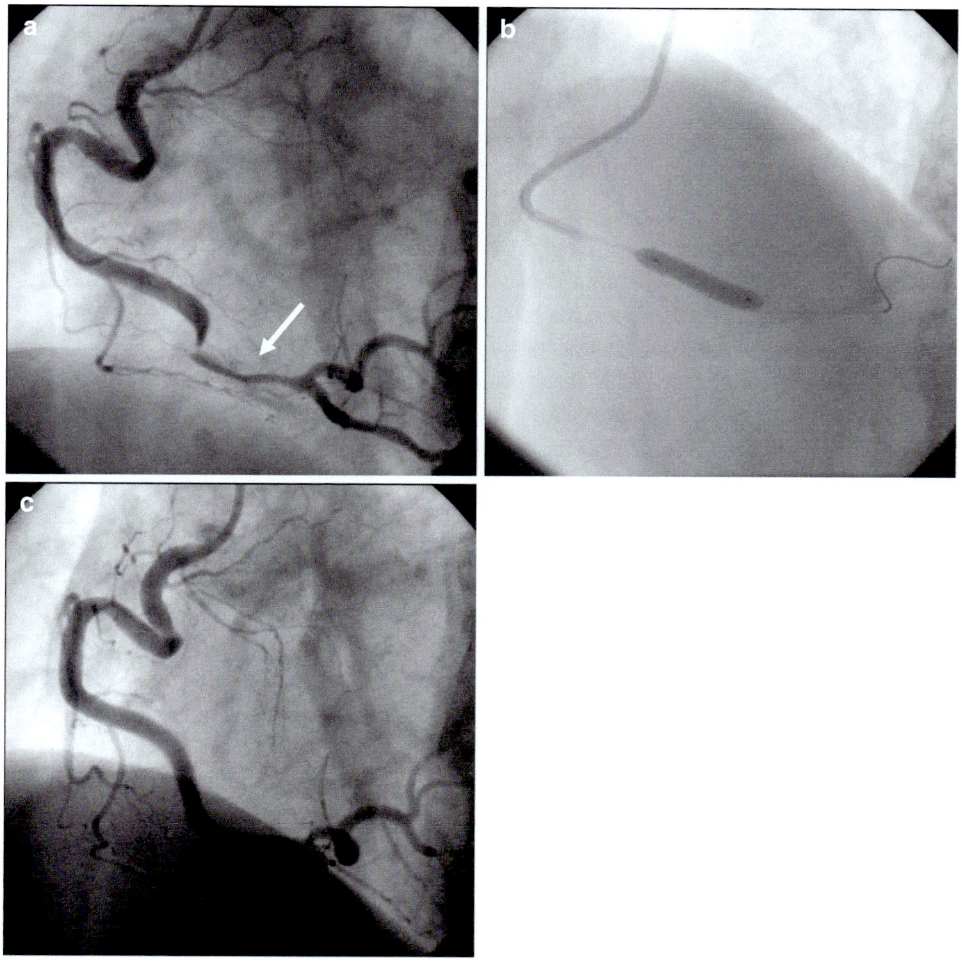

Fig. 20.3 Stent placement in a very tortuous RCA lesion through the deep engagement technique using 6Fr. Wave 3S. Severe tortuosity is seen in the proximal RCA (**a**). Through balloon anchoring, deep engagement to the mid portion of the RCA was possible (**b**). Angiogram after stent placement (**c**)

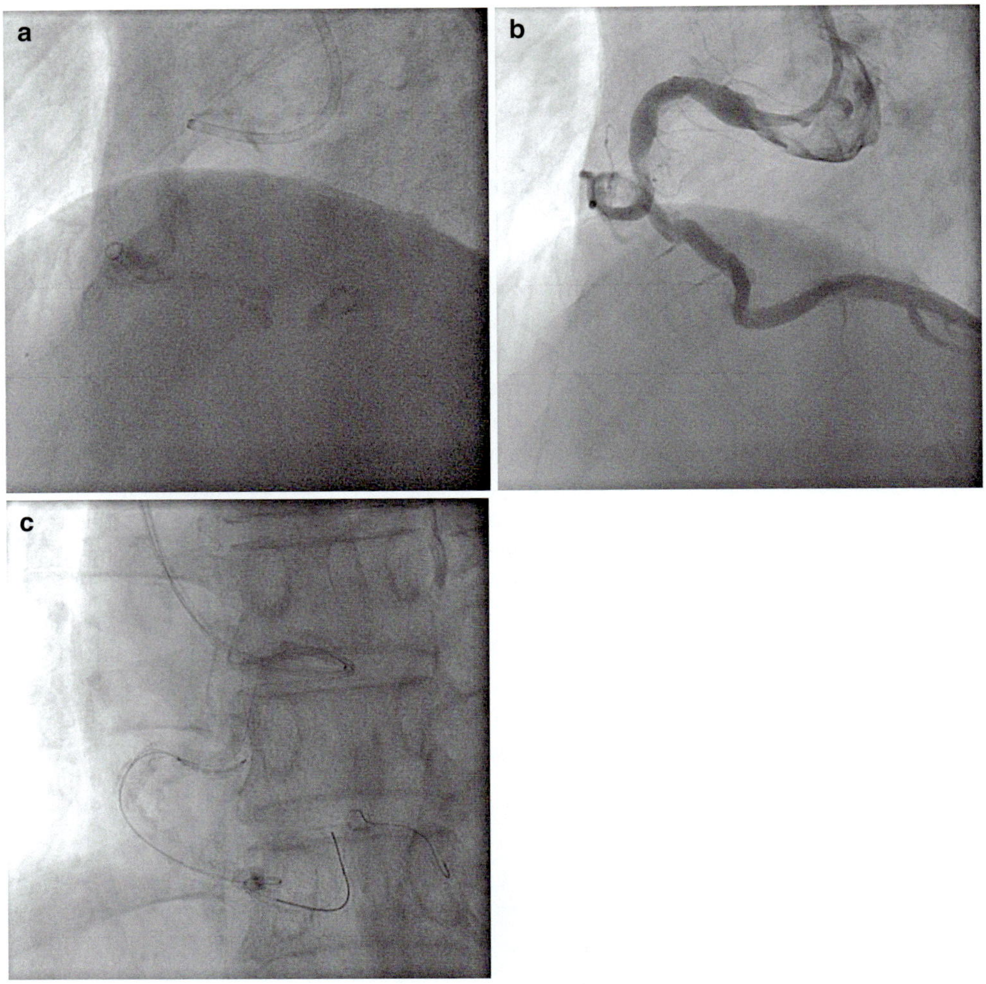

Fig. 20.4 A case where the parallel wire technique was not successful. A lesion that is both severely calcified and tortuous is seen in the mid portion of the RCA. (**a**) before contrast injection, (**b**) after contrast injection). The tortuous portion would not straighten even when using the parallel wire technique, making stent delivery extremely difficult (**c**) stacking of the stent in front of the lesion. In a case like this, another technique to increase backup support should be taken

In addition, in TRI, which often uses a 6 Fr GC with a smaller inner diameter than a 7 Fr, the effects of the parallel wire technique could be diminished through an entanglement of the wires. To prevent this from occurring, insertion of the second wire should be done with a minimum amount of torque (Fig. 20.5). This is also an extremely important cautionary point in the balloon anchoring technique, which will be explained in the next section.

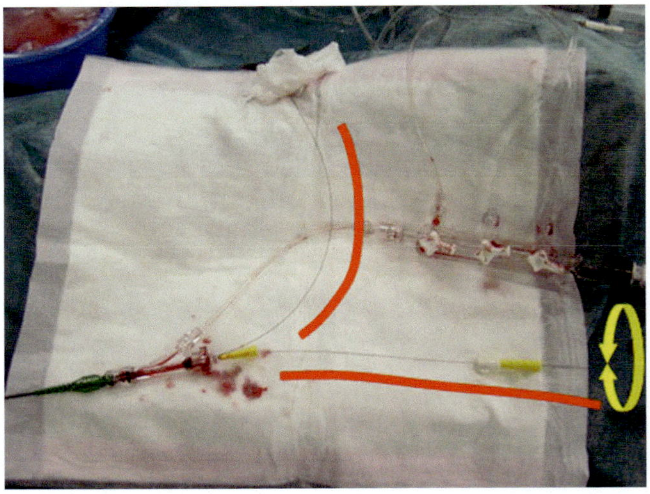

Fig. 20.5 How to prevent entanglement of guidewires in the parallel wire technique. Clearly keep the first wire separate, and anchor the wire using moist gauze. Be careful not to apply more than 360° of torque in one direction to the second wire

20.4 Balloon Anchoring Technique

The balloon anchoring technique aligns with the mother-child catheter technique (explained in the next section) as one of most effective techniques that can be taken in the treatment of severely calcified lesions and tortuous lesions by TRI, and is believed to be a technique that operators should by all means master. The procedure basically consists of inserting a wire into a side branch proximal to the target lesion, and while inflating a balloon in the side branch,

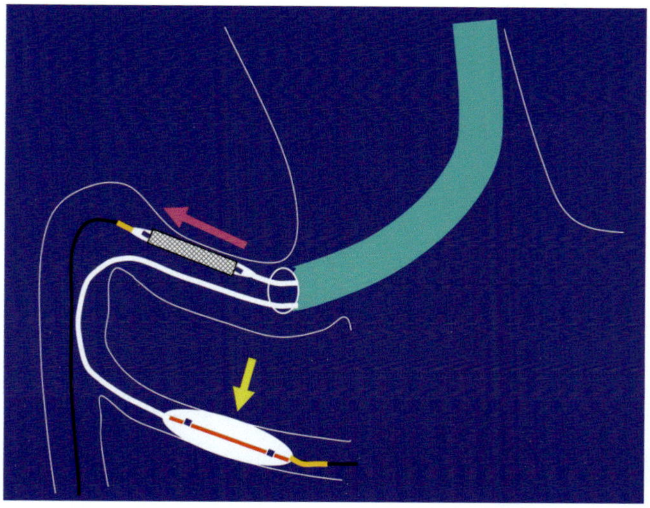

Fig. 20.6 Basic balloon anchoring technique. A wire is inserted into a side branch proximal to the target lesion, and while a balloon is inflated in the side branch, the stent (device) is advanced to the target lesion. Sufficient anchoring effects can be achieved in most cases at lower than regular inflation pressure in the side branch

advancing the stent (device) to the target lesion (Figs. 20.6 and 20.7). Even if the balloon used for anchoring is inflated at low pressures, it will be effective in most cases. Whenever possible, anchoring should take place in a section clear of lesions in order to prevent dissection in the side branch. In addition, in cases when the device cannot cross the lesion, its rebound may cause the wire in the side branch to slip deeply into the vessel, resulting in possible perforation of the vessel. Thus, the use of hydrophilic guidewires, tapering wires, and intermediate or stiffer wires as anchoring wires should be avoided whenever possible. Moreover, as was mentioned above, since entanglement of the wires will reduce the inherent effects of the balloon anchoring technique as well, insertion of the second wire must be done with a minimum amount of torque.

If there is no suitable side branch proximal to the target lesion, there are cases where it is effective to have one more wire inserted in the target vessel for anchoring in the distal portion of the target lesion (Fig. 20.8).

However, in this kind of anchoring, the shaft of the anchor balloon could hinder the passage of the device. Because of this it is often not effective in patients with small vessel diameter.

20.5 Mother-Child Catheter Technique

In 6 Fr TRI, although strong backup support can be achieved through the deep engagement technique, its indications are limited because of possible damage to the coronary ostium by the GC. There are also cases where the catheter will not be able to be inserted very deeply due to reasons including calcification at the origin of the coronary artery and the course of the artery.

The mother-child catheter technique uses a catheter that has a smaller diameter than a 6 Fr GC as an inner catheter. The GC can be inserted more deeply and more safely into the coronary artery than in the case of direct deep engagement, making this an extremely effective technique in the treatment of highly tortuous lesions and calcified lesions. Basically, a GC of 6 Fr or larger is used for the outer catheter and a straight 5 Fr or smaller GC is used for the inner catheter. We often use the 4 Fr KIWAMI (Terumo, Heartrail II) as the inner catheter (KIWAMI is approved only in Japan). Figure. 20.9 shows a 5 Fr GC (ST-01 Terumo) placed in a 6 Fr GC.

The GC used as the inner catheter is basically one that can be inserted into a 6Fr GC, and is a straight type with no curved tip, with an effective length of about 120 cm.

A hemostatic value is attached to the GC serving as the outer catheter, and the inner catheter is passed through it. If the inner catheter is to be inserted during the procedure, in order to facilitate this process, the attached Y-connector can be removed from the 3-way manifold and closed with a stopcock, and a Y-connector can be attached anew to the 5 Fr GC. This also makes it easier to reconnect the 3-way manifold to the original GC when the 5 Fr GC no longer becomes necessary. Because, however, the length of the Y-connector attached to the outer catheter equals the length that the inner catheter cannot be inserted, decision on whether or not to remove the outer catheter's Y-connector should depend on how deeply the operator wishes to insert the inner catheter. There are cases where the small diameter straight catheter generally used as the inner catheter can be deeply engaged by the support of the GC alone, but if a balloon can be inflated in the coronary artery, the balloon should first be advanced and inflated when necessary to serve as an anchor for deep engagement (Fig. 20.10). To prevent damage to the coronary artery wall by the GC tip, there is also the technique of inflating the balloon right outside the tip of the GC, and while deflating it, use it as an inserter and anchor.

An experiment has been reported to show that backup support equivalent to that of a 7 Fr GC can be achieved by just extending a 5 Fr inner catheter by about 50 mm beyond the tip of a 6 Fr GC [1]. However, generalizations on how many millimeters the inner catheter should be extended cannot be made because it will depend upon the degree of calcification or tortuosity. For instance, in the case of tortuosity near the coronary ostium, if the inner catheter can cross over this area, it would clearly be easier to deliver the stent as compared to conventional engagement using a 7 Fr GC. On the other hand, in

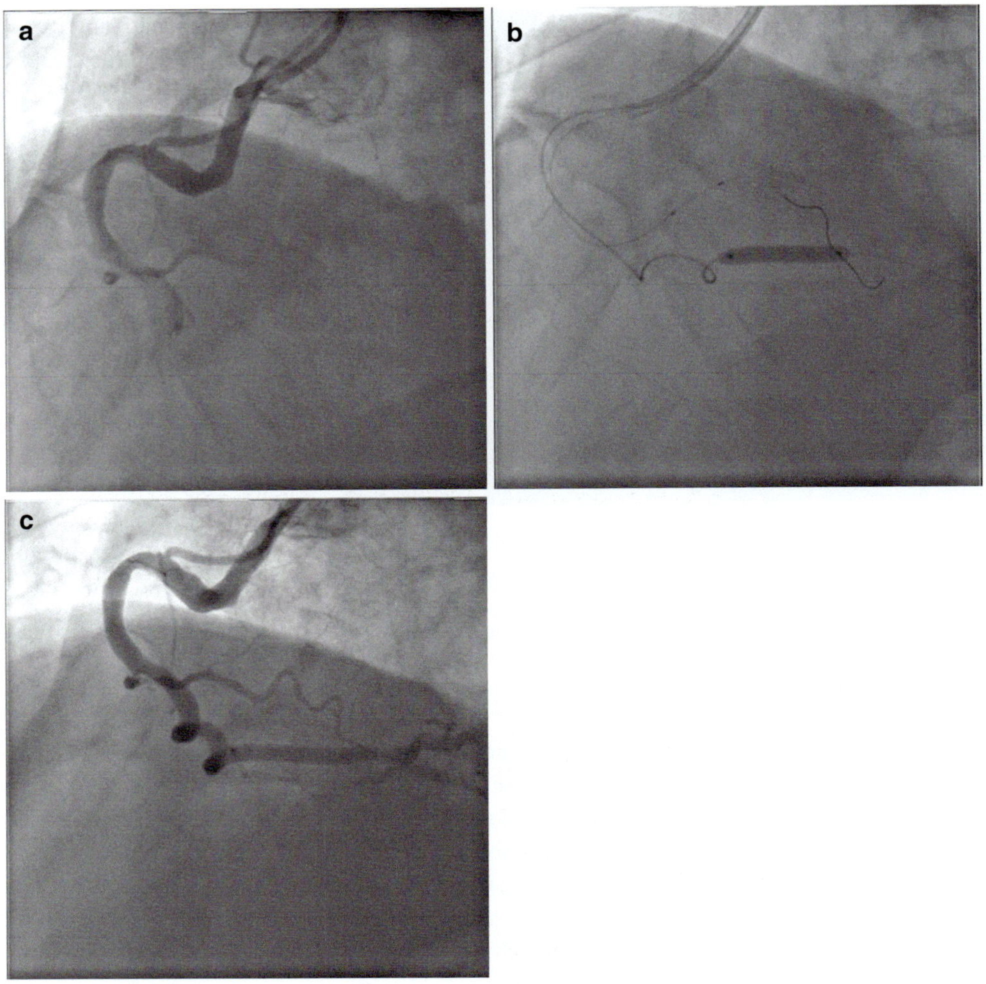

Fig. 20.7 Balloon anchoring technique in a highly tortuous RCA lesion. A total occlusion is seen in the RCA mid portion in the pre-procedure angiogram (**a**). Since it was not possible to deliver a stent by a conventional method, a 2.0 mm balloon was inflated for anchoring in the RV branch, and a Driver 3.0/18 mm was advanced to successfully cross the lesion (**b**). Final angiogram (**c**). A 7 Fr GC was used in this case. The stent delivery system that was employed had a large outer diameter that made it impossible to use a 6 Fr GC. Currently, nearly all stent delivery systems, for both DES and BMS, can be used for balloon anchoring technique through a 6 Fr. GC

severely calcified lesions, there are cases where stent delivery will be difficult unless the inner catheter is advanced beyond the lesion.

After deep engagement of the inner catheter, sufficient caution must be taken against drawing air into the coronary artery when introducing the device. Pressure dampening by the inner catheter often occurs; in other words, coronary blood flow is interrupted, and withdrawal of the balloon from the inner catheter results in negative pressure within the circuit. Pressure dampening for a short time will not be a problem if the procedure is done quickly. Indeed, there are times when the procedure is continued in the presence of dampening because backup support will, of course, be weakened if the GC is removed from its pressure dampening position. However, in such a case, since air in the circuit cannot be confirmed through backward flow from the Y connector, it must be confirmed before dampening occurs that the circuit is free of air. Moreover, extreme caution must be taken to prevent air from being drawn in when a device is introduced. Once the device has crossed the lesion, the GC is promptly removed from the pressure dampening position. If there is no dampening, or if removal of the GC from the pressure dampening position will make the next step difficult, the procedure is continued without GC removal if ischemic symptoms and hemodynamics permit. In any case, this technique must be done as quickly as possible while avoiding the admission of air into the coronary artery.

The GuideLiner catheter (Vascular Solutions, Inc.) (Fig. 20.11) has been introduced clinically as a device for use as an inner catheter [2], and its efficacy in TRI has also been reported [3]. From its structural features, it is much easier to use than a conventional inner catheter when the system is assembled during the procedure. However, since its outer diameter is larger than that of a 4 Fr GC, sufficient understanding of the device as compared to conventional small diameter GCs is necessary in using it. This includes difficulty in extreme deep engagement and the possibility that a stent might get lodged on the proximal edge of the catheter during delivery (Fig. 20.12).

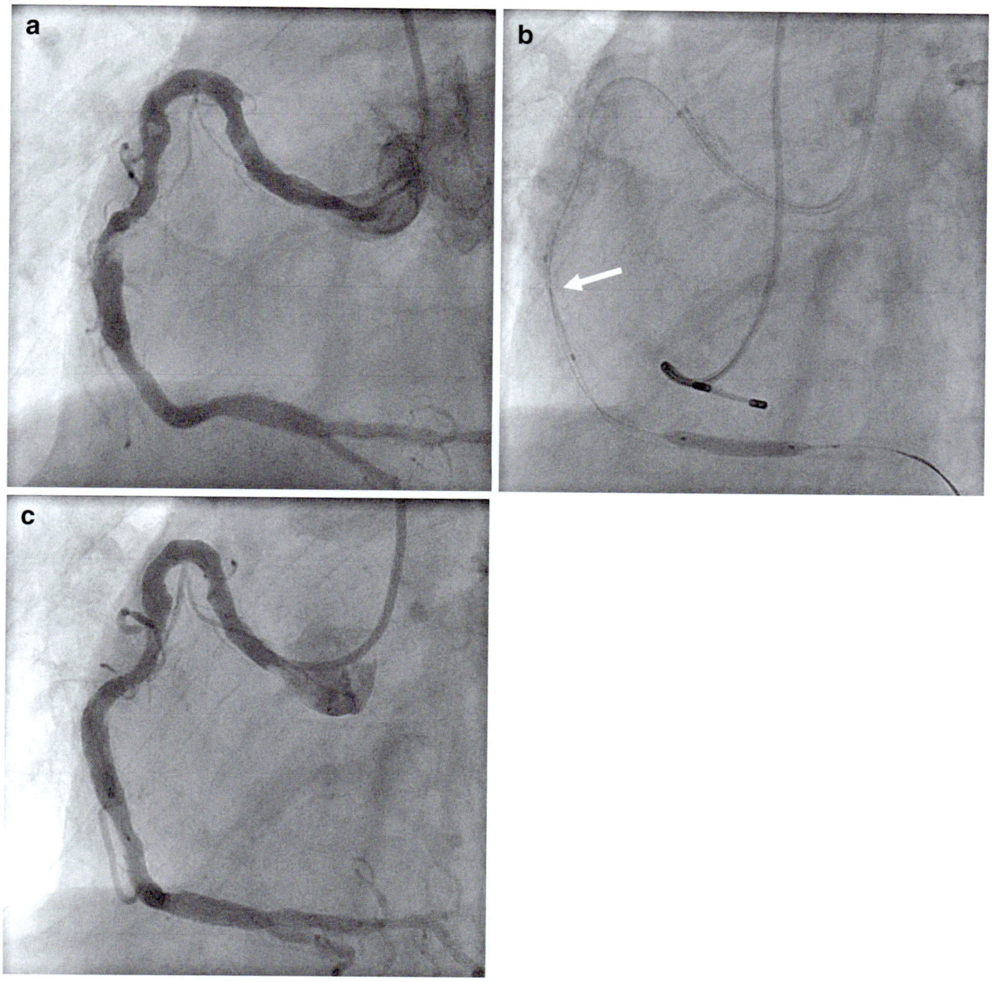

Fig. 20.8 Balloon anchoring technique in a case with no suitable side branch. A severely stenotic lesion with calcification is seen in the RCA mid portion (**a**). Since there was no side branch in front of the lesion that was suitable for anchoring, anchoring was undertaken at the distal RCA, resulting in successful passage of the stent (*white arrow*) (**b**). Final angiogram (**c**)

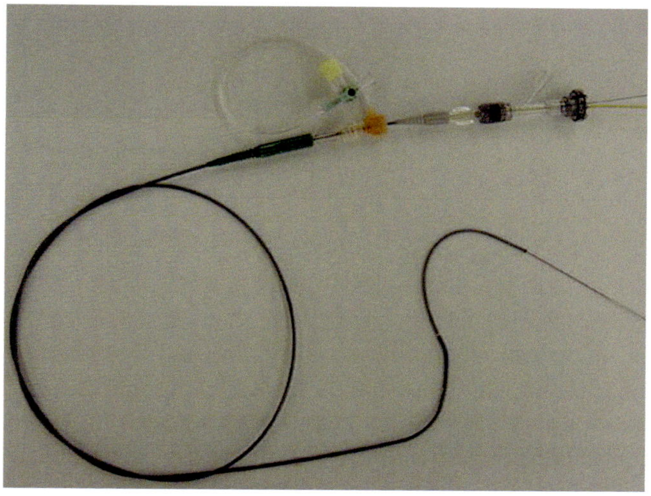

Fig. 20.9 Complete view of the 5-in-6 system using the Terumo Heartrail 5 Fr Straight (ST-01)

20.5.1 Difference Between Balloon Anchoring Technique and Mother-Child Catheter Technique

Both the balloon anchoring technique and the mother-child catheter technique are extremely effective methods for calcified lesions and tortuous lesions, but proper differentiation between the techniques will be necessary as each technique will have lesions that pose difficulty, and lesions or conditions that should be avoided. First, as was previously mentioned, the balloon anchoring technique generally requires a side branch for anchoring. Similar to the kissing balloon technique, all the procedure requires is insertion of the wire and balloon, making it relatively easy to perform compared to the mother-child catheter technique. But on the other hand, forced delivery of the stent in a severely calcified lesion could result in deformation or drop-off of the stent.

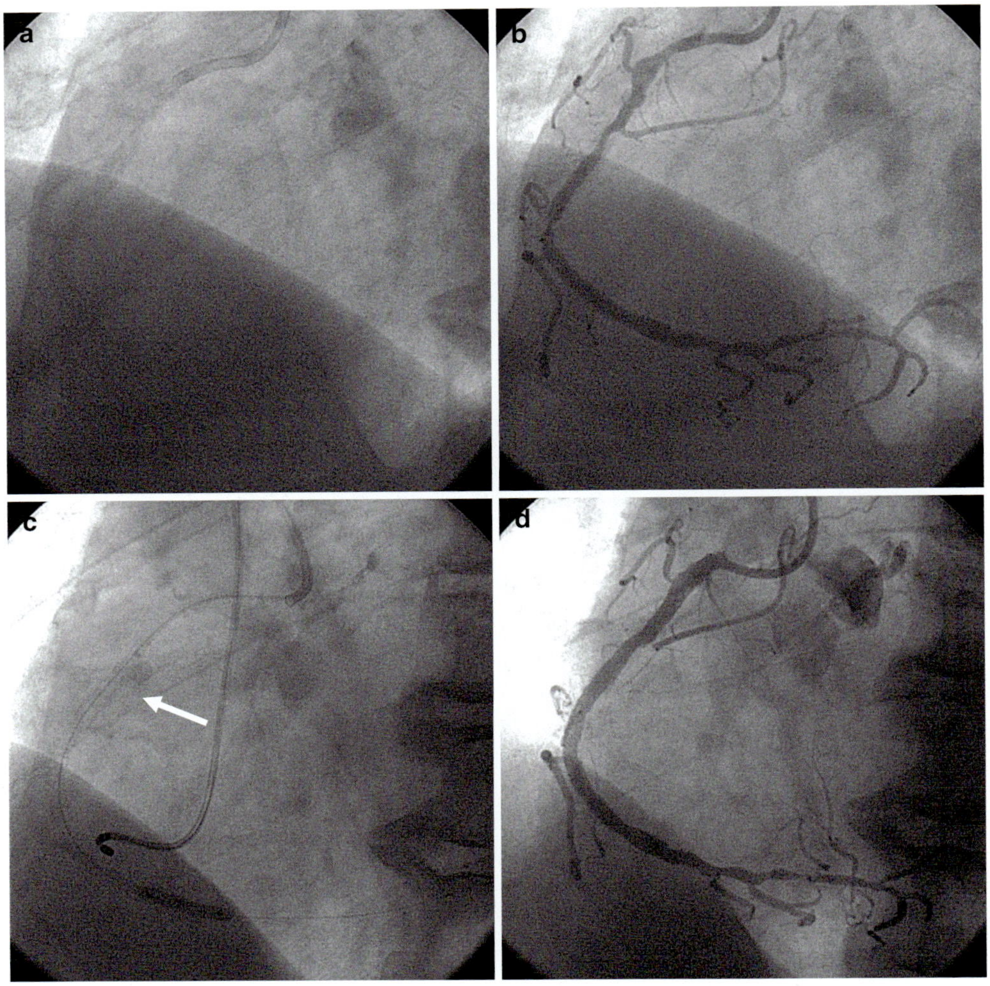

Fig. 20.10 Mother-child catheter technique. Severe calcification is seen extensively in the right coronary artery (**a**), and a diffuse lesion is seen from mid portion to proximal (**b**). Stent delivery was attempted with a 6Fr AL1, but it failed to cross the lesion. The GC was exchanged to a 6Fr Wave 3, and with anchoring by a 3.0 mm balloon, a 4Fr inner catheter (KIWAMI, Terumo Heartrail II) was advanced through the 6 Fr catheter (*white arrow* indicates tip of the inner catheter) (**c**). This made stent delivery possible and good dilatation was achieved (**d**)

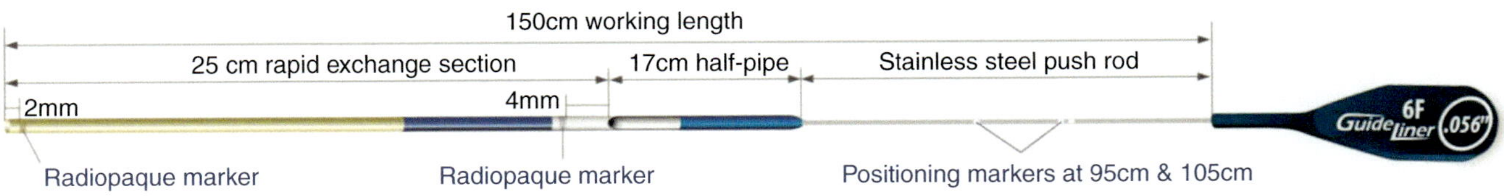

Fig. 20.11 Overall view of the GuideLiner (Version 3). (Version 3 has not received approval in some countries at the time of this publication)

In the mother-child catheter technique, especially when a 4 Fr GC with a flexible tip is used as the inner catheter, the inner catheter can be advanced to a point just before or past the target lesion. The inner catheter also acts as a protective sheath, making more sure delivery of the stent possible by also preventing drop-off of the stent in a calcified lesion. However, protection of the side branch is basically not possible, and it cannot be performed in cases needing a 2-stent technique for a bifurcation lesion (Fig. 20.13). When this technique is used during a PCI procedure, there are problems such as a somewhat complicated assembly of the system; the possibility of inducing ischemia during the time the inner catheter is in the coronary artery; cases where the inner catheter has to be removed when more than one stent needs to be delivered; and inability to confirm the positioning of the stent by angiography when pressure dampening by the inner catheter occurs. But both techniques are extremely important in the treatment of severely calcified lesions and tortuous lesions by 6 Fr TRI.

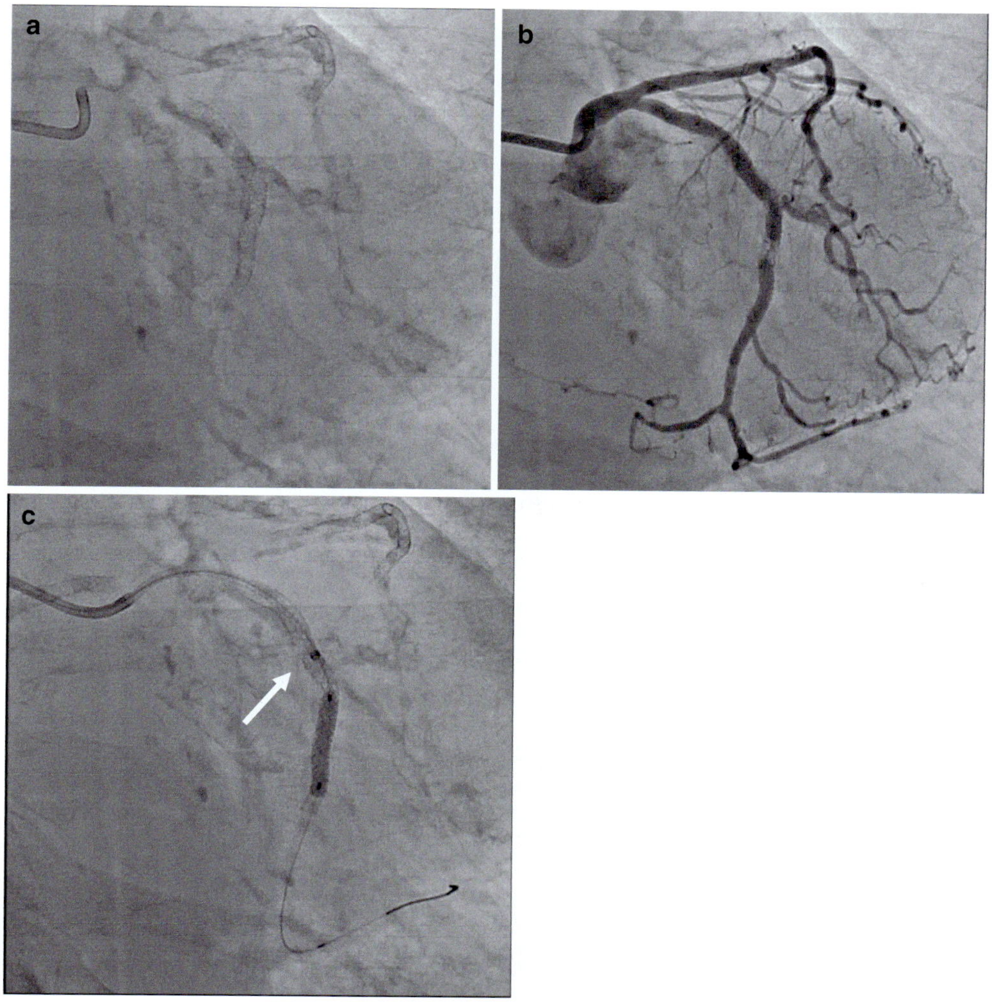

Fig. 20.12 Dilatation by a DCB using GuideLiner (Version 2) for in-stent restenosis with severe calcification noted in the proximal portion of the lesion. Severe calcification is seen throughout the coronary artery (**a**). Enlargement of the aorta made GC engagement by both the extra back-up type and Amplatz type difficult. GC engagement was possible using a 6 Fr JL4.5, but because of poor backup support, the mother-child catheter technique using GuideLiner (Ver.2) was taken to treat the in-stent restenosis in the LCx midportion (**b**). Through balloon anchoring, GuideLiner was inserted up to the OM bifurcation (*white arrow*), and a drug-coated balloon (3.0/15 mm SeQuent Please, B Braun) was successfully delivered (**c**). (Some devices, including the SeQuent Please used in this case, are not recommended for use with GuideLiner, because their specifications make it difficult to pass through the guide catheter extension)

20.6 High-Speed Rotational Atherectomy by TRI

High-speed rotational atherectomy (Rotablator™ (Boston Scientific Co.)) is effective for severely calcified lesions and when it can be performed, it would be an extremely effective option for implementation by TRI as well.

Burrs up to 1.75 mm can be used if a 6 Fr GC is employed. However, if, with the introduction of DES, the main purpose of Rotablator becomes not the opening of the vessel through ablation of the calcified portion, but the modification of the lesion to facilitate balloon expansion and stent delivery, in most cases a 1.5 mm burr would be sufficient for ablation purposes. Therefore, when Rotablator can be used, it would be possible to treat many severely calcified lesions by 6 Fr TRI. Once the operator becomes proficient in this technique, there will be no difference between the clinical outcomes of TRI and TFI [4], and from the fact that quite a few of the patients with severely calcified coronary artery lesions—the targets of Rotablator—also have calcification in the peripheral vessels, TRI's inherent advantage of reducing bleeding complications at the puncture site will be highlighted as well.

In the use of Rotablator, the Rotawire is rarely used from the start of the procedure due to problems with its maneuverability, and this makes it necessary to exchange from a conventional guidewire to the Rotawire. There will be times when difficulty is then encountered in the exchange of guidewires because the microcatheter conventionally used is unable to cross the lesion due to calcification. We often use

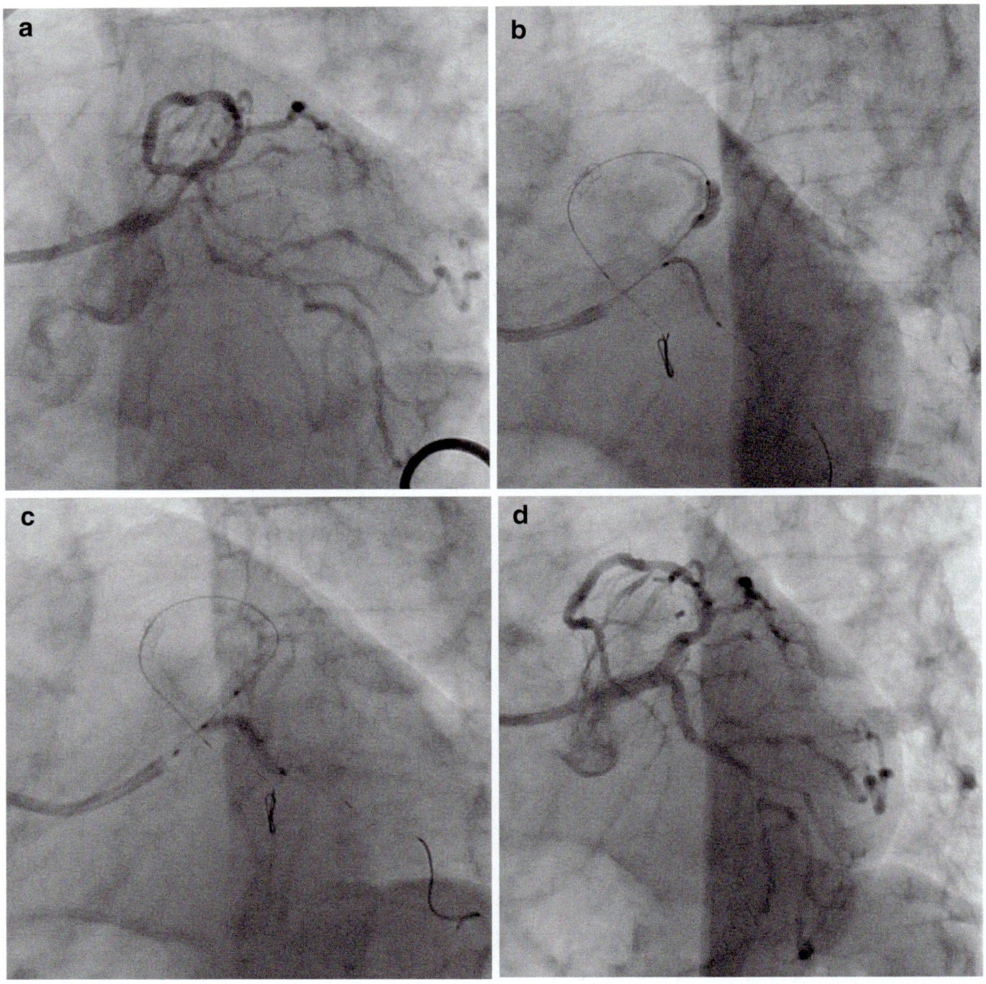

Fig. 20.13 Mini-crush technique taken for a LMT true bifurcation. An LMT bifurcation lesion with severe calcification is seen (**a**). Conventional stent delivery to the LCx was not possible, so the balloon anchoring technique was taken to attempt stent delivery (**b**). The stent was placed at the ostium of the LCx (**c**), and following this, the proximal portion of the stent was crushed with a balloon, and a stent was implanted from the LMT to LAD. Finally, KBT was performed in the LMT, and good dilatation was achieved (**d**). In this case, the balloon anchoring technique was taken because if stent delivery were to be done by the mother-child catheter technique, we would not be able to insert a balloon to crush the proximal portion of the stent

Corsair (ASAHI INTECC) as the microcatheter for exchange to the Rotawire but a problem with Corsair is that it sometimes cannot be inserted past the lesion because of its somewhat large outer diameter. Tornus (ASAHI INTECC) is effective in calcified lesions that present difficulty for balloon crossover, and can be used with no problem in TRI with a 6 FR GC, and it is, at times, effective as a microcatheter for wire exchange when Rotablator is used. However, Tornus does not have a very smooth wire lumen and as resistance can often be felt when inserting and removing the wire, sufficient caution must be taken to prevent kinking of the wire.

Even when Rotablator can be used, many operators generally prefer 7 Fr. TFI for the treatment of severely calcified lesions. However, if they become proficient in using the aforementioned balloon anchoring technique and mother-child catheter technique for stent delivery, almost all cases can be treated with a 6 Fr GC, and they will no longer feel the necessity of 7 Fr TFI.

As shown in the case in Fig. 20.14, it is highly possible that stent delivery by conventional methods will be difficult after Rotablator, even for 7 Fr TFI, especially in calcified lesions with tortuosity in the proximal portion of the lesion. In such a case, if the procedure is undertaken by assuming that the mother-child catheter technique will be used, the procedure time can also be reduced. A large percentage of hemodialysis patients, who often have severely calcified lesions, have occlusion or calcification of the peripheral arteries and often have bleeding complications at the puncture site. If these patients can be treated by TRI, such post-procedure bleeding complications could be prevented.

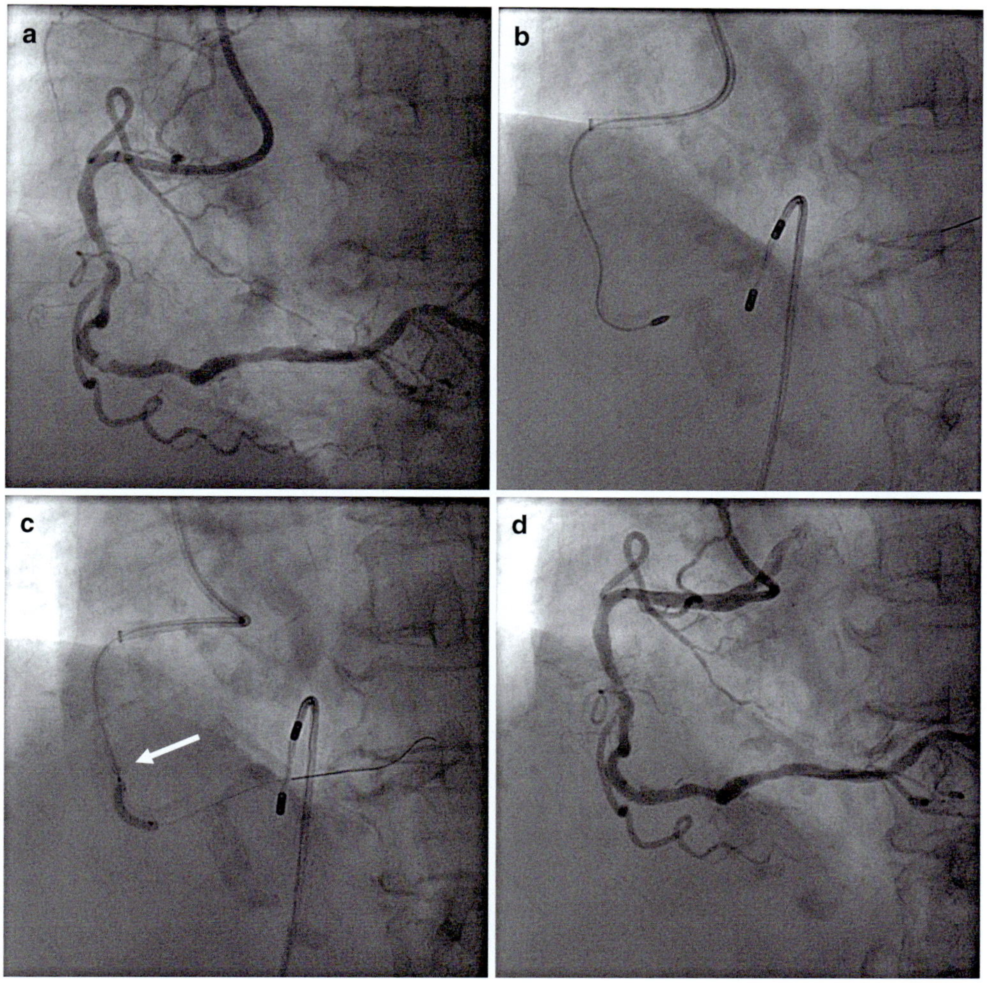

Fig. 20.14 Rotablator for severely calcified RCA lesion. A severely calcified lesion is seen in the RCA mid portion (**a**). Ablation with a 1.5 mm burr was performed (**b**), and with anchoring by a 2.5 mm balloon, a 4 Fr inner catheter was advanced just proximal of the lesion (indicated by the *white arrow*) (**c**). This allowed delivery of the stent and good dilatation of the lesion was achieved (**d**)

20.7 Other Considerations

The tips and tricks for calcified lesions and tortuous lesions have been explained. The issue common to both types of lesions is how to achieve GC backup support, and each of these two types of lesions has its unique technical problems. In many cases, even in highly tortuous lesions, no special technique would be necessary if the coronary artery is flexible and can straighten out through insertion of the guidewire. But when both severe calcification and tortuosity are present at the same time, quite a few cases will be difficult to treat if these respective techniques are conducted independently. It would thus be necessary to prepare plans before the procedure that assume a combination of the Rotablator and the mother-child catheter technique or the balloon anchoring technique like a case in Fig. 20.14.

20.8 Summary

The treatment of calcified lesions and tortuous lesions by TRI was outlined and explained by showing actual cases. When TRI was first introduced, the inner lumen of 6 Fr GCs was narrow, and on top of this, the outer diameters of balloons and stent delivery systems were large. The techniques that could be used were thus limited and it naturally followed that TRI could not be used for highly difficult, severely calcified and tortuous lesions. However, the inner diameters of GCs have now increased and the balloon and stent delivery systems are becoming smaller. As mentioned above, it has become possible to select techniques and devices that can supplement the lack of GC backup support in 6 Fr TRI, and it no longer appears necessary to use 7 Fr TFI. A learning curve is, of course, necessary for techniques to be taken in severely calcified lesions and tortuous lesions, and key techniques should be mastered through staged studies of such lesions.

References

1. Takeshita S, Takagi A, Saito S. Backup support of the mother-child technique: technical considerations for the size of the mother guiding catheter. Catheter Cardiovasc Interv. 2012;80: 292–7.
2. Kumar S, Gorog DA, Secco GG, Di Mario C, Kukreja N. The GuideLiner"child" catheter for percutaneous coronary intervention — early clinical experience. J Invasive Cardiol. 2010;22: 495–8.
3. Eddin MJ, Armstrong EJ, Javed U, Rogers JH. Transradial interventions with the GuideLiner catheter: role of proximal vessel angulation. Cardiovasc Revasc Med. 2013;14:275–9.
4. Watt J, Oldroyd KG. Radial versus femoral approach for high-speed rotational atherectomy. Catheter Cardiovasc Interv. 2009;74: 550–4.

Transradial Approach for Patients with Prior CABG

21

Marcelo Sanmartin and Carlos Moreno-Vinues

Abstract

Patients with previous coronary artery bypass graft (CABG) surgery represent a high-risk population with specific challenges to transradial access ,especially with saphenous vein grafts (SVG) intervention. In this chapter we review several specific problems related to cannulation of bypass grafts for diagnostic and intervention purposes through the radial artery. We also provide specific technical "tips and tricks" that might be helpful to overcome most common difficulties.

21.1 Introduction

The transradial approach is the best option for the majority of patients undergoing coronary angiography or intervention [1–3]. Its main advantages are the low rate of access site vascular and bleeding complications and the possibility of earlier ambulation without closure devices, improving patient's comfort and minimizing overall costs [4]. However, patients with previous coronary artery bypass graft (CABG) surgery represent a a high-risk population with specific challenges to transradial access [5–7]. For this reason, post-CABG patients have been typically excluded or underrepresented in many transradial access studies [1, 3]. Previous surgical revascularized patients, especially with saphenous vein grafts (SVG), represent challenging cases even to the moderately experienced transradial operator [7].

In this chapter we review several specific problems related to cannulation of bypass grafts for diagnostic and intervention purposes through the radial artery. We also provide specific technical "tips and tricks" that might be helpful to overcome most common difficulties.

M. Sanmartin, MD, PhD, FESC (✉) • C. Moreno-Vinues, MD
Cardiology Department, Hospital Universitario Ramon y Cajal, Madrid, Spain
e-mail: msanfer@telefonica.net

21.2 Patient Preparation

Pre-procedural evaluation of patient's peculiarities including a careful review of past medical history and current clinical status is of paramount importance to a successful procedure. Particularly, getting knowledge of the number, type and location of previous grafts helps to speed up the whole procedure, minimize radiation and avoid complications related to excess of contrast media. If possible, clinical information should be coupled with previous review of all angiographic recordings or even noninvasive CT images (if available). Gaining insight from a previous echocardiogram or MRI regarding global and segmental left ventricular function is also advisable.

As in every cardiac catheterization procedure, assessment of the quality of radial, as well as ulnar and femoral artery pulsations should be obtained. Past history of anatomical variations, such as radial loops or severe subclavian tortuosity should be taken into account.

The left radial artery is our preferred option in most cases [8]. Going through the left arm will allow easy access to the left internal mammary artery (LITA) graft and also to SVG. Selective cannulation of a contralateral thoracic graft is possible, although sometimes it can be cumbersome [9, 10]. Assessing the descending thoracic aorta to subselective cannulation of the rare case of gastroepiploic arterial graft to left posterior descending artery is also easier through the left arm [11].

Y. Zhou et al. (eds.), *Transradial Approach for Percutaneous Interventions*, DOI 10.1007/978-94-017-7350-8_21

Reasons to avoid transradial approach in patients with previous CABG are exposed in Table 21.1.

21.3 Diagnostic Coronary Angiography

In general, start with native coronary angiography. Complete occlusion of a native vessel that supply blood flow to a contractile left ventricular segment without collaterals or a competitive ("to-and-fro") flow mean that there is a patent graft that should be selectively cannulated later on. On the other hand, clear visualization of distal segments of a native coronary artery tells you that the graft has no or minimal anterograde flow.

21.3.1 Catheter Selection

Multipurpose catheters, such as TIG, Brachial type K curves can be used for native coronary angiography, but in general are not useful for graft cannulation. Sometimes the AL1 curve allows both native and SVG selective angiography, but it is not our initial default strategy. The JL 3.5 catheter also allows easy access to both coronary ostia in most cases and occasionally engages SVG with a high take-off in ascending aorta. JL or TIG shapes can be useful in selective contralateral subclavian artery cannulation. Table 21.2 summarizes catheter selection for selective engagement of bypass grafts

Our routine strategy is starting with a JL 3.5 catheter. After selective left coronary imaging, the catheter is gently pulled back and, after straightening its primary curve with the help of a conventional 0,035' wire it is rotated clockwise and advanced for selective right coronary angiography. Once native coronary artery imaging is finished, a short try of engaging a SVG to left circumflex system with the JL catheter can be done applying a careful pull-back and small rotation while in LAO 45° view. Most commonly, a different catheter will be necessary as explained below.

21.4 Saphenous Vein Grafts

Saphenous vein grafts (SVGs) are commonly used in patients with multivessel coronary disease. In general, patients have one or two proximal aortic anastomoses. Right coronary SVG are more anterior and have a slightly lower take off compared to left coronary SVG. We recommend using the left radial approach for selective engagement of SVG for diagnostic or intervention purposes.

If your usual choice for right coronary artery cannulation is a Judkins Right (JR) catheter, it is a good advice to try it also for SVG imaging. In general, it is not difficult to engage the SVG to distal right coronary territory through the left arm with a JR or MP catheters. Coming from the right arm, these catheters usually are less useful. For SVGs originating from less anterior or the left side of the aorta, that is, those oriented to the left circumflex or left descending coronary artery, Amplatz left catheters represent usually a better option (Fig. 21.1). Our default strategy is AL 1 shape, both for diagnostic and interventions in SVG. Sometimes an AL 2 curve is a better option, especially from the right arm or in

Table 21.1 Reasons to avoid transradial approach for diagnostic or intervention in patients with previous bypass grafts

Absence of bilateral radial pulsations
Dialysis fistulae
Known difficult anatomic variations (radial loops, lusoria artery)
Need for large-bore guiding catheters (≥7 French)
During learning curve

Table 21.2 Catheter selection for bypass grafts engagement during diagnostic and intervention procedures

Free aorto-coronary grafts	Right radial	Left radial
To RCA	JR4, JL3.5, multipurpose, AL1, AR2	JR4, multipurpose, AL1, AR2
To Cx	AL1, AL2, extra-backup	AL1, AL2
To LAD/diagnonal	AL1, AL2, multipurpose	AL1, AL2
Pedicled grafts		
LIMA	JL3.5 or TIG or Simm then exchange IMA or JR4	LIMA, JR4, Williams 3D
RIMA	IMA, JR4, Williams 3D	Simm then exchange IMA or JR4 or Vertebral

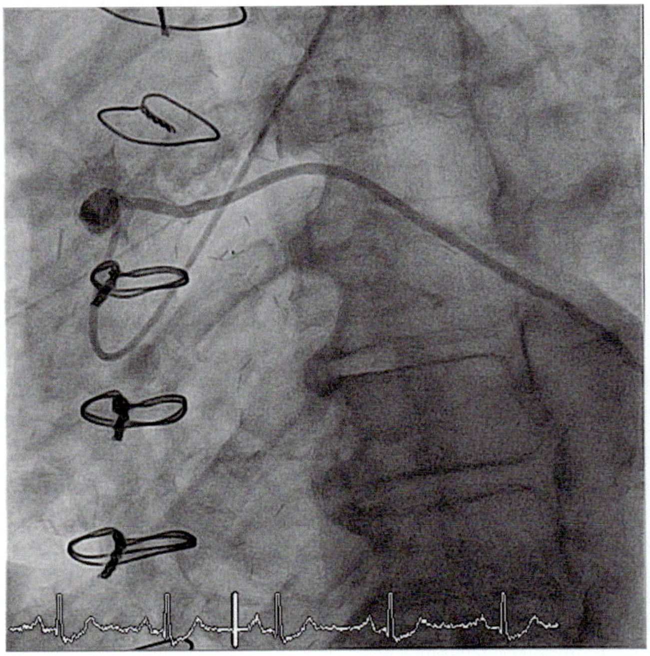

Fig. 21.1 Selective angiography of saphenous vein graft to obtuse marginal branch using AL 1 catheter

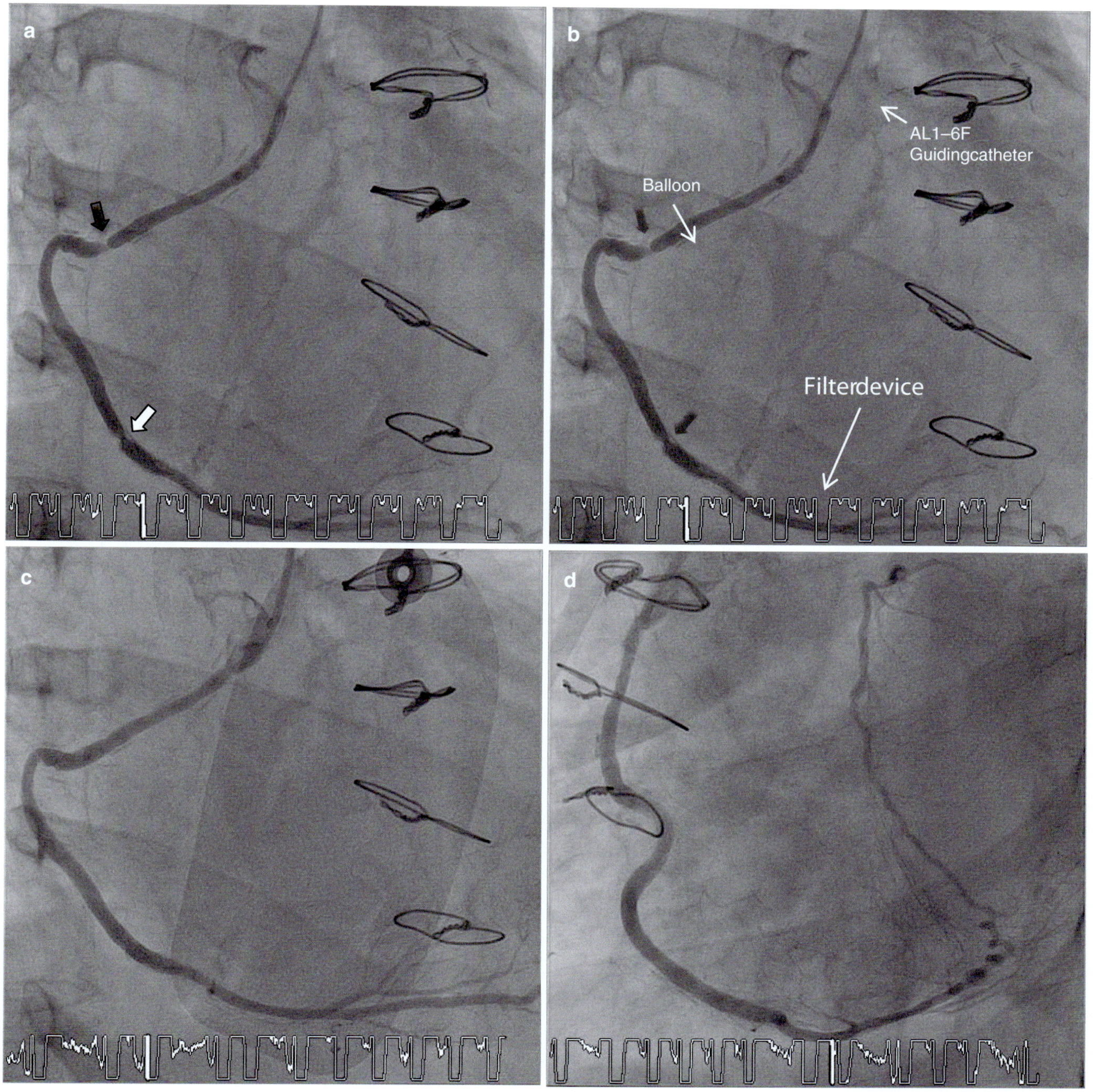

Fig. 21.2 Complex PCI of saphenous vein graft (*SVG*) to distal right coronary artery disease treated by left radial approach. Coronary angiography had shown chronic total occlusion of left main, total occlusion of the left internal thoracic graft and severely and diffusely disease of left marginal branches. Patient was in cardiogenic shock and was considered not suitable for a third revascularization surgery and PCI of restenotic SVG was performed. Severely diseased femoral and iliac arteries precluded intraaortic balloon insertion. Panel **a**: baseline angiography taken with a 5 F Judkins Left 3.5 diagnostic catheter showing severe stenosis at proximal third (*black arrow*) and focal in-stent restenosis (*white arrow*). Panel **b**: the same angiographic view showing perfect alignment of a 6 F AL1 guiding catheter and distal protection device in place. Panels **c** and **d**: final result after placing to everolimus-eluting stents showing adequate expansion and no signs of distal embolization. Recovery of good collateral flow to left descending artery was achieved.

case of significant aortic dilatation. Moving from a typical LAO view to a RAO view trying to visualize lateral take-off of these left-oriented aortocoronary grafts are sometimes helpful in challenging cases.

The selection of an appropriate guiding catheter is a key point for transradial approach in presence of SVG. A good support is often needed to overcome complex lesions and need for distal filters. Accordingly, we recommend 6 F guiding catheters and the left radial approach. AL 1 is the usual choice for SVG to left coronary territories and JR4 or multipurpose guiding catheters for right coronary SVG. In some cases, AL1 offers better support also for right coronary SVG (example in Fig. 21.2). Another solution could be using extra-backup curves typically used for left coronary interventions by reshaping the primary curve with the straight part of the 0.035' wire (that never should be pushed outside the catheter during this procedure). Finding a good support from your guiding catheter is usually the "Achilles heel" of transradial interventions on SVG, compared to native vessels. Fortunately, lesser support from guiding catheters can sometimes be overcome using catheter extensions such as Heartrail™ or GuideLiner™ [12].

21.5 Internal Mamary Artery Grafts

There is no doubt about the long-term benefit of a LIMA graft to the left anterior descending artery. Use of both IMAs for CABG and total arterial revascularization has become standard in many centers. An interesting statement by some cardiac surgeons related to BIMA (bilateral internal thoracic artery) grafts is: "twenty minutes more of surgery for twenty years more of survival". Frequently, BIMA is performed using the right IMA a T-side graft from the pedicled LIMA, which obviously facilitate transradial operators' task.

The are two possibilities of transradial approach to intubate ITAs: homolateral and contralateral accesses:

Homolateral transradial access
It represents the easiest and fastest way to get to ITA grafts, even compared to transfemoral approach, so it is the preferred route for many operators (Fig. 21.3). The preferred catheter to selectively intubate the ITA is the standard femoral internal thoracic artery curve catheter but frequently the JR4 achieve adequate imaging and support. It usually depends on the take-off angle in the subclavian artery and the place of implantation. The angle between distal subclavian and ITA is usually acute so coming from homolateral radial artery, ITA is not always the ideal catheter and a wider choice of curves can be considered, such as JR and Williams' 3D right catheter with its angulated and longer tip.

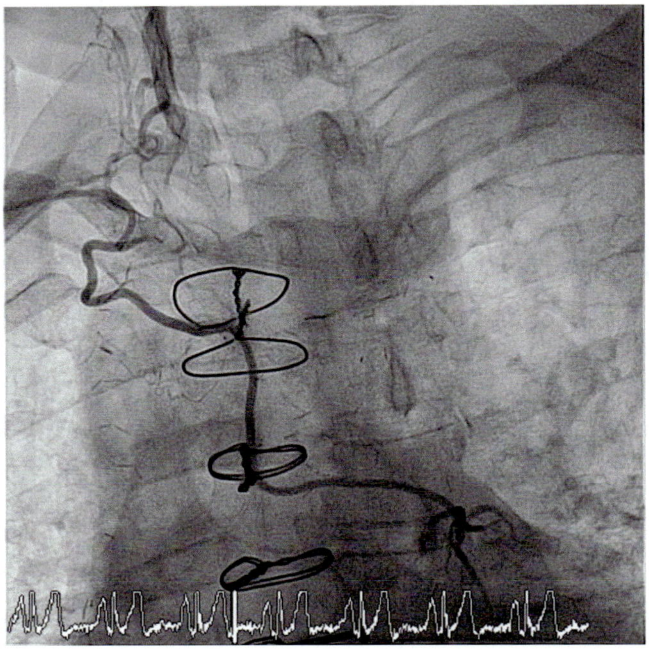

Fig. 21.3 Selective right internal thoracic artery graft to left anterior descending artery performed with standard IMA catheter through homolateral access

Native coronary intervention through the LITA is not unusual. In these frequently complex procedures, we consider the left radial approach an additional advantage, because it is easier to achieve an extra support by deep cannulation of the ITA graft. This should be done carefully and in a stepwise approach, preferably with a 5 F guiding catheter and/or using a small/deflated balloon to provide some tapering between the tip of the guiding catheter and the 0,014' guidewire. Using a soft-tip guiding catheter will also minimize the risk of dissection through this maneuver.

Contralateral transradial access
The presence of a pedicled LITA graft is not a contraindication for a right radial catheterization. The safety and feasibility of LITA angiography from a right radial access has been demonstrated even with fewer catheters and success rates similar to a transfemoral or homolateral transradial approach [9, 10]. In addition, BITA grafting is often performed because of higher durability and longevity of arterial grafts and improved late outcomes.

The first step is catheterization of the contralateral subclavian artery. This can be accomplished by pulling back a Judkins left or Tiger catheters through the ascending aorta. Operators should have Simmons 1 or 2 curves for more difficult cases and be familiar with manipulation of these catheters. After correct orientation and selective cannulation, a hydrophilic 0,035' guidewire is advanced through the distal subclavian, preferably to distal brachial or even the radial artery for additional support (Fig. 21.4). Once the guidewire is positioned the catheter is advanced over the wire to the mid-subclavian portion. Additional support can be gained by wire-anchoring through simple tricks: (1) inflating a pressure cuff over the contralateral arm surrounding the guidewire; (2) asking the patient to bend his arm while advancing the catheter with the wire in place or; (3) by simply manual compression of the humeral or radial artery (Fig. 21.5) [13]. Sometimes, high quality images can be obtained by nonselective injection in proximal subclavian artery having a blood-pressure cuff inflated to a supra-systolic pressure on the same arm. Finally, JR 4 or ITA catheters allow selective cannulation of ITA for selective angiography. Thus, for operators not comfort with the left radial approach or that does not have a viable left radial access, engaging LITA grafts from right radial approach may not be a complex task with appropriate expertise and material.

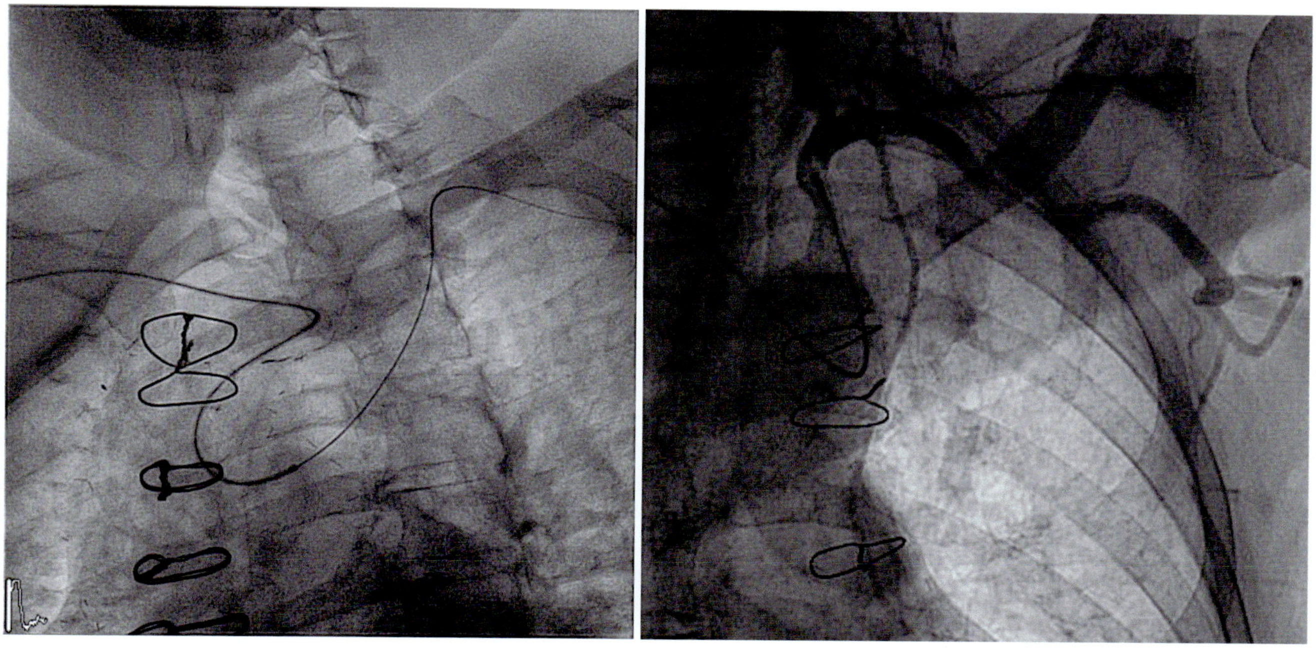

Fig. 21.4 Contralateral subclavian access through right radial approach. Non-selective subclavian angiography with a pneumatic cuff inflated on the left arm achieved diagnostic left internal thoracic graft imaging

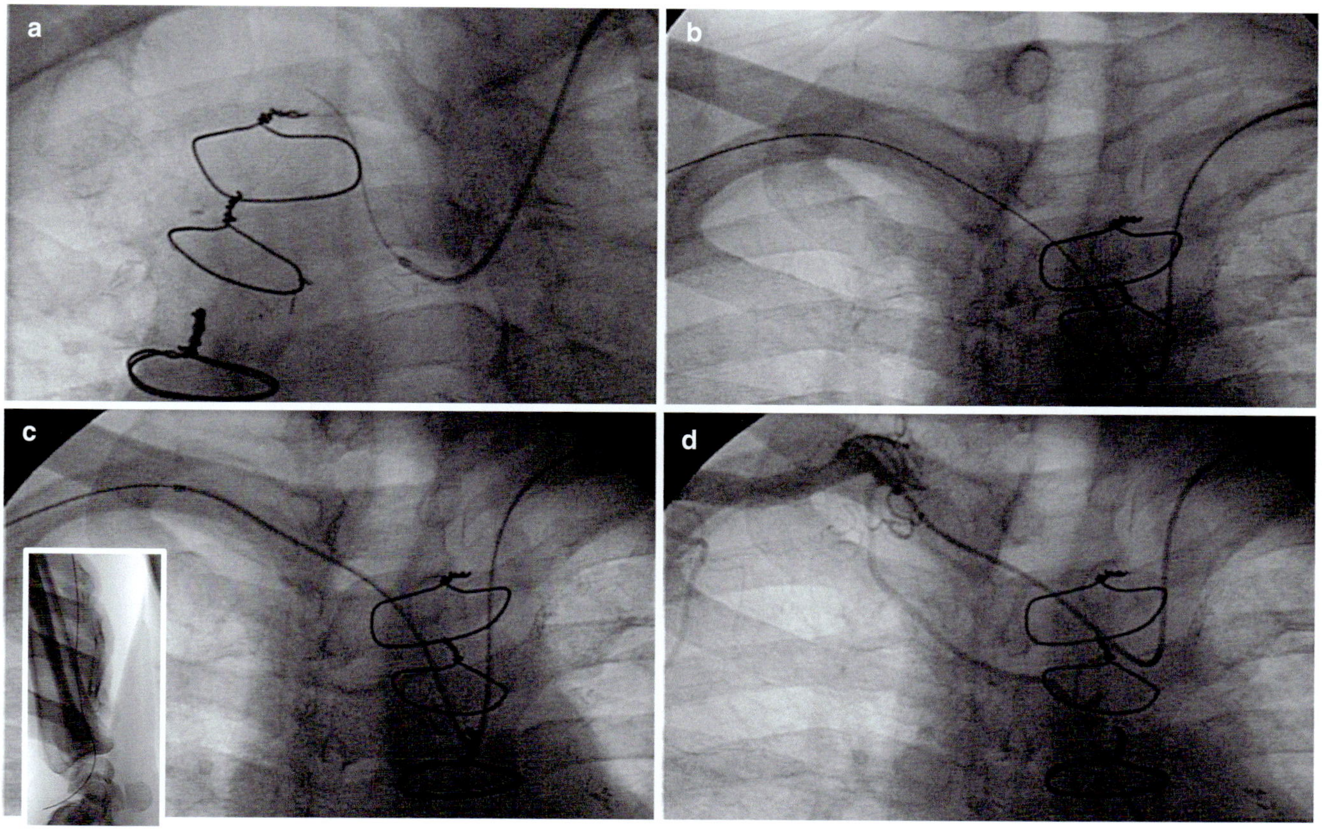

Fig. 21.5 Gaining support for contralateral subclavian cannulation. Panel **a**: a long 280 cm hydrophylic 0,035' wire is carefully advanced using a diagnostic 5 F IMA catheter for orientation. Panel **b**: the 0,035' guidewire is advanced distally through contralateral brachial artery but there is insufficient support for advancement of the diagnostic catheter. Panel **c**: further advancement of the guidewire allows anchoring the system by external contralateral radial compression. The catheter can be progressed to the subclavian artery, distal to the take off of right internal thoracic artery. Panel **d**: non-selective angiography of right internal thoracic artery with diagnostic images. In case of non-selective imaging a pneumatic blood-pressure cuff inflated to suprasystolic pressure can be used to improve image quality

Conclusions

The transradial technique has become standard of care for reducing bleeding complications, improving patient comfort and reducing overall costs for coronary percutaneous catheterization. Patients with previous surgical revascularization represent a specially difficult subgroup, albeit also benefit from transradial approach. With accumulated experience and knowledge of several anatomical peculiarities and a few technical tricks, operators can significantly reduce the amount of contrast dye, radiation exposure, spasm and ultimately the number of failed transradial attempts.

References

1. Kiemeneij F, Laarman GJ, Odekerken D, Slagboom T, van der Wieken R. A randomized comparison of percutaneous transluminal coronary angioplasty by the radial, brachial and femoral approaches: the access study. J Am Coll Cardiol. 1997;29(6):1269–75.
2. Rao SV, Cohen MG, Kandzari DE, Bertrand OF, Gilchrist IC. The transradial approach to percutaneous coronary intervention: historical perspective, current concepts, and future directions. J Am Coll Cardiol. 2010;55(20):2187–95.
3. Bertrand OF, Belisle P, Joyal D, Costerousse O, Rao SV, Jolly SS, et al. Comparison of transradial and femoral approaches for percutaneous coronary interventions: a systematic review and hierarchical Bayesian meta-analysis. Am Heart J. 2012;163(4):632–48.
4. Sanmartin M, Cuevas D, Goicolea J, Ruiz-Salmeron R, Gomez M, Argibay V. Vascular complications associated with radial artery access for cardiac catheterization. Rev Esp Cardiol. 2004;57(6):581–4.
5. Dehghani P, Mohammad A, Bajaj R, Hong T, Suen CM, Sharieff W, et al. Mechanism and predictors of failed transradial approach for percutaneous coronary interventions. JACC Cardiovasc Interv. 2009;2(11):1057–64.
6. Abdelaal E, Brousseau-Provencher C, Montminy S, Plourde G, MacHaalany J, Bataille Y, et al. Risk score, causes, and clinical impact of failure of transradial approach for percutaneous coronary interventions. JACC Cardiovasc Interv. 2013;6(11):1129–37.
7. Michael TT, Alomar M, Papayannis A, Mogabgab O, Patel VG, Rangan BV, et al. A randomized comparison of the transradial and transfemoral approaches for coronary artery bypass graft angiography and intervention: the RADIAL-CABG Trial (RADIAL Versus Femoral Access for Coronary Artery Bypass Graft Angiography and Intervention). JACC Cardiovasc Interv. 2013; 6(11):1138–44.
8. Sanmartin M, Cuevas D, Moxica J, Valdes M, Esparza J, Baz JA, et al. Transradial cardiac catheterization in patients with coronary bypass grafts: feasibility analysis and comparison with transfemoral approach. Catheter Cardiovasc Interv Off J Soc Cardiac Angiography Interv. 2006;67(4):580–4.
9. Burzotta F, Trani C, Hamon M, Amoroso G, Kiemeneij F. Transradial approach for coronary angiography and interventions in patients with coronary bypass grafts: tips and tricks. Catheter Cardiovasc Interv Off J Soc Cardiac Angiography Interv. 2008;72(2):263–72.
10. Burzotta F, Trani C, Todaro D, Romagnoli E, Niccoli G, Ginnico F, et al. Comparison of the transradial and transfemoral approaches for coronary angiographic evaluation in patients with internal mammary artery grafts. J Cardiovasc Med. 2008;9(3):263–6.
11. Sharma GL, Louvard Y, Tavolaro O, Lefevre T, Loubeyre C, Dumas P, et al. Less invasive PTCA of a gastroepiploic artery combining the transradial approach and 5 Fr guiding catheter: a case report. Catheter Cardiovasc Interv Off J Soc Cardiac Angiography Interv. 2002;56(4):494–7.
12. Farooq V, Mamas MA, Fath-Ordoubadi F, Fraser DG. The use of a guide catheter extension system as an aid during transradial percutaneous coronary intervention of coronary artery bypass grafts. Catheter Cardiovasc Interv Off J Soc Cardiac Angiography Interv. 2011;78(6):847–63.
13. Garcia-Touchard A, Fernandez-Diaz JA, Francisco DO, Goicolea-Ruigomez J. Intraarterial guidewire external compression: a simple technique for successful LIMA angiography through the right radial approach. J Interv Cardiol. 2008;21(2):175–7.

Part IV

Miscellaneous Issues in Transradial Intervention

Slender PCI via Transradial Approach

22

Ferdinand Kiemeneij, Shigeru Saito, and Wei Liu

Abstract

The less invasive radial access for percutaneous coronary intervention (PCI) has gained the favour of interventionists for its advantage in reducing access site complications, improving patient comfort and reducing mortality. However, due to the smaller diameters of radial artery, the catheter size is therefore too large for some patients, which makes this technique painful, cumbersome and sometimes unsafe, also sets a limitation for complex PCI. In addition, radial artery occlusion (RAO) is more common when guides are large in comparison to the radial artery. This led to the development of series of downsized equipment and corresponding techniques to overcome this problem, which was so called "Slender" for this new approach.

22.1 Introduction of Slender TRI

The greatest advantage of transradial intervention compared to transfemoral intervention is the reduced bleeding complications. Bleeding complications are associated with an increased mortality rate in PCI, thus TRI has shown to improve the survival rate in coronary intervention [1, 2]. As of 2013, the European Society of Cardiology (ESC) and the Society for Coronary Angioplasty and Intervention (SCAI) have officially recommended TRI as the preferred approach for coronary intervention [3, 4].

Electronic supplementary material The online version of this chapter (doi:10.1007/978-94-017-7350-8_22) contains supplementary material, which is available to authorized users.

F. Kiemeneij, MD, PhD (✉)
Department of Cardiology, Tergooi Hospital, Blaricum, The Netherlands
e-mail: f.kiemeneij@gmail.com

S. Saito, MD, FACC, FSCAI, FJCC
Division of Cardiology & Catheterization Laboratories, Shonan Kamakura General Hospital, Kamakura, Japan
e-mail: cto.expert@gmail.com

W. Liu
Department of Cardiology, Beijing Anzhen Hospital, Capital Medical University, Beijing, China
e-mail: Liuwei525@hotmail.com

The normal inner lumen diameter of the radial artery ranges from 1.5 to 4 mm. Standard TRI is generally performed using a 6 Fr catheter that has an outer lumen (O.R) diameter of 2 mm, along with a corresponding sheath that has an O.R. of 2.7 mm. This shows that traditional catheter, sheath and interventional device sizing needs to be miniaturized [5]. The sizing of standard interventional equipment is not only painful for the patient, but can be unsafe due to the increased radial artery occlusion (RAO) and radial artery spasm (RAS). This leads to a general decrease in the feasibility and success rate of TRI.

A study done by Dr Shigeru Saito in Japan quantifies the issues with traditional interventional catheter sizing compared to radial artery sizing, especially in japan and other Asian countries. 250 Japanese patients undergoing TRI had their radial artery diameter measured. The results (Fig. 22.1) shows that less than 45 % of male patients and 30 % of female patients had a radial artery diameter large enough to accommodate an 8 Fr catheter, which is the only way of allowing some complex interventional techniques for specific lesions using multiple large interventional devices in traditional TRI.

The evolution of interventional equipment and materials has been led by the Slender Club Japan (SCJ) which was initiated by Dr Fuminobu Yoshimachi. They have revolutionized TRI and created a plethora of innovative manoeuvers, which has sprouted the new field of TRI called "Slender TRI" [6].

Y. Zhou et al. (eds.), *Transradial Approach for Percutaneous Interventions*, DOI 10.1007/978-94-017-7350-8_22

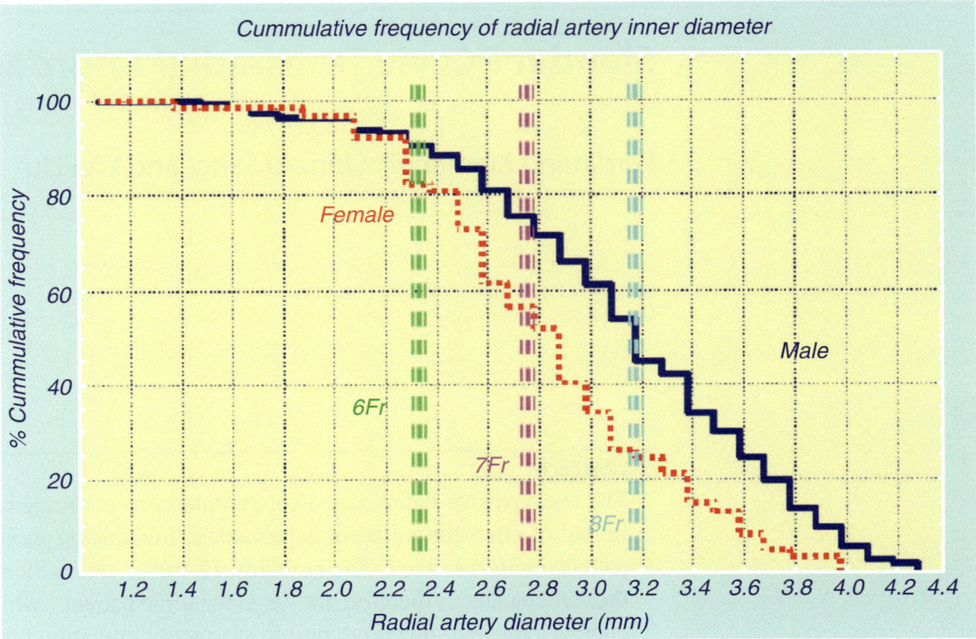

Fig. 22.1 Distribution of radial artery diameters of 250 Japanese patients, along with the percentage of males and females eligible for surgery with 6 Fr, 7 Fr, and 8 Fr catheters respectively

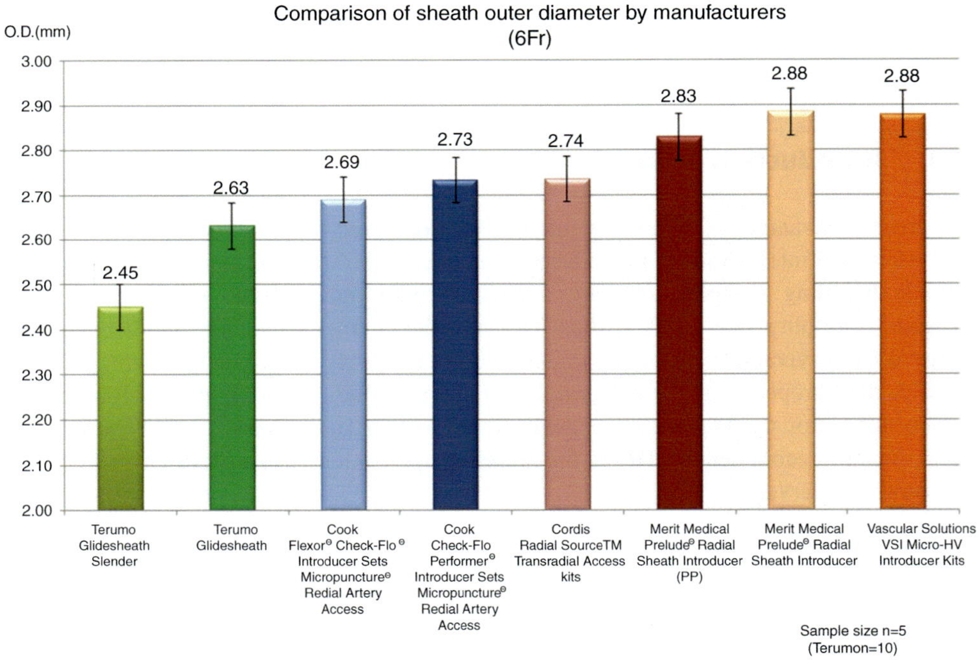

Fig. 22.2 Comparison of Terumo Glidesheath Slender® O.D. to other industry available sheaths

22.2 Slender Techniques

Slender PCI encompasses a range of techniques and miniaturization of devices and materials. Slender PCI can be categorized into miniaturization of materials (such as sheaths, catheters and wire and balloon catheters), sheathless coronary intervention, guideless coronary intervention and back-up improving techniques.

22.2.1 Miniaturization of Sheaths

In traditional TRI, the sheath is first inserted into the radial artery to house the guiding catheter. The thickness of the sheath is essential in determining how large the outer diameter of the GC can be. The Terumo Corporation recently made a sheath that can accommodate a 6 Fr catheter, but has an O.D. similar to that of a traditional sheath that can house a 5 Fr catheter. This was accomplished by reducing the thickness of the sheath from 0.20 to 0.12 mm, making the Terumo Glidesheath Slender® one of thinnest sheaths on the market (Fig. 22.2). Professor Kamiar Aminian conducted a report in which 114 patients under TRI using the Terumo Glidesheath Slender®. The report showed a 99.1 % procedural success rate and a 4.4 % occurrence of radial artery spasm (RAS) [7].

22.2.2 Miniaturization of Guiding Catheter

Recently, a coronary accessor has been developed by KIWAMI, Heartrail II, TERUMO, Tokyo, Japan. It can access the coronary artery and advance the coronary stents. The outer diameter of the catheter is 1.43 mm, allowing the catheter to be inserted into a 4 Fr introducer sheath and the inner diameter is1.27 mm (0.050 in.), which can accommodate most currently available coronary stents.

Manipulation of 4 Fr guiding catheter is different from 6 Fr or 5 Fr guiding catheter.

The advantage of this system is minimally invasive angioplasty and early ambulation, even when used with the transfemoral approach, without using any haemostatic devices. Also it leads to less consumption of contrast dye. With this technique a conventional 0.014″ guide wire can also be used.

However some disadvantages include the limited size of the devices used and there is less support for the guiding catheter as this is a coronary accessor. For some patients manipulation of the GC is more difficult and also sometimes the device gets damaged due to friction in the small inner lumen [8]. For female operator we need power injectors and also any IVUS cannot be used in this system. The coronary accessor can be used for complex lesions like CTO in RCA using 3 mm size of stent.

The clinical NAUSICA trial, explains the feasibility of this system comparing 4 Fr and 6 Fr systems with 80 patients in each group. Eligible patients were randomly assigned in a 1:1 ratio to undergo either 4-Fr or 6-Fr TRI.

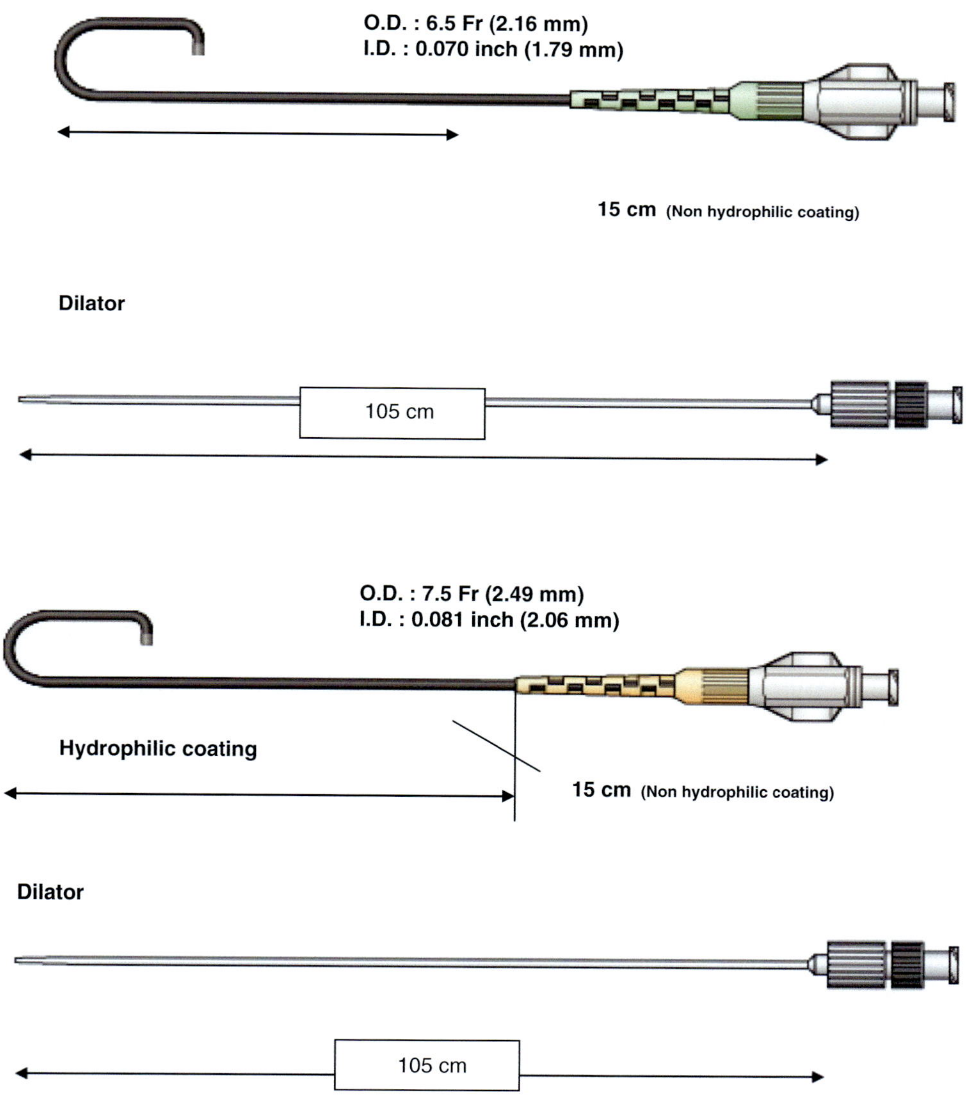

Comparison between 6 Fr and 4 Fr showed, significantly lower incidence of access-site complication (0 % vs 5 %). And also numerically low but statistically no significant incidence of radial artery occlusion (0 % vs 4 %). Compare to 6 Fr system, 4 Fr system had significantly shorter Haemostasis time (3.9 h vs. 5.3 h) but procedural time and fluoroscopy time were similar between these groups. This data shows that the 4 Fr coronary accessory system is feasible [9].

22.2.3 Sheath Less Technique

The Sheathless Eaucath (Asahi Intecc Co., Japan) is a coronary guiding catheter that has been recently developed and makes it possible to perform PCI without using an introducer sheath.

In the Normal System, in order to introduce a 6 French guiding catheter, first we have to insert a 6 French introducer into the radial artery. The outer diameter of a 6 French introducer is as similar as an 8 French guiding catheter. In the Sheathless System: The outer diameter of a 5 French sheathless guiding catheter is equivalent to a 3 French introducer. By putting "3 French" system, we can achieve 0.059-in. diameter in inner lumen. This is the concept of "Virtual" 3 French System.

The Advantages of this sheathless system include less traumatic to the radial arteries, achievement of the bigger lumen for the guiding catheter in a limited size of the radial artery and possible improvement in the preservation of the radial pulse. How the insertion of catheter through skin and arterial wall may be difficult, plus catheter stabilization is poor and catheter exchange is not easy, which needs to be further improved.

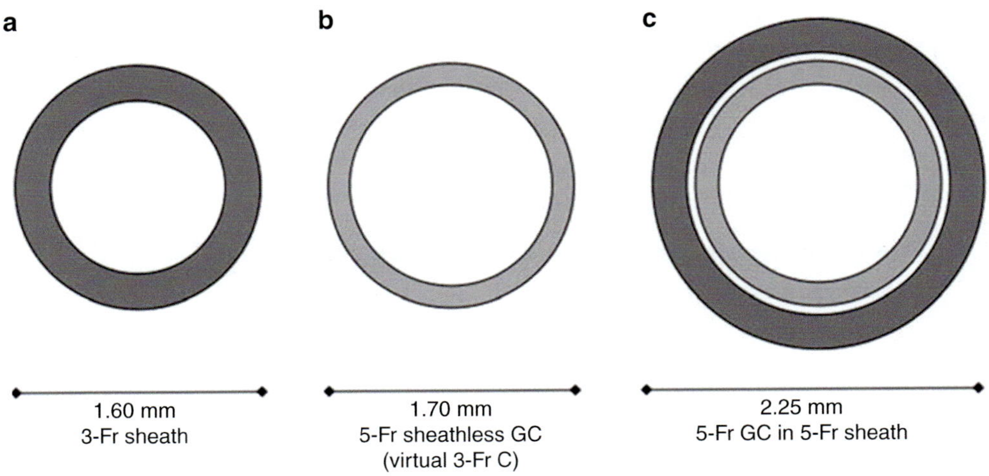

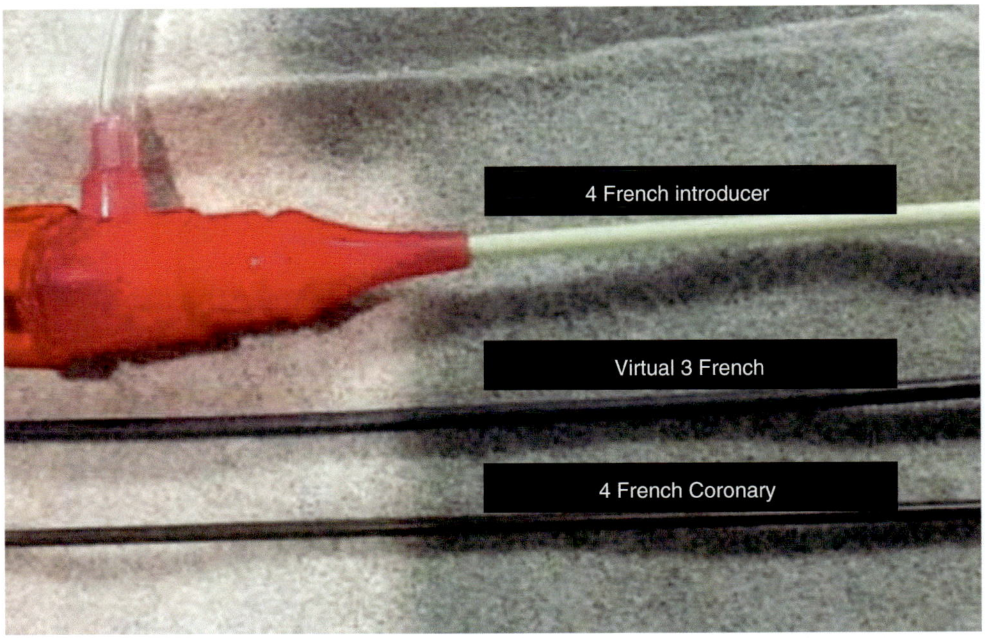

22.2.3.1 Procedures of Inserting a Sheathless Guiding Catheter

First give a local anesthesia to make an incision,then insert the angiograph wire for the sheath introducer. While advancing the angiography guide wire to the brachial artery, check the tip of the wire under fluoroscopy to make sure that it is not entering to the side branches. When the angiography wire reaches the brachial artery, insert a sheath introducer and exchange a guide wire for 220 cm angiography guide wire. We need 4 F sheath introducer for 6.5 sheath less catheter because the catheter is thinner than a 5 F sheath introducer. For a 7.5 F sheath less catheter, a 5 F sheath introducer should be used. Advance the 220 cm angiography guide wire to the ascending aorta by carefully observing it under fluoroscopy (Refer to video 1).

Incise the puncture side approximately by 1 mm to reduce resistance of the sheath less catheter and remove the sheath introducer to insert the sheath less catheter. Before you insert the sheath less catheter over the 220 cm angiographic guide wire, you need to dock the dilator with sheath less catheter. In order to avoid deformation of the distal shape of the sheath less catheter, please insert the dilator with the sheath less catheter just before the insertion into the body. After inserting the dilator into the sheath less catheter it should be locked by the docking device at the end of the dilator. By turning it clockwise, you can see the tip of the dilator coming out of sheath less catheter. Insert the system over the angiographic guide wire under this condition. Have an assistant holding angiographic guide wire while you insert the system into the body. If the insertion resistance is considerable you can make another incision. If the catheter is not sufficiently wet there could be considerable resistance, so wet the surface of the catheter with saline solution by using a syringe to allow smooth insertion. Because the sheath less catheter has a hydrophilic coating except the last 15 cm from the connector it would be very slippery when its surface is wetted with saline solution. Another way to enhance lubricity is to hold the piece of gauze of saline solution in your left hand while inserting the catheter. Keep inserting until it reaches the ascending aorta. When the sheath less catheter reaches the ascending aorta release the dilator lock and angiography guide wire. Connect the catheter to a Y connector and release air. As for the rest continue the procedure as usual. Cases of haemorrhage have not occurred according to our knowledge (Refer to the video 2).

First pull back the tip of sheathless catheter from the coronary artery. Disconnect the Y connector and advance the 220 cm guide wire into the body to the ascending aorta. Insert the dilator by advancing the guide wire first before the dilator. Dock the dilator to the catheter with the docking device and pull back the system to the brachial artery. Remove the angiographies guide wire first and then remove the entire system and stop bleeding. This method prevents the anterior vessel to be damaged by the catheter (Refer to the video 3).

22.2.4 Extra Back Up Techniques

With the miniaturization of catheters, the lack of back up force can be an issue. The thin walls increase the catheter flexibility, but could cause the catheter to slip back as other interventional devices are pushed through. These manoeuvers and techniques allow for a greater back-up force, while still maintaining the flexibility of slender catheters.

Loops – A loop is created by using exaggerated force while simultaneously giving a clock-wise or counter clock-wise rotation, forcing the catheter to twist and form a loop. This loop pushes up against the opposing wall of the aorta, creating a greater coaxial back-up force for other interventional devices. There are three different types of loops; the α-loop used for LAD lesions, the γ-loop used for CX lesions and ε-loop used for RCA lesions.

Anchor wire – Also known as the dummy wire technique, the anchor wire technique is when a secondary guidewire is inserted into a non-target coronary artery. This allows for an extra anchor point, increasing back-up force [10].

Anchor Balloon – This technique is very useful when deep engagement is required. A balloon is inflated in the target artery, distal to the lesion. The balloon is then retrieved and a stent can be delivered to the lesion site. The original anchor technique dictated that the balloon remain in the artery while a secondary wire with the stent be advanced into the guiding catheter. This required the use of a 6 Fr or 7 Fr GC, while the slender version of the anchor balloon technique can be done using a 4 Fr or 5 Fr GC [11].

Parallel wire – In this technique, two wires are advances simultaneously into the target artery, allowing for greater back-up force. It is particularly useful for complex lesions such as CTOs.

Mother and Child – A smaller catheter is inserted into the guiding catheter to increase back-up force. It is a commonly used technique amongst interventionists who practice Slender TRI [12].

22.3 Limitations

The innovations that have come out of Slender TRI have pushed the boundaries of material science in respect to percutaneous coronary intervention. The theoretical benefits are evident on a small scale, but for Slender TRI to achieve true validity and feasibility, large scale randomized testing needs to be undertaken. A limitation of the thin walled catheters are the lack of durability, and their tendency to be damaged.

Due to the flexibility, they are also harder to manipulate and position. It also results in poor back-up force.

Due to the inherent size of 5 Fr guiding catheters, larger interventional devices such as thrombus aspiration catheters, ≥3.0 mm cutting balloons, BVS >3 mm, IVUS imaging catheters, or ≥1.5 mm rotablator burrs cannot be used, so patient selection is critical as not all lesions can be treated.

Inexperience and careless patient selection can lead to prolonged fluoroscopy and procedural times, along with subpar treatment success due to inadequate visualization and interpretation of coronary pathology in smaller 3 Fr and 4 Fr catheters.

Procedural costs may increase due to the rising cost of new and innovative catheters, sheaths and interventional devices along the increased use of advanced techniques (such as the anchor wire, anchor balloon, parallel wire and mother and child techniques) which requires the use of multiple interventional devices, pushing the cost of Slender TRI beyond convention.

Slender TRI is also associated with a longer learning curve, which is already problematic when dealing with transradial intervention as a whole.

The popularity of TRI, and subsequently Slender TRI, has risen significantly over the last few decades. This rise will inevitably continue, bringing forth more in depth large scale studies along with a decrease in the limitations of Slender TRI.

Case 22.1

CTO of RCA treated by retrograde approach using bi-radial virtual 4 French guiding catheters (Fig. 22.3).

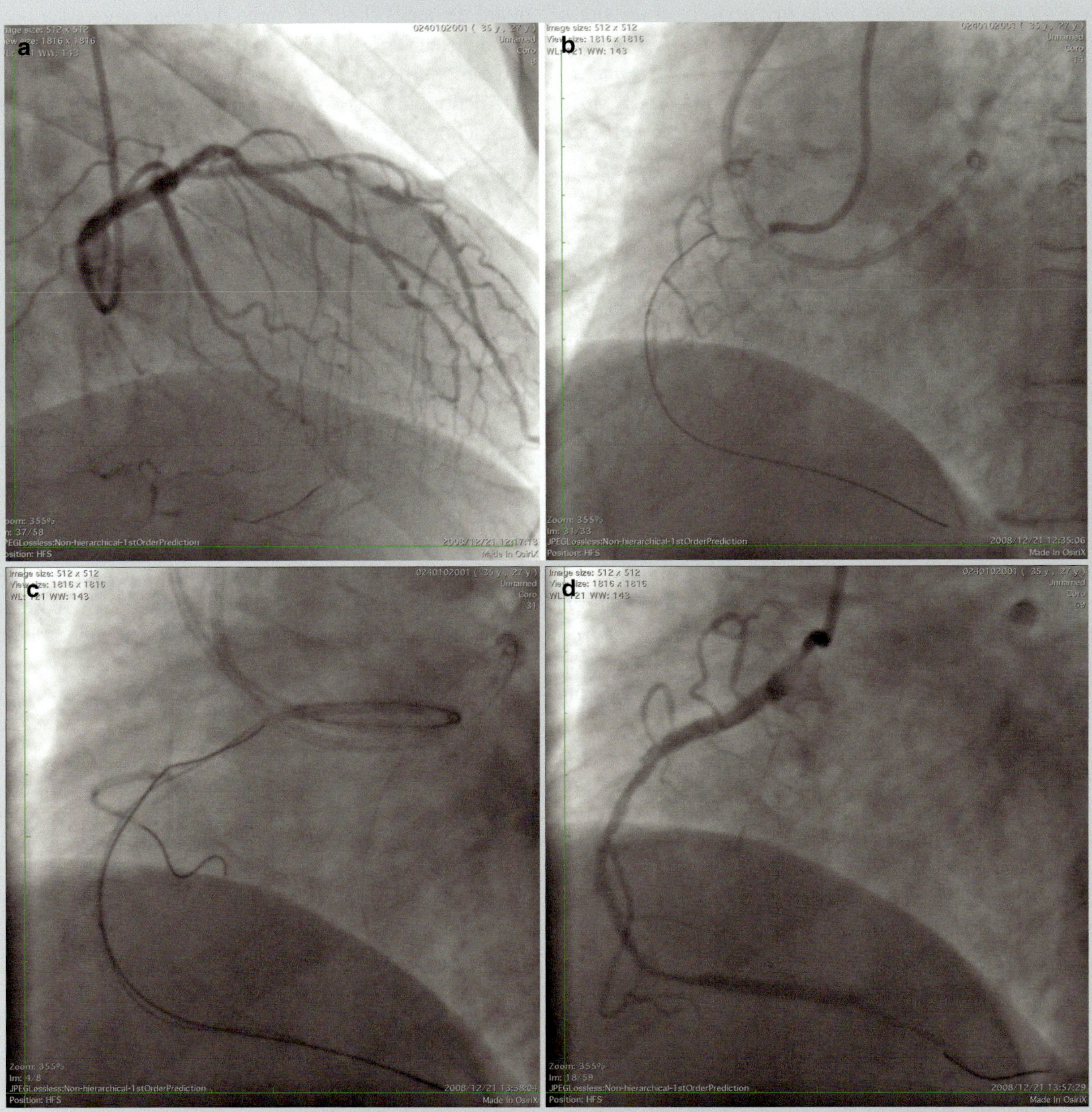

Fig. 22.3 *Left* (**a**): a wire passed to a septal channel (6-Fr EBU3.5 guiding catheter without introducer [Launcher, Medtronic]). *Right* (**b**): retrograde wire reached distal end of RCA CTO lesion (6-Fr SAL1.0 guiding catheter without introducer [Launcher, Medtronic]). Sion-Blue guidewire (ASAHI) reached distal end of CTO lesion through septal channel from LAD. *Left* (**c**) : retrograde and antegrade wires passed through the CTO lesion. Miracle-3 guidewire (ASAHI) passed through CTO lesion with the guidance by retrograde wire. *Right* (**d**) Final angiogram

Case 22.2

CTO of RCA treated by antegrade approach through a 4 French guiding catheter from right radial approach (Fig. 22.4).

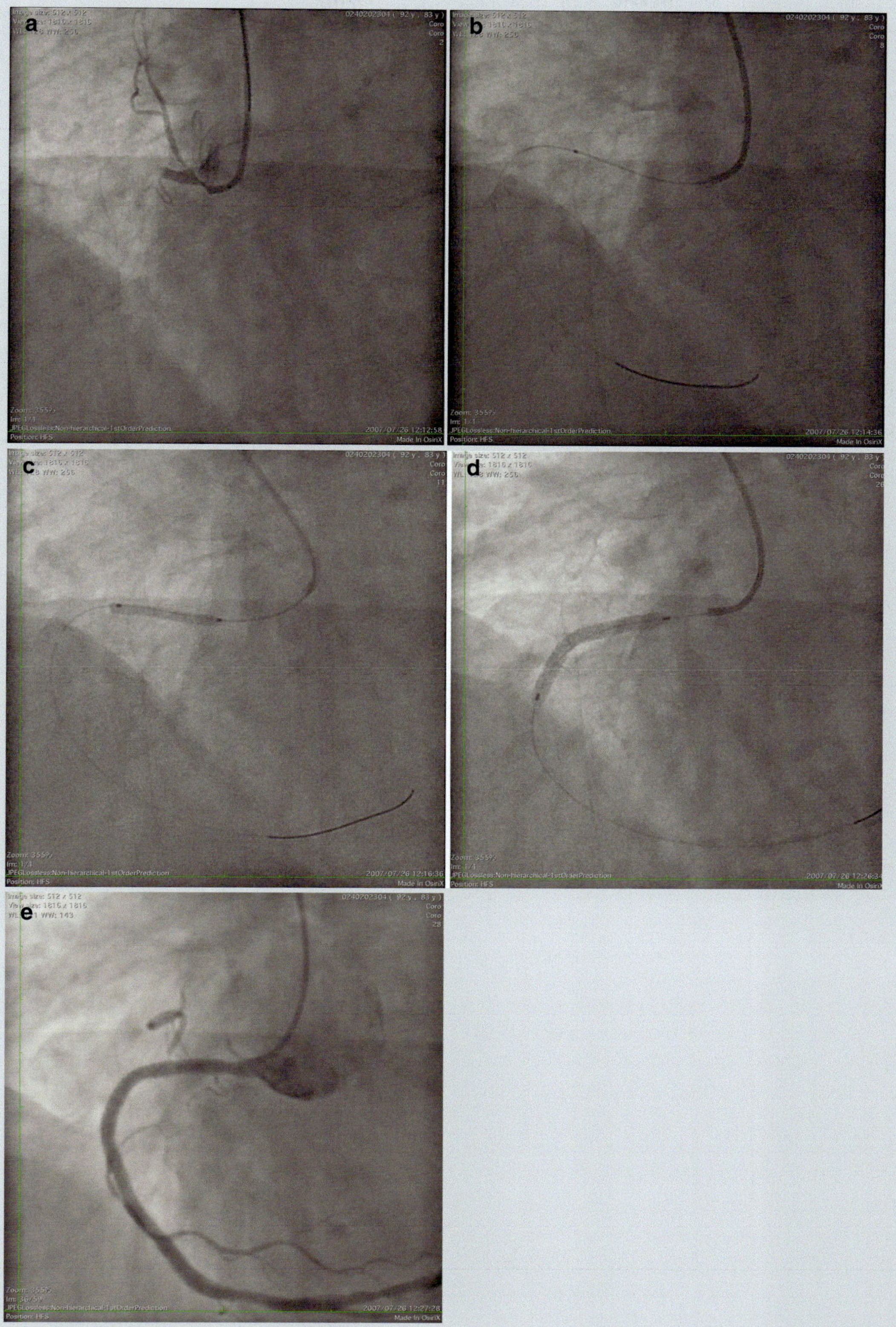

Fig. 22.4 *Left* (**a**): Initial RCA angiogram. TERUMO 4-French JR4 guiding catheter (KIWAMI, TERUMO). *Right* (**b**) a stiff wire passed through the CTO lesion assisted by microcatheter support. Choice-PT guidewire (Boston) passed through CTO lesion with the assistance of Finecross microcatheter (TERUMO). *Left* (**c**): 2.5 × 20 mm Maverick balloon dilatation (Boston). (**d**): 3.0 × 28 mm DES implantation (Xience-V, Abbott). (**e**) Final angiogram

References

1. Chase AJ, Fretz EB, Warburton WP, et al. Association of the arterial access site at angioplasty with transfusion and mortality: the M.O.R.T.A.L study (Mortality benefit Of Reduced Transfusion after percutaneous coronary intervention via the Arm or Leg). Heart. 2008;94:1019–25.
2. Jolly SS, Yusuf S, Cairns J, et al. Radial versus femoral access for coronary angiography and intervention in patients with acute coronary syndromes (RIVAL): a randomised, parallel group, multicentre trial. Lancet. 2011;377:1409–20.
3. Hamon M, Pristipino C, Di Mario C, et al. Consensus document on the radial approach in percutaneous cardiovascular interventions: position paper by the European Association of Percutaneous Cardiovascular Interventions and Working Groups on Acute Cardiac Care** and Thrombosis of the European Society of Cardiology. EuroIntervention J EuroPCR Collaboration Working Group Interv Cardiol Eur Soc Cardiol. 2013;8:1242–51.
4. Rao SV, Tremmel JA, Gilchrist IC, et al. Best practices for transradial angiography and intervention: a consensus statement from the society for cardiovascular angiography and intervention's transradial working group. Catheter Cardiovasc Interv Off J Soc Cardiac Angiography Interv. 2014;83:228–36.
5. Saito S, Ikei H, Hosokawa G, Tanaka S. Influence of the ratio between radial artery inner diameter and sheath outer diameter on radial artery flow after transradial coronary intervention. Catheter Cardiovasc Interv Off J Soc Cardiac Angiography Interv. 1999; 46:173–8.
6. Kiemeneij F, Yoshimachi F, Matsukage T, et al. Focus on maximal miniaturisation of transradial coronary access materials and techniques by the Slender Club Japan and Europe: an overview and classification. EuroIntervention J EuroPCR Collaboration Working Group Interv Cardiol Eur Soc Cardiol. 2015;10:1178–86.
7. Amoroso G, van Dullemen A, Westgeest P, van Duinen M. "Virtual" 3 Fr transradial coronary stenting with the 5 Fr Meito Masamune sheathless guiding catheter: feasibility and safety in an outpatient setting. J Invasive Cardiol. 2016;28:109–14.
8. Tonomura D, Shimada Y, Yano K, et al. Feasibility and safety of a virtual 3-Fr sheathless-guiding system for percutaneous coronary intervention. Catheter Cardiovasc Interv Off J Soc Cardiac Angiography Interv. 2014;84:426–35.
9. Takeshita S, Asano H, Hata T, et al. Comparison of frequency of radial artery occlusion after 4Fr versus 6Fr transradial coronary intervention (from the Novel Angioplasty USIng Coronary Accessor Trial). Am J Cardiol. 2014;113:1986–9.
10. Hamood H, Makhoul N, Grenadir E, Kusniec F, Rosenschein U. Anchor wire technique improves device deliverability during PCI of CTOs and other complex subsets. Acute Card Care. 2006;8:139–42.
11. Fujita S, Tamai H, Kyo E, et al. New technique for superior guiding catheter support during advancement of a balloon in coronary angioplasty: the anchor technique. Catheter Cardiovasc Interv Off J Soc Cardiac Angiography Interv. 2003;59:482–8.
12. Takahashi S, Saito S, Tanaka S, et al. New method to increase a backup support of a 6 French guiding coronary catheter. Catheter Cardiovasc Interv Off J Soc Cardiac Angiography Interv. 2004;63: 452–6.

0.010-inch Guidewire in Slender Intervention

23

Takashi Matsukage

Abstracts

0.0010-in. guidewire, so called "ten wire" is a guide-wire whose diameter is 0.010-in. throughout. Historically speaking, 0.014-in. guidewires have been used most commonly. However, it may be about time to reconsider if the diameter of guidewires needs to be 0.014-in. since devices of PCI such as guidewires, balloons, stents, etc. are getting more and more sophisticated as medical technology advances.

Even for basic coronary lesions, the use of 8Fr guide catheter was important for stenting during the 1990s. Nowadays, 4, 5 or 6 Fr. guiding catheter via radial approach is good enough to implant a stent to a simple lesion. It has already proved that smaller diameter size of guide catheters provides patients to less vascular complications [1, 2], reduced amounts of contrast media [3], and optimizing patient ease [4]. Therefore, we should advance technology of PCI in the direction of routine usage of smaller size guide catheters. However, there still exists some limitation of PCI with 5 or 6 Fr. guiding catheters to deal with complex lesions because smaller size guide catheters sometimes don't have enough room to accommodate usual devices. Then, 0.010-in. guidewire is useful to overcome this limitation.

Kissing balloon technique (KBT) through 5 Fr. guiding catheter is impossible with 0.014-in. guide-wires. 6 Fr. or lager guiding catheter is required to perform KBT with 0.014-in. guidewires. Yoshimachi et al. reported in 2007 [5] that use of 0.010 in. guidewires and specialized balloons for a 0.010 in. guidewire (Ikazuchi-X produced by Kaneka Medix, Tokyo, Japan) make KBT through 5 Fr. guiding catheter possible. The Ikazuchi-X PTCA balloon system is compatible with a 0.010 in. guidewire and consists of a regular rapid-exchange balloon catheter component. The maximum external diameter of the balloon is 2.1 Fr., though it is 2.4 Fr. with the smallest 0.014 in.-compatible balloons. Therefore making it likely to pass two balloons over two wires through a 5 Fr. guiding catheter. In this manuscript of 2007, we showed feasibility of KBT through 5 Fr. guiding catheter based on the results of In vitro experiments and animal experiments and reported the first case of KBT with 5 Fr. guide catheter, which was performed to protected left main disease. Nowadays, at some hospitals in Japan, KBT through 5Fr. guiding catheter is routinely performed replacing 6 Fr. guiding catheter.

Trifurcation lesions are challenging to treat due to difficulty in branch's ostium's patency preservation. Concurrent triple-balloon inflation can result in improvement of these difficulties, consistent with the need of kissing balloon technique for bifurcation lesion. However, simultaneous triple-balloon inflation technique requires 8 Fr. or larger guiding catheter if 0.014-in. guidewires are used because the guide catheter has to accommodate three guidewires and balloons simultaneously. Therefore, trans-radial approach is almost impossible with the technique using 0.0014-in. guidewires. Matsukage et al. reported two cases of trifurcation lesions involving a left main coronary artery (LMCA) stenosis treated with stent implantation and simultaneous triple-balloon inflation technique through 6 Fr. guiding catheter with 0.010-in. guide wires and its compatible balloons treated via radial approach. It also shows simultaneous triple-balloon inflation is to obtain an almost complete round circle at the LMCA by intravascular ultrasound imaging.

In addition that 0.010-in. guidewires are able to save space for a smaller guide catheter, the guidewire are good to pass coronary arteries in some situations thanks to its

T. Matsukage, MD, PhD
Tokai University Hachioji Hospital, Tokyo, Japan
e-mail: ptc@b03.itscom.net

Y. Zhou et al. (eds.), *Transradial Approach for Percutaneous Interventions*, DOI 10.1007/978-94-017-7350-8_23

Table 23.1 0.010-inch guidewire specification

Manufacturer	Guidewire	Tip stiffness (g)	Coating characteristics
Asahi Intecc	Decillion FL	0.8	Coil with hydrophilic; Tip 80 mm
	Decillion HS	1.5	Polymer coated; Tip 120 mm
	Decillion MD	3.0	Coil with hydrophilic; Tip 80 mm
	RG3; 300 mm	0.8	For bidirectional approach use
Japan Life Line	Slender 01	0.9	Coil with hydrophilic; Tip 30 mm
	Slender support	1.3	Coil with hydrophilic; Tip 30 mm
	eel slender	1.5	Polymer coated; Tip 115 mm
Kaneka Medix	TEN-NYO NL	0.75	Coil with hydrophilic; Tip 200 mm
	TEN-NYO HT	0.75	Coil with hydrophilic; Tip 300 mm

thinness. The area of 0.010-in. guidewire is 51 % smaller than one of 0.014-in. guidewire. One report shows management for a side branch with total occlusion after efficacious implantation of a stent in the target lesion with a 0.010-in. system even after failure of 0.014-in. guidewires [7]. Table 23.1 presents the specifics of the 0.010-in. guidewires.

When it comes to crossing chronic total occlusion (CTO), 0.010-in. guidewires seem to have potential tremendous power. In the the Prospective Multicenter Registry of IKAzuchi-X for CHronic Total OcclUsion (the PIKACHU registry), we show the welfare and efficiency of a 0.010-in. guidewire and a balloon catheter for management of CTO [8]. The PIKACHU registry is a prospective, multicenter registry study. A 0.010-in. guidewire was used as the primary guidewire to try to pass the CTO lesion. The primary endpoint included: success using a 0.010 system. The outcomes are as follows. 141 patients with one lesion each were registered. The average period of occlusion was 9 months (range 3–156). A 6 Fr. guiding catheter used in 72 cases (51.1 %) and TRI was 76.6 %. CTOs between 10 and 20 mm long, observed in 53 occlusions. There were 107 lesions (75.9 %) with bending of more than 45°. Calcification presented in 91 lesions (64.5 %). A 0.010-in. guidewire was successfully passed through in 97 of 141 lesions (68.8 %). A 0.010-in. guidewire compatible balloon catheter was passed in 87 of the 97 lesions (88.7 %) and final PCI success was achieved in all the cases. The overall experimental success rate was 87.9 % (124/141). No major adverse cardiac events (MACE) or bleeding complications were observed. This concludes the 0.010-in. catheter to be safe and practical for managing CTO lesions.

As reviewed so far, 0.010-in. guidewire have tremendous potential. To use the guidewires routinely, the safety and feasibility of the system should be confirmed. We perfumed the IKATEN Registry for assessment of this system as the main device for treating PCI [9]. The registry is a prospective, multicenter, nonrandomized registry study. Patients undergone PCI with 0.010-in. guidewire and associated balloon as the main device were registered. The co primary end- points included clinical and device success rates, the secondary endpoints were MACE and bleeding complications. The outcomes were as follows. A total of 133 patients with 148 lesions were enrolled. The majority were male (75.3 %), and mean age was 69 ± 10 years. Type B2/C lesions comprised 60 % of the lesions, CTO was 16.9 %, and bifurcation lesions were found in 22.3 % of patients. A transradial approach was used in 79.7 % of patients, and the average guiding catheter size was 5.1 ± 0.4 Fr. Clinical success rate was 99.2 %, and device success rate was 99.3 %. Device failure took place in one case of chronic total occlusion due to ineffective guidewire passage. MACE and bleeding complications were not presented besides small hematoma at the puncture site in a single patient. Stent delivery success rate on 0.010-in. guidewire was 93.9 % because of failure of stent balloon to pass eight lesions. To close, it suggests that the 0.010-in. system is without risk and is viable for routine PCI (bifurcation and CTO lesions).

We as interventional cardiologists have been so accustomed to using 0.014-in. guide wires that manipulating 0.010-in. guidewires may feel somehow difficult. Devises of PCI have been being improved and sophisticated routinely, and trans-radial approach is spreading all over the world. We as interventional cardiologist should get accustomed to using 0.010-in. guidewires to apply the wires in accordance with suitable lesions, and it may be high time to consider what diameter of guidewires is appropriate for today.

Case Report

A 60-year-old male patient was admitted to our hospital because of chest pain on effort (CCS class III). His coronary risk factors included diabetes, hypertension and dyslipidemia. Coronary angiography revealed significant stenosis in the mid potion of left anterior descending artery (LAD) and the ostium of diagonal branch (Fig. 23.1).

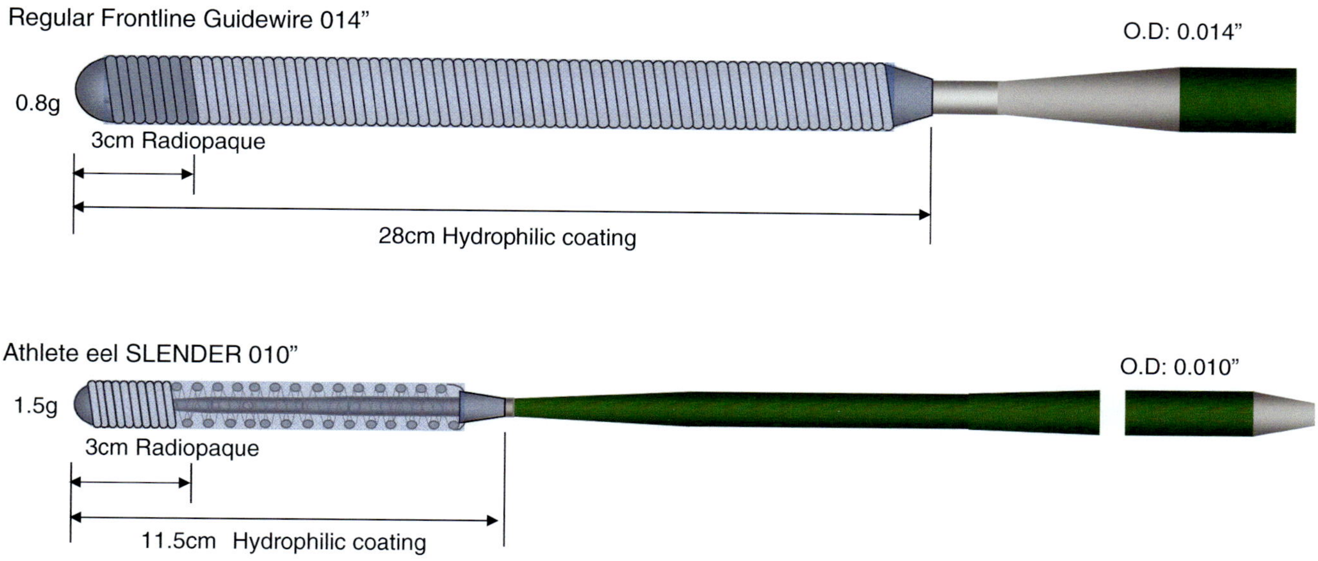

Fig. 23.1 Schema of 0.014-in. and 0.010-in. guidewire

We therefore performed elective percutaneous coronary intervention with the following procedural steps. A 6-Fr-sized sheath introducer was inserted into the right radial artery and a 6-Fr Heartrail-II SL 4.0 guiding catheter (Terumo, Tokyo, Japan) was inserted into left coronary artery. Initially two guidewires, Sion (Asahi Intecc, Nagoya, Japan) and Runthrogh Hypercoat (Terumo, Tokyo, Japan) were advanced into the LAD and the diagonal branch, respectively. A Xience Prime stent (3.5 × 28 mm; Abbott Vascular, IL, USA.) was implanted from the LAD crossing over the diagonal branch at an inflation pressure of 16 atmosphere (atm) after balloon dilatation of Sapphire II (OrbusNeich, Wanchai, Hong Kong) (Fig. 23.2). We try to re-crossed the guidewire to the diagonal branch through the stent strut. However, a regular guidewire did not cross the strut of stent to diagonal branch after a stent implantation (Fig. 23.3). A guidewire passed side branch to change the Athlete eel slender (Japan Life Line, Tokyo, Japan) in 0.010-in. sized. A 0.010-in. guidewire advanced the strut of jailed stent smoothly. Finally, Kissing Balloon Technique was undergone in 0.010 & 0.014-in. combinations to the LAD and the diagonal branch (Fig. 23.4).

The final angiography revealed excellent results as shown in Fig. 23.5.

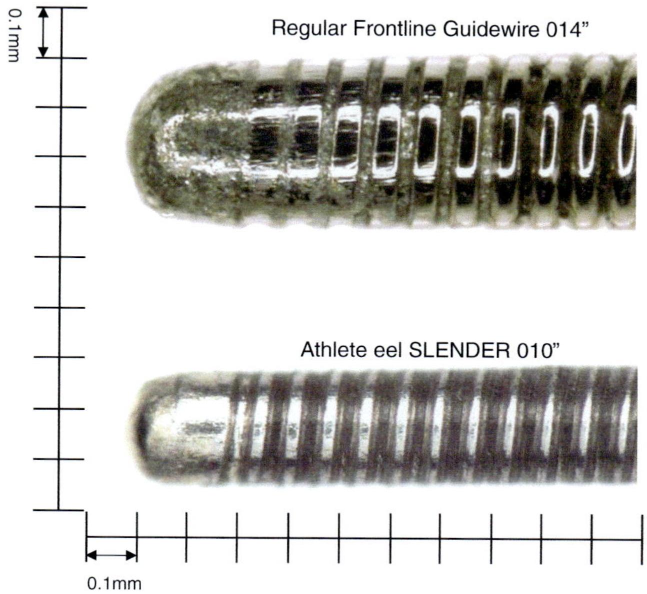

Fig. 23.2 Close up picture of tip of 0.014 and 0.010-inchguidewire

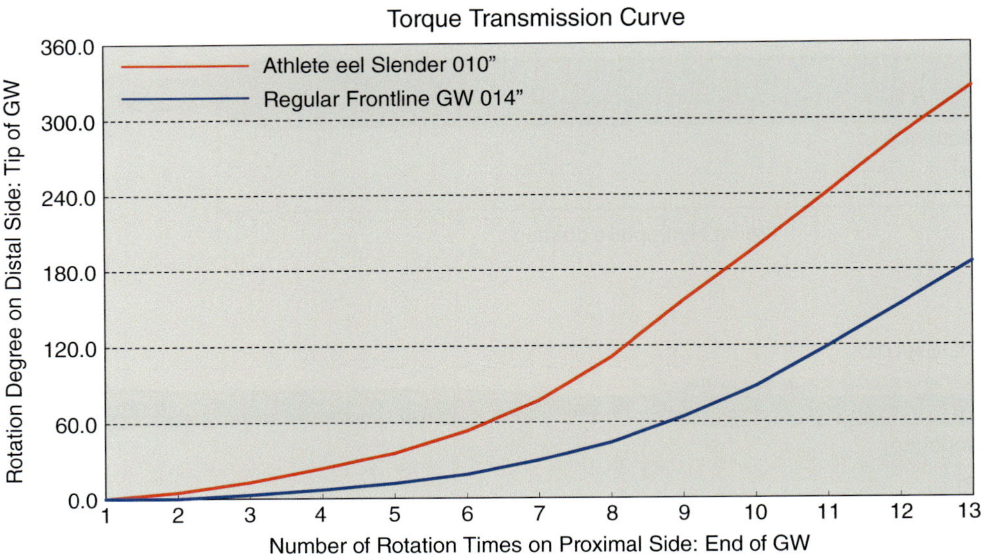

Fig. 23.3 Torque transmission curve: comparison of 0.014-in. with 0.010-in. guidewire

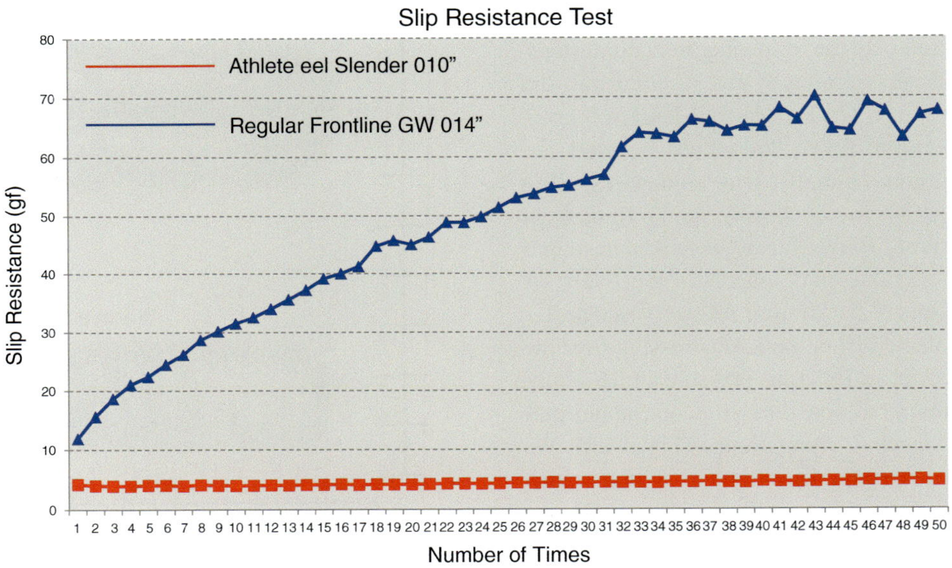

Fig. 23.4 Slip resistance : comparison of 0.014-in. with 0.010-in. guidewire

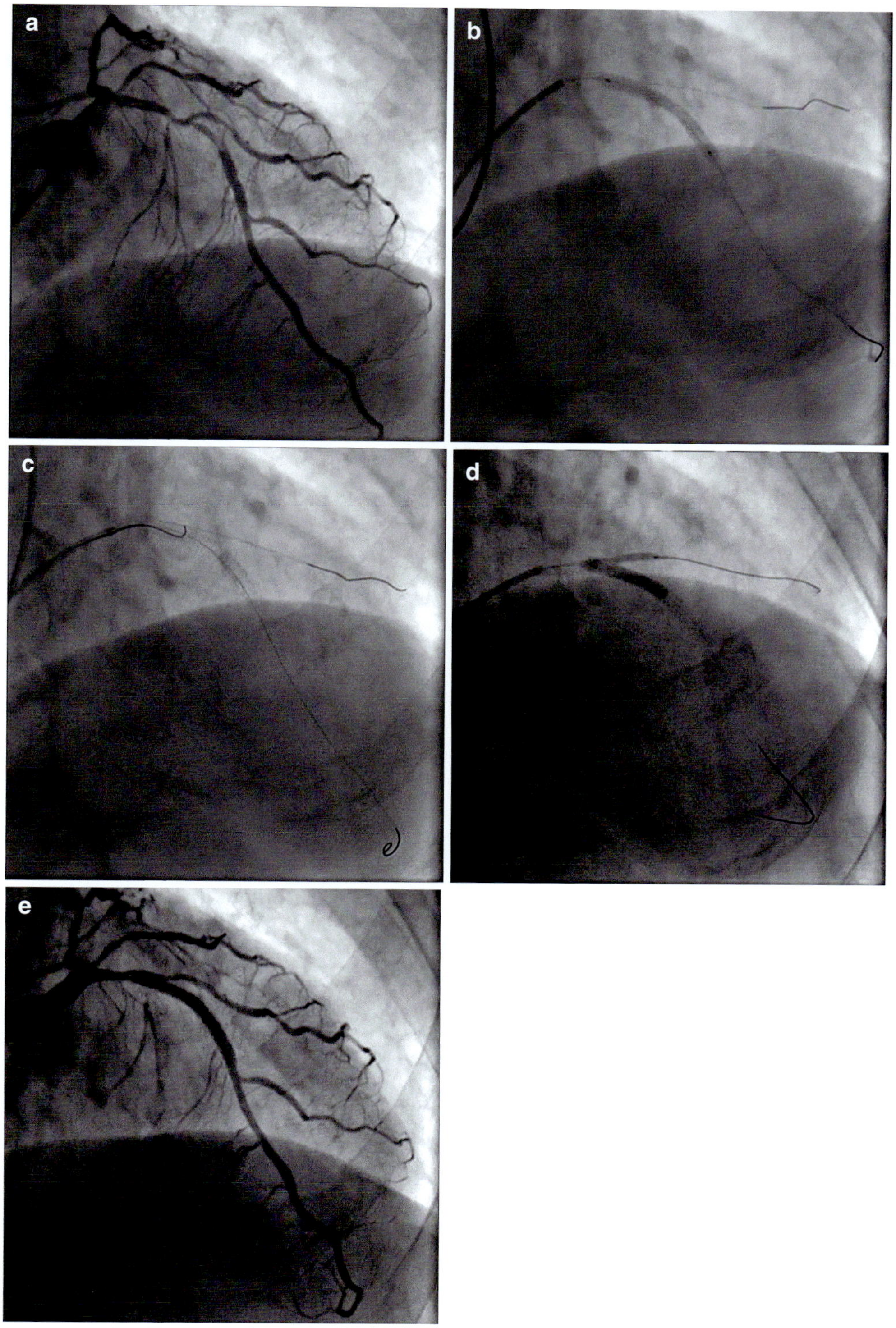

Fig. 23.5 (**a**) A control angiography showing tight stenosis of the mid portion of LAD involving large diagonal branch. (**b**) A EES was deployed in the LAD after regular 0.014-inch guidewires were advanced into the LAD and diagonal branch. (**c**) A regular 0.014-inch guidewire did not advance through the strut of stent. However, a 0.010-inch guidewire was smoothly advanced the strut. (**d**) The final kissing balloon technique was performed to LAD and diagonal branch. (**e**) Final angiography of the left coronary artery

References

1. Saito S, Ikei H, Hosokawa G, et al. Influence of the ratio between radial artery inner diameter and sheath outer diameter on radial artery flow after transradial coronary intervention. Catheter Cardiovasc Interv. 1999;46:173–8.
2. Nagai S, Abe S, Sato T, et al. Ultrasonic assessment of vascular complications in coronary angiography and angioplasty after transradial approach. Am J Cardiol. 1999;83:180–6.
3. Metz D, Meyer P, Touati C, et al. Comparison of 6Fr with 7Fr and 8Fr guiding catheters for elective coronary angioplasty: results of a prospective, multicenter, randomized trial. Am Heart J. 1997;134:131–7.
4. Saito S, Miyake S, Hosokawa G, et al. Transradial intervention in Japanese patients. Catheter Cardiovasc Interv. 1999;46:37–41.
5. Yoshimachi F, Masutani M, Matukage T, et al. Kissing balloon technique within a 5 Fr guiding catheter using 0.010 inch guidewires and 0.010 inch guidewire- compatible balloons. J Invasive Cardiol. 2007;19(12):519–24.
6. Matsukage T, Masuda N, Ikairi Y. Simultaneous triple-balloon inflation technique within a 6 Fr guiding catheter for a trifurcation lesion. J Invasive Cardiol 2008;20:E210–E214.
7. Otsuka Y. A novel 0.010-inch guidewire for crossing jailed sidebranches. Catheter Cardiovasc Interv. 2009;73:346–9.
8. Matsukage T, Masutani M, Yoshimachi F, et al. A prospective multicenter registry of 0.010-inch guidewire and compatible system for chronic total occlusion: the PIKACHU registry. Catheter Cardiovasc Interv. 2010;75:1006–12.
9. Matsukage T, Yoshimachi F, Masutani M, et al. A new 0.010-inch guidewire and compatible balloon catheter system: the IKATEN registry. Catheter Cardiovasc Interv. 2009;73:605–10.

Trans Radial Excimer Laser Coronary Atherectomy Application During Complex PCI

24

John Rawlins, Jehangir Din, Suneel Talwar, and Peter O'Kane

24.1 Introduction

Use of lasers for treating atherosclerotic vascular disease began in the 1980s when it was initially utilized in treating critical limb ischemia [1]. The absorption properties of laser light by atherosclerotic material created the hypothesis that laser could resolve a range of coronary and peripheral occlusions [2]. The application of laser to debulk or ablate coronary atherosclerosis followed and laser gained momentum as a potential method to remove atherosclerosis and reduce the rate of vessel restenosis and occlusion that accompanied coronary balloon angioplasty [3], prior to the advent of stents.

Several large scale successful clinical trials during early experience suggested a prominent role for laser in interventional cardiology [4, 5]. However, the application of laser energy was limited due to the size of the machine, prolonged warmup and calibration time. The laser catheters were very rigid, restricting their deliverability. Lasing technique was rudimentary, with a tendency for quickly going thought the catheters of the target lesions, which have not allow enough absorption of the laser energy within the irradiated plaque and thus did not yield the maximum ablative potential of the device. As such, initial experience was marred with early frequency of significant complications including abrupt vessel closure, thrombosis and vessel dissection [6, 7]. The coronary interventional community turned away from the technology. However, following modifications in newer catheter design permitting smaller laser generators [8] and introduction of safe lasing techniques emphasizing slow debulking and concomitant injections of saline [9, 10] have led to important improvement in clinical results [11]. The indications for laser atherectomy are now well defined, and the procedure is becoming well established within modern interventional practice.

The development of smaller diameter laser catheters have progressed alongside the adoption of the transradial approach for percutaneous coronary intervention (TRI). Advantages of this approach are explored in detail throughout this book. Importantly the radial access offers improved safety, efficacy and better patient experience compared to transfemoral procedures. It is therefore not surprising that TRI has become the default route of vascular access site for the mainly of percutaneous coronary interventions (PCI). The purpose of this chapter is to describe the principles and practice of Excimer laser coronary atherectomy (ELCA) and specifically its application during TRI. The indications for ELCA are described, and illustrated with cases performed exclusively from the radial artery.

24.2 Excimer Coronary Laser Atherectomy (ECLA)

Laser devices harness light of a specific wavelength to generate a unidirectional beam of high-intensity light that can be directed towards on object of interest. The wavelength of the emitted light is used to categorize the type of laser (Table 24.1). The depth of penetration of the laser is directly related to its wavelength, with laser in the ultraviolet range (shorter wavelength) having less depth of penetration, less heat production, and less unwanted tissue damage. Excimer lasers use rare gas and halogen to generate pulses of short wavelength, high-energy ultraviolet light (Fig. 24.1). Upon electrical discharge, energy immersed by atoms causes their high energy state. Electronic excitation of each atom leads to bonding with other atomic species (argon, krypton, xenon). And this results is the formation of an excimer. Upon the molecule's return to prior state, short wavelength ultraviolet radiation is produced.

J. Rawlins, BSc, MBBS, MRCP, MD • J. Din, MBBS, MRCP, MD • S. Talwar, MBBS, MRCP, MD
Dorset Heart Centre Royal Bournemouth Hospital Bournemouth, Dors, Bournemouth, UK
e-mail: John.Rawlins@rbch.nhs.u

P. O'Kane, BSc, MBBS, FRCP, MD(Res) (✉)
Dorset Heart Centre, Royal Bournemouth Hospital, Bournemouth, Dorset BH7 7DW, UK
e-mail: Peter.O'Kane@rbch.nhs.uk

Y. Zhou et al. (eds.), *Transradial Approach for Percutaneous Interventions*, DOI 10.1007/978-94-017-7350-8_24

Table 24.1 Different types of laser categorized by emitted light wavelength

Laser type	Wavelength (nm)	Absorption depth (mm)	Absorption mechanism
XeCl[a] (Excimer)	308	0.05	Protein-lipids
Nd:YAG[b]	1060	2.0	Protein-water
Dye	480	0.5	Protein
Argon	488	0.5	Protein
Ho:YAG[c]	2060	0.3	Water
Nd:YAG	1320	1.25	Water

[a]Xenon chloride
[b]Neodymium-doped yttrium aluminium garnet
[c]Holmium yttrium aluminium garnet

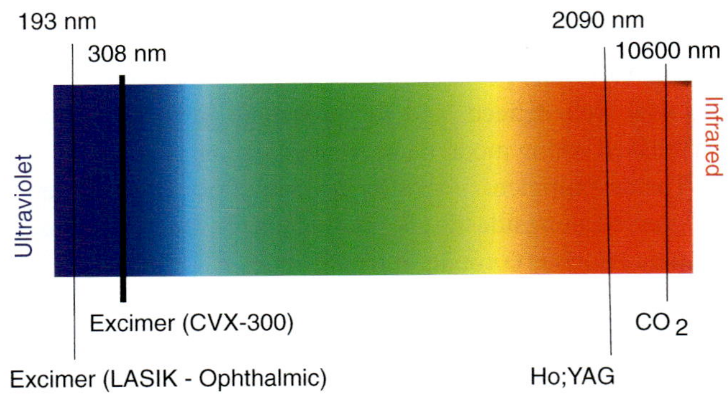

Fig. 24.1 The spectrum of light. The wavelength of light emitted from a laser is determined by the lasing medium and it is an important factor in determining the properties of the system. Laser light emitted from the Spectranectics CVX-300 excimer (XeCl) laser system is "Cool" (308 nm) which is similar to laser light employed for LASIK (193.3 nm) used in Ophthalmic surgery. In contrast to infrared lasers, the excimer laser has a shallow penetration of depth (50 um) and ablates tissue precisely without excessive heat production and minimises inadvertent tissue damage

Excimer laser tissue ablation is mediated through three distinct mechanisms: photochemical, photo-thermal, and photomechanical. UV light is rapidly and effectively absorbed by intravascular tissue and thrombus, and the absorbed light breaks carbon-carbon bonds, weakening the structure of the cells (photochemical). In addition, laser light elevates the temperature of intracellular water, eventually producing water vapor causing the cells to rupture. The generation of a vapour bubble cloud at the tip of the catheter enables controlled disruption of the atherosclerotic material (photo-thermal). Expansion and implosion of these vapor bubbles generates the photomechanical effect as the pressure is released from the vapour bubble, further disrupting the obstructive intravascular material as well as sweeping the freed particles downstream (photomechanical). The vast majority of the fragments released during laser atherectomy are >10 microns in diameter and are easily filtered by the reticuloendothelial system downstream which avoids microvascular obstruction and no-reflow phenomena.

The minimum energy needed to penetrate the UV light into the adjacent tissue and consequent creation of a steam bubble called "fluence" (range 30–80 mJ/mm^2). "Pulse repetition" is the amount of pulses produced during 1 s. "Pulse width" is the length of each pulse. Pulse width can be adjusted according to needs of the lesions (Fig. 24.2).

24.2.1 Excimer Laser Equipment and General Technique

The CVX-300 cardiovascular laser excimer system (Spectranetics, Colorado Springs, CO, USA, Fig. 24.2) uses Xenon chloride (XeCl) as the active medium. Consequently, the light produced is pulsed and remains in the ultraviolet B (UVB) region of the spectrum with a wavelength of 308 nm and a tissue penetration depth between 30 and 50 microns. The excimer laser light is produced by a transportable generator that is powered by mains electricity with a standard plug suitable for each country. Its is the only device currently available with FDA approval.

ELCA catheters are delivered using a monorail segment that is well-matched with any standard 0.014″ guidewire and are presented in four diameters for use in the coronary artery 0.9 mm, 1.4 mm, 1.7 mm, and 2.0 mm sizes. The catheters most commonly used have a concentric array of laser fibres at the tip. Alternatively eccentric laser catheters are available where the laser fibres are focused toward one hemisphere of the catheter tip which potentially serves as a better device for debulking In-stent Restenosis (ISR – Fig. 24.2). The larger diameter devices (1.7 mm & 2.0 mm catheters, and the eccentric catheters) are primarily used in straight sections of large diameter vessels for example in treating saphenous vein grafts. They necessitate 7 F and 8 F guide catheters correspondingly, which limits their deliverability via the radial route. The remainder can be used effectively via a 6 F guiding system. From the radial route, care should be taken to select a guiding catheter that provides adequate support, and that remains coaxial during lasing. The use of sheathless large calibre guides (eg Ashai sheathless 7.5 F system, Japan) is a solution for when large calibre laser catheters are being considered.

It is essential that certain safety procedures should be observed in the catheter lab when performing laser atherectomy. Prior to the excimer laser being activated all persons in the room, even the patient, must wear protective tinted spectacles to minimize the risk of retinal exposure to the ultraviolet light and all windows should be covered and the doors should be locked. Following this safety checklist, the laser unit is warmed up and then the selected catheter is plugged into the generator and calibrated prior to being introduced into the body. Even when the catheter is in-vivo, all staff in the vicinity should wear eye protection in case the laser catheter breaks

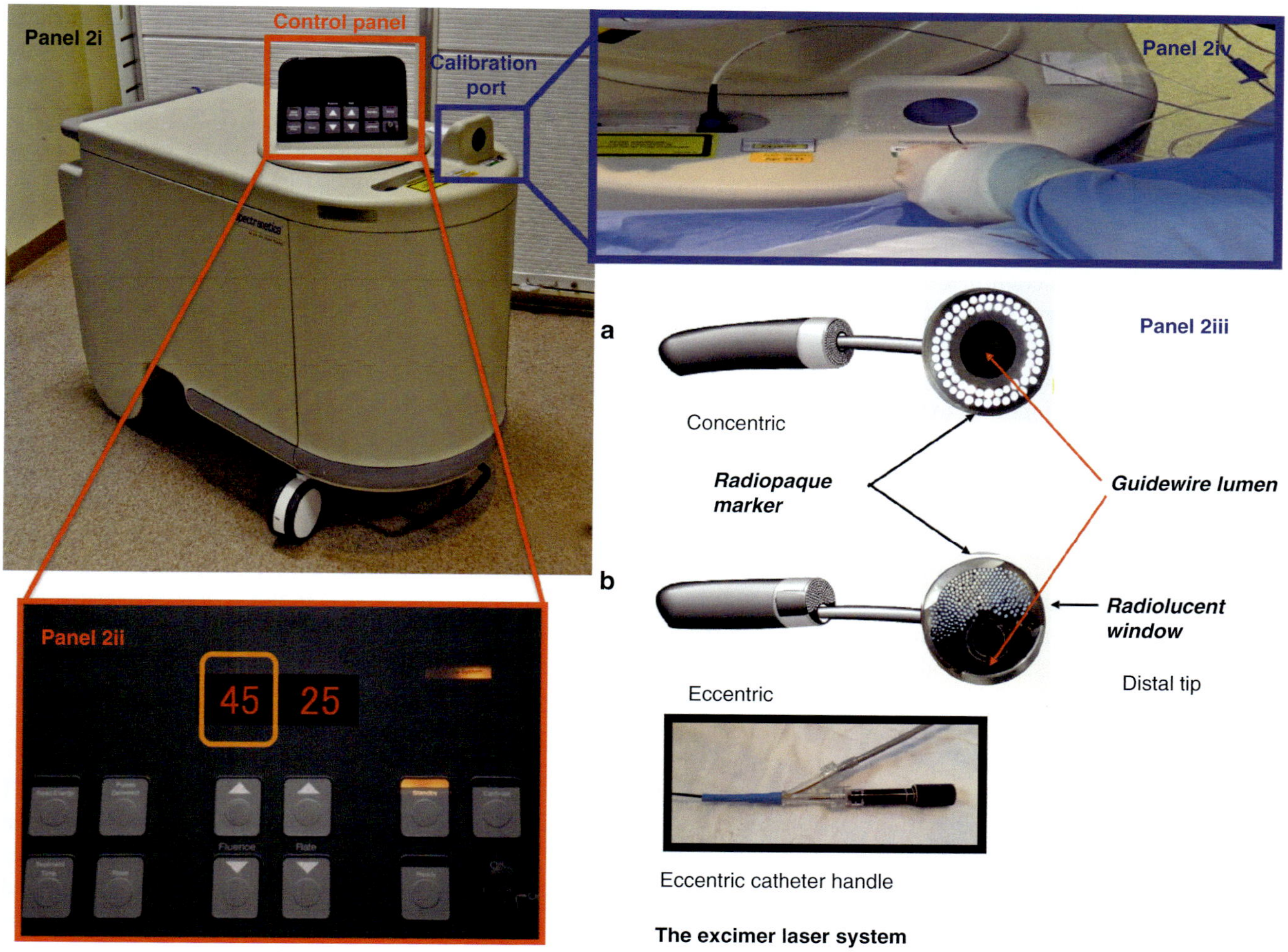

Fig. 24.2 The Spectranetics CVX-300 Excimer laser system. Panel **i** illustrates the pulse generator. The controls are located on the top of the device, and illustrated in panel **ii**. Two numbers are visible, with fluence on the left (indicated with an *orange box*, in this case set at 45 mJ/mm^2), and pulse repetition frequency on the right (in this example, 25Hz). Panel **iii** illustrates the two available configurations of laser catheter – concentric and eccentric – referring to the orientation of the laser fibres within the catheter. These are directed at the calibration port (Panel **iv**) before being introduced into the body

and releases UV light. Laser catheter size selection is primarily based on (a) the severity of the lesion, (b) the reference vessel diameter, and (c) consistency of the target material [12].

The selected catheter is advanced to the lesion over a standard 0.014″ guide wire which is supportive and well placed in the distal coronary vessel, Lasing can commence with the catheter on or just proximal to the lesion. Both the 0.9 mm and 1.4 mm are 6 F compatible catheters, along with the 0.9 mm, X-80 ELCA catheter. This device is constructed to enhance deliverability as the radio-opaque marker is set back from the tip, containing 65 fibers of 50 μm diameter. In general the 0.9 mm X80 catheter is used in non-crossable, non-dilatable fibro-calcific lesions given it's deliverability characteristics and because this catheter can emit the most power (80 mJ/mm^2) at the highest repletion rate (80 Hz) necessary for 'balloon resistant' coronary lesions. The larger (1.4–2.0 mm) catheters are used in larger diameter vessels with straight segments and are therefore particularly useful when dealing with heavy intra-coronary thrombus or in the treatment of saphenous venous grafts (SVG). In some circumstances more than one catheter may be required, gradually increasing size based on the result obtained from the initial laser procedure.

24.2.2 Saline Infusion Technique

Both blood and iodinated contrast media, in comparison to water or saline, absorb the majority of delivered excimer laser energy. If not removed from the catheter tip, this results in the formation of cavity micro-bubbles at the site of energy delivery. This can potentiate the effect of the pressure waves at the catheter tip, and this increases the likelihood of traumatic vessel dissection [13]. In order to keep the tip free from contrast/blood during lasing. it is recommended that a saline flush/infusion technique is used [14]. This maximizes the delivery of laser energy directly into the atherosclerotic material, limiting vascular dissection rates [15].

In order to clear blood from the catheter/tissue interface, a 1 l bag of 0.9 % saline is connected to the manifold via a three-way tap, and a clean 20 ml Leur-lock syringe replaces the standard contrast syringe. Once contrast has been cleared from the flush tubing, confirmed by direct screening whilst purging the system with saline, 5 ml of saline should be infused prior to laser activation followed by a slow injection continued at a rate of 2–3 ml/s throughout the lasing process (usually 5–10 s). It is important to ensure that the guide catheter is well intubated into the coronary artery to ensure saline delivery to the laser catheter tip. It is important to directly visualize under fluoroscopy that all contrast is flushed from the guide catheter in the selected starting position for lasing, and that the saline does not get mixed with contrast. For the coronary catheters the duration of each lasing train is preset so for the standard catheters activation will automatically stop after 5 s with a 10 s rest period before the next laser train can commence. The X80 0.9 mm catheter permits 10 s activation and 5 s rest period reflecting its use in more complex lesions subsets. Continue the lasing, until the catheter has gone through the lesion or enough alteration has been made to allow balloon expansion.

The excimer laser energy is carried in pulses as the catheter is slowly [0.5 mm/s] advanced through the lesion. Since the depth of the excimer laser penetration is shallow [35–50 micron] the slow progression along the target lesion provides enough absorption of the emitted light energy into the lesion and subsequent ablation of the atherosclerotic plaque and thrombus. Upon completion of several trains of emission along anterograde laser propagation the laser catheter should perform retrograde lasing particularly in severe lesions when there is resistance for anterograde crossing. Continuous saline flushes accompany all stages of the procedure to reduce adverse expansion of acoustic shock waves from interaction between the contrast media or blood and the laser light. Application of laser in blood or contrast media is rarely performed in certain specific situations, but should only be undertaken by experienced operators (see later sections).

24.2.3 Specific Radial Considerations

When planning ELCA via the radial approach, there are a number of a factors that should be considered:

1. Route of access – In general, the native coronary vessels can be easily accessed from the right radial approach. Access to vein grafts anastomosed onto the ascending aorta can be technically challenging from this route, with guide support often poor. The left radial approach is these circumstances offers more guide support, and in general preferred for patients in whom graft intervention is being undertaken.
2. Size of the Laser catheter: its diameter being employed will determine the diameter of the guiding catheter that should be used. Both 0.9 mm and 1.4 mm catheters can be used via a 6 F guiding system, with the 1.7 mm and 2.0 mm requiring 7 F and 8 F diameter guiding catheters respectively. If it is felt that a larger diameter is required, then solutions for delivery of large calibre guiding systems include the use of sheathless guides or balloon tracking to deliver such equipment to the aortic root.
3. Shape of the guide – In general, a supportive guide is preferred. It must align co-axially with the coronary ostium to allow adequate flow of saline during injection. Operators should gain experience in PCI using the radial approach and selecting appropriate guiding catheters prior to embarking upon complex lesion subsets that may require ELCA.

24.2.4 Contraindications

Laser coronary atherectomy can be safely performed in PCI institutions without on-site cardiothoracic surgery but as with all PCI procedures, arrangements for offsite surgical cover must be in place. Other than lack of informed consent and unprotected left main disease [a relative contraindication] there are no absolute coronary contraindications to laser.

24.2.5 Avoiding Complications – Tips and Tricks (Fig. 24.3)

ELCA complications are on the whole similar to those encountered during routine PCI. Specific issues arise from interruption of the continuous saline flush/contamination with contrast, which can generate excessive heat, and increase the risk of vascular perforation. ELCA is not recommended when the operator is conscious of presence of large length sub-intimal guidewire positioning (as is the case in typical dissection re-entry case). In such cases, any anterograde injection may lead to propagation of a dissection plane and ultimately resulting in a longer length of stenting if not immediate no-reflow phenomena. Furthermore the saline infusion is unlikely to reach the intended target given the lack of run off from the lesion and will be therefore ineffective. In addition, ELCA catheters are relatively indiscriminate in performing tissue ablation and will essentially ‘modify’ any tissue in their field of delivery. Within the sub-intimal space the catheter would lie in closer proximity to the media and adventitia of the vessel that may cause per-

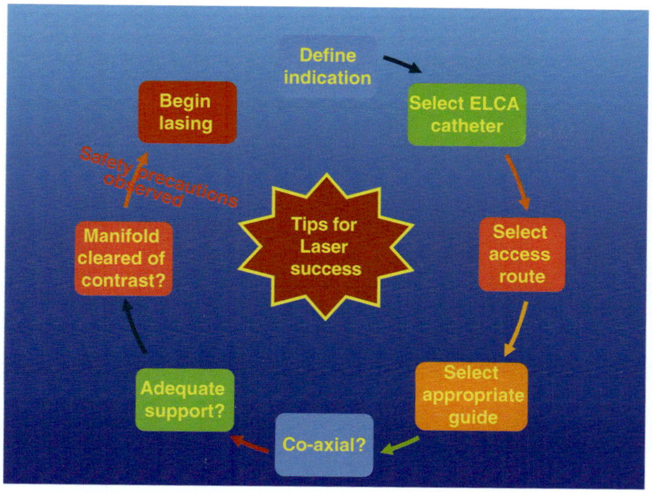

Fig. 24.3 Tips and tricks for successful laser atherectomy. Once the indication for laser has been defined, the appropriate catheter selected, the access route can be determined. Almost all devices can be delivered via the radial route, although delivery of an 8 F catheter (or equivalent sheathless guide) requires care and many need techniques such as balloon tracking. Once an appropriate coaxial guide has been selected, that maintains good co-coaxial support, then ELCA can be undertaken once adequate safety precautions have been employed

foration. This should be reserved for operators experienced in both CTO and ELCA intervention.

24.3 Clinical Indications for ELCA

As the application of ELCA has been refined, a number of indications have emerged for the technique. These are summarised below, with a brief summary of the evidence that underpins the use of ELCA. Each indication is illustrated with a case, with ELCA being applied via the radial route.

24.3.1 Acute Coronary Syndromes and Myocardial Infarction

Patients presenting with acute myocardial infarction (AMI) represent a medical emergency. There is marked activation of the clotting cascade with production of large amounts of platelet and fibrin rich thrombus within the coronary arterial vasculature. In most developed countries the recommended treatment for AMI associated with ST segment elevation on the ECG is immediate emergent PCI (Primary PCI) [16, 17]. The preferred route of access in primary PCI should be radial, with a mortality advantage being demonstrated in a number of randomised trials and meta-analysis [18]. In such circumstances, ELCA may be a beneficial revascularisation modality given its potential for effective thrombus removal [19], promotion of fibrinolysis [20], platelet stunning effects [21], and concomitant plaque debulking [22].

However, randomized clinical data regarding for the use of ELCA in AMI remains limited. The largest study to date, The CARMEL [Cohort of Acute Revascularization of Myocardial infarction with Excimer Laser] [23] multicenter registry, registered 151 AMI patients from 6 centers in the USA, 1 in Canada and 1 in Germany. One in five cases involved a SVG, and large thrombus burden was present in IRA in 65 % of the patients. Adjunctive glycoprotein IIb/IIIa inhibitor (GPI) was administered in 52 % of the cases. Following ELCA, TIMI flow grade was significantly increased from 1.2 to 2.8, with an associated reduction in angiographic stenosis (83–52 %). Overall a 91 % procedural success rate, a 95 % device success rate and a 97 % angiographic success rate were reported [23]. There was a low rate (8.6 %) of associated major adverse coronary events (MACE) (3 % dissection, with just 0.6 % rate of distal embolization and associated no-reflow). The greatest laser effect was observed in lesions associated with a outsized angiographic thrombus burden. Further data has suggested that ELCA is accomplished of removing up to 80 % of the thrombus burden from the treated targets [24]. Two other small registries examining the effects of ELCA in ACS suggested a greater outcome with regards to TIMI flow and myocardial blush grade compared with manual thrombus aspiration devices [25, 26]. There is a single randomized trial, the Laser AMI study. This included just 66 patients, and demonstrated safety and feasibility. A second, larger Laser AMI study is ongoing in patients treated with Primary PCI, with a 1:1 randomization to either ELCA or manual thrombus aspiration followed by standard PCI strategies. The primary endpoint in this study will be MACE at 6 months follow-up and is due to report in 2016 [27].

In the majority of cases, a 6 F guide catheter is most frequently used catheter diameter when treating AMI. This immediately limits the choice of ELCA catheter to either the 0.9 mm or 1.4 mm diameter device. Practically, a longer lasing duration (10 s) is preferred due to the enhanced thrombus ablation that occurs. Therefore, the 0.9 mm X80 catheter is often used in preference to the 1.4 mm device due to its ability to deliver a longer duration of Laser pulses, for relatively little loss in luminal diameter (Fig. 24.4).

24.3.2 ELCA for Non-crossable/Non-dilatable Lesions (Balloon Failure)

In contemporary PCI practice and with an expanding elderly patient cohort, it is not unusual to find that a coronary lesion can be crossed with a 0.014″ guidewire but either a low profile balloon fails to cross or once across the lesion fails to fully expand. This situation is considered as balloon failure, and a situation where ELCA may be applied. The success rate in uncross able or un dilatable stenoses is high, approaching 90 %, using the X80 catheter. However, when these targets are calci-

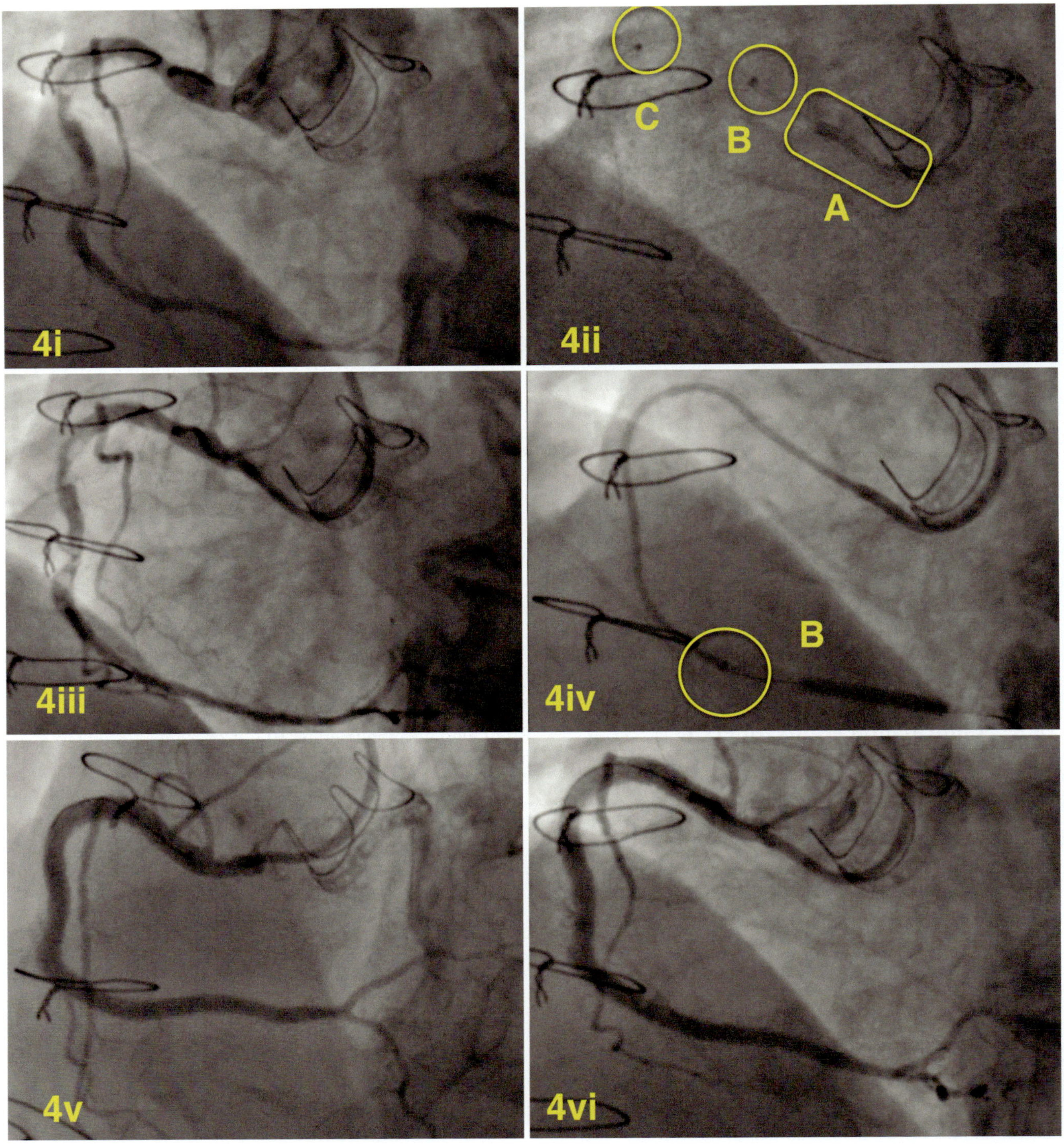

Fig. 24.4 ELCA for thrombus (and calcium). The use of ELCA in intra-coronary thrombus. This 68 year old male presented with inferior ST elevation myocardial infarction having previously had a tissue aortic valve replacement 6 years before. Primary PCI was undertaken form the right radial artery. Panel **i** illustrates a large dominant right coronary artery (RCA) containing a large amount of organised thrombus associated with calcific culprit tandem lesions. Noting the tortuous nature of the proximal vessel, the guide was switched for an amplatz shape (*box A*), and a guideliner (*box B*) was used to deliver the 0.9 mm laser catheter(*box C*) to the lesion. The effect of laser can been seen in panel **iii**, with a dramatic reduction in organised thrombus. The additional benefit of laser was also to modify the calcified lesions to permit balloon and subsequent stent passage to complete the case. The guideliner was then engaged deeply into the vessel to allow delivery of overlapping drug eluting stents, with an excellent overall final result (panels **v** and **vi**)

fied, the response is less favourable to laser debulking than that of non calcified lesions [79% vs. 96%, p<0.05] [28, 29].

However, in cases of balloon failure, the default technique for the majority of PCI operators remains rotational atherectomy (RA). Even for the proficient ELCA user, RA would be preferred if there was heavy calcification as it is more effective at debulking. This method necessitates delivery of a dedicated 0.009″ guidewire (Rotawire™) into the distal coronary vessel. This wire is less deliverable directly, and it may not be possible either independently or through a microcatheter exchange system when the lesion is very stenotic/calcific. Here, ELCA can be used upstream to modify the lesion and create a channel through which a Rotawire™ can be delivered distally (usually via a micro catheter) and RA then used for lesion debulking. We first termed the combination of ELCA and RA as the RASER technique and we have developed this use of combined atherectomy devices to great clinical effect in a number of challenging cases [30]. It is particularly effective for non-crossable, non-dilatable calcified stenosis and has been demonstrated to have a low complication rate in experienced hands [30, 31].

The application of such techniques can be achieved through the radial approach. If it is anticipated that such a situation may be encountered during a case, then a passive supporting guiding catheter choice up-front is preferred although active guide support can also be effective for laser atherectomy. The X80 0.9 mm catheter is selected in the vast majority of balloon failure cases since this catheter provides the widest range of power and repetition rate to maximise the chance of procedural success. Since this catheter only requires a 6 F guiding system it can be readily utilised during TRI. Other techniques that can be used to facilitate the PCI include the use of Guideliner™ for the delivery of the ELCA, although care should be taken to retract the device prior to commencing lasing as often the comprise to flow from obstruction of the lumen can lead to ischemia. Support strategies that require the use of additional wires (anchor wires/balloons etc) can also be used given that it is possible to safely laser with an second wire in place (Fig. 24.5).

24.3.3 ELCA for Chronic Total Occlusions

Chronic total occlusions CTO are thought-provoking atherosclerotic stenoses that are regularly difficult to traverse with a guide wire, respond unfavourably to balloon angioplasty and resist stent deployment. There have been significant advances in CTO techniques in recent years with adoption of anterograde dissection re-entry (ADR) systems [32] increasing utilisation of retrograde approach [33]. The success of trans radial CTO has improved as techniques have evolved. The role of ELCA is in resistant lesions, when equipment is incapable to go through the lesion despite attaining distal wire position – through whichever approach. In addition, ELCA may have extra valuable properties than simply being able to go through or sufficiently debulk the resistant lesion. Its ablative effect is conveyed through the lesion architecture, potentially weakening bonds between the constituent components of the CTO, facilitating equipment delivery. In addition, the anti-thrombotic [19, 20] and platelet suppressive [21] effects of ELCA may reduce the risk of thrombotic complications during disobilteration. A success rate of 86–90 % for ELCA in CTO cases has been reported [34, 35]. From a technical perspective saline is often not used at the laser-lesion interface for CTO cases as antegrade injections are usually not desirable to avoid hydraulic pressure extending sub-intimal planes and extending areas of dissection into the potential re-entry zone.

The only catheter used in CTO intervention is the 0.9 mm X90 catheter, due to its deliverability and the high power and fluence rates that can be delivered over a 10 s lasing interval. There are no specific considerations when undertaking ELCA within this context from the radial route, as the catheter can be easily delivered via a standard 6 F guide. The determinants of success relate more to the specific characteristics of the lesion and the general principles and techniques that may be used in arterial recanalisation (eg. use of the retrograde approach or ante-grade dissection re-entry etc). Within a CTO it remains mandatory to use ELCA over a guide wire that traverses the lesion and not to just apply laser energy to the proximal cap. The latter would be unpredictable and carry a significant risk of vessel perforation (Fig. 24.6).

24.3.4 ELCA in Under Expanded Stents

Under expanded coronary stents pose a important risk for stent thrombosis and subsequent opposing clinical outcomes. There are some PCI options available when confronted with these cases and in most situations where this is encountered, maximal balloon dilatation in terms of diameter and pressure have already been undertaken without success. The phenomenon usually results from the presence of resistant atheroma and inadequate lesion preparation prior to stent delivery. To allow full expansion, modification of the plaque that surrounds the under-expanded stented segment is required. RA although, an option, risks metal fragment embolisation and stalling of the burr. In addition it will often be less effective at ablating the resistant material behind the stent, the substrate that is usually responsible for the under expansion. Compared to RA, in this setting ELCA is both a safe and effective therapy. Indeed, ELCA remains the only technique that is able to accomplish stent expansion without disrupting the stent architecture. Bench model testing has confirmed that ELCA can be performed through stented segments without disturbing the strut configuration [36, 37]. The effect of

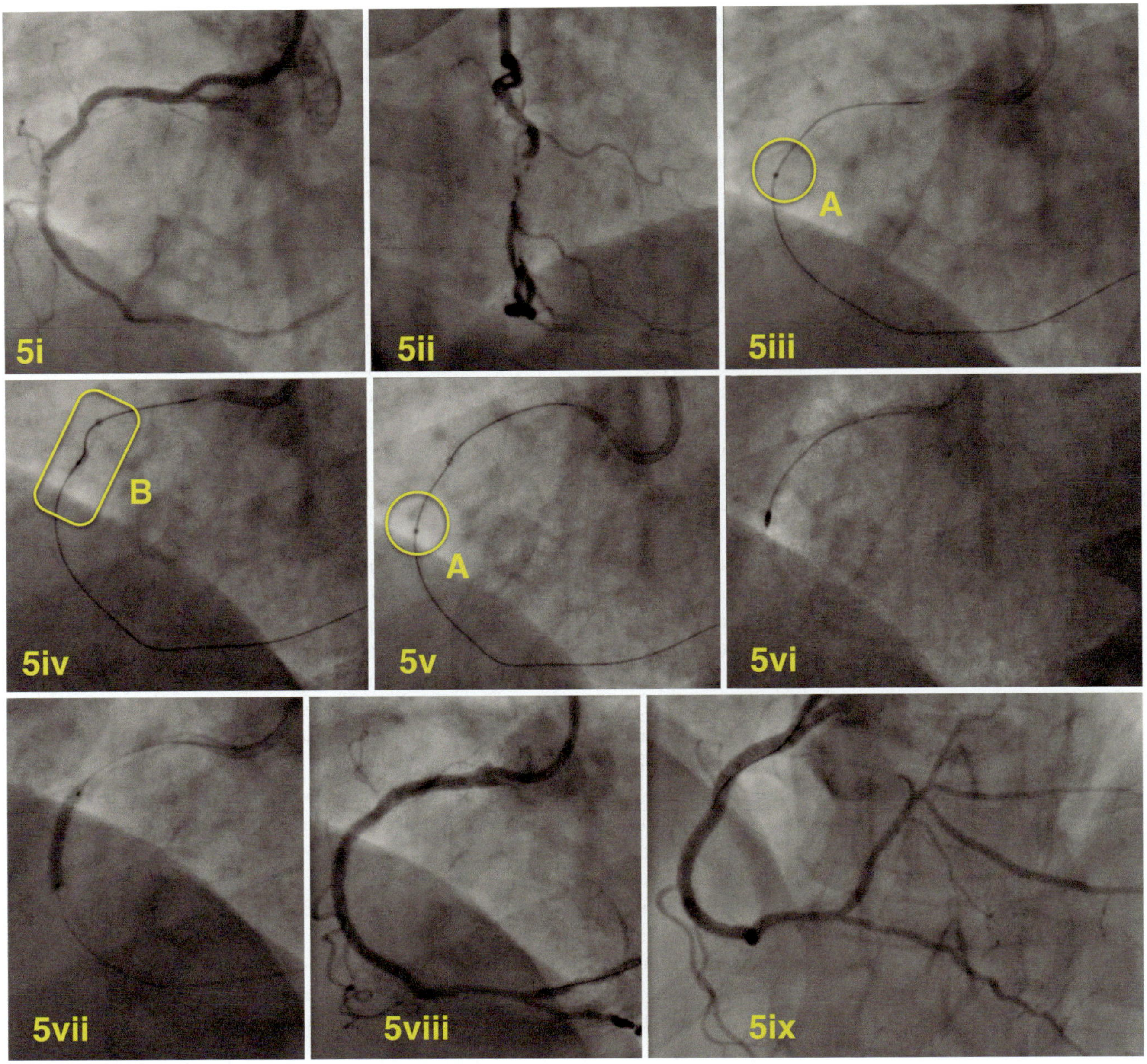

Fig. 24.5 ELCA for an uncrossable lesion. The use of ELCA in a calcific uncrossable lesion. Panels **i** and **ii** illustrate a critical lesion in a dominant RCA. Using a 7 F Amplatz 7 F guiding catheter via the right radial artery the lesion was wired with a tapered tip 0.014″ guidewire (Fielder XT). it was not possible to cross the lesion with the lowest profile balloon nor micro catheter. It was also not possible to wire the vessel independently with a rotawire to facilitate rotational atheterectomy. ELCA was used (panel **III**) to ablate a passage to facilitate crossing and subsequent delivery of a rotawire. Despite an initial delivery of 5000 pulses (panel **iii**), it was still not possible to advance a low profile balloon (Panel **iv**, *box B*). Further ELCA, with the aid of a guideliner for support (panel **v** *box A*), eventually traversed the lesion with the laser catheter, allowing rotawire delivery and susequent rotatational atheterectomy (panel **vi**). After expansion of appropriate non-compliant balloons (panel **viii**), the case was completed with overlapping drug eluting stents (Panels **viii** and **ix**)

laser on the polymer and drug coated on a stent is less well known which sometimes would necessitate a further DES when laser therapy is successfully applied to an newly deployed under expanded stent.

The ablative capabilities of ELCA are established on absorption of its energy in the atheroma, and subsequent lesion modification and ablation. As such, presence of a stent does not restrict the application of ELCA energy into the surrounding constrictive tissue on the abluminal stent surface. Importantly, even if the target lesions are not directly in the focus of laser beam, the application of ELCA energy in blood vessels induces acoustic shock waves that can propagate into the surrounding structures. By high power energy (80 mJ/mm^2/80 Hz), the 0.9 mm X-80 catheter can be advanced across even heavily calcified resistant lesions, and used to deliver energy into the under-expanded section of stent. We

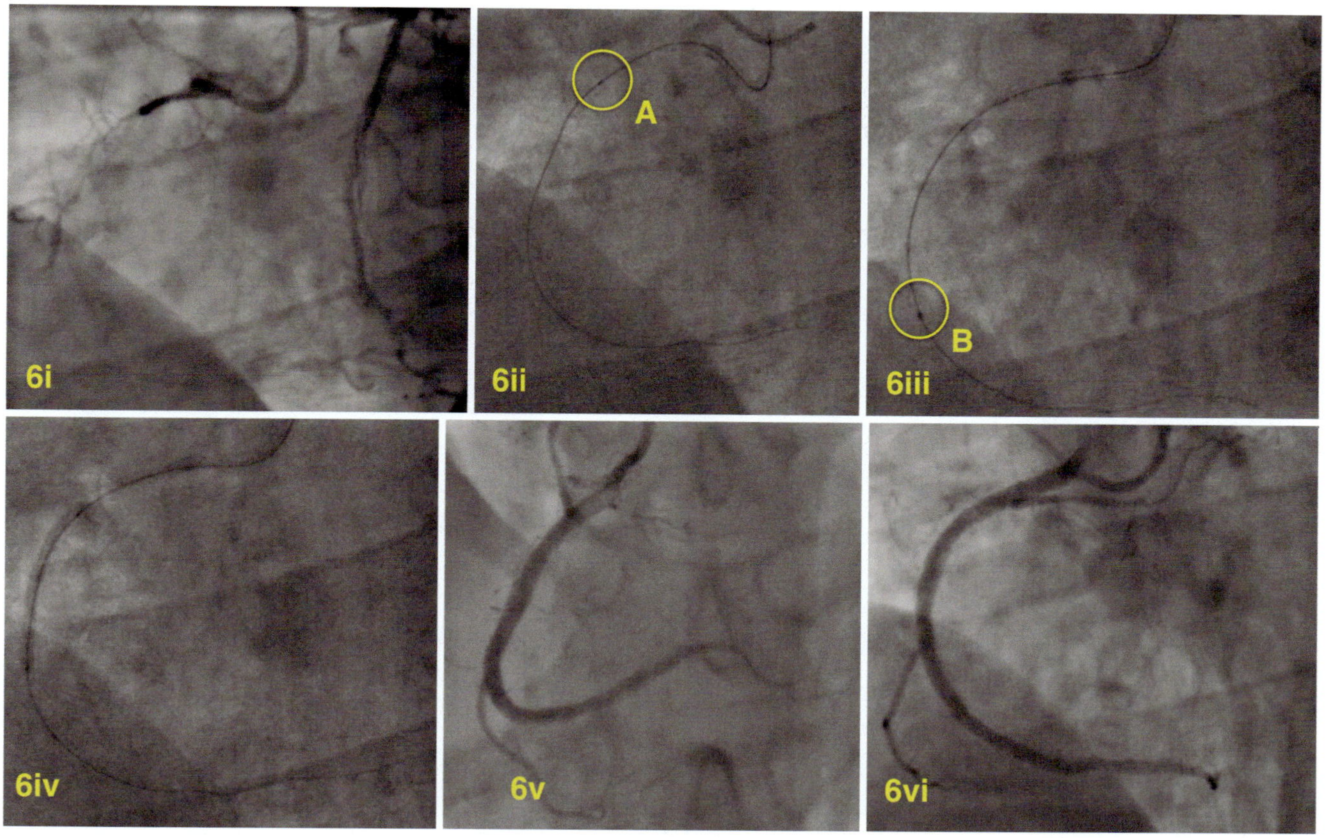

Fig. 24.6 ELCA for chronic total occlusions. The use of ELCA in a chronic total occlusion (CTO). Panel **i** demonstrates a CTO of the right coronary artery in a male patient. Access was obtained using bi-radial approach (6 F in left coronary, 7 F in RCA). After successful antegrade wiring with a polymer jacket 0.014″ guidewire (Pilot 200), it was not possible to cross the proximal cap with the lowest profile balloon/microcatheter (Panel **ii**, with *box A* illustrating the most distal balloon position achieved). Using an 0.9 mm X80 Excimer laser catheter, it was possible to traverse the lesion (Panel **iii**, with *box B* illustrating the distal laser catheter position). After appropriate non-compliant balloon pre-dilatation (Panel **iv**, demonstrating full balloon expansion), the case was completed with overlapping drug eluting stents, with an excellent final result (panels **v** and **vi**)

have found that delivering laser at these settings in the absence of saline, or indeed with contrast injection, amplifies the effect and increases the chance of success. Using laser for this indication is the ONLY exception to normal losing practice whereby saline is used as explained before. Within a stented environment "contrast-mileu" lasing appears to be safe. The modification induced facilitates high pressure balloon angioplasty, allowing full stent expansion [38–41].

This technique has been analytically evaluated in the ELLEMENT registry of 28 patients [40]. Using an increase of 1 cm^2 on IVUS or an increase of at least 10 % in minimal stent diameter by QCA as a definition of procedural success, this was achieved in 96.4 % (27/28) of cases. Peri-procedural MI occurred in 7.1 %, with transient slow-flow in 3.6 % and ST elevation in 3.6 %. There were no cases of perforation or tamponade. At follow up, there was a single cardiac death and a TLR rate of 6.7 %. Overall, this study confirmed that the use of ELCA in the treatment of an stent under-expansion is a harmless and effective technique, with a low complication rate. The authors do not comment on the access route used for the PCI but from our experience of 16 patients combined with three other UK centres, 44 % of laser procedures for under expanded stents were performed transradially using either a 6 F or 7 F guiding system (Fig. 24.7).

24.3.5 In Stent Restenosis

In spite of significant improvements in drug eluting stents (DES), target lesion revascularization (TLR) remains a restriction of PCI, with significant angiographic ISR evident of up to 10 % in those with DES [42] reported in one registry.

ELCA is a safe and effective technique in the treatment of ISR [43]. Examination of 107 re-stentoic lesions in 98 patients, with both IVUS and quantitative angiography (QCA), showed that lesions treated with ELCA, compared to balloon angioplasty (POBA) alone, had a greater cross sectional area and luminal gain, with more intimal hyperplasia ablation. Removal of this excess tissue may allow better stent expansion, and there was a trend towards a less frequent need

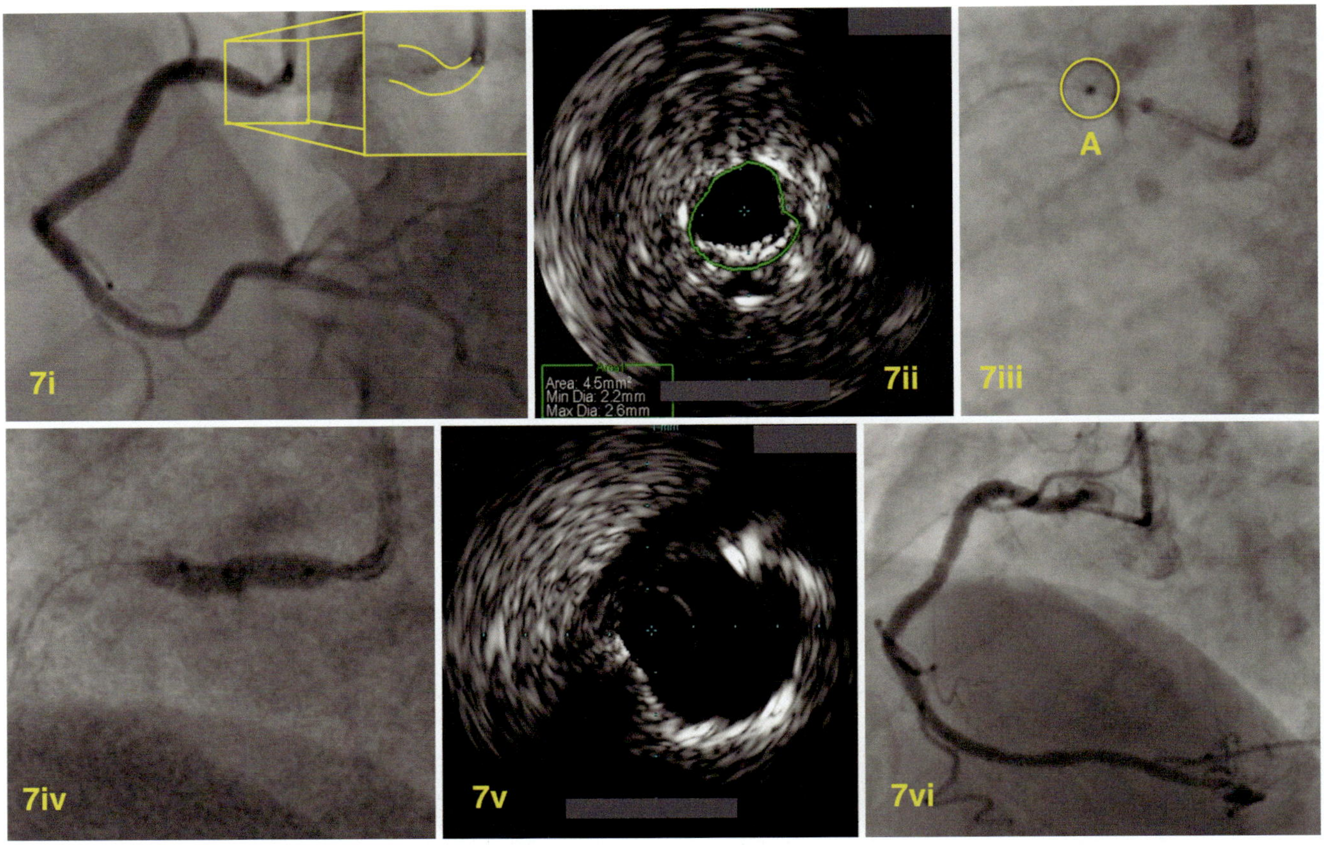

Fig. 24.7 ELCA for stent under-expansion. Panel **i** illustrates severe stent under-expansion in the ostium of a large dominant RCA from a female patient who has previously undergone PCI. The minimal MLA is shown in panel **ii**. From the right radial artery and using a 7 F guiding catheter along with a guideliner extension, the lesion was treated with 0.9 mm X80 ELCA catheter. 7000 pulses were delivered, and this facilitated balloon angioplasty, with full expansion o f an NC balloon being illustrated in panel **iv**. The final angiographic and IVUS result is shown in panel **vi** and **v** respectively, with full stent expansion having been achieved

for target vessel revascularization (TVR) at 6 months, but this did not make it to statistical significance (TVR 21 % vs. 38 % p=0.083) [43].

Catheter choice is determined by the size of the artery that is being treated, and this should be considered when establishing the access route. There are no other specific issues when using ELCA for ISR via the radial route. In general, adequate lesion debulking can be achieved with a 1.4 mm catheter via a 6 F guide catheter, but in aggressive large calibre re-stenosis, or with dense neo-intima the use of 1.7 mm or 2 mm catheters (delivered via an appropriate guide) can be effective. A dual catheter strategy may be adopted when treating large calibre arteries. An alternative can be the use of eccentric catheters, with the laser fibres oriented in an offset arrangement around a monorail delivery tube. Rotation of the catheter in a quadrantic fashion allows targeted ablation of re-stenotic tissue and may allow a greater luminal gain, although the two techniques (eccentric vs. concentric) have not been compared directly. The eccentric devices necessitate a large calibre guiding catheter, and accordingly this should be considered when embarking on such a case (Fig. 24.8).

24.3.6 Saphenous Vein Grafts

Obstructions in old saphenous vein grafts regularly contain of diffuse or multifocal plaques often containing thrombus [44, 45] (OCT paper reference) These lesions are progressive and prone to distal embolization leading to microvascular obstruction and the no reflow phenomenon, which is associated with adverse clinical outcomes [46]. Therefore, distal protection devices (DPD) are promoted when attempting SVG-PCI [45]. However, it is often not possible to advance a DPD beyond a very severe lesion due to the bulky nature of such systems. Additionally, the friable nature of such lesions can itself account for distal embolization resulting purely the from passage of such bulky equipment. ELCA is a safer alternative, and ability of laser to provide foreseeable debulking of these grafts even in the setting of AMI and in the presence of a heavy thrombus burden which has been documented [47, 48]. Furthermore, the remarkably low rate of distal embolization during ELCA of degenerative bypass grafts (1–5 %) impedes the need for routine adjunct distal protection device (DPD) in the majority of cases where the excimer laser is used [47]. However, when OCT has been used to visualise the effects of

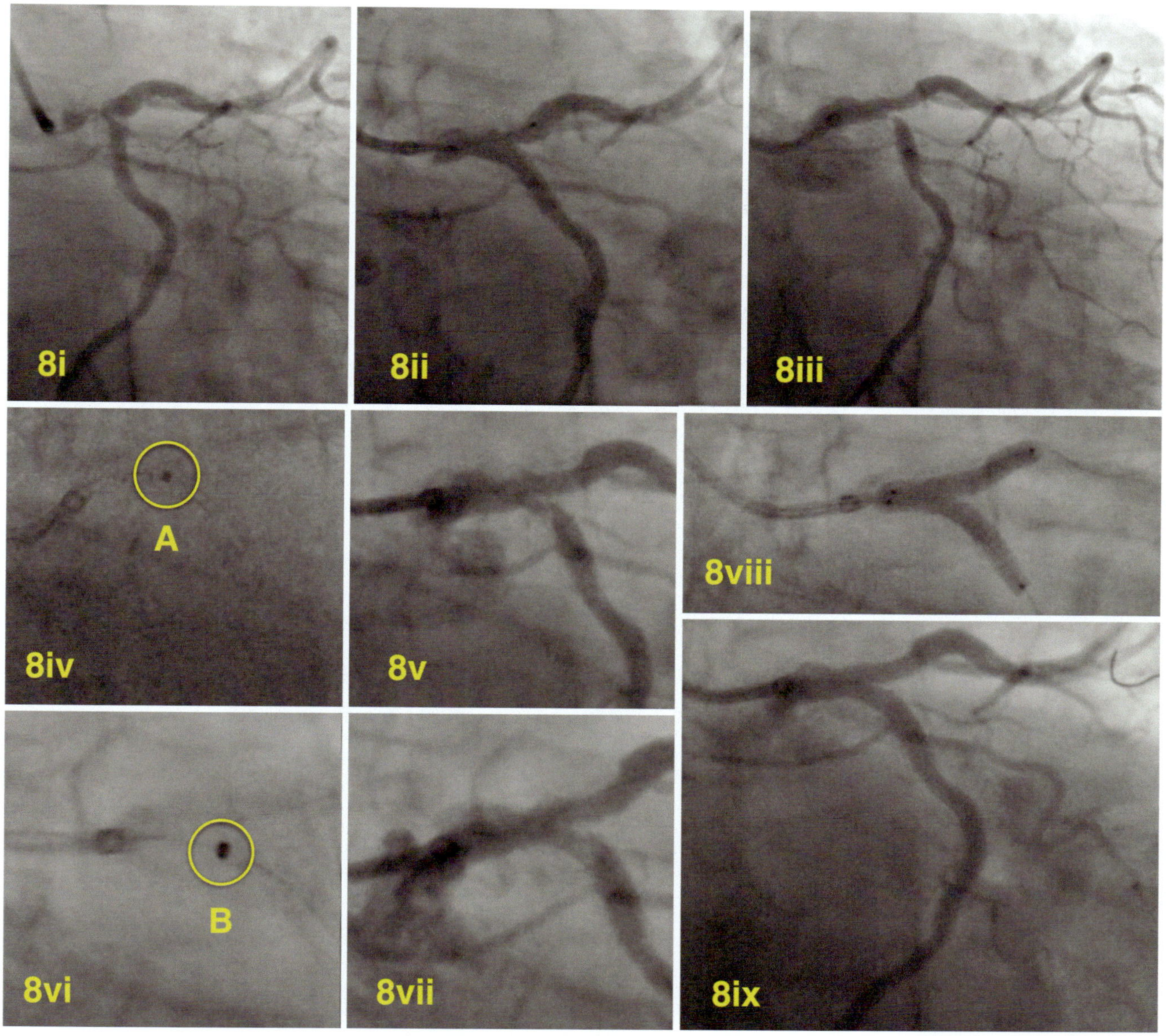

Fig. 24.8 ELCA for in-stent restenosis. Panel **i** illustrates a severe distal Left main-stem bifurcation lesion in a 78 year old male patient that was treated using a two-stent cullotte strategy with DES and final kissing balloon. Although an immediate excellent final result was achieved (panel **ii**), the patient presented 6 months later with angina and coronary angiography demonstrated severe in-stent restenosis at the ostium of the left circumflex. From a right radial approach using a 7 F guiding system the Excimer laser (**vi**), was used to debulk the lesion using a two catheter strategy (0.9 mm and 1.7 mm), with the appearance post laser being illustrated in panels **v** and **vii** respectively. Full balloon expansion was achieved, and the case completed with kissing drug coated balloon inflations (**viii**). There was an excellent final angiographic and IVUS appearance

ELCA in SVG PCI, it is clear that there remain friable fragments that could embolise and cause no reflow [49]. Where a lesion is too severe for initial DPD passage, one application of ELCA in SVG PCI is purely to create a small channel to deliver a DPD. Alternatively, a larger calibre laser catheter can then be used to maximally debulk the lesion prior to stenting. Indeed, laser atherectomy can be so effective in a degenerative vein graft that the option of not completing the case with a stent can be a good alternative (Fig. 24.9).

When approaching SVG PCI from the radial route, ideally the left radial approach should be adopted as it offers favourable angulation for adequate guide catheter support from the contra-lateral aortic wall, often well suited to an amplatz left coronary guiding conformation. PCI of left sided vein grafts is possible from the right radial approach, but obtaining adequate guide catheter support is often challenging. These principles also apply for both ELCA and DPD delivery, when a supportive catheter position if preferred. If lesion de-bulking with a large calibre ELCA device is considered, then this will require a larger calibre guide (either 7 F(1.7 mm catheter) or 8 F(2.0 mm catheter)) that may limit deliverability from the radial route, as discussed above (Table 24.2).

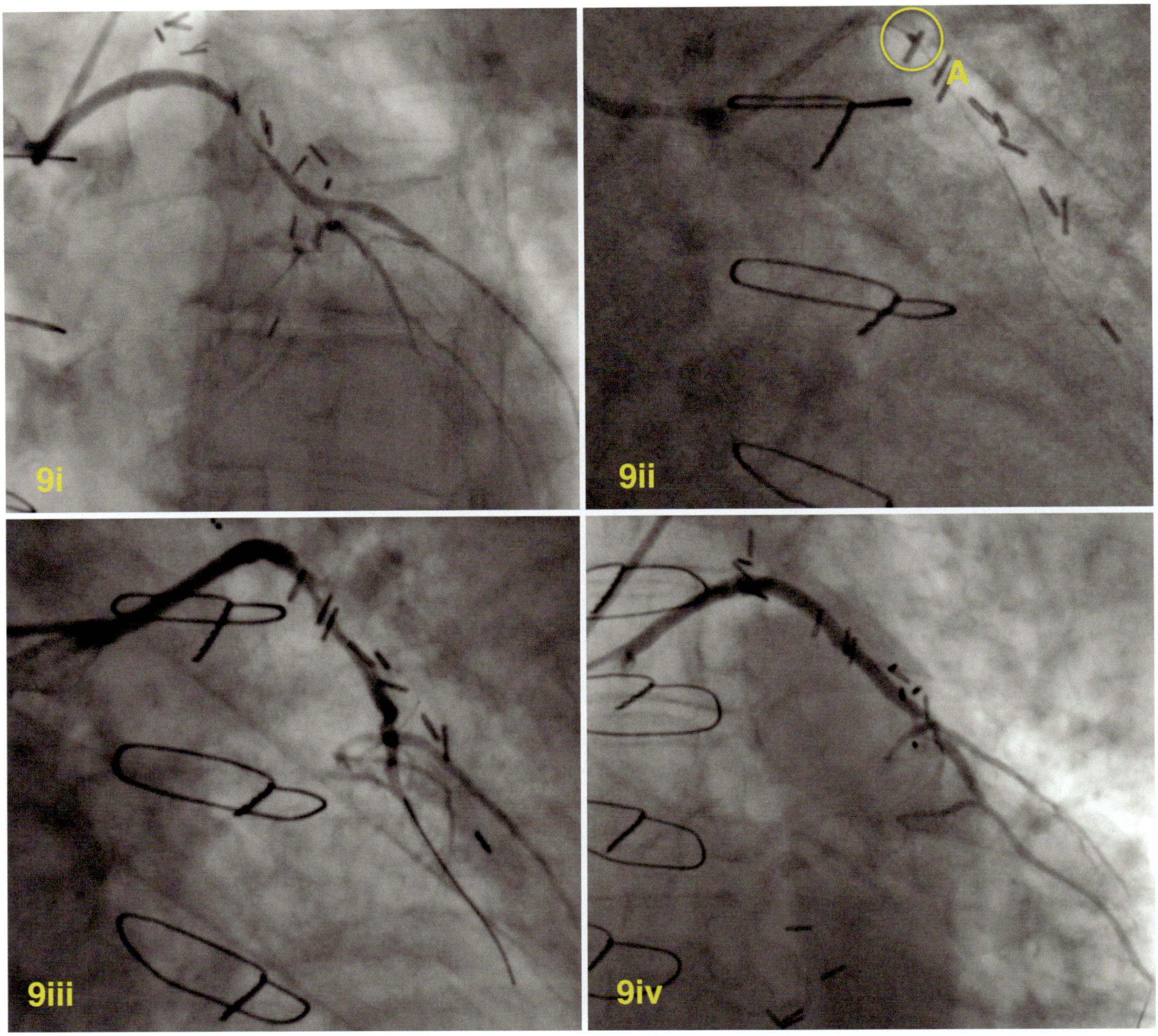

Fig. 24.9 ELCA for Saphenous vein grafts intervention. A 92 year old man with severe chest pain and lateral ischaemia on 12 lead ECG presented to the catheter lab. Coronary angiography from the left radial artery demonstrated a severe lesion in the degenerative vein graft. Here, a 1.4 mm Excimer laser catheter was used to debulk the graft, with an excellent result (Panel **iii**). The case was completed with overlapping drug eluting stents

Table 24.2 Clinical Indications for ELCA with optimal catheter selection

Indication for ELCA	Laser catheter prefered
Acute MI/Intra-coronary thrombus	0.9–1.4 mm catheter
Uncrossable lesions	0.9 mm X80
Chronic total occlusions	0.9 mm X80
Under-expanded stent	0.9 mm X80
Instent restenosis	0.9–2.0 mm catheters (concentric or eccentric)
Saphenous vein grafts	0.9–2.0 mm catheters

Conclusions

These six clinical situations describe the existing warnings for the use of Excimer Laser atherectomy in modern interventional practice. A detailed description of the ELCA technique and its application via the radial route has been supplemented with a number of cases. These illustrate key points that apply to both the use of the radial route in complex intervention and the use of ELCA specifically within the coronary circulation. This technology provides a solution to a variety of problems that may be encountered, including massive intra-coronary thrombus, an uncrossable lesion and stent under expansion. All applications are accessible via the radial route, and even the delivery of large calibre devices can be achieved with planning and the selection of appropriate guiding catheter technologies. Careful case selection, proper use of the laser equipment and integration of a safe, effective lasing technique plays a vital role in effective laser interventions.

References

1. Choy DSJ. History and state-of-the-art of lasers in cardiovascular disease. Laser Med Surg News Adv. 1988:34–8.
2. Cook SI, Eigler NL, Shefer A, et al. Percutaneous excimer laser coronary angioplasty of lesions not ideal for balloon angioplasty. Circulation. 1991;84:632–43.
3. Koster R, Kahler J, Brockhoff C, Munzel T, Meinhurtz T. Laser coronary angioplasty: history, present and future. Am J Cardiovasc Drugs. 2002;2(3):197–207.
4. Bittl JA, Sanborn TA, Tcheng JE. Clinical success, complications and restenosis rates with excimer laser coronary angioplasty. Am J Cardiol. 1992;70:1553–9.
5. Geschwind HJ, Dubois-Rande JL, Zelinsky R, et al. Percutaneous coronary mid-infrared laser angioplasty. Am Heart J. 1991;122:552–8.
6. Bittl JA, Ryan TJ, Keaney JF. Coronary artery perforation during excimer laser coronary angioplasty. J Am Coll Cardiol. 1993;21:1158–65.
7. Topaz O. Whose fault is it? Notes on "true" versus "pseudo" laser failure. Editorial. Cathet Cardiovasc Diagn. 1995;36:1–4.
8. Taylor K, Reiser C. Large eccentric laser angioplasty catheter. In proceedings of lasers in surgery: advanced characterization, therapeutics and systems. SPIE. 1997;2970:34–41.
9. Tcheng JE. Saline infusion in excimer laser coronary angioplasty. Semin Interv Cardiol. 1996;1:135–41.
10. Topaz O. A new safer lasing technique for laser facilitated coronary angioplasty. J Interv Cardiol. 1993;6:297–306.
11. Topaz O. Coronary laser angioplasty. In: Topol EJ, editor. Textbook of interventional cardiology. Philadelphia: WB Saunders Company; 1995. p. 235–55.
12. Topaz O, Safian RD. Excimer laser coronary angioplasty. In: Safian RD, Freed MS, editors. Manual of interventional cardiology. 3rd ed. Royal Oaks: Physicians Press; 2001. p. 681–91.
13. Baumbach A, Haase KK, Rose C, Oberhoff M, Hanke H, Karsch KR. Formation of pressure waves during in vitro excimer laser irradiation in whole blood and the effect of dilution with contrast media and saline. Lasers Surg Med. 1994;14:3–6.
14. Tcheng JE, Wells LD, Phillips HR, Deckelbaum LI, Golobic RA. Development of a new technique for reducing pressure pulse generation during 308-nm excimer laser coronary angioplasty. Cathet Cardiovasc Diagn. 1995;34:15–22.
15. Deckelbaum LI, Natarajan MK, Bittl JA, Rohlfs K, Scott J, Chisholm R, Bowman KA, Strauss BH. Effect of intracoronary saline infusion on dissection during excimer laser coronary angioplasty: a randomized trial. The percutaneous excimer laser coronary angioplasty (PELCA) investigators. J Am Coll Cardiol. 1995;26:1264–9.
16. The Task Force on the management of ST-segment elevation acute myocardial infarction of the European Society of Cardiology (ESC). ESC guidelines for the management of acute myocardial infarction in patients presenting with ST-segment elevation. Eur Heart J. 2012;33:2569–619.
17. American College of Cardiology Foundation/American Heart Association Task Force on Practice Guidelines. 2013 ACCF/AHA guideline for the management of ST-elevation myocardial infarction. J Am Coll Cardiol. 2013;61:e78–140.
18. Karrowni W, Vyas A, Giacomino, B, Schweizer M, Blevins A, Girotra S, Horwitiz P. Radial versus femoral access for primary percutaneous interventions in ST-Segment elevation myocardial infarction patients a meta-analysis of randomized controlled trials. JACC Cardiovascular Interventions. 2013;6(8):814–23.
19. Dahm JB, Topaz O, Woenckhaus C, et al. laser facilitated thrombectomy: a new therapeutic option for treatment of thrombus–laden coronary lesions. Catheter Cardiovasc Interv. 2002;56:365–72.
20. Topaz O, Minisi AJ, Morris C, Mohanty PK, Carr Jr ME. Photoacoustic fibrinolysis: pulsed-wave, mid infrared laser-clot interaction. J Thromb Thrombolysis. 1996;3:209–14.
21. Topaz O, Minisi AJ, Bernardo NL, McPherson RA, Martin E, Carr SL, Carr Jr ME. Alterations of platelet aggregation kinetics with ultraviolet laser emission: the "stunned platelet "phenomenon. Thromb Haemost. 2001;86:1087–93.
22. Topaz O, Bernardo NL, Shah R, et al. Effectiveness of excimer laser coronary angioplasty in acute myocardial infarction or in unstable angina pectoris. Am J Cardiol. 2001;87:849–55.
23. Topaz O, Ebersole D, Das T, Alderman EL, Madyoon H, Vora K, Baker JD, Hilton D, Dahm JB. Excimer laser angioplasty in acute myocardial infarction [the CARMEL multicenter study]. Am J Cardiol. 2004;93:694–701.
24. Topaz O, Shah R, Mohanty PK, McQueen RA, Janin Y, Bernardo NL. Application of excimer laser angioplasty in acute myocardial infarction. Lasers Surg Med. 2001;29:185–92.
25. Niccoli G, Belloni F, Cosentino N, Fracassi F, Falcioni E, Roberto M, Panico RA, Mongiardo R, Porto I, Leone AM, Burzotta F, Trani C, Crea F. Case-control registry of excimer laser coronary angioplasty versus distal protection devices in patients with acute coronary syndromes due to saphenous vein graft disease. Am J Cardiol. 2013;112(10):1586–91.
26. Shishikura D, Otsuji S, Takiuchi S, Fukumoto A, Asano K, Ikushima M, Yasuda T, Hasegawa K, Kashiyama T, Yabuki M, Hanafusa T, Higashino Y. Vaporizing thrombus with excimer laser before coronary stenting improves myocardial reperfusion in acute coronary syndrome. Circ J. 2013;77(6):1445–52.
27. Dorr M, Vogelgesang D, Hummel A, et al. Excimer laser thrombus elimination for prevention of distal embolisation and no-reflow in patients with acute ST elevation myocardial infarction: results from the randomised LaserAMI study. Int J Cardiol. 2007;116:20–6.
28. Bittl JA. Clinical results with excimer laser coronary angioplasty. Semin Interv Cardiol. 1996;1:129–34.
29. Bilodeau L, Fretz EB, Taeymans Y, Koolen J, Taylor K, Hilton DJ. Novel use of a high energy excimer laser catheter for calcified and complex coronary artery lesions. Catheter Cardiovasc Interv. 2004;62:155–61.
30. McKenzie DB, Talwar S, Jokhi PP, O'Kane PD, Osherov A, Strauss B, Dahm J. How should I treat severe coronary artery calcification when it is not possible to inflate a balloon or deliver a RotaWire? EuroIntervention. 2011;6(6):779–83.
31. Fernandez JP, Hobson AR, McKenzie D, Shah N, Sinha MK, Wells TA, Levy TM, Swallow RA, Talwar S, O'Kane PD. Beyond the balloon: excimer coronary laser atherectomy used alone or in combination with rotational atherectomy in the treatment of chronic total occlusions, non-crossable and non-expansible coronary lesions. EuroIntervention. 2013;9(2):243–50.

32. Werner GS, Schofer J, Sievert H, Kugler C, Reifart NJ. Multicentre experience with the BridgePoint devices to facilitate recanalisation of chronic total coronary occlusions through controlled subintimal re-entry. EuroIntervention. 2011;7:192–200.
33. Joyal D, Thompson CA, Grantham JA, Buller CE, Rinfret S. The retrograde technique for recanalization of chronic total occlusions: a step-by-step approach. JACC Cardiovasc Interv. 2012;5:1–11.
34. Topaz O. Laser for total occlusion recanalization. In: Waksman R, Saito S, editors. Chronic total occlusions: a guide to recalization. West Sussex: Blackwell Publishing; 2009.
35. Holmes Jr DR, Forrester JS, Litvack F, et al. Chronic total obstructions and short term outcome: the excimer laser angioplasty registry experience. Mayo Clin Proc. 1993;68:5–10.
36. Papaioannou T, Yadegar D, Vari S, Shehada R, Grundfest WS. Excimer laser (308 nm) recanalisation of in-stent restenosis: thermal considerations. Lasers Med Sci. 2001;16:90–100.
37. Burris N, Lippincott RA, Elfe A, Tcheng JE, O'Shea JC, Reiser C. Effects of 308 nanometer excimer laser energy on 316 L stainless-steel stents: implications for laser atherectomy of in-stent restenosis. J Invasive Cardiol. 2000;12:555–9.
38. Lam SC, Bertog S, Sievert H. Excimer laser in management of under expansion of a newly deployed coronary stent. Catheter Cardiovasc Interv. 2014;83:E64–8.
39. Sunew J, Chandwaney RH, Stein DW, et al. Excimer laser facilitated percutaneous coronary intervention of a nondilatable coronary stent. Catheter Cardiovasc Interv. 2001;53:513–7.
40. Latib A, Takagi K, Chizzola G, Tobis J, Ambrosini V, Niccoli G, Sardella G, DiSalvo ME, Armigliato P, Valgimigli M, Tarsia G, Gabrielli G, Lazar L, Maffeo D, Colombo A. Excimer Laser LEsion modification to expand non-dilatable stents: the ELLEMENT registry. Cardiovasc Revasc Med. 2014;15(1):8–12.
41. Egred M. A novel approach for under-expanded stent: excimer laser in contrast medium. J Invasive Cardiol. 2012;24(8):E161–3.
42. Dangas GD, Claessen BE, Caixeta A, Sanidas EA, Mintz GS, Mehran R. In-stent restenosis in the drug-eluting stent era. J Am Coll Cardiol. 2010;56:1897–907.
43. Mehran R, Mintz GS, Satler LF, et al. Treatment of in-stent restenosis with excimer laser coronary angioplasty: mechanisms and results compared with PTCA alone. Circulation. 1997;96:2183–9.
44. Webb JG, Carere RG, Virmani R, et al. Retrieval and analysis of particulate debris after saphenous vein graft intervention. J Am Coll Cardiol. 1999;34:468–75.
45. Baim DS, Wahr D, George B, et al. Randomized trial of a distal embolic protection device during percutaneous intervention of saphenous vein aorto-coronary bypass grafts. Circulation. 2002;105:1285–90.
46. Bittl JA, Sanborn TA, Yardley DE, et al. Predictors of outcome of percutaneous excimer laser coronary angioplasty of saphenous vein bypass graft lesions. The Percutaneous Excimer Laser Coronary Angioplasty Registry. Am J Cardiol. 1994;74:144–8.
47. Giugliano GR, Falcone MW, Mego D, et al. A prospective multicenter registry of laser therapy for degenerated saphenous vein graft stenosis: the COronary graft Results following Atherectomy with Laser (CORAL) trial. Cardiovasc Revasc Med. 2012;13:84–9.
48. Ebersole D, Dahm JB, Das T, et al. Excimer laser revascularization of saphenous vein grafts in acute myocardial infarction. J Invasive Cardiol. 2004;16:177–80.
49. Rawlins J, Talwar S, Green M, O'Kane P. Optical coherance tomography following percutaneous coronary intervention with excimer laser coronary atherectomy. Cardiovasc Revasc Med. 2014;15(1):29–34.

25 Mechanical Circulatory Support in Transradial or Transbrachial Intervention for Acute Coronary Syndrome

Hon-Kan Yip and Cheuk-Man Yu

25.1 Introduction & History Review

Although transfemoral arterial approach (TFA) was the first developed method for coronary angiography and percutaneous coronary intervention (PCI), it has its own disadvantages, including the need for the bed rest for the requirement of puncture site compression after the procedure, vascular complications of local hematoma, psoas hematoma, arterio-venous fistula and pseudoaneurysm, as well as difficult access due to tortuous aorta or occlusion of femoral-iliac-aortic route [1–7]. Thus, to develop an alternative modality with easily approach, lesser vascular complications and comparable safety as the femoral arterial approach for PCI is of utmost importance. Transradial arterial approach (TRA) for coronary angiography and PCI is therefore developed as an alternative and even well-accepted first line approach. In fact, TRA which is a reasonably simple route of vascular access [8–10] for catheter-based coronary intervention, and has been developed for almost 20 years. As the safety and efficacy of this method has already been extensively discussed and validated for a long time by many clinical studies worldwide [8, 10], TRA is currently one of the most popular approaches, especially in Asia, for elective PCI [10–15]. Additionally, clinical studies have further proved that TRA is safe and efficacious in elective coronary angiographic study on an out-patient basis [15], elective left main coronary intervention [16], cerebral angiographic study, and vertebral or carotid stenting [17, 18]. Furthermore, while TRA for primary PCI is already a daily practice for hemodynamic stable patients in many medical centers of the world, in particular in Asia [19, 20], how to utilize the TRA for coronary intervention for acute ST-segment elevation myocardial Infarction (STEMI), non-STEMI and unstable angina with hemodynamic instability with the requirement of circulatory/mechanical support is an important issue that should be realized in our clinical practice.

H.-K. Yip (✉) • C.-M. Yu
Cardiology, Kaohsiung Chang Gung Memorial Hospital, Kaohsiung, Taiwan, Republic of China

Cariology department Prince of Wales Hospital, The Chinese University of Hong Kong, Hong Kong, China
e-mail: han.gung@msa.hinet.net; cmyu@cuhk.edu.hk

25.2 Promptly Evaluate the High-Risk Patients with Hemodynamic Instability

The current guidelines have been clearly shown how to stratify the risk early for patients with presentation of acute chest pain syndrome [21–23]. With respect to those high risk patients with hemodynamic instability, the minimally required information should include clinical presentation, patient's medical history, vital sign upon presentation, chest X-ray, electrocardiogram, Thrombolysis In Myocardial Infarction (TIMI) score [24] or "EuroSCORE"/"EuroSCORE II" [25, 26], laboratory findings especially renal function, and transthoracic echocardiography findings if available.

25.3 Careful Plan for Vascular Access Site

Prior to perform the catheter-based coronary intervention, the first priority is to find out which is the most suitable vascular access. In fact, there are six peripheral vascular accesses that can be approached, including right and left femoral, radial and brachial arteries.

In acute coronary syndrome (ACS) patients with hemodynamic instability, the mechanical circulatory support, such as intra-aortic balloon pump (IABP), should be considered using a TFA approach (Fig. 25.1). It usually improves hemodynamic status. This circulatory support can help interventional cardiologists to more easily to find the radial pulse and therefore facilitate TRA for PCI (Fig. 25.1). The challenging situation is that both femoral arterial pulses are not palpable, or both iliac arteries have already occluded, i.e., both left and right TFA approach is impossible. In this way, the right or left brachial arterial approach is the final resort for the patient.

Y. Zhou et al. (eds.), *Transradial Approach for Percutaneous Interventions*, DOI 10.1007/978-94-017-7350-8_25

25.4 Indication of TRA for PCI in ACS Patients with Hemodynamic Instability

In ACS patients with hemodynamic instability, their hemodynamic condition may get worse and develop profound cardiogenic shock prior to or during PCI [27]. In this situation, not only the IABP support is required (Fig. 25.2), but the extra-corporeal membrane oxygenator (ECMO) (Fig. 25.2) [28, 29] or other left ventricular assistant devices (LVADs) [30] may be required to promptly stabilize the patient's blood pressure. In this way, the both femoral arterial routes will be utilized for these circulatory mechanical supports and PCI must be performed from TRA. In case the radial artery diameter is too small, it may mean that the ulnar artery may be the dominant artery of the forearm and ulnar arterial access should be considered. Finally, if the ulnar artery approach is difficult, then brachial arterial approach should be considered.

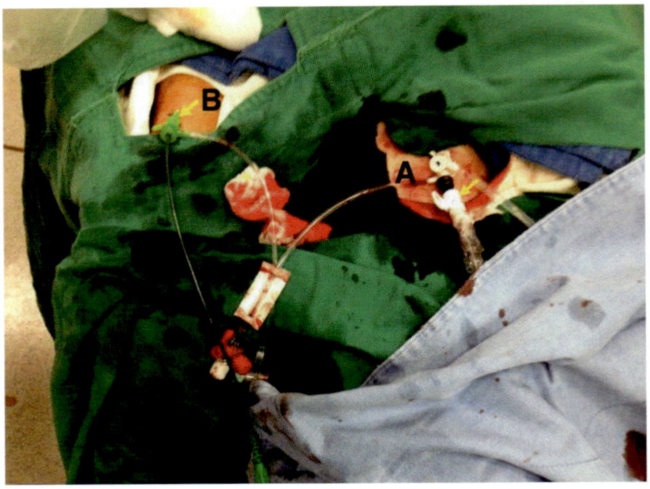

Fig. 25.1 Illustrating the indications for both transfemoral and transradial arterial approaches for hemodynamic unstable patient. A male patient experienced acute coronary syndrome and unstable hemodynamic condition was identified. Therefore, transfemoral arterial approach for intra-aortic balloon pump support was performed (**a**, *yellow arrow*), followed by transradial arterial approach (**b**, *yellow arrow*) for percutaneous coronary intervention

25.5 Some Techniques are Required to Overcome the Difficulties of Arterial Route Access

Correct needle puncture into the right position of the radial artery is no doubt the first step of the successful procedure. However, even if the puncture needle is already inside the radial artery, the guide wire that comes with the sheath system may not be able to be advanced into the true lumen of the artery. In this way, the operator can try to use 0.014″ PCI wire (Fig. 25.3a), followed by utilization of the 6 French (Fig. 25.3b) (but not the 7 French) Terumo arterial sheath (TERUMO Interventional systems).

In some cases, the communication between the proximal end of right radial artery and the distal end of the right brachial artery is very tortuosity or even forms a loop. In this situation, operator can utilize a suitable fluoroscopic view, followed by contrast injection to identify the anatomy of the vessels. The 0.035″ hydrophilic Terumo wire (TERUMO Interventional systems) should be used first to attempt crossing the anatomical difficulty. If fails, a PCI 0.014″ coronary guide wire can be used to solve the problem. After the guide wire crossed the anatomical difficulty, a smaller and soft guiding catheter should be used along the guide wire and advance gently with a twisting action to cross the anatomical difficulty. The 0.014″ guide wire are then be replaced by the 0.035″ wire to support the advancement of the guiding

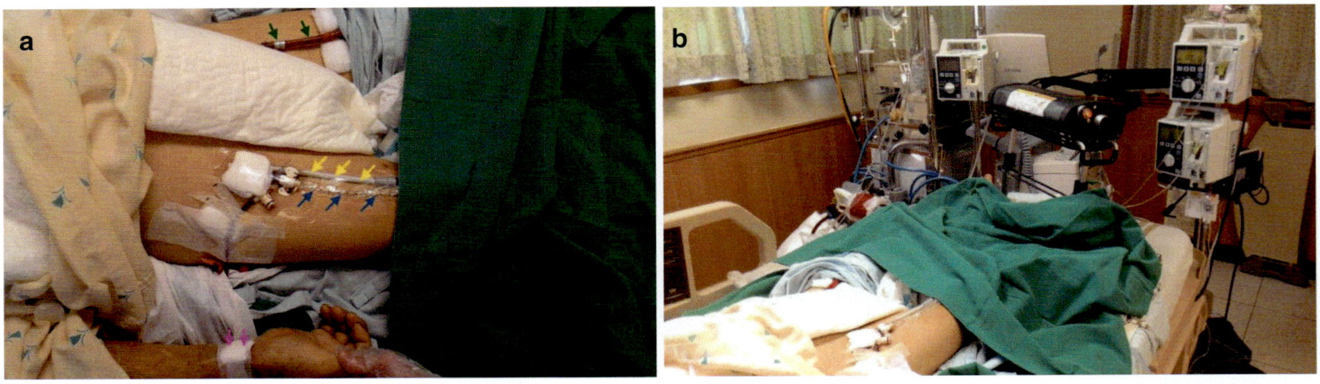

Fig. 25.2 Illustration of intra-aortic balloon pump (IABP) support and extracorporeal membrane oxygenator (ECMO) implantation for a female patient who experienced acute anterior ST-segment elevation myocardial infarction complicated by profound cardiogenic shock undergoing primary percutaneous coronary intervention (PCI). (**a**) Right femoral venous sheath (*yellow arrows*) and left femoral arterial sheath (*green arrows*) of ECMO implantation, right femoral arterial sheath (*blue arrows*) of IABP implantation, and transradial approach for primary PCI (*pink arrows*). (**b**) Figure illustrating the IABP and ECMO machines for life support in this patient

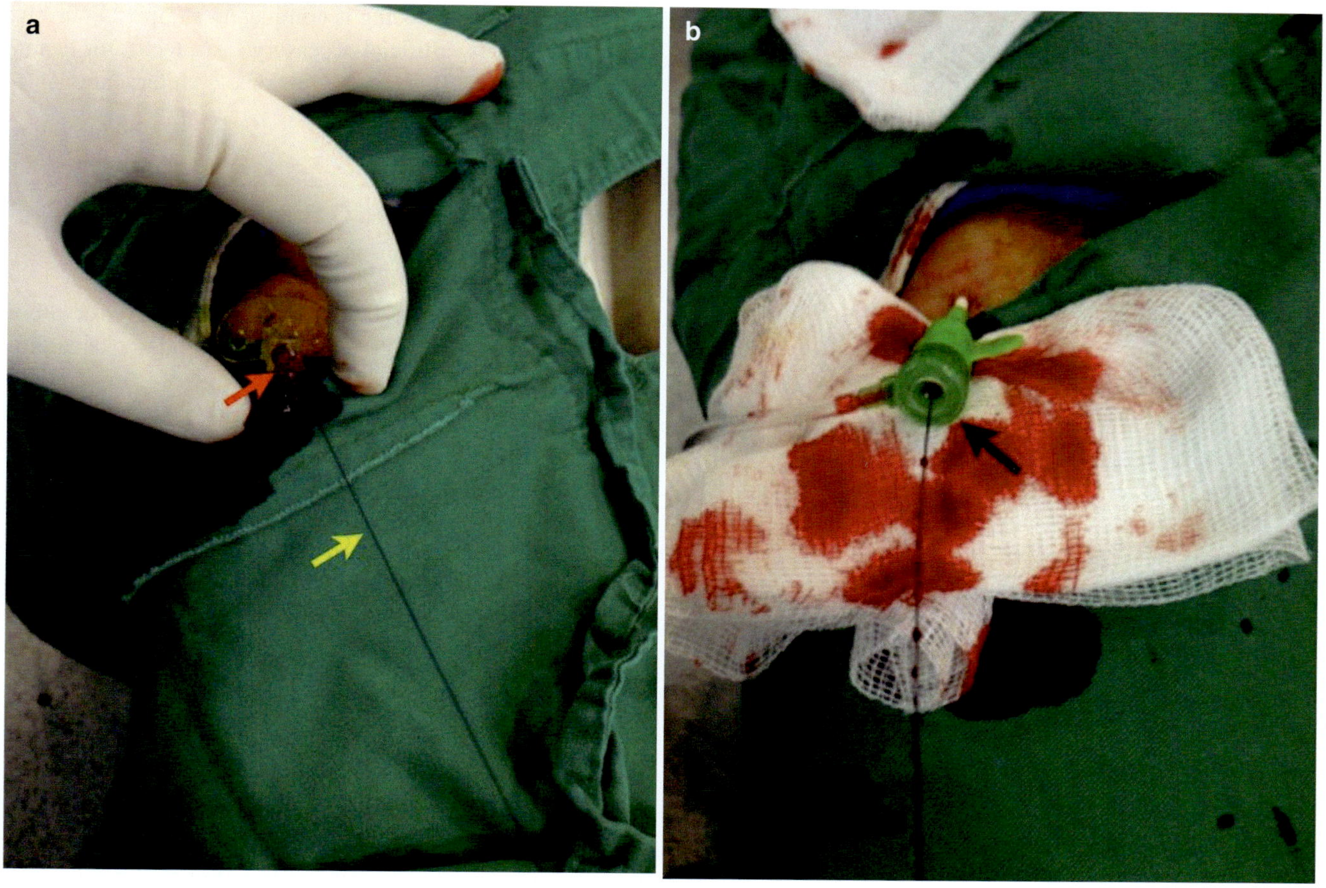

Fig. 25.3 Techniques are required to overcome the difficulties of arterial route access. (**a**) Illustrating the 0.014″ PCI guidewire (*yellow arrow*) to be utilized for crossing the puncture needle (*red arrow*) and went into the radial artery without difficulty. (**b**) A 6 French arterial sheath was utilized along the 0.014″ PCI guidewire and inserted into the radial artery (*black arrow*)

catheter to the ascending aorta for engagement of left and right coronary arteries.

In some cases, especially in those very thin and obese patients with history of hypertension, tortuosity at the proximal end of innominate artery often occurs. In this situation, the using the 0.035″ hydrophilic Terumo wire and taking a deep breath by patient is usually an effective method for the wire to cross the tortuosity and entrances into the ascending aorta, followed by advancing the guiding catheter along the wire into the destination. Sometimes, a big angulation may appear at the aortic root when left TRA is utilized. This situation will increase the difficulty in engaging the coronary arteries. A soft guiding catheter along a hard guide wire is recommended in this situation.

25.6 Guiding Catheter Selection

Whether the PCI procedure can be successfully achieved, the first key step is that the guiding catheter is able to offer a good support. Therefore, how to select a suitable guiding catheter is extremely important. Currently, many new guiding catheters with different purposes have been developed. Thus how to choose a good guiding catheter for the PCI procedure is mainly dependent on the operators' experience and the available instruments in their catheterization laboratories. Some centers would like to use the Kimny (Boston Scientific), Ikari (Boston Scientific), Amplatz (Medtronic, INC.) guiding catheters for right coronary artery intervention and Kimny (Boston Scientific), Ikari (Boston Scientific), Amplatz (Medtronic, INC.) and Launcher (EBU 3.5, 3.75 or 4.0) (Medtronic INC.) guiding catheters for left-side coronary artery intervention since these guiding catheters often offer good support interventional tools.

25.7 Indication and Strategy of Homeostasis for Brachial Artery Approach (Fig. 25.4)

In the setting of unstable hemodynamic condition, femoral arterial approach of circulatory mechanical support is usually required [28–31]. These mechanical circulatory supports, for example: simultaneous IABP and ECMO have

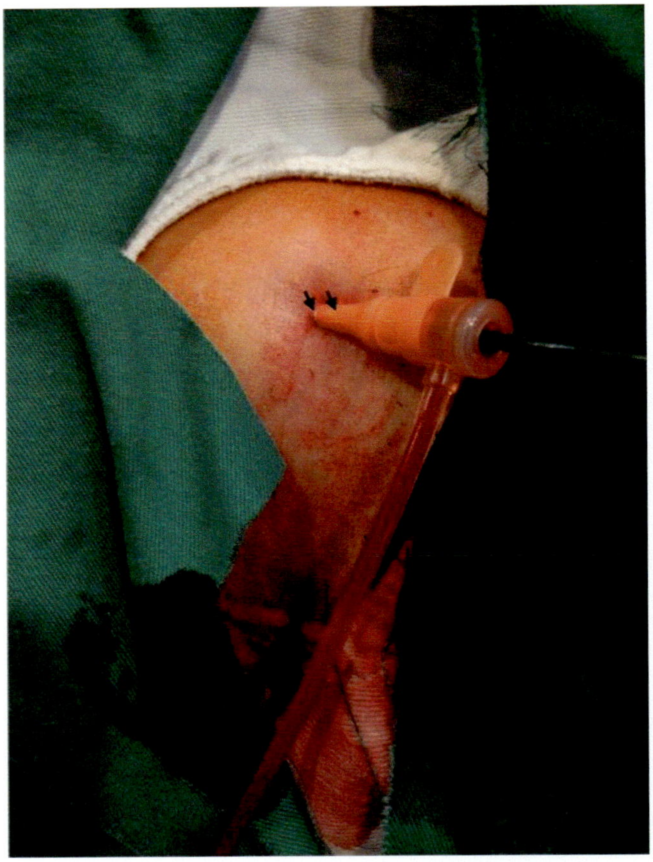

Fig. 25.4 Indication and technique for brachial arterial approach for PCI. Both radial pulses were too weak in a patient with angina pectoris who underwent percutaneous coronary angiographic study. Transbrachial artery approach was used for the patient (*black arrows*)

already occupied both femoral arterial routes [28–31]. Furthermore, both radial artery pulses may be too weak that are difficult to be found due to hypoperfusion or had severe atherosclerotic stenosis in some patients. In this circumstances, the brachial arterial approach (i.e., at the level of elbow area) would be the last resort for arterial access. Furthermore, in our clinical practice, it is not rare to find that patients would have both common iliac or femoral artery occlusion as well as unstable hemodynamic condition. In this situation, the right brachial artery approach for implantation of IABP is also the only arterial access for the patients [32].

Anatomically the brachial area is surrounded by abundant soft tissue. Thus, if the method of homeostasis is not appropriate, the puncture site will develop vascular complication with extremely swelling and even haematoma formation [33]. Several methods could be used to avoid these complications. Firstly, try to avoid the puncture needle passing through the posterior wall of the artery. Secondly, the physician should check the ACT and administer an appropriate dosage of protamine for reversing the heparin effect prior to remove the arterial sheath. Thirdly, the puncture site should be compressed manually (i.e., compressed by applying a firm finger pressure) until the bleeding is completely stopped. Fourthly, utilization of new artificial accessory instrument, for example, Hemostatic Bandage (QuickClot[R] Interventional[TM], Z-Medica LLC), could be useful.

25.8 Indication and Optimization of IABP Support

Mechanically-supported PCI is widely accepted for those ACS patients with unstable hemodynamic condition or cardiogenic shock upon presentation [27–31, 34–36]. In addition, prophylactic IABP support (i.e., as a bridge) for left main or multiple-vessel coronary intervention has recently been shown to offer an additional benefit for those patients who have left ventricular systolic dysfunction (i.e., ejection fraction ≤35 %) with or without congestive heart failure [31]. The results of these observational studies have provided good experience as the reference for our clinical practice [27–31, 34–36].

In order to get the maximal arterial pulse augmentation by IABP, the tip of balloon should be placed at the end of the aortic arch (i.e., at the beginning of the thoracic descending aorta). Also, the arterial waveform should be checked after implantation of IABP and optimized by adjusting the deflation and inflation button. If the waveform is not clear, then normal saline flushing is required. The electrocardiogram leads must be firmed attached in the appropriate positions to provide good synchronization of the balloon timing.

25.9 Complications of Implantation of IABP

Some particular complications that may occur during the implantation of IABP must be detected early. Firstly, perforation of femoral, external iliac or common iliac arteries will more likely to occur in those patients with very tortuous arterial access route over the inguinal region or lower abdominal aorta. Such complication will cause acute blood loss, retroperitoneal hematoma and deterioration of blood pressure. Thus, careful and gentle approach for arterial puncture and IABP sheath implantation should always be exercised even at the emergent procedure to avoid these complications. Secondly, arterial venous fistula is not infrequent to occur, especially in some patients who's anatomical distribution of femoral artery and femoral vein may overlap (i.e., the femoral vein goes above the femoral artery) or very close of each other. Quick vascular ultrasound assessment will be helpful if there is any doubt in the location of the femoral vein in relation to the femoral artery. Thirdly, venous sheath or IABP sheath may pass through both femoral vein and artery simultaneously. This is the result of a rare complication that the puncture needle goes through the vein and artery that could be discovered under the fluoroscopy guidance. Lastly, it is not uncommon to find critical ischemia of the lower limb after IABP implantation. This is almost always due to the result of severe iliofemoral atherosclerosis and/or obstruction of IABP sheath implantation site. All of these complications should be promptly identified and dealt with by the active input of vascular surgeons.

25.10 How to Take Care Patients After Receiving IABP Support

Patients put on IABP support should be taken care according to the guidelines and protocols of the coronary care units. These include regular follow up of the vital signs, urine output, the biochemistry (renal and liver function, electrolytes), complete blood count with differential count, chest X-ray, 12-lead electrocardiogram, cardiac enzymes, transthoracic echocardiography, oxygen saturation, and pulmonary capillary wedge pressure measurement by the Swan-Ganz catheter, as well as paying attention to bleeding complications. Furthermore, wound care, early identification and treatment of infection, as well as regular assessment of the perfusion of the lower extremities are particular important.

25.11 Timing for Removal of IABP

In those patients undergoing PCI with prophylactic IABP supported, the IABP should be removed a few hours or at least within 24 h after PCI. In this situation, early removal of IABP is safe to the patients. In those patients who have ACS with unstable hemodynamics or cardiogenic shock undergoing early or primary PCI, timing for IABP weaning/removal should be individualized and is mainly dependent on the clinical condition of the patient. Serial assessment of left ventricular function by echocardiograph, pulmonary capillary wedge pressure, cardiac output/cardiac index, urine output and chest X-ray are the important parameters that guide the optimal timing of weaning of IABP. In general, 3–5 days after PCI may be a suitable time line for weaning of IABP as this is the critical time interval of recovery from myocardial stunning. Of various parameters, the clinical information is the utmost important guide for weaning of IABP.

25.12 Prediction of Recurrent CHF After Removal of IABP

Some patients may promptly develop congestive heart failure (CHF) and acute pulmonary edema after removing the IABP support. The commonest period of developing acute pulmonary edema usually occurs at days 3–5 after removing IABP. There are some clinically relevant parameters may provide important information for predicting CHF, including severe left ventricular dysfunction, difficultly in weaning off the IABP, increased left ventricular end-diastolic pressure/pulmonary capillary wedge pressure, pulmonary hypertension, ischemia-related mitral regurgitation, atrial fibrillation, decrease in urine output, hypotension, low cardiac index, and advance age of >80 years old.

25.13 Indications for ECMO Support

Previous studies have revealed that in STEMI patients complicated by profound cardiogenic shock, IABP-supported primary PCI did not improve clinical outcome when compared with non-IABP-assisted primary PCI [27]. On the other hand, study has demonstrated that early ECMO-assisted primary PCI improved 30-day outcome in AMI patients complicated by cardiogenic shock [28]. Growing evidence have also supported the concept that ECMO offered additional benefit for improving the prognosis in ACS patients with compromised hemodynamics who underwent PCI [37–40].

Clinical observational study has revealed that not all the cardiogenic shock patients undergoing primary PCI will benefit from ECMO support, but only seen in those with profound cardiogenic shock [28]. Thus, ECMO support is highly selected for patients profound cardiogenic shock undergoing primary PCI, or in the setting of acute refractory heart failure and post-cardiac arrest [41–43].

Definitions of cardiogenic shock and profound shock have been described in the previous report [27]. In brief, patients who experience cardiogenic shock upon presentation or to be observed at catheterization laboratory meet the following prospectively defined criteria for early cardiogenic shock: (1) Chest X-ray showing pulmonary edema with systolic blood pressure (SBP)<90 mmHg, or, (2) Persistent hypotension with SBP<90 mmHg associated with low cardiac output and clear lung fields, not related to cardiac arrhythmia, showing no response to adequate fluid supply, and requiring inotropic infusion. Profound cardiogenic shock was defined as SBP<75 mmHg despite intravenous inotropic infusion and IABP support which is associated with altered mental status and respiratory failure [27, 28].

Observational studies have strongly recommended that early and rapid ECMO implantation along with IABP support for those patients with profound cardiogenic shock was crucial for life-saving [28, 29, 31, 37–40]. It was further emphasized that early implantation of ECMO means that whenever the patients fulfilled the criteria of profound cardiogenic shock, ECMO should be implanted without [28]. Therefore, ECMO implantation at both emergency room or cardiac catheterization laboratory is recommended [28].

25.14 How to Collaborate Between Cardiovascular Surgeons and Interventional Cardiologists

In order to maximize the change of saving the life, ECMO implantation has been recommended to be completely set up within 15 min [28]. Thus an experienced heart team with 24 h standby who works harmoniously and proficiently for implantation of ECMO support is essential. Such multidisciplinary work should consist of cardiovascular surgeon, interventional cardiologists, bypass-team members, technicians and nursing specialist.

25.15 Benefits of ECMO-Supported Primary PCI

In ACS patients with profound cardiogenic shock, complete revascularization is usually difficult and the chance of achieving a normal blood flow (i.e., TIMI-3) in the target vessel is relatively low. This is mainly attributed to the very unstable blood pressure in these patients. On the other hand, with the use of ECMO support, patients' hemodynamic condition become stable [28]. Thus, operators will have enough time to completely revascularize the infarct-related artery with significantly lower stress during the procedure [28]. Of particular importance is that combined IABP & EMCO-supported PCI would offer dual benefits, i.e., stabilized the hemodynamics and increased coronary artery perfusion [28]. In this way, the chance of having normal blood flow in the target vessel will be maximized.

25.16 Complications of ECMO Implantation

Although implantation of ECMO can be performed in many settings such as Emergency Room, ordinary ward, operating theatre or intensive cardiac care, cardiac catheterization laboratory remains the mostly recommended venue. The latter setting has the obvious advantage of fluoroscopy guidance, and therefore complication of vessel perforation could be avoid, especially in those with very tortuous vessels.

When left femoral vein and artery are the access routes for ECMO implantation, particular attention should be paid to the tortuosity of common iliac artery and/or vein, and the angulation between common iliac artery and abdominal aorta (i.e., at the aortic bifurcation) or between common iliac vein and inferior vena cava. Although it is not a frequent complication, vessel perforation caused by the ECMO sheath may happen at these areas. Several methods could be utilized to avoid this complication. Firstly, the procedure should be performed under fluoroscopy guidance. Secondly, the sheaths should be advanced gently into the vessels. Thirdly, the use of a more stiff guide wire, for example 260″ Teflon wire, can provide a better support when the sheaths are being advanced to the right atrium or abdominal aorta.

In fact, most of the complications that happen during implantation of IABP can occur at implantation of ECMO. Among them, infection and upper gastrointestinal tract bleeding are the most frequently encountered complications.

25.17 Management and Timing to Remove the ECMO Support

Management of ECMO The entire ECMO system and all the related instruments for vascular access should be placed on a mobile cart so as to facilitate rapid transportation to the cardiac catheterization laboratory or other places. The ECMO is usually set up through the femoral venoarterial route by the percutaneous puncture method. In case of difficulty in percutaneous puncture, surgical incision and cut-down procedure can be performed.

During implantation, the tip of the arterial cannula is recommended to reside just above the aorto-iliac junction, whereas the tip of the venous cannula is placed at the middle level of the right atrium. Fluoroscopy should be used to confirm the positions of the cannulas. A catheter is placed for antegrade reperfusion to protect the lower extremity from acute critical limb ischemia if distal limb perfusion is inadequate. Heparinization should be used continuously and the activated clotting time (ACT) should be kept at about 150 to <180 s if no bleeding was observed in order to avoid blood clot formation in the filter.

The pump flow was initially set up at about 2–3 L/min with a mean blood pressure to be kept to ≥55 mmHg. Dopamine or other inotropic agents should be used if the mean blood pressure is <55 mmHg. A few minutes after the ECMO system operates normally, the flow can then be increased to a full flow of 3.5–4.0 L/min so as to maintain mean blood pressure >70 mmHg.

The circuit, including pump head and oxygenator, should be changed under the following conditions: a marked plasma leak, hemoglobinuria or blood-clot formation in the circuit system. It is recommended to measure serial cardiac enzymes and transthoracic echocardiography should be performed every day to assess the recovery of left ventricular function.

ECMO Weaning Protocol In consideration of the duration and extensiveness of myocardium stunning after a major ischemic attack, all patients with ECMO support should be maintained for at least 72 h before weaning is attempted unless complications occur. If the patient's hemodynamic and clinical conditions are stable and echocardiography shows an improvement of left ventricular systolic function (ejection fraction >40 %), the inotropic agent can be stepped down carefully. Of note, oxygen saturation is an important parameter which should be continuously monitored. When the mixed venous oxygen saturation is ≥70 % and there is no evidence hemodynamic deterioration, pump flow can then be reduced gradually to 500 mL/min. Eventually, ECMO is removed when patient's hemodynamic status is persistently stable.

Conclusion

Patients with ACS and cardiogenic shock usually carried a grave prognosis with high in-hospital mortality. Although PCI is the only option of coronary revascularization to salvage the infarcting myocardium and hopefully saving lives, mortality remains high without any adjunctive mechanical hemodynamic support. With the introduction of IABP and ECMO, they provide circulatory support to maintain more stable blood pressure, coronary perfusion and oxygenation. They also facilitate an optimized and early time window for transradial PCI. However, the cardiology team should be well trained and prepared for incorporating these tools, in particular the indications, vascular access, complications, maintenance and timing of removal of the mechanical supports. A heart team with multidisciplinary approach is the key to success if urgent and rapid ECMO service is to be contemplated.

References

1. Rich MW, Crecelius CA. Incidence, risk factors, and clinical course of acute renal insufficiency after cardiac catheterization in patients 70 years of age or older. Arch Intern Med. 1990;150:1237–42.
2. Spaulding C, Lefevre T, Funck F, Thebault B, Chauveau M, Hamda B, et al. Left radial approach for coronary angioplasty: results of a prospective study. Cathet Cardiovasc Diagn. 1996;39:365–70.
3. Sievert H, Ensslen R, Fach A, Merie H, Rubel C, Spies H, et al. Brachial artery approach for transluminal angioplasty of the internal carotid artery. Cathet Cardiovasc Diagn. 1996;39:421–3.
4. Friedman HZ, Cragg DR, Glazier SM, Gangadharan V, Marsalese DL, Schreiber TL, et al. Randomized prospective evaluation of prolonged versus abbreviated intravenous heparin therapy after coronary angioplasty. J Am Coll Cardiol. 1994;24:1214–9.
5. Oweida SW, Roubin GS, Smith RB, Salam AA. Post-catheterization vascular complications associated with percutaneous transluminal coronary angioplasty. J Vasc Surg. 1990;12:310–5.
6. Bittl JA. Comparative safety profiles of hirulog and heparin in patients undergoing coronary angioplasty. Am Heart J. 1995;130:658–65.
7. Nasser TK, Mohler ER, Wilensky RL, Hathaway DR. Peripheral vascular complications following coronary interventional procedures. Clin Cardiol. 1995;18:609–14.
8. Wu CJ, Lo PH, Chang KC, Fu M, Lau KW, Hung JS. Transradial coronary angiography and angioplasty in Chinese patients. Cathet Cardiovasc Diagn. 1997;40:159–63.
9. Galli M, Zerboni S, Politi A, Paone R, Ferrari G. Transradial approach for coronary procedures: initial experience and results. G Ital Cardiol. 1998;28:767–73.
10. Shibata Y, Doi O, Goto T, Hase T, Kadota K, Fujii M, et al. New guiding catheter for transradial percutaneous transluminal coronary angioplasty. Cathet Cardiovasc Diagn. 1998;43:344–51.
11. Chen YH, Wu CJ, Chang HW, Fang CY, Chen CJ, Yu TH, et al. Effects and safety of intracoronary thrombectomy using transradial application of PercuSurge distal balloon protection system in patients with early or recent myocardial infarction. Cardiology. 2004;102:206–14.
12. Yip HK, Wu CJ, Yang CH, Chang HW, Fang CY, Hung WC, et al. Serial changes in circulating levels of soluble CD40 ligand and C-reactive protein in patients with unstable angina undergoing coronary stenting: role of inflammatory mediators in predicting late restenosis. Circ J. 2005;69:890–5.
13. Yip HK, Wu CJ, Hang CL, Chang HW, Hung WC, Yeh KH, et al. Serial changes in platelet activation in patients with unstable angina following coronary stenting: evaluation of the effect of clopidogrel loading dose in inhibiting platelet activation. Circ J. 2005;69:1208–11.
14. Yang CH, Guo BF, Yip HK, Hsieh K, Fang CY, Chen SM, et al. Bilateral cardiac catheterizations: the safety and feasibility of a superficial forearm venous and transradial arterial approach. Int Heart J. 2006;47:21–7.
15. Wu CJ, Hung WC, Chen SM, Yang CH, Chen CJ, Cheng CI, et al. Feasibility and safety of transradial artery approach for selective cerebral angiography. Catheter Cardiovasc Interv. 2005;66:21–6.
16. Cheng CI, Wu CJ, Fang CY, Youssef AA, Chen CJ, Chen SM, et al. Feasibility and safety of transradial stenting for unprotected left main coronary artery stenosis. Circ J. 2007;71:855–61.
17. Yip HK, Youssef AA, Chang WN, Lu CH, Yang CH, Chen SM, et al. Feasibility and safety of transradial arterial approach for simultaneous right and left vertebral artery angiographic studies and stenting. Cardiovasc Intervent Radiol. 2007;30:840–6.
18. Wu CJ, Cheng CI, Hung WC, Fang CY, Yang CH, Chen CJ, et al. Feasibility and safety of transbrachial approach for patients with severe carotid artery stenosis undergoing stenting. Catheter Cardiovasc Interv. 2006;67:967–71.
19. Yip HK, Wu CJ, Chang HW, Fang CY, Yang CH, Chen SM, et al. Effect of the PercuSurge GuardWire device on the integrity of microvasculature and clinical outcomes during primary transradial coronary intervention in acute myocardial infarction. Am J Cardiol. 2003;92:1331–5.
20. Youssef AA, Change LT, Hang CL, Wu CJ, Cheng CI, Yang CH, et al. Level and value of interleukin-18 in patients with acute myocardial infarction undergoing primary coronary angioplasty. Circ J. 2007;71:703–8.
21. Amsterdam EA, Wenger NK, Brindis RG, et al. 2014 AHA/ACC Guideline for the management of patients with non-ST-elevation acute coronary syndromes: a report of the American College of Cardiology/American Heart Association Task Force on Practice Guidelines. J Am Coll Cardiol. 2014;64:e139–228.
22. Amsterdam EA, Wenger NK, Brindis RG, et al. 2014 AHA/ACC Guideline for the management of patients with non-ST-elevation acute coronary syndromes: executive summary: a report of the American College of Cardiology/American Heart Association Task Force on Practice Guidelines. Circulation. 2014;130:2354–94.
23. Amsterdam EA, Wenger NK, Brindis RG, et al. 2014 AHA/ACC Guideline for the management of patients with non-ST-elevation acute coronary syndromes: a report of the American College of Cardiology/American Heart Association Task Force on Practice Guidelines. Circulation. 2014;130:e344–426.
24. Antman EM, Cohen M, Bernink PJ, et al. The TIMI risk score for unstable angina/non-ST elevation MI: a method for prognostication and therapeutic decision making. JAMA. 2000;284:835–42.

25. Michel P, Roques F, Nashef SA, EuroSCORE Project Group. Logistic or additive EuroSCORE for high-risk patients? Eur J Cardiothorac Surg. 2003;23:684–7.
26. Hernández-Vaquero D, Díaz R, Meana B, Morís C. External validation of the EuroSCORE II risk stratification model in the USA. Eur J Cardiothorac Surg. 2015;48:177.
27. Yip HK, Wu CJ, Chang HW, Chen MC, Hang CL, Fang CY, Hsieh YK, Yang CH, Yeh KH, Fu M. Comparison of impact of primary percutaneous transluminal coronary angioplasty and primary stenting on short-term mortality in patients with cardiogenic shock and evaluation of prognostic determinants. Am J Cardiol. 2001;87:1184–8.
28. Sheu JJ, Tsai TH, Lee FY, Fang HY, et al. Early extracorporeal membrane oxygenator-assisted primary percutaneous coronary intervention improved 30-day clinical outcomes in patients with ST-segment elevation myocardial infarction complicated with profound cardiogenic shock. Crit Care Med. 2010;38:1810–7.
29. Chung SY, Sheu JJ, Lin YJ, Sun CK, et al. Outcome of patients with profound cardiogenic shock after cardiopulmonary resuscitation and prompt extracorporeal membrane oxygenation support. A single-center observational study. Circ J. 2012;76:1385–92.
30. Seyfarth M, Sibbing D, Bauer I, Fröhlich G, Bott-Flügel L, Byrne R, Dirschinger J, Kastrati A, Schömig A. A randomized clinical trial to evaluate the safety and efficacy of a percutaneous left ventricular assist device versus intra-aortic balloon pumping for treatment of cardiogenic shock caused by myocardial infarction. J Am Coll Cardiol. 2008;52:1584–8.
31. Lee WC, Tsai TH, Chen YL, et al. Safety and feasibility of coronary stenting in unprotected left main coronary artery disease in the real world clinical practice--a single center experience. PLoS One. 2014;9:e109281.
32. Smith TB, Shridhar P, Khalil R, Lasorda DM. Prolonged duration of transbrachial intra-aortic balloon pump as bridge to heart transplantation. BMJ Case Rep. 2015;5:2015.
33. Gan HW, Yip HK, Wu CJ. Brachial approach for coronary angiography and intervention: totally obsolete, or a feasible alternative when radial access is not possible? Ann Acad Med Singapore. 2010;39:368–73.
34. Prondzinsky R, Lemm H, Swyter M, Wegener N, Unverzagt S, Carter JM, Russ M, Schlitt A, Buerke U, Christoph A, Schmidt H, Winkler M, Thiery J, Werdan K, Buerke M. Intra-aortic balloon counterpulsation in patients with acute myocardial infarction complicated by cardiogenic shock: the prospective, randomized IABP SHOCK Trial for attenuation of multiorgan dysfunction syndrome. Crit Care Med. 2010;38:152–60.
35. Truby L, Naka Y, Kalesan B, Ota T, et al. Important role of mechanical circulatory support in acute myocardial infarction complicated by cardiogenic shock. Eur J Cardiothorac Surg. 2015; 48:322–8.
36. Altayyar S, Rochwerg B, Alnasser S, Al-Omari A, Baw B, Fox-Robichaud A, Alhazzani W. Intra-aortic balloon pump in patients with cardiogenic shock complicating myocardial infarction: a systematic review and meta-analysis of randomized trials (protocol). Syst Rev. 2014;3:24.
37. Abu-Omar Y, Tsui SS. Mechanical circulatory support for AMI and cardiogenic shock. J Card Surg. 2010;25:434–41.
38. Tsao NW, Shih CM, Yeh JS, Kao YT, Hsieh MH, Ou KL, Chen JW, Shyu KG, Weng ZC, Chang NC, Lin FY, Huang CY. Extracorporeal membrane oxygenation-assisted primary percutaneous coronary intervention may improve survival of patients with acute myocardial infarction complicated by profound cardiogenic shock. J Crit Care. 2012;27:530.e1–11.
39. Kim H, Lim SH, Hong J, Hong YS, Lee CJ, Jung JH, Yu S. Efficacy of veno-arterial extracorporeal membrane oxygenation in acute myocardial infarction with cardiogenic shock. Resuscitation. 2012; 83:971–5.
40. Chung ES, Lim C, Lee HY, Choi JH, Lee JS, Park KH. Results of extracorporeal membrane oxygenation (ECMO) support before coronary reperfusion in cardiogenic shock with acute myocardial infarction. Korean J Thorac Cardiovasc Surg. 2011; 44:273–8.
41. Chen YS, Lin JW, Yu HY, et al. Cardiopulmonary resuscitation with assisted extracorporeal life-support versus conventional cardiopulmonary resuscitation in adults with in-hospital cardiac arrest: an observational study and propensity analysis. Lancet. 2008;372: 554–61.
42. Tsuneyoshi H, Rao V. The role of extracorporeal membrane oxygenation (ECMO) therapy in acute heart failure. Int Anesthesiol Clin. 2012;50:114–22.
43. Wu MY, Lee MY, Lin CC, Chang YS, Tsai FC, Lin PJ. Resuscitation of non-postcardiotomy cardiogenic shock or cardiac arrest with extracorporeal life support: the role of bridging to intervention. Resuscitation. 2012;83:976–81.

Transradial Intracoronary Spasm Provocation Test

26

Seung-Woon Rha and Harris Abdullah Ngow

Abstract

An important cause of pain with normal coronary vessels is coronary artery spasm (CAS). Undiagnosed coronary artery spasm can lead to significant cardiovascular morbidity and mortality. Many of these patients endure recurrent angina in spite of optimal medical therapy, causing impairment to their quality of life. In addition, this has profound impact on the cost of healthcare as many of these patients have repeated hospital admissions or multiple visits to the healthcare professionals.

According to numerous publications, half of the symptomatic patients undergoing coronary angiography revealed normal or non-obstructive coronary arteries, despite coronary angiography being the gold standard for assessing coronary arteries (Sharaf et al. Am J Cardiol 87:937–941, 2001). The transient nature of coronary artery spasm may explain the difficulty in diagnosing this vasospastic syndrome in conventional angiography study. A provocative diagnostic strategy has been used in several centres to induce vasospasm during coronary angiography. There are many pharmacological and non-pharmacological agents that had been studied in the past. Although the use provocation test is limited due to scarcity of clinical evidence or safety study, several agents have been used in some cardiac centres especially in Korea and Japan. Acetylcholine (Ach) and Ergonovine (Erg) are two agents that are more widely used in these centers. There is no published guideline available for the provocation test, but centre specific-protocols have been established, individualized and published. Transradial route has been seen as advantageous due to its lower risk for access site complications, slender system for quick recovery, shorter procedure time and convenience for both physician and patients.

26.1 Aetiology of Coronary Spasm

The novel heart syndrome that mimics atherosclerotic coronary artery disease was initially described by Prinzmetal et al. in 1959 [1, 2]. It was first illustrated as a variant form of angina which predominantly occurred at rest and usually related with transient ST-segment elevation myocardial infarction on the electrocardiogram. The angina resulted from occlusive or sub-occlusive epicardial artery that underwent spasm [3]. Although older published studies suggest that the prognosis for patients with coronary artery spasm is rather benign and excellent, contemporary reports indicate that this syndrome has been associated with dismay outcome such as prolong ischemia, acute coronary syndrome, arrhythmias and sudden cardiac death [4–8]. The vasospastic mechanism was thought to originate at or near the site of atherosclerotic plaque initially [8–10]. However, this is found to be not true in vast majority of patients as many have been found to be related to dysfunctional endothelial vasomotor system. The risk factors for atherosclerotic coronary artery disease have been broadly investigated for the past three decades. On the other hand, very limited studies have been performed on the risk factors and predictors of coronary artery spasm. It was

S.-W. Rha (✉) • H.A. Ngow
Cardiovascular Center, Korea University Guro Hospital, Seoul, Korea
e-mail: swrha617@yahoo.co.kr; harrisngow@gmail.com

Y. Zhou et al. (eds.), *Transradial Approach for Percutaneous Interventions*, DOI 10.1007/978-94-017-7350-8_26

hypothesized that the risk factors and forecasters of this syndrome are not the same as traditional risk factors of coronary atherosclerotic disease such as diabetes mellitus, hypertension, dyslipidaemia, old age, smoking and present of family history of coronary artery disease [11]. In coronary artery spasm, the risk factors are thought to employ its results on disturbing the endothelial function and impairing the vasomotor response of the coronary artery through endothelium derive relaxing factor (EDRF). This leads to vasoconstrictive response by reversing or abolishing the vasodilatory response of acetylcholine [12]. Diagnosis can be difficult at time, given the transient nature of coronary artery spasm, and might require a battery of more sophisticated provocative diagnostic strategy. Therefore it is imperative to perform a provocative test to induce spasm in patients with normal coronaries or in patients with insignificant coronary artery lesions to account for the angina symptoms [13].

26.2 Vaso-Provocative Agents

In the current contemporary practice, it seems provocation testing in the cardiac catheterization laboratory is increasingly performed in Korea and Japan. In the contrary, this procedure is performed less frequently in the western world including the US though the exact quantitative data are available on scientific literature. Previously, many stimulating tests have been performed for detecting coronary artery spasm [14, 15]. These tests may be a pharmacological challenge test or non-pharmacological tests. Numerous agents have been described in the laboratory for spasm provocation testing such as: acetylcholine (Ach), ergonovine (Erg), neuropeptide-y and dopamine [16–20]. For instance, ergonovine maleate was most widely used previously [13]. However, it has many disadvantages due to administration route via IV that can cause widespread diffuse vasospasm in all coronary trees at the same time. Moreover, it has propensity to induce severe prolonged coronary artery spasm leading to hazardous adverse effects. As a result of these disadvantages, newer provocative agent like acetylcholine has been increasingly used as an alternative replacing ergonovine [19, 21, 22].

In clinical practice, a relative larger body of clinical evidence supports the use of acetylcholine as a provocative agent to induce coronary artery spasm, as compared to ergonovine. Acetylcholine induces vasodilatation in the regular coronary arteries by releasing endothelium-derived relaxing factor (EDRF) [23]. In the atherosclerotic artery, acetylcholine can prompt coronary artery spasm due to direct effect on the vascular smooth muscle cells [24]. Acetylcholine acts on the endothelium and smooth muscle via the muscarinic receptor. In healthy endothelium, acetylcholine activation results in vasodilatation. In case of endothelial dysfunction, endothelial cells fail to produce sufficient amount of nitric oxide (NO), a powerful smooth muscle relaxant therefore resulting in blood vessel vasoconstriction rather than vasodilatation [25, 26]. Several adverse effects of acetylcholine include hypotension, bradycardia, dyspnoea and occasionally flushing [27]. Intracoronary acetylcholine can precipitate bradyarrhythmias during the provocation test especially in the right coronary testing or dominant left circumflex artery. Nevertheless, this risk can be avoided with temporary cardiac pacing or by simple measure with induced cough. The most serious reactions include ventricular tachycardia; shock and cardiac tamponade are rare nowadays [28, 29].

The other pharmacological agent that's often used clinically in vasospastic provocation test is ergonovine. This agent acts on the smooth muscle cells mainly through the activation of the serotonergic (5-HT2) receptors to produce blood vessel contraction [30]. Endothelial activation by ergonovine also causes release of inhibitory prostanoid substances thereby leading to profound vasoconstriction in those patients with endothelial dysfunction. Ergonovine predominantly metabolized by the hepatic enzyme cytochrome CYP3 4A. The adverse reactions of ergot include ischemia, angina, arrhythmias, myocardial infarction, nausea, ergotism and anaphylaxis reactions [31]. The absolute contraindications for ergonovine are; pregnancy, severe left ventricular dysfunction, severe hypertension (BP >180/110 mmHg), moderately severe to severe aortic stenosis and high grade stenosis in the left main stem artery [32].

Both acetylcholine and ergonovine is widely used in Korea and Japan as a provocation agent for the diagnosis of coronary artery spasm [33–35]. However, both agents are not approved by the U.S. Food and Drug Administration for the indication of coronary artery provocation test yet [36].

26.3 Protocol of Coronary Vasospasm Testing

A pharmacological agent induced vasospasm provocation test is performed to diagnose coronary artery spasm for patients presenting chest pain syndrome with a diagnostic coronary arteriography presenting normal or near-normal vessels. The provocation test can be done with intracoronary administration of acetylcholine or ergonovine. Various testing protocol is available using intracoronary or intravenous administration have been described depending on the logistic and expertise of the specialized center. The important distinction of induction of spasm by intravenous ergonovine is the ability of this agent to induce diffuse multivessel contraction resulting in hemodynamic instability thus rendering the arteriography hard to obtain and interpret. Furthermore, intracoronary vasodilator like nitroglycerine or verapamil may be required to relieve the spasm. As a result, most experts would recommend intracoronary administration compare to the conventional intravenous administration of ergonovine as this is safer in current perspective.

Table 26.1 Vasospasm testing dosing protocols around the regions

First author	Ergonovine	Acetylcholine
Invasive testing		
Japanese Circulation society [33]	Ergonovine 20–60 ug (LCA, IC)	20–100 ug (LCA, IC)
	Ergonovine 20–60 ug (RCA, IC)	20–50 ug (RC, IC)
Okumura et al. [19]	200 ug IV	20–100 ug (LCA, IC)
		20–50 ug (RCA, IC)
Song et al. [35]	Ergonovine 1–30 ug IC	10–100 ug IC
Sueda et al. [38]	Ergonovine 64 ug (LCA, IC)	20–100 ug (LCA, IC)
	Ergonovine 40 ug (RCA, IC)	20–50 ug (RCA, IC)
Takagi et al. [41]	Ergonovine 20–60 ug (LCA, IC)	20–100 ug (LCA, IC)
	Ergonovine 20–60 ug (RCA, IC)	20–50 ug (RCA, IC)
Yasue et al. [42]	NA	Suspected vessel 10–100 ug IC
		Contralateral vessel: 20–200 ug (LCA, IC) 20–50 ug (RCA, IC)
Rha et al. [34, 43]	NA	20, 50, 100 ug (LCA, IC) 20–50 ug (RCA, IC)

IC Intracoronary, *IV* Intravenous, *LCA* Left coronary artery, *RCA* Right coronary artery, *NA* Not applicable

Intracoronary administration also allows separate administration of the agent in the right and left coronary artery. No doubt intravenous administration of the ergonovine has good sensitivity approaching 100 % when angina is the diagnostic criteria and sensitivity of 94 % when electrocardiographic ST-segment elevation is documented, latest reports showed that the frequency of provoking coronary spasm with intracoronary ergonovine is 2.2–2.6 times higher than the intravenous mode [37, 38]. The specificity of intravenous or intracoronary testing is nevertheless similarly high at>90 % [16, 39]. In spite of the high sensitivity, false negative results have been reported too. Thus, a negative ergonovine result cannot completely exclude the diagnosis of coronary spasm and the operator shall interpret such finding with care [40]. Table 26.1 describes the various protocol and practice of vasospasm provocation test around the regions.

In our center, this test has been performed for the past 10 years in over 6000 patients presented with unexplained chest pain syndrome with normal and near-normal coronary artery anatomically (<30 % stenosis). Acetylcholine provocation test results are more sensitive for the typical patients of vascospastic angina despite less specific response than the ergonovine test. It means that it is safe to treat patients according to acetylcholine provocation results and there will be limited chance of false negative results. The usual dose of acetylcholine provocation test is described as in Table 26.1.

26.4 Pathophysiology of Vasospastic Angina

Several mechanisms have been described in the pathogenesis of this vasospastic syndrome though the mechanisms are poorly defined and likely multifactorial. Generally, the mechanisms of vasospasm have been postulated to involve either the vascular endothelial cells or the hyperreactive vascular smooth muscles. Patients have spontaneous angina episodes associated with reversible tightening of focal segment or segments of the coronary artery leading to functional obstruction of the blood flow causing myocardial ischemia. In this vasospastic syndrome, intracoronary acetylcholine induces spasm at high frequency without compromising hemodynamic status [42]. Usually acetylcholine expands blood vessels when the endothelium is normal, but it contracts blood vessels when there is endothelial detachment or injury. The potent smooth muscle relaxant, nitric oxide (NO), is secreted from the endothelial cells when the endothelium is normally intact [26, 44]. In healthy endothelium, NO is produced by reactive NO species (eNOS) when it is activated by various cellular signals. Elevation of intracellular calcium level due to mechanical shear stress in turn activates eNOS activity via calmodulin thereby promotes NO release and hence vasodilatation. This receptor mediated vasodilatation is induced by many vasoactive physiological mediators including acetylcholine, bradykinin, G proteins, and phospholipase C in vascular endothelium leading to inositol triphosphate production and release of stored ionic calcium in the cells. As a result of this receptor activation, cellular calcium inflow is promoted via the ionic channels. Further stimulation by physiological active substances like acetylcholine, insulin, and bradykinin coupling with the mechanical shear stress on vascular wall also enhance release of eNOS activity [45]. NO stimulates soluble guanylate cyclase in vascular smooth muscle to increase the level of cyclic guanosine monophosphate (cGMP) and hence vasodilatation. Under standard conditions, NO is produced and released from healthy endothelial cells. In vasospastic coronary arteries, this hypereactivity to nitroglycerine is perhaps owing to the absence of baseline production and release of NO from the healthy endothelium present in the arteries [46].

The mechanism of vascular smooth muscle cells contraction has recently been described [47, 48]. Under the influence of vasoconstrictive substance, G protein coupling with phospholipase C (PLC) in smooth muscle cells is stimulated to release inositol triphosphate (IP3). IP3 opens calcium ion channel in the sarcoplasmic reticulum. Ionic calcium is released into the cytoplasm resulting in increased intracellular calcium concentration. In addition, calcium channels are also present on the cell membrane that opens under various physiological stimuli. The additive effect is the sudden surge of intracellular calcium concentration. Intracellular calcium ions bind to calmodulin to form Calcium/calmodulin complexes. These complexes will then bind to the catalytic subunit of myosin light chain kinase (MLCK) converting it to its active form. Phosphorylation of the myosin light chain (MLC) by the active MLCK activates Magnesium-ATPase in the head of myosin by actin. This results in vascular smooth muscle cells contraction. Following that, the intracellular calcium level falls, calcium/calmodulin complex dissociates and MLCK becomes inert. The activity of myosin light chain phosphatase (MLCPh) become predominant, MLC will undergo phosphorylation and resulting in vascular smooth muscle relaxation [49]. MLC phosphorylation is encouraged by MLCK but suppressed by MLCPh. Rho-kinase has been shown to suppress MLCPh activity [50]. Rho-kinase controls the balance between contraction and relaxation of the vascular smooth muscle. Its action is not dependent on intracellular calcium level. Once activated by vasoactive substances, Rho, a low molecular weight G protein, is activated by the G-protein-coupling receptor. At the same time, the target protein, Rho-kinase, is activated. Rho-kinase inhibits the phosphorylation of MBS, rendering MLCPh inactive. This produces imbalance between MLCK's and MLCPh's activity therefore promoting phosphorylation of MLC and resulted in exaggerated contraction of vascular smooth muscle [50, 51].

Therefore, the cellular basic of hyperactive coronary vascular smooth muscle cell consist of the end substrate for the evolution of coronary artery spasm. The pathogenesis of this condition is likely to be multifactorial and heterogeneous among different population. Several other pathophysiological factors also have an important role in the genesis of this vasospastic entity including the autonomic nervous system, endothelial dysfunction, systemic inflammation, oxidative stress and genetics. Other environmental factors, for instance, smoking, metabolic abnormalities, and alcohol consumption may too contribute to its genesis. Racial variations in the incidence have been reported with higher prevalence in Korea and Japan suggesting a genetic influence [52]. Lastly, the interplay among these factors in the evolution of coronary spasm is rather elusive and poorly defined.

26.5 Transradial Provocation Testing

Transradial route has been increasingly used as the preferred access route for coronary intervention. The most compelling reason for adopting transradial access is the increased patient safety that results from virtually elimination of access site vascular complications and bleeding [53]. Besides, transradial route has the advantage of early sheath removal, faster recovery, patient's comfort and lower cost compared to femoral access [54]. With that in mind, we have been performing vasospasm provocation test in our center since the initial inception of the invasive cardiovascular center in 2004. To date, we have been performing more than 6000 patients for the past 10 years.

In our usual workflow for intracoronary spasm provocation test, the patient with chest pain syndrome will undergo a routine coronary angiography via the transradial route as mentioned in the prior chapter. All vasodilators or vasoconstrictor are withheld for at least 72 h prior to coronary angiography. Routine coronary angiography is performed early in the morning and if the angiography is normal or near-normal; Acetylcholine provocation test ensues immediately after the arteriography via the 4 F transradial diagnostic catheter. Control angiography of the left and right coronary arteries is performed. The best angiography projection is taken to ensure separation of each of the branches of the vascular trees. The angiography is then repeated after acetylcholine injection at the same projection again. Upon completion of the procedure, nitrate is administered and angiography is performed at the same projection again while the coronary is maximally dilated. RAO cranial or AP cranial view was routinely evaluated for the observation of combined myocardial bridge (MB).

Currently, we are using 4 F transradial diagnostic catheters for this purpose. There are three different types of 4 F single catheters for bilateral engagement (both left and right coronary arteries) in our center that can be used for the provocation test either with ergonovine or acetylcholine. They are 4 F RM (Rha-Moon) catheter (Jung Sung Medical, JSM, Korea), 4 F CR (Cheon-Rha) catheter (Jung Sung Medical, JSM, Korea), 4 F Tiger catheter (Terumo, Japan). The descriptions for the procedure are illustrated in Figs. 26.1, 26.2 and 26.3.

Coronary artery spasm is prompted by intracoronary injection of acetylcholine after diagnostic angiography. Acetylcholine is injected by 20 (A1), 50 (A2) and 100 (A3) μg/min into the left coronary artery over a 1 min period with 5 min intervals to the maximum tolerated dose under constant monitoring of electrocardiogram (ECG) and blood pressure. Angiography is then repeated after each acetylcholine dose until significant vasoconstriction (70 %) response. Intracoronary infusion with 0.2 mg nitroglycerine is given after completing the acetylcholine provocation test.

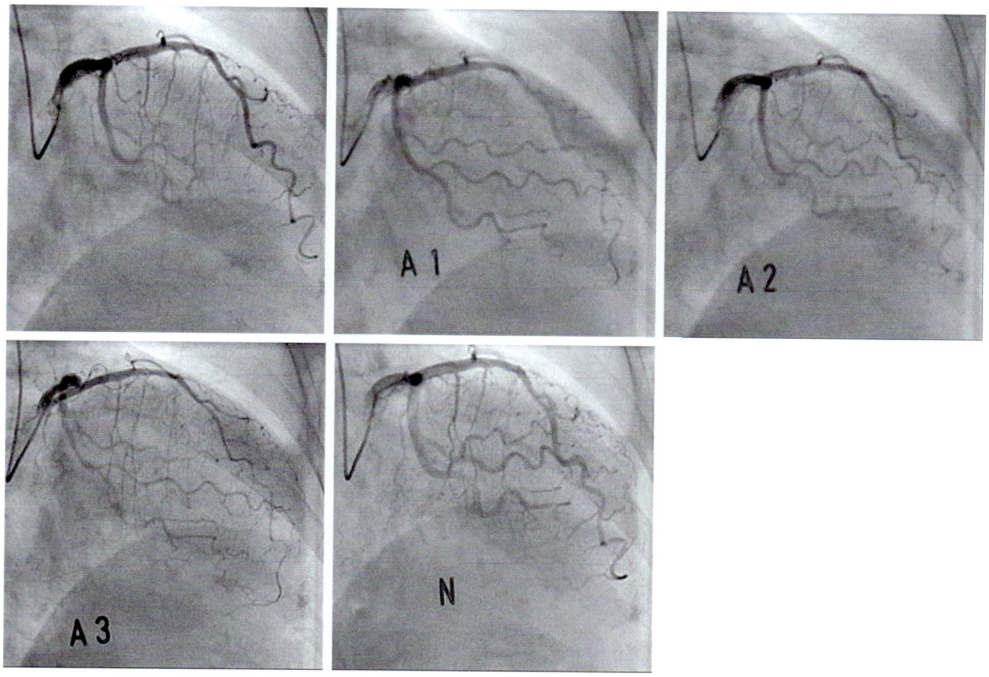

Fig. 26.1 Acetylcholine provocation test with 4 F RM catheter. Coronary Arteriogram of the left coronary artery was performed in right anterior oblique projection via the right radial route with 4 F RM catheter. A control angiography was taken at baseline. Subsequently, an incremental dose of intracoronary Acetylcholine was administered. In this patient, the third dose (100 ug) of acetylcholine induced left anterior descending artery spasm. A completion angiography was repeated with administration of nitroglycerine 200 mcg at the same projection. Interpretation was performed by comparing the A3 to the final angiography after nitrate administration. (*A1* Acetylcholine 20 ug, *a2* Acetylcholine 50 ug, *A3* Acetylcholine 100 ug, *N* nitroglycerine 200 ug)

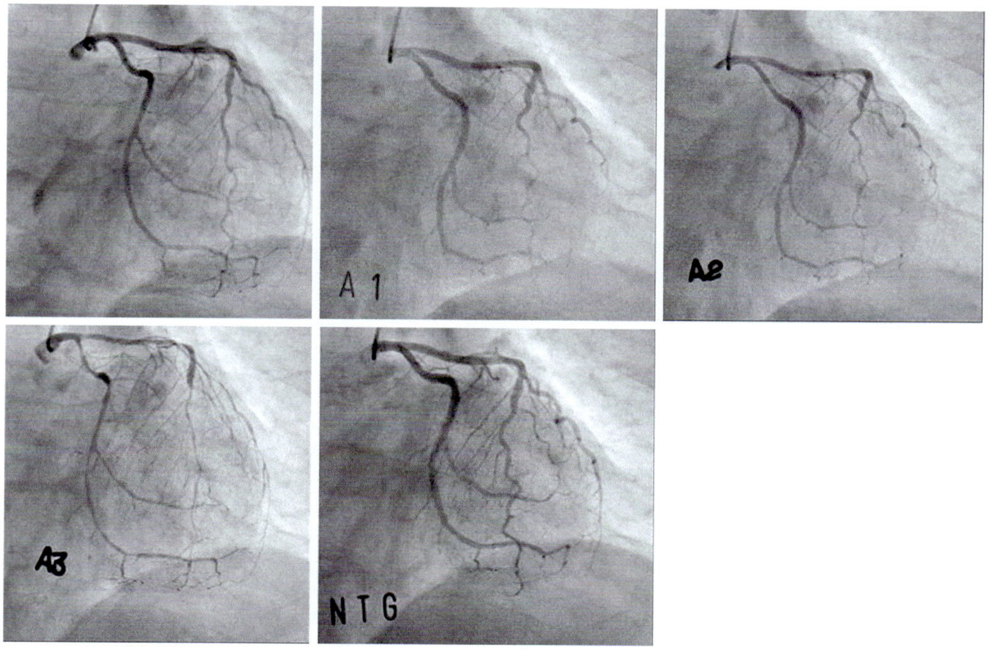

Fig. 26.2 Acetylcholine provocation test with 4 F CR catheter. Coronary Arteriogram of the left coronary artery was performed in right anterior oblique projection via the right radial route with 4 F CR catheter. A control angiography was taken at baseline. Subsequently, an incremental dose of intracoronary Acetylcholine was administered. In this patient, the mid-distal portion of the left anterior descending artery looked vasospastic after the first dose of acetylcholine but this was not clinical significant without angina or dramatic electrocardiographic changes. After the third dose (100 ug) of intracoronary acetylcholine injection, this induced a significant left anterior descending artery spasm. A completion angiography was repeated with administration of nitroglycerine 200 mcg at the same projection which showed maximal vasodilatation. Interpretation was performed by comparing the A3 to the final angiography after nitrate administration. (*A1* Acetylcholine 20 ug, *A2* Acetylcholine 50 ug, *A3* Acetylcholine 100 ug, *N* nitroglycerine 200 ug)

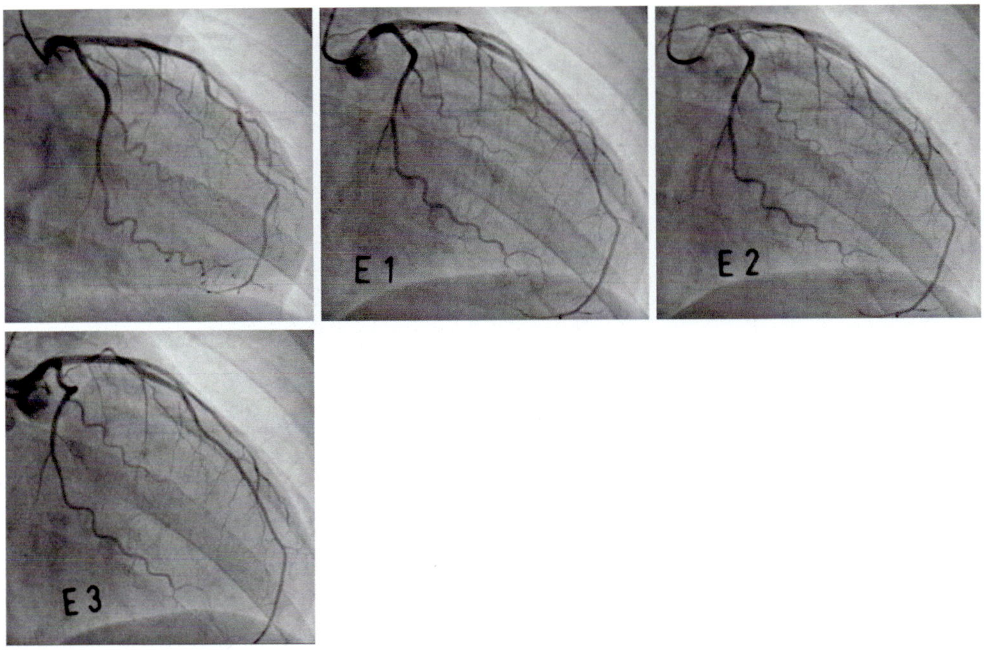

Panel a

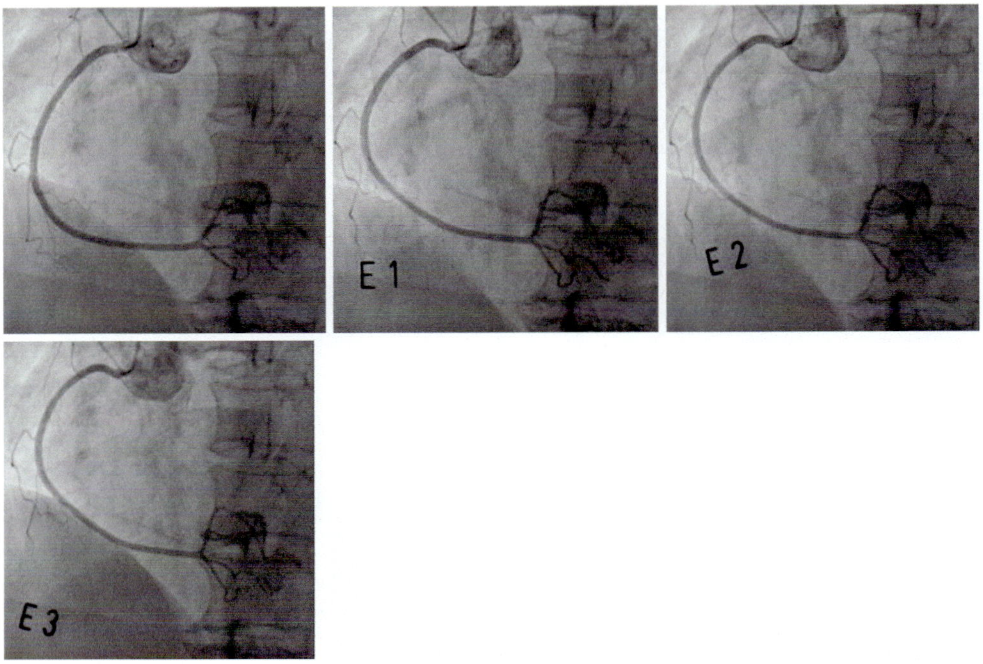

Panel b

Fig. 26.3 Intracoronary Ergonovine provocation test (**Panel a** and **b**). Coronary angiogram of the left coronary artery was performed in right anterior oblique projection via the right radial route with *4 F Tiger catheter*. A control angiography was taken at baseline. Subsequently, an incremental dose of intracoronary Ergonovine was administered. In this patient, the Ergonovine challenge test failed to induce vasospasm of the left anterior descending artery (**Panel a**) and right coronary artery (**Panel b**) despite repeated at incremental maximal doses. Nevertheless, due to high clinical suspicious, a repeat test was performed using Acetylcholine in **Panel c**. (*E1* Ergonovine 10 ug, *E2* Ergonovine 20 ug, *E3* Ergonovine 50 ug). Subsequent intracoronary acetylcholine provocation test after negative ergonovine provocation test (**Panel c**). An immediate repeat test was performed with Acetylcholine. Baseline control coronary arteriogram of the left coronary artery was performed in right anterior oblique projection via the right radial route with 4 F Tiger catheter. An incremental dose of intracoronary Acetylcholine was administered after failing Ergonovine challenge test. In this patient, a diffuse left anterior descending artery spasm was induced with 50 ug of intracoronary Acetylcholine (A2 dose). The test was aborted when coronary spasm was induced and intracoronary nitroglycerine 200 ug was administered to reverse the vasospastic effect. A completion angiography was repeated with administration of nitroglycerine 200 mcg at the same projection which showed maximal vasodilatation. Interpretation was performed by comparing the A2 to the final angiography after nitrate administration. (*A1* Acetylcholine 20 ug, *A2* Acetylcholine 50 ug, *N* nitroglycerine 200 ug)

Fig. 26.3 (continued)

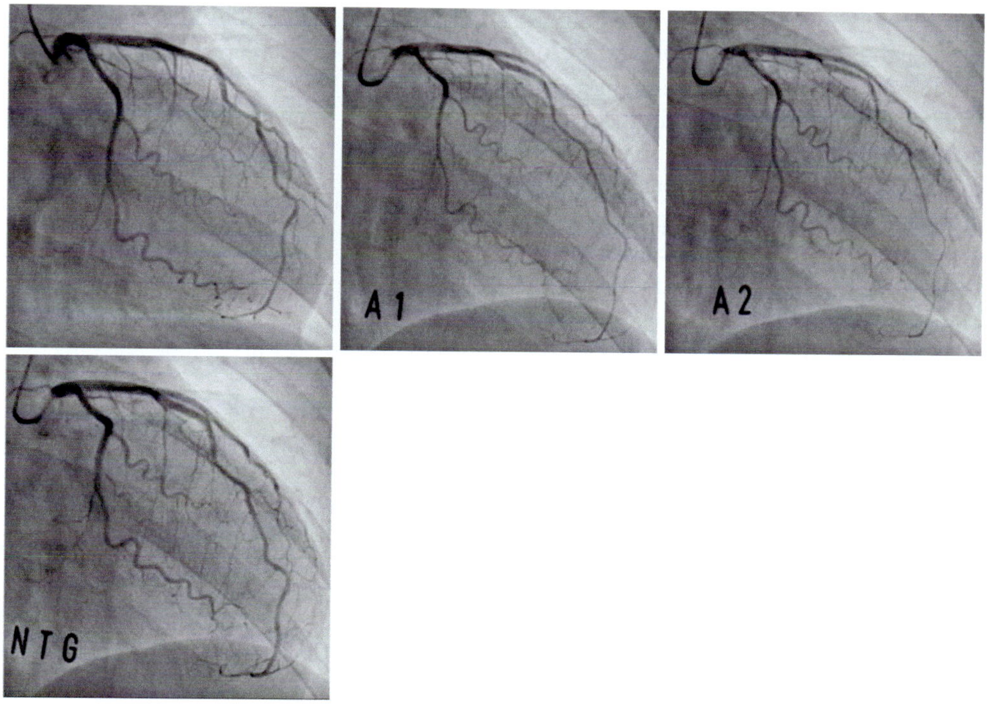

Panel c

Angiography is then performed 2 min later. If focal or diffuse significant vasoconstriction of coronary arteries is induced with any dose of acetylcholine by visual assessment, the procedure is stopped. End systolic images for each segment of the left coronary artery are chosen according to the corresponding points on the electrocardiographic trace (QRS onset or end of T wave) and analysed using the proper quantitative coronary angiographic (QCA) system of the catheterization laboratory (FD-20, Phillips, Amsterdam, The Netherlands). The coronary artery diameters are measured with QCA before and after the administration of acetylcholine at the site that show the greatest changes following drug administration. Reference diameter is measured at the proximal and distal portion of each artery before and after the intracoronary acetylcholine infusion and the mean reference diameter is used to assess the diameter narrowing.

During the coronary angiography and acetylcholine provocation test, significant CAS is defined as focal or diffuse severe transient luminal narrowing (>70 %) by visual assessment with or without chest pain or ischemic ECG change such as ST-T segment elevation, depression (≥1 mm) or T wave inversion. The normal coronary appearance is defined as less than 20 % luminal narrowing on coronary angiogram that is measured with QCA. Multi-vessel spasm (MVS) is defined as significant CAS of ≥2 major epicardial coronary arteries. The presence of baseline spasm is defined as focal or diffuses narrowing more than 30 % in diameter on the angiogram before the acetylcholine provocation test in comparison to final angiogram after intracoronary nitroglycerine infusion. Diffuse CAS is defined as significant CAS site length ≥30 mm.

In our center, intracoronary ergonovine provocation test is rarely performed nowadays in our patients due to its adverse effect and safety issues as described earlier. An example of ergonovine challenge test is illustrated in Fig. 26.3 in which it failed to induce vasoconstriction in one such patient and subsequent acetylcholine provocation test performed was positive.

26.5.1 Safety and Practice Guidelines

From our experience, transradial intracoronary spasm provocation test is generally safe and feasible. We have not encountered any untoward conventionally described detrimental effects in our patients such as prolonged ischemia, refractory ventricular tachyarrhythmia, myocardial infarction or even death. This is consistent with the contemporary reports that provocation testing is relatively safe [41]; though prolonged ischemia, MI, tachyarrhythmia and death has been reported in the older scientific literatures as a result of prolonged refractory spasm or recurrent spasm after testing [55, 56]. The safer results in our center coming from the modified (+) provocation test criteria as transient luminal narrowing greater than 70 % instead of traditional transient total or subtotal occlusion.

We believe that the obstacles to the performance of transradial invasive coronary spasm provocation test are the relatively steep learning curve of transradial catheter handling and the occasionally unfriendly radial route anatomy. Therefore interventional cardiologists shall be more open to change and with the correct attitude, this test can be safely adopted and performed in the vast majority of the patients.

Guidelines recommendations differ among the society for coronary artery spasm testing. Prior ACC/AHA guidelines support limited use of provocation testing for spasm nonetheless the current guidelines does not address this issue specifically whereas other practice guidelines do [33, 57–59].

Besides, routinely in our invasive cardiac catheter laboratory, a positive coronary spasm test after acetylcholine or ergonovine provocation test is defined as transient significant >70 % luminal narrowing with/without ischemic ST-T Change or chest pain. Other operators may arbitrarily defined as >50 % luminal narrowing compare to control arteriography. In the literature, a standard definition of coronary spasm after provocation test is defined as transient, total or subtotal (>90 %) luminal narrowing of a coronary with signs or symptoms of myocardial ischemia manifested as angina-like pain and ischemic electrocardiographic changes on the ST-T segment [33]. Due to this variation in our practice and interpretation of test results, a closer appraisal of the current available data is needed to arrive at a more meaningful evidence-based practice and recommendations.

We have recently reported the safety and efficacy of intracoronary acetylcholine provocation test, mostly via transradial intracoronary provocation test and evaluated for long-term clinical outcomes in this particular subset of patients [60]. We assessed the pervasiveness of coronary artery spasm and the influence of coronary artery spasm on 5-year clinical outcomes in a series of Asian coronary artery spasm patients documented by intracoronary acetylcholine provocation test.

1413 patients without significant coronary artery disease undergone acetylcholine provocation test between Nov. 2004 and Oct. 2008 were enrolled. Significant coronary artery spasm was defined as>70 % of narrowing by incremental intracoronary injection of 20, 50 and 100 μg. Patients were divided into two groups based on the presence of significant coronary artery spasm (the non-coronary artery spasm group: n = 640, the coronary artery spasm group; n = 773). To adjust probable confounders, a propensity score matched (PSM) analysis was performed using the logistic regression model. A total of 54.7 % (773/1413) patients were diagnosed as coronary artery spasm documented by acetylcholine provocation test. After PSM analysis, two propensity-matched groups (451 pairs, n = 902, C-statistic = 0.677) were formed. Despite the similar incidence of individual hard endpoints including mortality, myocardial infarction and revascularization, the coronary artery spasm group presented with higher trend of recurrent angina requiring follow up angiography than the non-coronary artery spasm group up to 5 years (HR; 1.56, 95 % C.I; 0.99–2.46, p = 0.054). The prevalence of coronary artery spasm was 54.7 %. Although the coronary artery spasm was not associated with increased incidence of major adverse clinical outcomes, the cumulative incidence of recurrent angina seems to be increased up to 5 years.

Conclusion

A diagnosis of coronary artery spasm cannot be directly established based on symptoms alone. Coronary angiography with intracoronary spasm provocation test is the only certain and effective method for the definite diagnosis of significant coronary artery spasm. Transradial provocation test did not differ methodologically from the conventional invasive testing and the only barrier to success is the steep learning curve of engaging and handling radial catheter, particularly bilateral engagement with single catheter. With the many advantages of transradial approach in comparison to transfemoral access, we predict it would become the preferred route for the intracoronary spasm provocation test in the future. Lastly, for a more meaningful and evidence-based guidelines with regards to the effectiveness and safety of provocation test, large ethnically diverse studies will be needed to help define the molecular pathways and develop more effective treatment for patients with significant coronary artery spasm.

References

1. Sharaf BL, Pepine CJ, Kerensky RA, Reis SE, Reichek N, Rogers WJ, et al. Detailed angiographic analysis of women with suspected ischemic chest pain (pilot phase data from the NHLBI-sponsored Women's Ischemia Syndrome Evaluation [WISE] Study Angiographic Core Laboratory). Am J Cardiol. 2001;87(8):937–41; a3.
2. Prinzmetal M, Kennamer R, Merliss R, Wada T, Bor N. Angina pectoris. I. A variant form of angina pectoris; preliminary report. Am J Med. 1959;27:375–88.
3. Maseri A, Mimmo R, Chierchia S, Pesola A, Parodi O, Severi S. Clinical coronarographic characteristics and pathogenetic mechanism of angina pectoris with s-t elevation (author's transl). G Ital Cardiol. 1976;6(1):13–25.
4. Yasue H, Takizawa A, Nagao M, Nishida S, Horie M, Kubota J, et al. Long-term prognosis for patients with variant angina and influential factors. Circulation. 1988;78(1):1–9.
5. Wang CH, Kuo LT, Hung MJ, Cherng WJ. Coronary vasospasm as a possible cause of elevated cardiac troponin I in patients with acute coronary syndrome and insignificant coronary artery disease. Am Heart J. 2002;144(2):275–81.
6. MacAlpin RN. Cardiac arrest and sudden unexpected death in variant angina: complications of coronary spasm that can occur in the absence of severe organic coronary stenosis. Am Heart J. 1993; 125(4):1011–7.
7. Togashi I, Sato T, Soejima K, Takatsuki S, Miyoshi S, Fukumoto K, et al. Sudden cardiac arrest and syncope triggered by coronary spasm. Int J Cardiol. 2013;163(1):56–60.

8. Takatsu F, Watarai M. Mild stenosis makes prognosis of vasospastic angina worse. Coron Artery Dis. 2011;22(1):1–5.
9. Maseri A, Davies G, Hackett D, Kaski JC. Coronary artery spasm and vasoconstriction. The case for a distinction. Circulation. 1990;81(6):1983–91.
10. Ngow HA, WMN WK. Coronary artery spasm: a quandary. Int Med J Malaysia. 2011;10(1):53–5.
11. Takaoka K, Yoshimura M, Ogawa H, Kugiyama K, Nakayama M, Shimasaki Y, et al. Comparison of the risk factors for coronary artery spasm with those for organic stenosis in a Japanese population: role of cigarette smoking. Int J Cardiol. 2000;72(2):121–6.
12. Werns SW, Walton JA, Hsia HH, Nabel EG, Sanz ML, Pitt B. Evidence of endothelial dysfunction in angiographically normal coronary arteries of patients with coronary artery disease. Circulation. 1989;79(2):287–91.
13. Adlam D, Azeem T, Ali T, Gershlick A. Is there a role for provocation testing to diagnose coronary artery spasm? Int J Cardiol. 2005;102(1):1–7.
14. Ajani AE, Yan BP. The mystery of coronary artery spasm. Heart Lung Circ. 2007;16(1):10–5.
15. Morikami Y, Yasue H, Okumura K, Horio Y, Fujii H, Matsuyama K. Effects of phentolamine and atropine on angina pectoris induced by handgrip test in patients with variant angina. Am J Cardiol. 1988;61(1):71–6.
16. Hackett D, Larkin S, Chierchia S, Davies G, Kaski JC, Maseri A. Induction of coronary artery spasm by a direct local action of ergonovine. Circulation. 1987;75(3):577–82.
17. Salomon P, Halawa B. Levels of neuropeptide Y and thromboxane B2 in patients with variant angina. Pol Arch Med Wewn. 1998;100(4):313–20.
18. Clarke JG, Davies GJ, Kerwin R, Hackett D, Larkin S, Dawbarn D, et al. Coronary artery infusion of neuropeptide Y in patients with angina pectoris. Lancet. 1987;1(8541):1057–9.
19. Okumura K, Yasue H, Horio Y, Takaoka K, Matsuyama K, Kugiyama K, et al. Multivessel coronary spasm in patients with variant angina: a study with intracoronary injection of acetylcholine. Circulation. 1988;77(3):535–42.
20. Crea F, Chierchia S, Kaski JC, Davies GJ, Margonato A, Miran DO, et al. Provocation of coronary spasm by dopamine in patients with active variant angina pectoris. Circulation. 1986;74(2):262–9.
21. Okumura K, Yasue H, Matsuyama K, Goto K, Miyagi H, Ogawa H, et al. Sensitivity and specificity of intracoronary injection of acetylcholine for the induction of coronary artery spasm. J Am Coll Cardiol. 1988;12(4):883–8.
22. Vita JA, Treasure CB, Nabel EG, McLenachan JM, Fish RD, Yeung AC, et al. Coronary vasomotor response to acetylcholine relates to risk factors for coronary artery disease. Circulation. 1990;81(2):491–7.
23. Chappell SP, Lewis MJ, Henderson AH. Effect of lipid feeding on endothelium dependent relaxation in rabbit aortic preparations. Cardiovasc Res. 1987;21(1):34–8.
24. Bossaller C, Habib GB, Yamamoto H, Williams C, Wells S, Henry PD. Impaired muscarinic endothelium-dependent relaxation and cyclic guanosine 5′-monophosphate formation in atherosclerotic human coronary artery and rabbit aorta. J Clin Invest. 1987;79(1):170–4.
25. Cacanyiova S, Dovinova I, Kristek F. The role of oxidative stress in acetylcholine-induced relaxation of endothelium-denuded arteries. J Physiol Pharmacol Off J Polish Physiol Soc. 2013;64(2):241–7.
26. Furchgott RF, Zawadzki JV. The obligatory role of endothelial cells in the relaxation of arterial smooth muscle by acetylcholine. Nature. 1980;288(5789):373–6.
27. Eshaghpour E, Mattioli L, Williams ML, Moghadam AN. Acetylcholine in the treatment of idiopathic respiratory distress syndrome. J Pediatr. 1967;71(2):243–6.
28. Sueda S, Saeki H, Otani T, Mineoi K, Kondou T, Yano K, et al. Major complications during spasm provocation tests with an intracoronary injection of acetylcholine. Am J Cardiol. 2000;85(3):391–4, a10.
29. Oshita A, Izoe Y, Kohno H, Fukuda H, Sueda S. Shock during spasm provocation tests with acetylcholine: four case reports. J Cardiol. 2007;49(1):41–7.
30. Suyama A, Kuriyama H. Mechanisms of the ergonovine-induced vasoconstriction in the rabbit main coronary artery. Naunyn Schmiedebergs Arch Pharmacol. 1984;326(4):357–63.
31. Srisuma S, Lavonas EJ, Wananukul W. Ergotism and factitious hypotension associated with interaction of ergotamine with CYP3A4 inhibitors. Clin Toxicol (Phila). 2014;52(7):674–7.
32. Scanlon PJ, Faxon DP, Audet AM, Carabello B, Dehmer GJ, Eagle KA, et al. ACC/AHA guidelines for coronary angiography. A report of the American College of Cardiology/American Heart Association Task Force on practice guidelines (Committee on Coronary Angiography). Developed in collaboration with the Society for Cardiac Angiography and Interventions. J Am Coll Cardiol. 1999;33(6):1756–824.
33. JCS Joint Working Group. Guidelines for diagnosis and treatment of patients with vasospastic angina (coronary spastic angina) (JCS 2008): digest version. Circ J Off J Jpn Circ Soc. 2010;74(8):1745–62.
34. Rha S-W, Choi BG, Choi SY, Park Y, Goud Akkala R, Lee S, et al. TCT-309 Impact of hyperuricemia on coronary artery spasm as assessed with intracoronary acetylcholine provocation test. J Am Coll Cardiol. 2013;62(18_S1):B99-B.
35. Song JK, Lee SJ, Kang DH, Cheong SS, Hong MK, Kim JJ, et al. Ergonovine echocardiography as a screening test for diagnosis of vasospastic angina before coronary angiography. J Am Coll Cardiol. 1996;27(5):1156–61.
36. Zaya M, Mehta PK, Merz CN. Provocative testing for coronary reactivity and spasm. J Am Coll Cardiol. 2014;63(2):103–9.
37. Waters DD, Szlachcic J, Bonan R, Miller DD, Dauwe F, Theroux P. Comparative sensitivity of exercise, cold pressor and ergonovine testing in provoking attacks of variant angina in patients with active disease. Circulation. 1983;67(2):310–5.
38. Sueda S, Ochi N, Kawada H, Matsuda S, Hayashi Y, Tsuruoka T, et al. Frequency of provoked coronary vasospasm in patients undergoing coronary arteriography with spasm provocation test of acetylcholine. Am J Cardiol. 1999;83(8):1186–90.
39. Bertrand ME, LaBlanche JM, Tilmant PY, Thieuleux FA, Delforge MR, Carre AG, et al. Frequency of provoked coronary arterial spasm in 1089 consecutive patients undergoing coronary arteriography. Circulation. 1982;65(7):1299–306.
40. Kim YG, Kim HJ, Choi WS, Im MS, Yoon CH, Suh JW, et al. Does a negative ergonovine provocation test truly predict freedom from variant angina? Korean Circ J. 2013;43(3):199–203.
41. Takagi Y, Yasuda S, Takahashi J, Tsunoda R, Ogata Y, Seki A, et al. Clinical implications of provocation tests for coronary artery spasm: safety, arrhythmic complications, and prognostic impact: multicentre registry study of the Japanese Coronary Spasm Association. Eur Heart J. 2013;34(4):258–67.
42. Yasue H, Horio Y, Nakamura N, Fujii H, Imoto N, Sonoda R, et al. Induction of coronary artery spasm by acetylcholine in patients with variant angina: possible role of the parasympathetic nervous system in the pathogenesis of coronary artery spasm. Circulation. 1986;74(5):955–63.
43. Kim JW, Park CG, Suh SY, Choi CU, Kim EJ, Rha SW, et al. Comparison of frequency of coronary spasm in Korean patients with versus without myocardial bridging. Am J Cardiol. 2007;100(7):1083–6.
44. Ignarro LJ, Buga GM, Wood KS, Byrns RE, Chaudhuri G. Endothelium-derived relaxing factor produced and released from artery and vein is nitric oxide. Proc Natl Acad Sci U S A. 1987;84(24):9265–9.
45. Dimmeler S, Fleming I, Fisslthaler B, Hermann C, Busse R, Zeiher AM. Activation of nitric oxide synthase in endothelial cells by Akt-dependent phosphorylation. Nature. 1999;399(6736):601–5.

46. Okumura K, Yasue H, Matsuyama K, Ogawa H, Kugiyama K, Ishizaka H, et al. Diffuse disorder of coronary artery vasomotility in patients with coronary spastic angina. Hyperreactivity to the constrictor effects of acetylcholine and the dilator effects of nitroglycerin. J Am Coll Cardiol. 1996;27(1):45–52.
47. Shimokawa H. Cellular and molecular mechanisms of coronary artery spasm: lessons from animal models. Jpn Circ J. 2000;64(1):1–12.
48. Katsumata N, Shimokawa H, Seto M, Kozai T, Yamawaki T, Kuwata K, et al. Enhanced myosin light chain phosphorylations as a central mechanism for coronary artery spasm in a swine model with interleukin-1beta. Circulation. 1997;96(12):4357–63.
49. Horowitz A, Menice CB, Laporte R, Morgan KG. Mechanisms of smooth muscle contraction. Physiol Rev. 1996;76(4):967–1003.
50. Kimura K, Ito M, Amano M, Chihara K, Fukata Y, Nakafuku M, et al. Regulation of myosin phosphatase by Rho and Rho-associated kinase (Rho-kinase). Science. 1996;273(5272):245–8.
51. Amano M, Ito M, Kimura K, Fukata Y, Chihara K, Nakano T, et al. Phosphorylation and activation of myosin by Rho-associated kinase (Rho-kinase). J Biol Chem. 1996;271(34):20246–9.
52. Murase Y, Yamada Y, Hirashiki A, Ichihara S, Kanda H, Watarai M, et al. Genetic risk and gene-environment interaction in coronary artery spasm in Japanese men and women. Eur Heart J. 2004; 25(11):970–7.
53. Jolly SS, Amlani S, Hamon M, Yusuf S, Mehta SR. Radial versus femoral access for coronary angiography or intervention and the impact on major bleeding and ischemic events: a systematic review and meta-analysis of randomized trials. Am Heart J. 2009;157(1):132–40.
54. Cooper CJ, El-Shiekh RA, Cohen DJ, Blaesing L, Burket MW, Basu A, et al. Effect of transradial access on quality of life and cost of cardiac catheterization: a randomized comparison. Am Heart J. 1999;138(3 Pt 1):430–6.
55. Pepine CJ, Feldman RL, Conti CR. Action of intracoronary nitroglycerin in refractory coronary artery spasm. Circulation. 1982; 65(2):411–4.
56. Pepine CJ. Ergonovine echocardiography for coronary spasm: facts and wishful thinking. J Am Coll Cardiol. 1996;27(5):1162–3.
57. Wright RS, Anderson JL, Adams CD, Bridges CR, Casey Jr DE, Ettinger SM, et al. 2011 ACCF/AHA focused update incorporated into the ACC/AHA 2007 Guidelines for the management of patients with unstable angina/non-ST-elevation myocardial infarction: a report of the American College of Cardiology Foundation/American Heart Association Task Force on Practice Guidelines developed in collaboration with the American Academy of Family Physicians, Society for Cardiovascular Angiography and Interventions, and the Society of Thoracic Surgeons. J Am Coll Cardiol. 2011; 57(19):e215–367.
58. Jneid H, Anderson JL, Wright RS, Adams CD, Bridges CR, Casey Jr DE, et al. 2012 ACCF/AHA focused update of the guideline for the management of patients with unstable angina/non-ST-elevation myocardial infarction (updating the 2007 guideline and replacing the 2011 focused update): a report of the American College of Cardiology Foundation/American Heart Association Task Force on Practice Guidelines. J Am Coll Cardiol. 2012;60(7):645–81.
59. Fox K, Garcia MA, Ardissino D, Buszman P, Camici PG, Crea F, et al. Guidelines on the management of stable angina pectoris: executive summary: the Task Force on the Management of Stable Angina Pectoris of the European Society of Cardiology. Eur Heart J. 2006;27(11):1341–81.
60. Choi BG, Park SH, Rha SW, et al. Five-year clinical outcomes in patients with significant coronary artery spasm; a propensity score-matched analysis. Int J Cardiol. 2015;184:533–9.

Transradial Peripheral Interventions

27

Dan Le and Ramesh Daggubati

Abstract

Peripheral arterial disease (PAD) is the consequence of atherosclerosis in the arteries of carotid, vertebral, abdominal mesenteric, renal, and extremity arteries. Patients presenting PAD are at significant threat of cardiovascular morbidity and mortality, primarily due to stroke (from cerebrovascular atherosclerosis) and myocardial infarction (from coronary atherosclerosis). The occurrence of PAD rises with age. Among U.S. individuals aged 40–59 years, 3 % will develop PAD; in those aged 60–69 years, 8 % will be affected; and in those above age 70, 19 % will develop PAD.

Percutaneous interventions are currently the first choice in patient with symptomatic PVD. Use of the radial artery for diagnostic and therapeutics is becoming taking on more popularity within the United States. The explanation for this intensified use is broadly published and includes less risk for access site complications, less costs, and higher patient ease compared to the traditional trans femoral approach (TFA) [1–2].

The purpose of this chapter is to discover the opportunity that the TRA can offer in the peripheral interventions.

27.1 Advantages of TRA for Peripheral Interventions

1. As RA is in superficial location, easy access, compressibility, easy control of bleeding, somewhat isolation from adjacent veins and dual palmar blood supply; hence, the common vascular difficulties present with the TFA, such as access-site bleeding, pseudoaneurysms, arterio-venous fistulas, and limb ischemia are markedly lower in TRA [3].
2. There are also particular anatomic benefits of the TRA for peripheral interventions (TRPI). For subclavian artery intervention the ipsilateral TRA permits excellent support. The right RA is the correct choice for circumstances when the left carotid artery ascends from the innominate artery, to evade trauma during passage of the catheter at the aortic arch. And, the angles of the mesenteric and renal arteries are more efficaous if advanced from the arm.
3. In patients with common femoral artery disease, TRA escapes extreme manipulation of the catheters in the aortas with atherosclerosis, through a diseased femoral artery, and the potential complications at the TFA site.
4. Finally, using TRA patient comfort is superior by the ability to sit up and ambulate early after the procedure that also reduces potential complications and expenses.

D. Le, MD • R. Daggubati, MD, FACC, FSCAI (✉)
Department of Cardiology, Brody School of Medicine, East Carolina University, Greenville, NC, USA
e-mail: daggur@yahoo.com

Y. Zhou et al. (eds.), *Transradial Approach for Percutaneous Interventions*, DOI 10.1007/978-94-017-7350-8_27

While it is not conclusive with large randomized trials, it is likely that patients undergoing peripheral vascular interventions would benefit more from TRA than those with coronary disease.

27.2 Disadvantages of TRA for Peripheral Interventions

Small RA size, arterial spasm, anatomic differences, and severe tortuosity at the subclavian artery may make procedural challenges for advancement of guide catheter or long introducer sheath.

The commonly used sheaths for traversing the length of the upper extremity and lengthy exposure of the RA can cause significant spasm. Thus, patient must receive spasmolytic cocktails and well sedation during procedures.

The size of the RA is important especially when a 7 Fr sheath is required for progressive peripheral equipment, since peripheral devices usually require larger sheath lumens.

27.3 Distance From Assess Site (RA) to the Target Artery

Due to the extended distance to different targets, the selection for sheath length must be adjusted. In general, the sheath should be measured to be 5–10 cm longer than the anticipated distance to the target vessel (Fig. 27.1).

27.4 General Considerations

Site of access is selected depending on the target vessel. Majority of the TRPI are achieved by left radial artery. The right radial artery is used for the right upper extremity, right vertebral artery and bilateral carotid procedures. Moreover, right radial artery can also be chosen in case of poor or absent left radial pulse triggers.

Access is attained regularly, with a short introducer sheath (1 Fr), inserted into the RA at the planned working site. Diagnostic angiography is completed after infusion of local vasodilators. For selective angiography, 140–150 cm vertebral-shaped catheters are the best options. To guide the wire into the descending aorta from the subclavian artery, Internal Mammary (IM) may be used. After familiarization with the anatomy, the size, shape, and length of the sheath can be chosen. 0.035-in. wire is left in place with the help of diagnostic catheter and then the working sheath may be brought to the target site. To avoid spam complications, it is advised to use moderate-to-deep sedation.

27.5 The Transradial Approach for Percutaneous Interventions of Supra-Aortic Arteries

27.5.1 Subclavian Artery Interventions

The TRA is considered effective not only because it presents with less complications attenuating the site of access, but they also for the stability provided by the guide support's help in the placing the sheath right next to the stenotic site (Fig. 27.2).

1. Access the RA with a short sheath and perform angiography with a 5 Fr, 100 cm multipurpose catheter.
2. After the anatomy is recognized, a 45 cm, 6 Fr or 7 Fr introducer sheath should be used for ipsilateral TRA, and brought right next to the lesion.
3. Go through the lesion with a 0.035 in. angled stiff, hydrophilic guidewire.
4. Pre-dilate the stenosis with an undersized balloon.
5. Progress with the 5 Fr Pigtail catheter into the transverse aorta to see the aorto-subclavian junction through aortography.
6. Finish the rest of the procedure traditionally by using bone markers for locating and placing the stent.

27.5.2 Carotid Artery Interventions

Carotid artery stenting is a recognized treatment method as a substitute for carotid endarterectomy in cases of revascularization of atherosclerotic internal carotid artery stenosis in those who are at high risk for surgery [4, 5].

Traditionally, the femoral approach is usually used. The TRA is challenged due to the acute angle between the common carotid artery and subclavian artery. Though, in consideration with presently accessible equipment, TRA in use of carotid stenting is suggested in the following situations.

- Treating right carotid artery via stent upon extremely diseased aortic arch.
- Treating left carotid artery via stent when the vessel rises from innominate artery,

1. Access the right RA with a 6 Fr, 90 cm Shuttle sheath and advance to the innominate artery.
2. Use of 5 Fr Simmons-1 catheters (Terumo Corporation) as the main catheter to assess the common carotid artery. For contralateral TRA, the 5 Fr Tig-1 Optitorque catheter (Terumo Corporation) is an alternative catheter.
3. Advance a 0.035″ Amplatz super-stiff wire into the external carotid artery or deep in the common

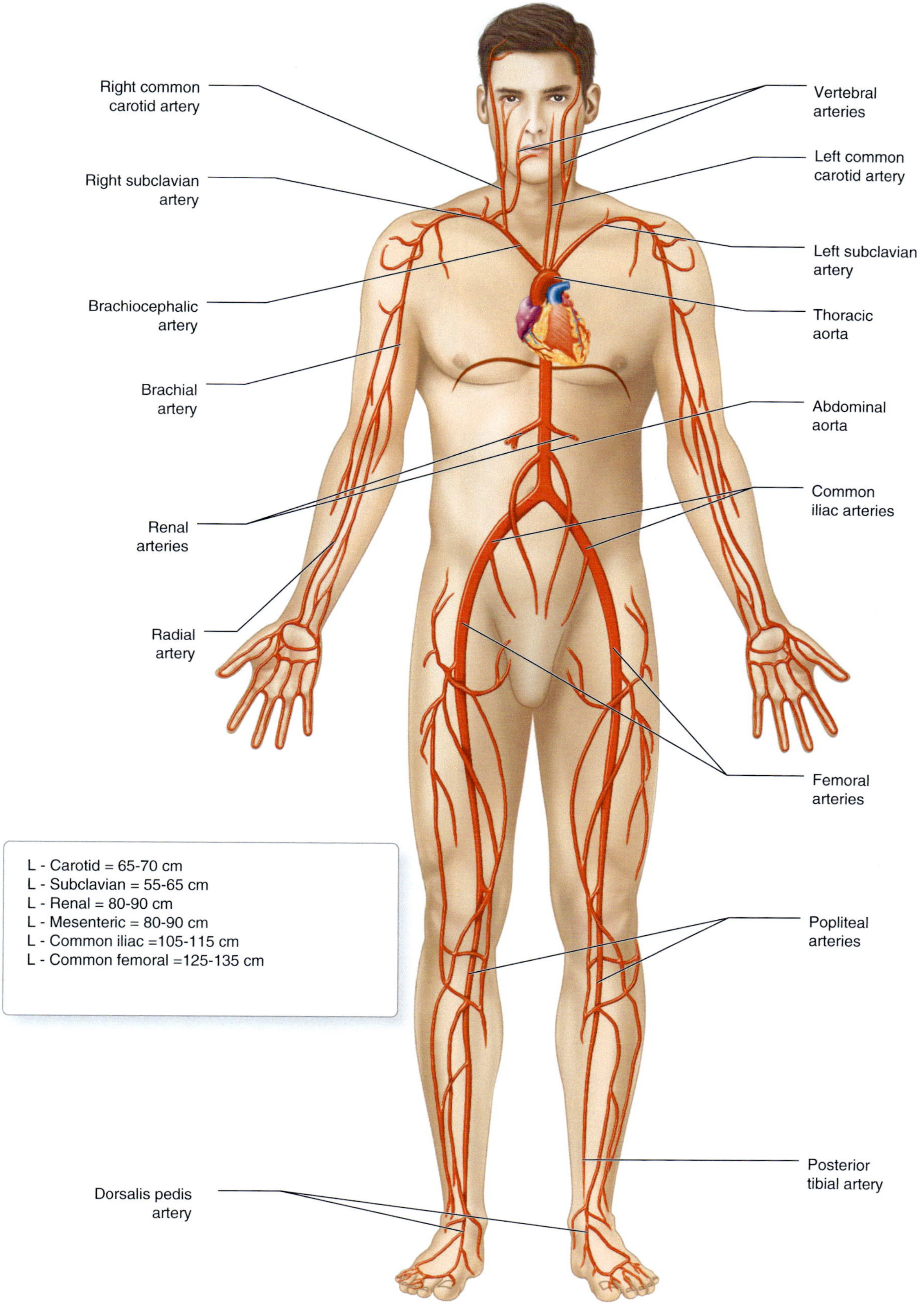

Fig. 27.1 The average distance from the left RA at wrist level (*L*) to the different target arteries

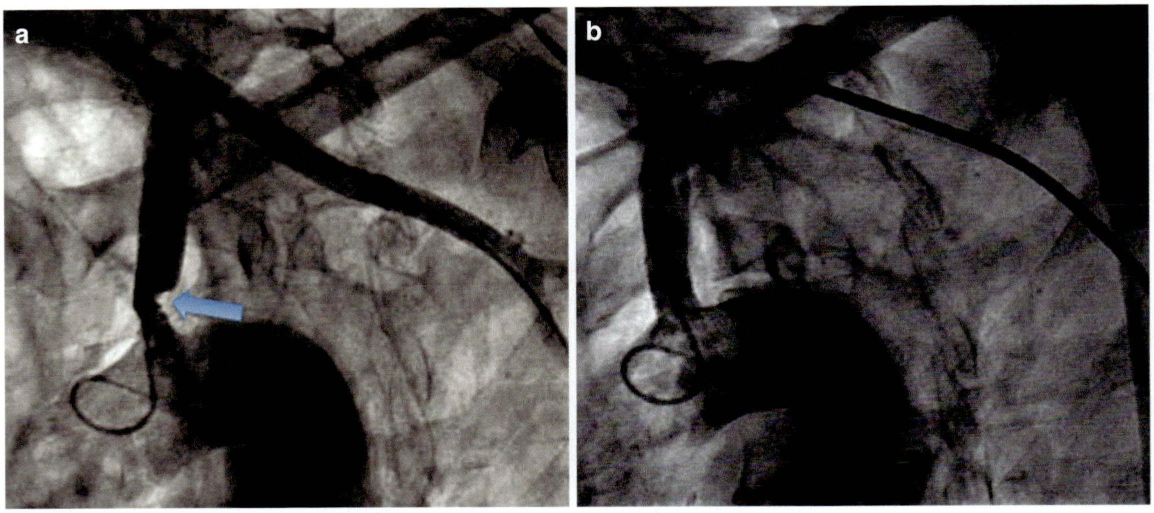

Fig. 27.2 Left TRA for left subclavian artery intervention. (**a**) Severe stenosis (*arrow*). (**b**) Stenting with optimal result

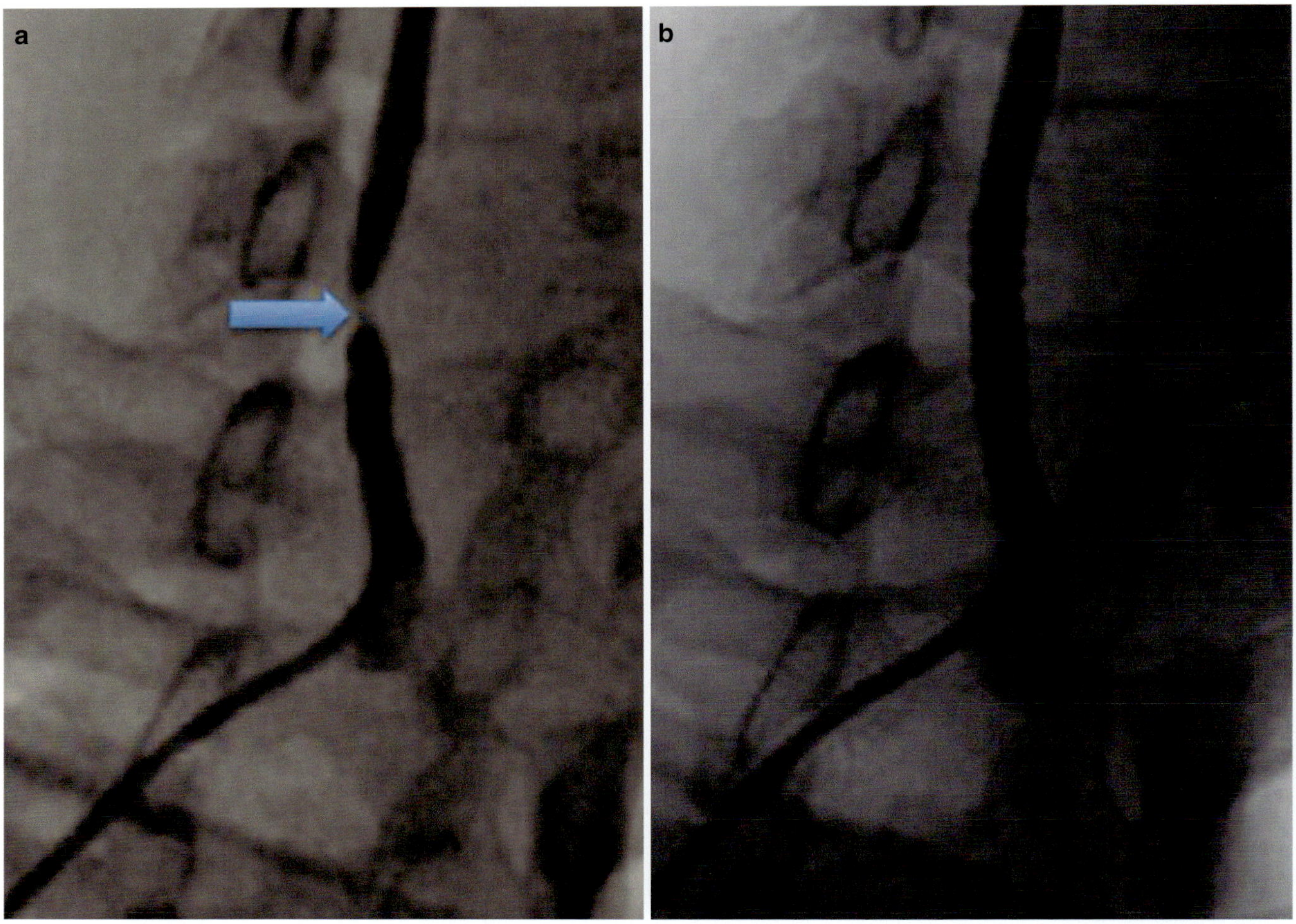

Fig. 27.3 TRA for vertebral artery intervention. (**a**) Severe stenosis (*arrow*). (**b**) Stenting with optimal result

carotid artery distant from the origin of the internal carotid artery.

4. Aim at ideal co-axial placement of a 6 Fr or 7 Fr carotid sheath of your choice for common carotid artery, the following part of the practice is achieved in standard manner.

27.5.3 Vertebral Artery Interventions

Vertebral artery stenosis angioplasty and stenting is a relatively new alternative modality of management (Fig. 27.3). A current study has documented the safety and effectiveness of the TRA to this intervention [6].

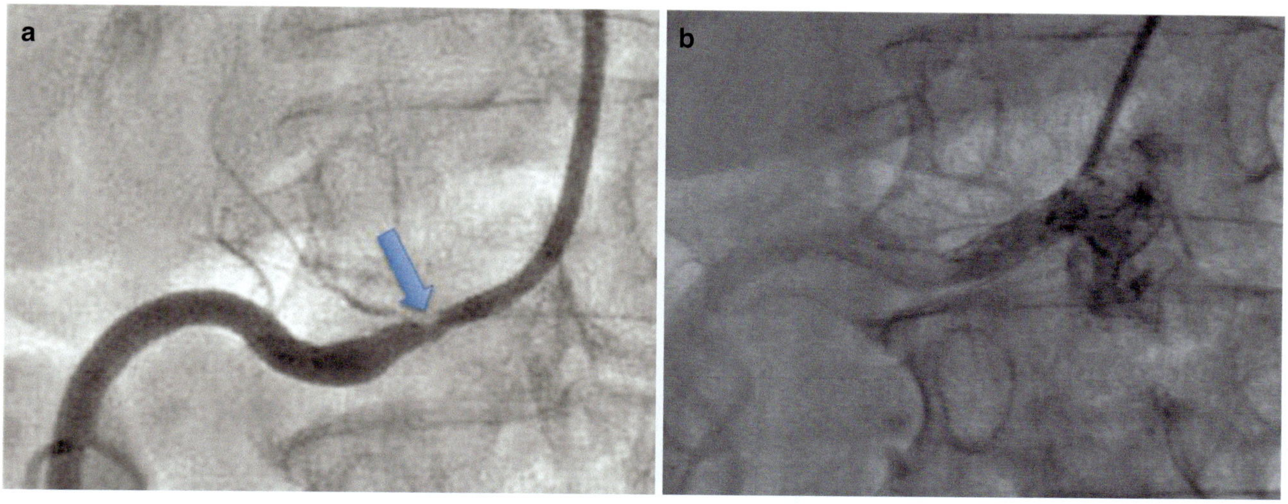

Fig. 27.4 TRA for right renal artery intervention. (**a**) Severe stenosis (*arrow*). (**b**) Stenting with optimal result

Ipsilateral TRA is the best choice for vertebral artery stent.

1. Access the ipsilateral RA with a 4 or 5 Fr, 90 cm long introducer sheath.
2. Position the tip of the sheath just distal to the take- off of the vertebral artery.
3. Regular PTCA guidewires, balloon catheters, and coronary stents should be acquired. Predilation of the lesion should be done with low pressure (between 4 and 6 atm). The stent should be deployed at low pressure (8–10 atm).

The procedure should be divided into two stages for intracranial vertebral or basilar artery occlusions. In the primary phase, the lesion should be dilated with 1.5 × 10 mm or 1.5 × 12 mm PTCA catheter at 4–6 atm in order to establish distal flow. In the second stage, the patient should be brought to the catheterization laboratory 24 h later and the lesion should be stented using a coronary stent at 8–10 atm. This strategy should be used to prevent hyper perfusion brain injury [6].

27.6 The Transradial Approach for Percutaneous Interventions of Renal and Mesenteric Arteries

A large number of patients undergoing renal artery stenting have uncontrolled hypertension despite high doses of antihypertensive medications (Fig. 27.4). Those with chronic mesenteric ischemia can undergo revascularization of the mesenteric arterial obstruction disease.

The aorto-ostial location which is common for both of these atherosclerotic stenoses leads to clinical viability of TRPI. The renal and mesenteric arteries most commonly points downward from the abdominal aorta (Fig. 27.5); thus, TRA offers more co-axial and less traumatic guide catheter assess as compared with TFA.

Left TRA should be preferred since the length of area to target is smaller and therefore a smaller amount catheter manipulation is commonly needed. This is due to lack of traversing at the aortic arch. Thus, practically both renal and mesenteric artery stenting procedures can be performed using regular-length multipurpose (MP) or Judkins Right (JR) guide catheters.

27.7 The Transradial Approach for Percutaneous Interventions of Iliac Artery

Iliac artery stenosis is common PVD that has traditionally been treated with surgery. However, angioplasty with stenting is a less invasive alternative management in patients with focal iliac artery stenosis [7] (Fig. 27.6).

Left TRA is preferred, because it avoids extra length and tortuosity of the aortic arch, allowing relatively easy tracking and deployment of a long 6 Fr sheath.

After obtaining left radial access with a 5 Fr introducer sheath, an internal mammary artery (IM) catheter is progressed over a long (300 cm) 0.035″ guidewire in the descending aorta, later the entire system is exchanged for a long (usually 100 cm or 110 cm) 6 Fr introducer sheath. The sheath is placed at the ostium of the culprit common iliac artery or in the distal aorta just above the bifurcation; the procedure is then performed in the standard manner. This TRA provides exceptional patient satisfaction and quick same day discharge.

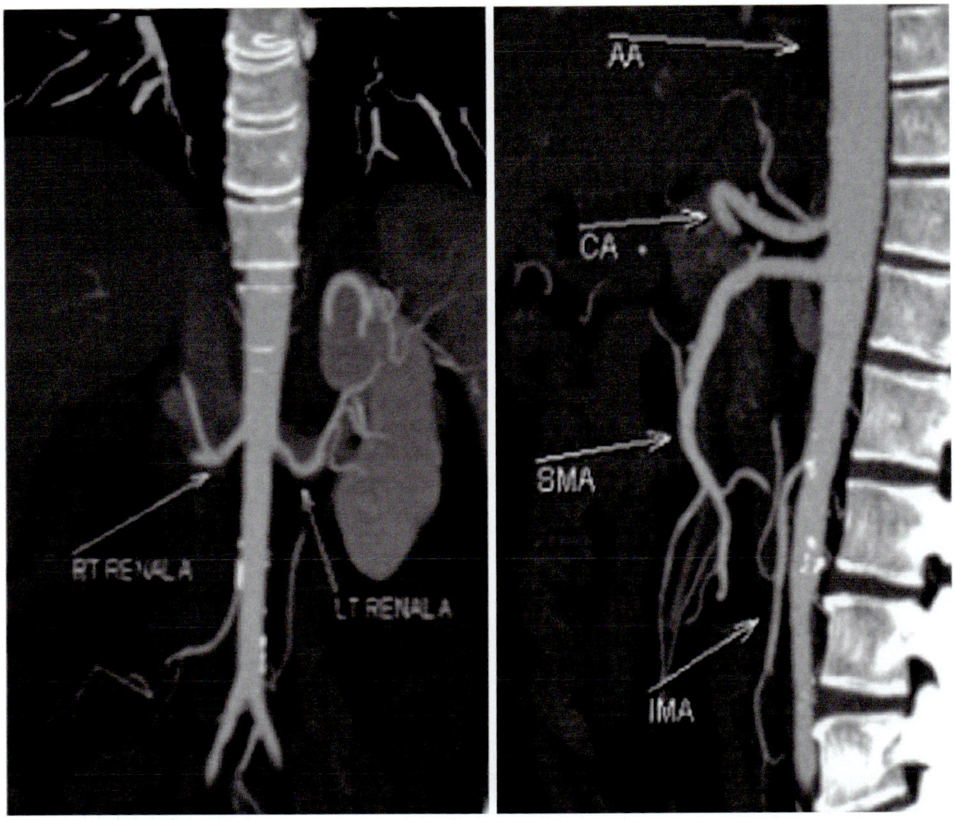

Fig. 27.5 Abdominal vessels. *AA* abdominal aorta, *CA* celiac artery, *SMA* superior mesenteric artery, *IMA* inferior mesenteric artery

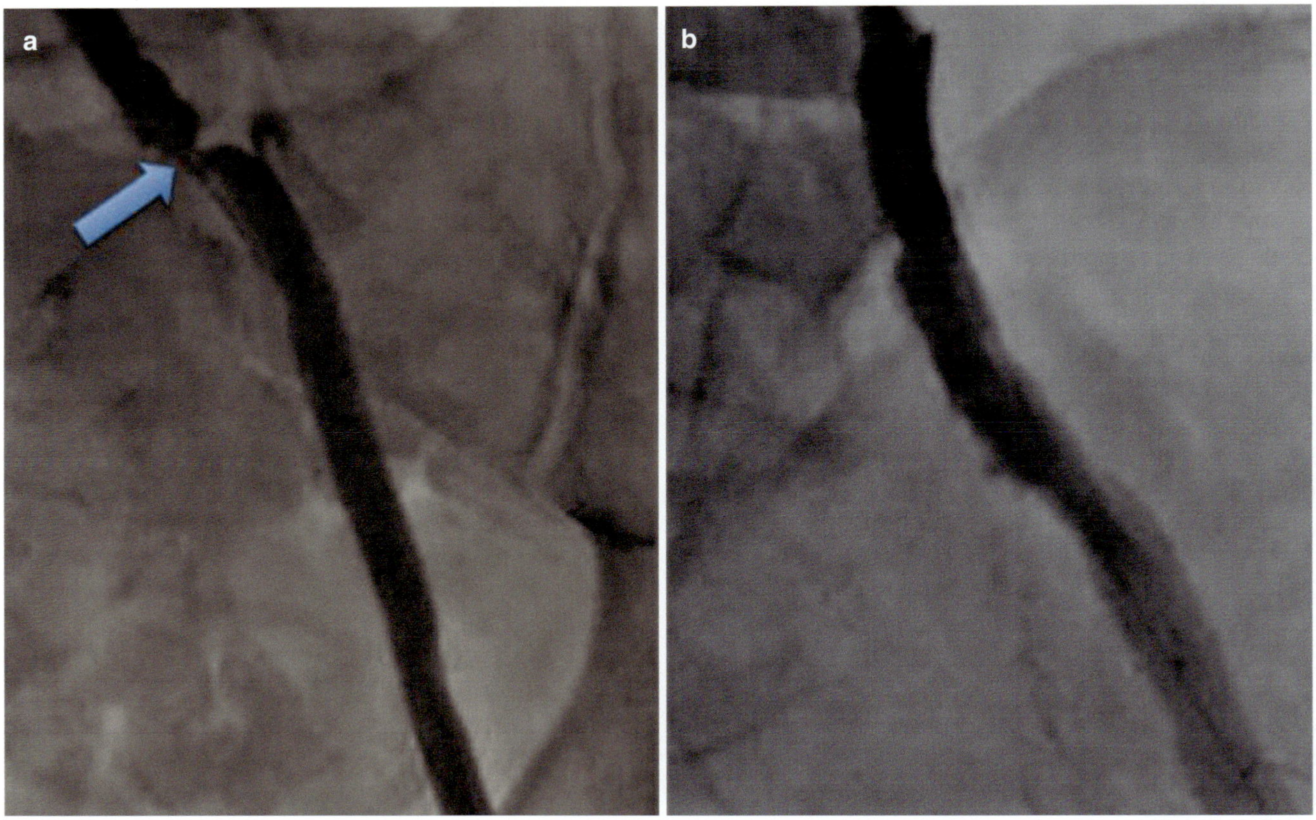

Fig. 27.6 TRA for left iliac artery intervention. (**a**) Severe stenosis (*arrow*). (**b**) Stenting with optimal result

27.8 Lower Extremity

TRA for low extremity interventions has been limited by the lack of adequate equipment as well as the very long distance from the access site to the target vessels.

27.9 The Summary Algorithm is Suggested for Access Selection for Peripheral Intervention

TRA is the approach of choice for stenting of the

- Subclavian artery
- Right carotid artery in the setting of a diseased arch
- Left carotid artery arising form the innominate artery
- Renal and mesenteric arteries
- Iliac arteries

TFA is still the first choice for stenting of the

- Right carotid artery (normal arch)
- Left carotid artery (normal takeoff)
- Low extremity arteries (CFA, SFA, Popliteal, below knee interventions)

Conclusions

Most peripheral vascular interventions are easily accessible from the TRA offering the several advantages, beside the already recognized decreased chance of post-procedural bleeding.

The us of the TRA for peripheral interventions is immensely supported. However, more transradial training programs, clinical trials and improvement of peripheral equipment are needed prior to use of this approach as standard procedure.

References

1. Agostoni P, Biondi-Zoccai GG, de Benedictis ML, et al. Radial versus femoral approach for percutaneous coronary diagnostic and interventional procedures; Systematic overview and meta-analysis of randomized trials. J Am Coll Cardiol. 2004;44: 349–56.
2. Jolly SS, Amlani S, Hamon M, Yusuf S, Mehta SR. Radial versus femoral access for coronary angiography or intervention and the impact on major bleeding and ischemic events: a systematic review and meta-analysis of randomized trials. Am Heart J. 2009;157:132–40.
3. Jolly SS, Yusuf S, Cairns J, et al. Radial versus femoral access for coronary angiography and intervention in patients with acute coronary syndromes (RIVAL): a randomized, parallel group, multicenter trial. Lancet. 2011;377:1409–20.
4. Patel T, Shah S, Ranjan A, Malhotra H, Pancholy S, Coppola J. Contralateral transradial approach for carotid artery stenting: a feasibility study. Catheter Cardiovasc Interv. 2010;75: 268–75.
5. Folmar J, Sachar R, Mann T. Transradial approach for carotid artery stent- ing: a feasibility study. Catheter Cardiovasc Interv. 2007;69:355–61.
6. Patel T, Shah S, Malhotra H, Radadia R, Shah L, Shah S. Transradial approach for stenting of vertebro basilar stenosis: a feasibility study. Catheter Cardiovasc Interv. 2009;74:925–31.
7. Staniloae CS, Korabathina R, Yu J, Kurian D, Coppola J. Safety and efficacy of transradial aortoiliac interventions. Catheter Cardiovasc Interv. 2010;75:659–62.